Atlas of Small Animal CT and MRI

Atlas of Small Animal CT and MRI

Erik R. Wisner, DVM, Dipl. ACVR
Professor of Diagnostic Imaging
School of Veterinary Medicine
University of California
Davis, CA

Allison L. Zwingenberger, DVM, MAS, Dipl. ACVR, Dipl. ECVDI
Associate Professor of Diagnostic Imaging
School of Veterinary Medicine
University of California
Davis, CA

WILEY Blackwell

This edition first published 2015 © 2015 by John Wiley & Sons, Inc

Editorial Offices

1606 Golden Aspen Drive, Suites 103 and 104, Ames, Iowa 50010, USA

The Atrium, Southern Gate, Chichester, West Sussex, PO19 8SQ, UK

9600 Garsington Road, Oxford, OX4 2DQ, UK

For details of our global editorial offices, for customer services and for information about how to apply for permission to reuse the copyright material in this book please see our website at www.wiley.com/wiley-blackwell.

Library of Congress Cataloging-in-Publication Data

Wisner, Erik R., author.

Atlas of small animal CT and MRI / Erik R. Wisner, Allison L. Zwingenberger.

    p. ; cm.

Atlas of small animal computed tomography and magnetic resonance imaging

Includes index.

ISBN 978-1-118-44617-1 (cloth)

1. Veterinary tomography. 2. Veterinary diagnostic imaging. 3. Magnetic resonance imaging. I. Zwingenberger, Allison L., author. II. Title. III. Title: Atlas of small animal computed tomography and magnetic resonance imaging.

[DNLM: 1. Dog Diseases–diagnosis–Atlases. 2. Cat Diseases–diagnosis–Atlases. 3. Magnetic Resonance Imaging–Atlases. 4. Tomography, Emission-Computed–Atlases. SF 991]

    SF757.8.W57 2015

    636.089′60757–dc23

2014049391

A catalogue record for this book is available from the British Library.

Wiley also publishes its books in a variety of electronic formats. Some content that appears in print may not be available in electronic books.

Cover images courtesy of Erik R. Wisner and Allison L. Zwingenberger

Set in 10.5/12.5pt Minion by SPi Publisher Services, Pondicherry, India

SKY10055192_091223

Contents

Preface

The first biomedical use of CT and MRI occurred in the 1970's and over the past three decades these imaging modalities have greatly advanced our ability to diagnose disorders of companion animals. The rapid clinical integration of CT and MRI since their introduction into veterinary medicine, coupled with continual advances in imaging technology and an ever-expanding body of literature, provide the inspiration for the *Atlas of Small Animal CT and MRI*.

This book is intended for residents and specialists in most any clinical specialty, motivated veterinary students, and any practicing veterinarian who routinely refers patients for advanced imaging. For those currently in training or new to CT and MRI, the text provides a broad, image-rich exposure to the subject. For more seasoned veterinary specialists, the book serves as both a refresher and as a quick reference.

This is the first textbook of veterinary cross-sectional imaging to present material in a comparative format and with correlation to other diagnostic tests and pathology. The book includes more than 700 patient-based figures composed of over 3000 individual images to illustrate most of the common, and a few uncommon, disorders diagnosed using CT and MRI. We have taken pains to use examples that have been definitively diagnosed, either histologically or cytologically, or by an overwhelming preponderance of clinical and other diagnostic evidence.

A text such as this is not written without the substantial support of many people. We would like to extend our appreciation to our diagnostic imaging, neurology, surgery, medicine and other colleagues whose expertise has informed the content of this atlas. We would also like to acknowledge our stellar residents and students whose inquiring minds have motivated us to author this text. Special thanks go to our technical staff, Rich Larson, Jason Peters, and Jennifer Harrison whose dedication and technical expertise over the years has been invaluable. We would also like to extend our gratitude to Michael French whose attention to detail has improved the quality of this work immensely, and to John Doval who conceived the overall book design. Our editors, Nancy Turner and Catriona Cooper, and project manager, Aileen Castell, were instrumental in ensuring our changes and suggestions were incorporated. Finally we would like to thank our loved ones, Gina, Tristan, Adriane, and Mike, whose support has given us the inspiration to complete this project.

Winston Churchill once wrote *"Writing a book is an adventure. To begin with, it is a toy and an amusement; then it becomes a mistress, and then it becomes a master, and then a tyrant. The last phase is that just as you are about to be reconciled to your servitude, you kill the monster, and fling him out to the public."* The origin of this book dates back to January 1, 2007 when the senior author, fortified with an ambitious new years resolution, drafted an initial outline and began archiving potential material for inclusion. Fast forward eight years and we too have finally reached the point at which we need to kill the monster, and fling him out to the public.

Erik R. Wisner
Allison L. Zwingenberger

How to use this Atlas

As shown in the sample images **a,b,c**, each figure in this atlas includes a header that identifies the figure number, the specific pathology illustrated, and the principal imaging modality. Immediately beneath each image is a string of either two or three abbreviations separated by commas which provide the reader with specific information about that image. The first abbreviation in the string generally specifies the imaging modality and specific image acquisition details. Remaining abbreviations provide information relating to image display, anatomic plane or orientation. The reader can refer to the comprehensive legend of figure abbreviations for details.

Figure 2.8.23   High-grade Oligodendroglioma (Canine)   CT & MR

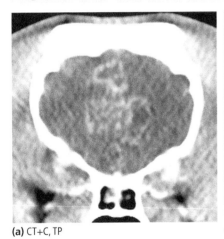 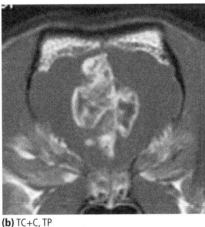 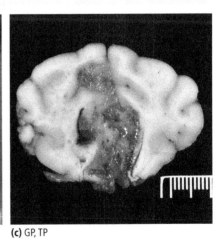

(a) CT+C, TP   **(b)** TC+C, TP   **(c)** GP, TP

5y French Bulldog with progressive neurologic signs referable to intracranial disease. There is an irregularly shaped, heterogeneously enhancing, bi-hemispheric mass evident on contrast-enhanced CT (**a**) and T1 MR (**b**) images. Post-mortem examination confirmed grade III oligodendroglioma (**c**).

Abbreviations

3D	Three-dimensional reformat	**LFB**	Luxol fast blue (stain)
ADC	Apparent diffusion coefficient	**LLAT**	Left lateral projection/view
ARTH	Arthrogram	**M**	Male
CAUD	Caudal view	**MC**	Male castrated
CC	Craniocaudal or caudocranial	**MED**	Medial projection/view
CRAN	Cranial view	**MIP**	Maximum-intensity projection
CT	Computed tomography	**MR**	Magnetic resonance
CT&MR	Computed tomography & magnetic resonance	**OBL**	Oblique view
		OP	Oblique plane
CT+C	CT with contrast medium	**PAS**	Periodic acid--Schiff (stain)
DORS	Dorsal view	**PD**	Proton density-weighted sequence
DP	Dorsopalmar or dorsoplantar	**RIGHT**	Right limb
DP	Dorsal plane	**RLAT**	Right lateral projection/view
DV	Dorsoventral projection	**SP**	Sagittal plane
DWI	Diffusion-weighted sequence	**SPGR**	Spoiled gradient recalled echo sequence
DX	Diagnostic radiography	**SSTSE**	Single-shot turbo spin-echo sequence
DX+C	Diagnostic radiography with contrast medium	**ST**	Short T1 inversion recovery (STIR)
		T1	T1-weighted sequence
ES	Endoscopy	**T1+C**	T1 with contrast medium
F	Female	**T1+C+FS**	T1 with contrast medium and fat saturation
FS	Female spayed		
FL	Fluid-attenuated inversion recovery sequence (FLAIR)	**T2**	T2-weighted sequence
		T2*	T2 star weighted sequence
GA	Gross anatomy	**TP**	Transverse plane
GP	Gross pathology	**US**	Ultrasound
IL	Illustration	**VD**	Ventrodorsal projection
LAT	Lateral projection/view	**VENT**	Ventral view
LEFT	Left limb	**XC**	External camera photography

Section 1
Head & Neck

1.1

Nasal cavity and paranasal sinuses

Normal anatomy

Symmetry of the thin, scrolled nasal turbinates is an important aid to detecting abnormalities in the nasal cavities. The turbinates are more densely formed rostrally and become thicker with more interspersed airspaces caudally. The turbinates are surrounded by mucosa but are themselves thin bone. Thin collimation is required to appreciate their structure in CT images. The nasal sinuses should be air filled with a thin or undetectable mucosal lining. A comparison of CT and MRI of the normal nasal cavities and paranasal sinuses to gross cross-sectional anatomy has been reported in mesaticephalic dogs (Figures 1.1.1, 1.1.2),[1] and computed tomography of the normal nasal cavity and nasolacrimal drainage system has been described in cats.[2,3]

Normal nasal cycle

The nasal cycle is a normal physiologic phenomenon with a periodicity of 2–3 hours, which has been described in dogs.[4,5] This frequent, alternating cycle is thought to allow nasal mucosa to recover from the minor trauma of conditioning inspired air. Many dogs with otherwise normal nasal CT or MR examinations will display asymmetry of the nasal mucosa reflected by apparent unilateral mucosal congestion (Figure 1.1.3). The asymmetry is due to unilateral vasoconstriction causing increased mucosal perfusion on the contralateral side resulting in mucosal thickening and increased resistance to airflow. In patients exhibiting the nasal cycle, the mucosal thickening on the affected side is uniform, and there is no evidence of underlying turbinate involvement.

Developmental disorders

The nasal septum and turbinates can occasionally appear asymmetrical in otherwise normal dogs and cats. These anomalies are often clinically insignificant but can sometimes lead to impaired airflow or obstruction. Brachycephalic dogs and cats may also have poorly developed or malformed turbinates and paranasal sinuses that predispose them to other sinonasal disorders. The sinuses may be partially developed, asymmetrical, or absent on one or both sides. Cats occasionally have marked distortion of turbinates that may represent abnormal growth resulting from severe viral rhinitis at an early age. Early trauma while skull growth is still occurring can also lead to distortion of nasal anatomy. Such patients are often prone to recurring rhinitis as adults. In brachycephalic cats, the nasal bones become dorsally rotated and reduced in size, and the course of the nasolacrimal duct becomes altered.[6]

Nasopharyngeal stenosis, a narrowing of the nasopharynx caudal to the choana, occurs most commonly as a congenital condition.[7] It may also be secondary to inflammation, trauma, or tumors. The regions of stenosis are very narrow and require thin-slice CT images to detect. Sagittal reformatted images are helpful for identifying and quantifying the stenosis (Figure 1.1.4).

Inflammatory disorders

Foreign body rhinitis

Imaging diagnosis of nasal foreign body rhinitis often depends on whether the foreign object can be directly visualized. When the object is not seen, as is often the

---

Atlas of Small Animal CT and MRI, First Edition. Erik R. Wisner and Allison L. Zwingenberger.
© 2015 John Wiley & Sons, Inc. Published 2015 by John Wiley & Sons, Inc.

case with plant awns or small wood fragments, diagnostic features include focal turbinate destruction, hyperplasia of the remaining overlying nasal mucosa, and regional accumulation of fluid or mucoid exudates.[8] Foreign body rhinitis is usually unilateral except when multiple foreign bodies are present, which can occur with plant awn inhalation. The severity of the secondary imaging findings can be related to the chronicity of the disorder as well as the inertness of the foreign material. In most patients, imaging abnormalities are limited to the nasal cavity or nasopharynx and do not usually involve the paranasal sinuses (Figures 1.1.5, 1.1.6, 1.1.7).[9]

Nonspecific rhinitis

Nonspecific rhinitis is a general term that includes inflammatory nasal disorders from viral, bacterial, parasitic, or allergic causes. Rhinitis may also occur as an extension of severe periodontal disease. The most common biopsy diagnosis in this category of disease is lymphocytic–plasmocytic rhinitis, which may also have a neutrophilic or predominantly eosinophilic component (Figures 1.1.8, 1.1.9). Rhinitis may also occur secondary to severe dental disease.

Radiographic findings may be normal, and cross-sectional imaging findings may range from minimal to marked. Exudative fluid is present bilaterally within the interstices of the nasal cavity, and fluid is generally present within the frontal and maxillary sinuses and the sphenoid recesses. The underlying nasal turbinate pattern is often unaffected, but turbinate atrophy, particularly the delicate bone of more peripheral turbinate regions, can occur with chronic or severe disease. Fluid can be distinguished from underlying hyperplastic mucosa on MRI and on contrast-enhanced CT. Mucosa is typically prominent and enhances intensely and uniformly. Dense bone of the nasal septum and nasal cavity margins is rarely affected, although productive reactivity of the maxillary and frontal bones can be seen with chronic disease.

Very rarely, canine patients may have much more aggressive appearing imaging findings, including mass lesions and dense bone destruction that appears consistent with neoplasia but has a biopsy diagnosis of eosinophilic rhinitis. These rare cases could be unusual nasal manifestations of eosinophilic granulomatous disease and, though inflammatory in etiology, are not typical of the imaging findings associated with nonspecific rhinitis. Up to a third of cats with nasal disorders of any type and many dogs with nasal disease also have secondary bulla effusion associated with auditory tube occlusion.

Nasal polyps are periodically encountered in association with chronic inflammatory disease. Depending on location, polyps may or may not be identified on cross-sectional images. Those polyps that extend into the air-filled nasopharynx are more likely to be identified (Figure 1.1.10). Nasal polyps occasionally ossify and can be mistaken for intranasal neoplasia, such as osteosarcoma (Figure 1.1.11).

Oronasal fistula

Oronasal fistulas may occur as developmental anomalies, secondary to trauma, or subsequent to severe dental disease or other inflammatory or neoplastic disorders. Large fistulas with discrete stomas are clearly evident on cross-sectional images. Smaller fistulas are more difficult to diagnose when mucosal margins are in close apposition (Figures 1.1.12, 1.1.13).

Mycotic rhinitis

Mycotic rhinitis is a common sinonasal disorder of dogs and occurs periodically in cats.[10] Aspergillosis is by far the most common organism responsible for canine mycotic rhinitis, but other less common organisms include *Cryptococcus*, *Rhinosporidium*, and *Blastomyces*. *Cryptococcus* is the most common causative agent in cats with mycotic rhinitis, but aspergillosis has also been reported.

Conventional radiographic abnormalities associated with aspergillosis include decreased nasal cavity opacity, loss of recognizable turbinate architecture and marginal remodeling, soft-tissue opacification within the frontal sinuses, and thickening of the frontal bone forming the frontal sinus margin.

In earlier phases of canine nasal aspergillosis, cross-sectional imaging characteristics often include a unilateral increase in nasal mucosal volume, presumably due to mucosal inflammation, hyperplasia, and associated exudates. With progressive disease, there is marked turbinate destruction and atrophy with resulting cavitation in the affected nasal cavity, which may be most evident in the rostral to mid nasal cavity. The nasal cavity may have a rim of soft-tissue thickening, peripherally consisting of fungal plaque and thickened mucosa. A soft-tissue mass component may be present in the caudal nasal cavity or frontal sinus. These fungal masses have characteristic features that include a nonuniform gas and fluid pattern. Frontal sinus epithelial lining thickening is routinely present, and affected frontal sinuses may contain fluid. In one study of 46 dogs, approximately 15% had disease primarily affecting the frontal sinus.[11] Affected maxillary, frontal, and vomer bones may become thickened with irregular margins due to reactivity. In some affected dogs, bone lysis also occurs. Erosion or overt destruction of the ethmoid bone (cribriform plate) resulting in communication with the cranial vault may also occur. This latter feature is important to evaluate since ethmoid destruction may affect therapeutic options and has been associated with a marked worsening of prognosis for successful treatment. In our experience, this parameter can be evaluated using either CT or MRI. However, thin-section CT viewed in both the transverse and reformatted dorsal planes seems to be more sensitive for detection of small, focal, destructive ethmoid fenestrations. Although the majority of patients have unilateral disease, some animals have bilateral imaging findings. In general, this constellation of cross-sectional imaging features, while not pathognomonic, is highly accurate for the diagnosis of canine aspergillosis (Figures 1.1.14, 1.1.15, 1.1.16).[11-15]

Feline aspergillosis is uncommon but occurs frequently enough that it must be included in a differential of feline nasal disease. In our clinical experience, imaging features include bilateral involvement, moderate to marked nasal turbinate destruction, and a greater degree of fluid and mucosal hyperplastic replacement compared to dogs. Maxillary and/or frontal bone remodeling and bone destruction can be seen. Contrast-enhanced images accentuate the difference between noncontrast-enhancing nasal exudates and adjacent contrast-enhancing nasal mucosa. Frontal sinus involvement is also seen, but sinus contents appear more fluid and fungal masses are not as prevalent. A common finding is the presence of a mass lesion in the nasopharynx, which on endoscopic exam is found to be granulomatous reactive tissue.[16]

Feline nasal cryptococcosis appears to occur in two forms. The first is that of localized rhinitis, and the second is that of nasal extension of more aggressive regional or systemic fungal disease. In cats with localized cryptococcal rhinitis, the disease is bilateral and nondestructive. Turbinates do not appear disrupted; however, the normally air-filled interstices between the turbinates appear fluid filled. In the more aggressive form, fungal granulomas can produce space-occupying masses that can erode adjacent bone and may extend caudally through the cribriform plate (Figure 1.1.17).

Neoplasia

Carcinomas are the most common nasal neoplasm in dogs, and lymphoma is the most common nasal tumor in cats. Most cats with nasal lymphoma are presented with localized stage I disease, although some may have nasal manifestations of multicentric lymphoma. Carcinomas include squamous, transitional, and adenomatous forms. Other tumor types periodically encountered include soft-tissue sarcomas, such as hemangiosarcoma; primary bone tumors, including chondrosarcoma, fibrosarcoma, osteosarcoma, and osteochondrosarcoma; and other round cell tumors, such as plasma cell tumor (Figures 1.1.18, 1.1.19, 1.1.20, 1.1.21, 1.1.22, 1.1.23, 1.1.24, 1.1.25, 1.1.26).

Virtually all patients with nasal neoplasia have a soft-tissue mass, although tumor margins are often poorly delineated because of summation with adjacent nasal mucosa and underlying disrupted turbinates. Discrete masses recognized on rhinoscopy may not be evident on cross-sectional imaging even when thin-section images are acquired. Mineralization may be evident either because of retention of turbinate remnants or, in the case of osteogenic tumors, from the presence of new tumor-related bone. Most nasal tumors are bilateral, although the distribution may be asymmetrical. Carcinomas typically arise in the mid to caudal aspect of the nasal cavity, while lymphomas are most often centered on the ventral nasal meatus and the nasopharynx. Neuroendocrine tumors arising from the nasal cavity typically arise on or adjacent to the cribriform plate of the ethmoid bone, extending both rostrally into the nasal cavity and caudally into the cranial vault.

Nasal tumor contrast enhancement is variable and often does not assist in delineating intranasal tumor margins because of the concurrent contrast enhancement of adjacent nasal mucosa. Contrast medium is more useful for delineating extranasal tumor margins in patients with extensive nasal cavity bone destruction or frontal sinus tumor extension.

Nasal tumors often extend into the sphenoid and frontal sinuses, but more often nasal masses cause obstructive frontal sinusitis because of occlusion of the communicating duct between the frontal sinus and nasal cavity. Tumor extension can be distinguished from obstructive sinus disease using contrast-enhanced imaging to differentiate vascularized mass from fluid or exudative sinus collections.

Ecto- and endoturbinate destruction is routinely present because of tumor mass replacement. Destruction of dense frontal, maxillary, vomer, and palatine bone is common and, in general, appears to be more pronounced with nasal carcinomas and soft-tissue sarcomas, although aggressive destruction occurs with lymphoma as well.

Cribriform plate destruction is a common feature of aggressive nasal tumors and should be carefully assessed since this has implications regarding therapeutic options and prognosis. Large destructive lesions are easily recognized. Smaller fenestrations are best evaluated using a combination of thinly collimated axial and dorsal plane reformatted images when CT is used and with thin dorsal plane 3D SPGR images using MR. Contrast-enhanced images can be useful when using either modality to detect meningeal enhancement in those patients with suspected intracranial encroachment.[9,17-20] CT and MRI are equally effective in diagnosing nasal neoplasia, although CT has a slight increase in sensitivity for detecting bone lysis.[21]

Figure 1.1.1 Normal Nasal Cavity (Canine)   CT

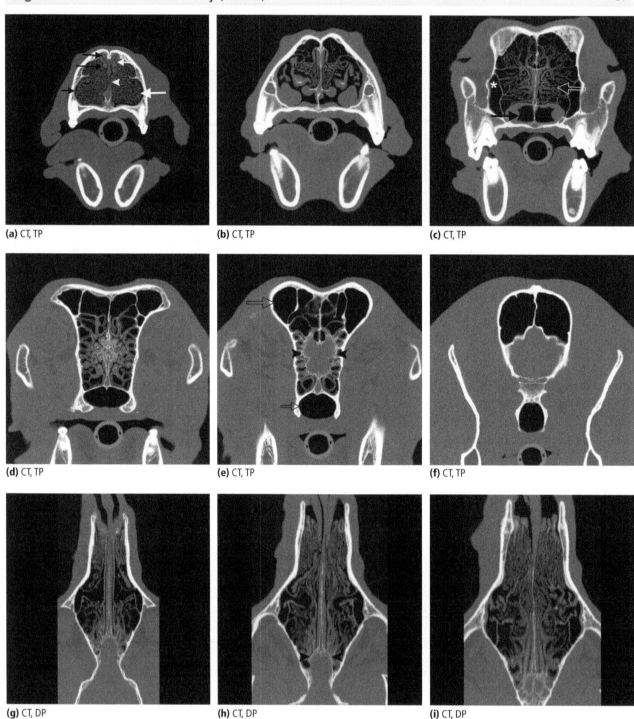

(a) CT, TP   **(b)** CT, TP   **(c)** CT, TP

(d) CT, TP   **(e)** CT, TP   **(f)** CT, TP

(g) CT, DP   **(h)** CT, DP   **(i)** CT, DP

2y MC Great Pyrenees mix. Representative transverse plane images of the nasal passages and paranasal sinuses ordered from rostral to caudal (**a–f**). Representative dorsal plane images ordered from dorsal to ventral (**g–i**). The dorsal (**a**: small white arrow) and ventral (**a**: large white arrow) nasal conchae are finely scrolled rostrally and become larger caudally as the ethmoidal conchae or ethmoturbinates (**c**: open arrow). The nasal septum (**a**: arrowhead) separates the left and right nasal cavities. The dorsal, middle, and ventral nasal meati (**a**: black arrows) allow airflow to the caudal nasal cavity. The nasal sinuses include the maxillary recess (**c**: asterisk), the frontal sinus (**e**: large open arrow), and the sphenoidal sinus (**e**: small open arrow). The nasopharyngeal meatus (**c**: black arrow) connects the nasal cavity to the pharynx. The cribriform plate (**e,h**: arrowheads) separates the nasal cavity from the calvarium.

Figure 1.1.2 Normal Nasal Cavity (Canine)   MR

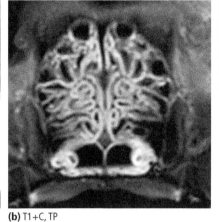

MR images of the nose provide good detail of the nasal turbinates. Normal turbinates are scrolled and symmetrical. They appear moderately intense on T1 images (**a**) and hyperintense on T2 (**c**), PD (**d**), and T1 contrast-enhanced (**b**) images.

(a) T1, TP

(b) T1+C, TP

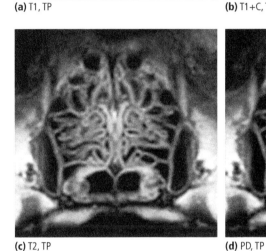

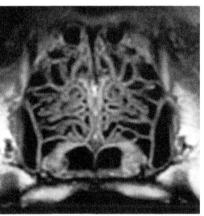

(c) T2, TP

(d) PD, TP

Figure 1.1.3 Normal Nasal Cycle (Canine)   CT

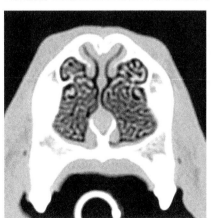

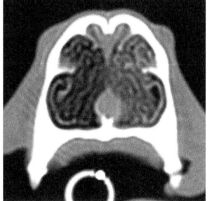

Typical appearance of normal ectoturbinates in the midnasal cavity (**a**). The nasal cycle results in turbinate asymmetry due to nonuniform mucosal perfusion (**b**). This is a normal physiologic phenomenon that is thought to accelerate the rate of nasal mucosal healing from minor injury due to nasal airflow. The nasal cycle has a periodicity of 2–3 hours in dogs.

(a) CT, TP

(b) CT, TP

Figure 1.1.4   Nasopharyngeal Stenosis (Canine)   CT

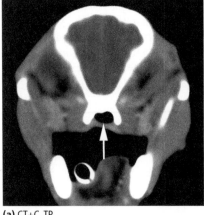

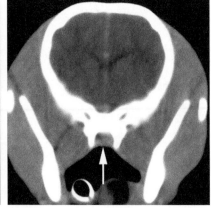

1y F Italian Greyhound with chronic nasal discharge. There is focal occlusion of the nasopharyngeal lumen near the level of the pterygoid processes and 1 cm caudal to the caudal margin of the hard palate (**b,d**: arrow). The pharyngeal lumen rostral and caudal to this focal lesion appears normal (**a,c**: arrow). The soft tissues associated with the occlusive lesion mildly contrast enhance (**b**). Nasopharyngeal stenosis was confirmed rhinoscopically, and biopsy revealed moderate chronic active neutrophilic, eosinophilic, and lymphoplasmacytic pharyngitis and rhinitis.

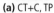

(a) CT+C, TP    **(b)** CT+C, TP

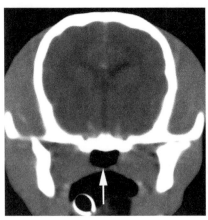

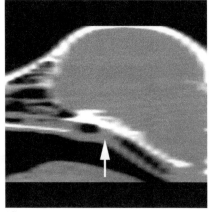

(c) CT+C, TP   **(d)** CT+C, SP

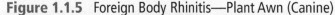

Figure 1.1.5   Foreign Body Rhinitis—Plant Awn (Canine)   CT

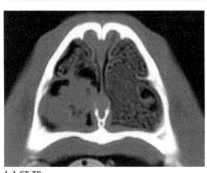

9y FS Labrador Retriever. The transverse plane image reveals unilateral regional nasal turbinate destruction. The fluid-attenuating mass represents a combination of remaining turbinates, mucosa, and accumulated exudate. The fragmented gas pattern suggests this is not a solid mass. A plant awn (foxtail foreign body) was removed at the time of rhinoscopy. Plant awns are usually not detected on CT or MRI, although the focal or regional inflammatory response is characteristic.

(a) CT, TP

Figure 1.1.6 Foreign Body Rhinitis—Tooth Fragment (Feline)

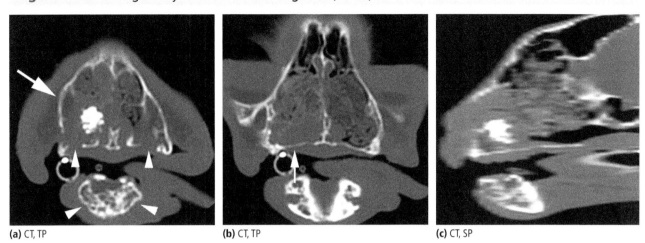

(a) CT, TP **(b)** CT, TP **(c)** CT, SP

16y MC Domestic Longhair with chronic right-sided nasal discharge, chronic renal failure, and multiple missing teeth (**a,c**). An irregularly margined mineral-attenuating mass is present in the rostral aspect of the right nasal cavity. This is associated with adjacent turbinate destruction and increased soft-tissue opacity, consistent with mucosal proliferation and exudates. There is also distortion of the right maxillary bone (**a**: arrow) that likely results from chronic rhinitis and concurrent metabolic bone disease due to chronic renal failure. Resorption of the right maxillary bone (**a**: arrow) and the hard palate caudal to the mass is also evident (**b**: arrow). The mineral opacity was a retained migrated tooth root with peripheral cementum proliferation. This cat also has many missing teeth, pronounced periodontal bone resorption, and proliferative bone remodeling seen with chronic dental disease (**a**: arrowheads).

Figure 1.1.7 Wood Foreign Body (Canine)

CT

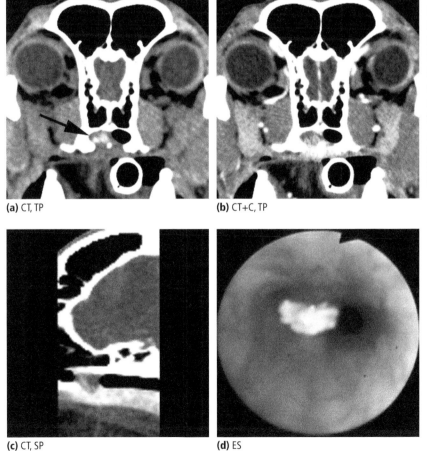

5y FS Australian Shepherd with reverse sneezing and respiratory distress. On unenhanced images, there is hyperattenuating material in the right caudal nasopharynx surrounded by soft tissue (**a**: arrow). On contrast-enhanced images, the soft tissue surrounding the foreign material is strongly enhancing (**b**), representing inflammation and granulomatous tissue. The material extends into the soft palate, which appears as a hyperattenuating structure (**c**). Endoscopy revealed a wood foreign body (stick) in the caudal nasopharynx (**d**). The stick was removed via endoscopy.

(a) CT, TP **(b)** CT+C, TP

(c) CT, SP **(d)** ES

Figure 1.1.8   Lymphocytic Plasmacytic Rhinitis and Sinusitis (Canine)   CT

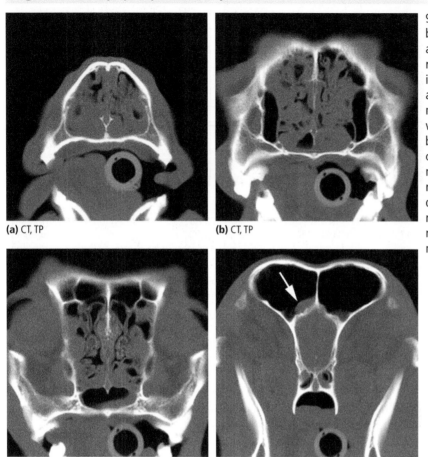

(a) CT, TP

(b) CT, TP

(c) CT, TP

(d) CT, TP

9y MC Australian Shepherd Dog with chronic bilateral nasal discharge. These are representative images of the sinonasal region from rostral to caudal. The normal turbinate pattern is partially obscured by mucosal proliferation and accumulated exudates. These findings are most pronounced rostrally and in the left ventral meatus. Although partially obscured by the increased fluid-opacity in the nasal cavity, there is evidence of nonuniform turbinate atrophy, which was confirmed with rhinoscopy. A small volume of dependent exudate is also seen in the ventral aspect of the right frontal sinus (**d**: arrow). Nasal biopsy revealed chronic lymphocytic plasmocytic neutrophilic rhinitis.

Figure 1.1.9 Eosinophilic Rhinitis and Sinusitis (Canine)   CT

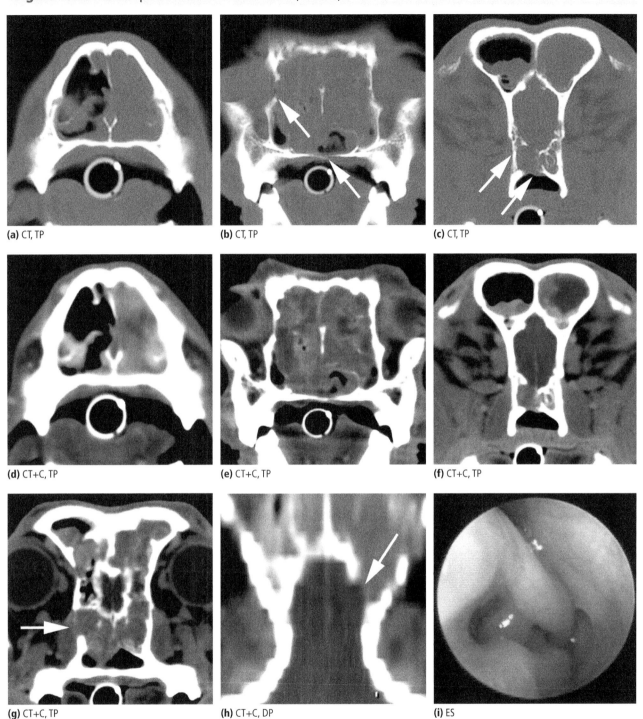

(a) CT, TP

(b) CT, TP

(c) CT, TP

(d) CT+C, TP

(e) CT+C, TP

(f) CT+C, TP

(g) CT+C, TP

(h) CT+C, DP

(i) ES

12y FS Australian Cattle Dog with a 5-year history of cough and mucopurulent nasal discharge. Images **a–c** are unenhanced, and images **d–f** are corresponding contrast-enhanced images. Images **g** and **h** are representative images of the cribriform plate and adjacent anatomy. There is soft-tissue opacification of the nasal cavity and frontal sinuses that heterogeneously contrast enhances. Marked bilateral turbinate destruction is seen with linear bony turbinate remnants evident in the mid-nasal cavity, best seen in image **b**. Multiple focal regions of cortical osteolysis are evident in bones comprising the sinonasal margins (**b**,**c**: arrows), and there is diffuse periosteal reaction involving the frontal bones. A biopsy acquired at the time of rhinoscopy revealed chronic eosinophilic, mastocytic inflammation consistent with allergic rhinitis. This is an unusually aggressive appearance for an immune-mediated rhinosinusitis. Although some features, such as the presence of cortical bone destruction and ill-defined mass effect, are consistent with neoplasia, the diffuse distribution of the soft tissue and bone destructive lesions and the persistence of some residual turbinate architecture are more indicative of inflammatory disease. The dog improved with medical management and had mild persisting signs referable to chronic nasal disease 2 years after the initial CT study was performed.

Figure 1.1.10 Suppurative Rhinitis—Inflammatory Nasal Polyp (Feline)

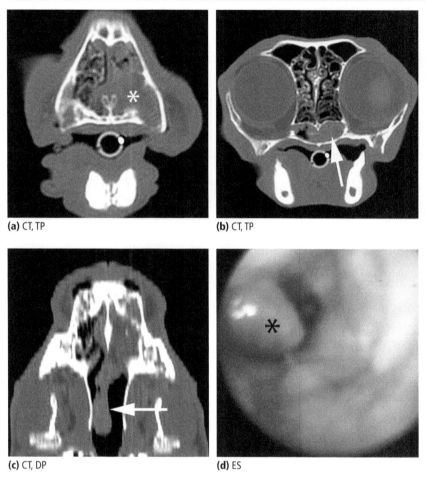

(a) CT, TP

(b) CT, TP

(c) CT, DP

(d) ES

13y MC Domestic Shorthair with a malodorous, brown mucoid left-sided nasal discharge. Multiple dental extractions had been performed 1 month prior to the CT scan. Multiple teeth are missing, and there is osteolysis of residual alveolar bone. Soft-tissue opacity is present within the left ventral nasal cavity and adjacent left maxillary canine alveolar cavity (a: asterisk). A pedunculated nasopharyngeal mass arises from the left nasal cavity (b,c: arrow). The full extent of the mass is appreciated in c, which includes a dorsal plane view of the nasopharynx. The polyp was excised at the time of rhinoscopy (d: asterisk). Although not determined from these images, an oronasal fistula was also present at the site of the canine tooth extraction.

Figure 1.1.11 Ossifying Inflammatory Nasal Polyp (Canine)

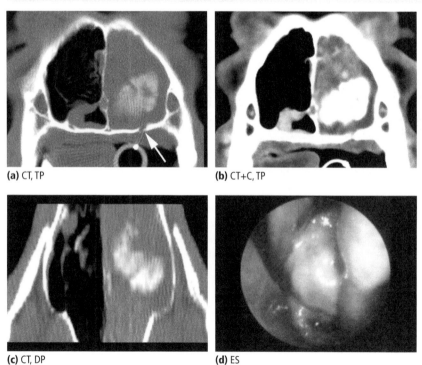

(a) CT, TP

(b) CT+C, TP

(c) CT, DP

(d) ES

13y MC Golden Retriever with left-sided epistaxis. A well-delineated, irregularly shaped mineralized mass is present in the left nasal cavity surrounded by uniform soft-tissue opacity (a). Nonuniform contrast enhancement of the nasal soft tissues suggests some preservation of the turbinates and overlying mucosa (b). The diameter of the left palatine foramen is increased (a: arrow), and the nasal septum is mildly deviated to the right. A well-demarcated mass was seen on rhinoscopic examination (d). Nasal biopsy revealed moderate diffuse chronic active rhinitis with reactive bone formation.

Figure 1.1.12 Oronasal Fistula (Canine)

CT

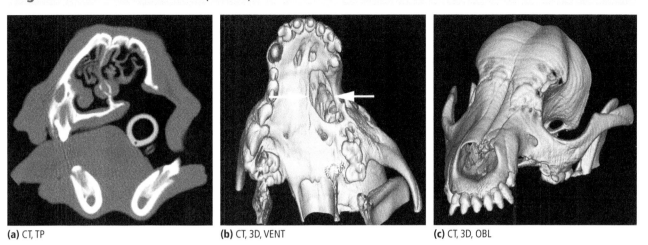

(a) CT, TP **(b)** CT, 3D, VENT **(c)** CT, 3D, OBL

6mo M Australian Shepherd with an oronasal fistula resulting from a bite injury at 1 week of age. Two attempts had been made to close the fistula. There is a large defect in the left palatine bone and maxilla seen on the transverse and 3D images (**b**: arrows). Multiple maxillary teeth are absent, and there is mild turbinate loss in the left nasal passage secondary to inflammation.

Figure 1.1.13 Oropharyngeal/Nasopharyngeal Fistula (Canine)

CT

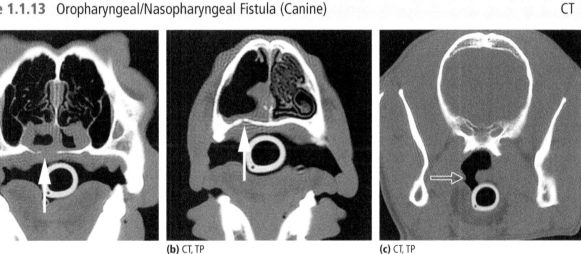

(a) CT, TP **(b)** CT, TP **(c)** CT, TP

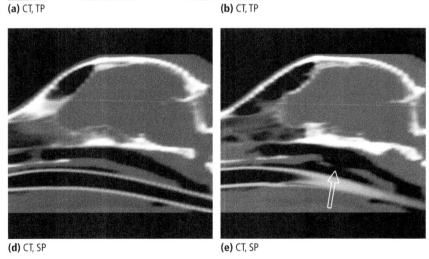

(d) CT, SP **(e)** CT, SP

15y FS German Shepherd Dog mix with 2-year history of nasal discharge. There is a focal defect in the right palatine bone (**a,b**: arrow). There is complete loss of the nasal turbinates in the right rostral nasal cavity (**b**). The soft palate is intact on midline (**e**), but on the right of midline there is a defect in the soft palate that allows communication between the nasal cavity, nasopharynx, oral cavity, and oropharynx (**c,e**: open arrow).

13

Figure 1.1.14 Mycotic Rhinosinusitis and Osteomyelitis—Aspergillosis (Canine)   CT

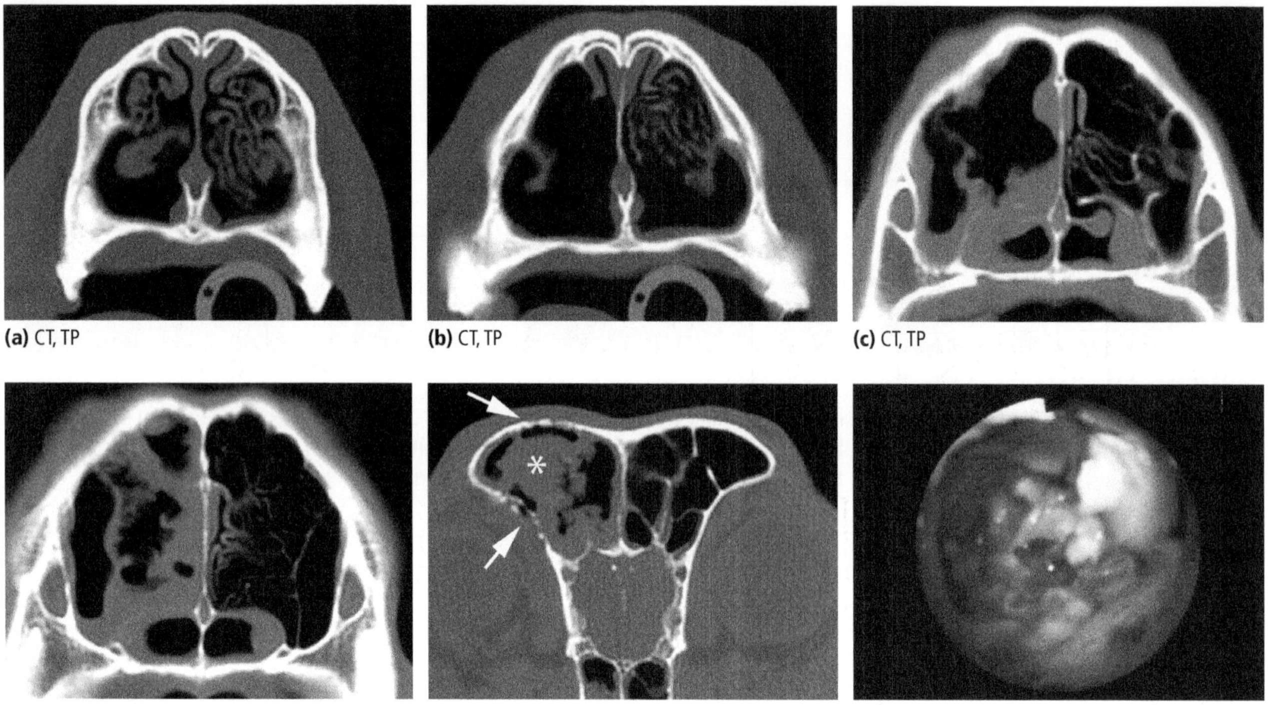

(a) CT, TP

(b) CT, TP

(c) CT, TP

(d) CT, TP

(e) CT, TP

(f) ES

8y MC Rottweiler with chronic right-sided nasal discharge. Images **a–e** are ordered from rostral to caudal. There is nearly complete right-sided turbinate destruction/atrophy with additional regional left-sided ventral turbinate atrophy (**a–c**). Amorphous soft-tissue opacity is present further caudally in the right nasal cavity and in the right frontal sinus (**c–e**). The heterogeneous soft-tissue mass in the frontal sinus, which contains fragmented gas and focal mineral opacities (**e**: asterisk), is characteristic of a fungus ball. Erosive destruction of the right frontal bone (**e**: arrows) is also seen as a result of chronic inflammation. The constellation of CT imaging findings is consistent with chronic mycotic rhinitis from *Aspergillus* species. Rhinoscopic findings included the presence of marked nasal mucosal hyperemia and fungal plaques (**f**). Right-sided nasal biopsy revealed severe suppurative and lymphofollicular rhinitis with fungal plaques.

Figure 1.1.15 Mycotic Rhinosinusitis and Osteomyelitis—Aspergillosis (Canine)   CT

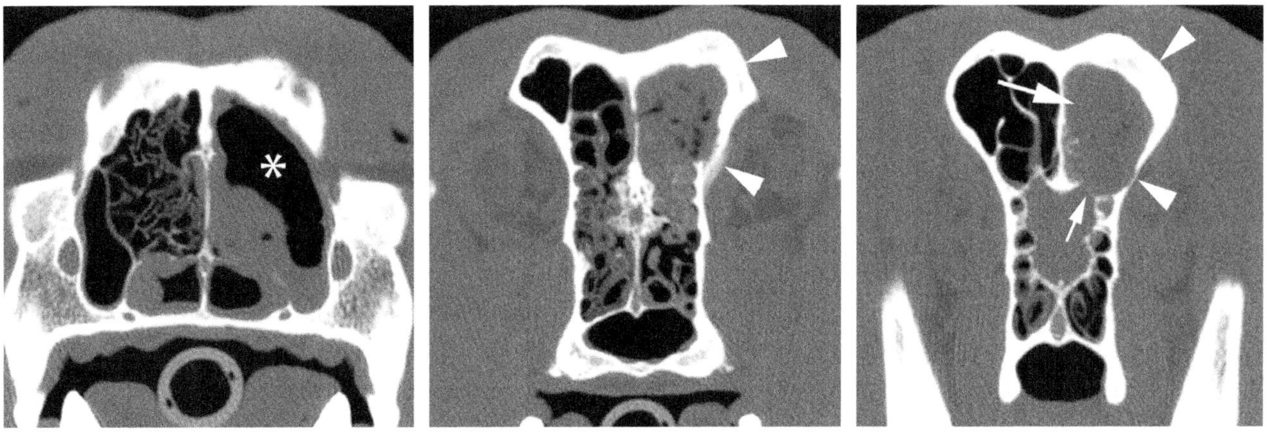

(a) CT, TP

(b) CT, TP

(c) CT, TP

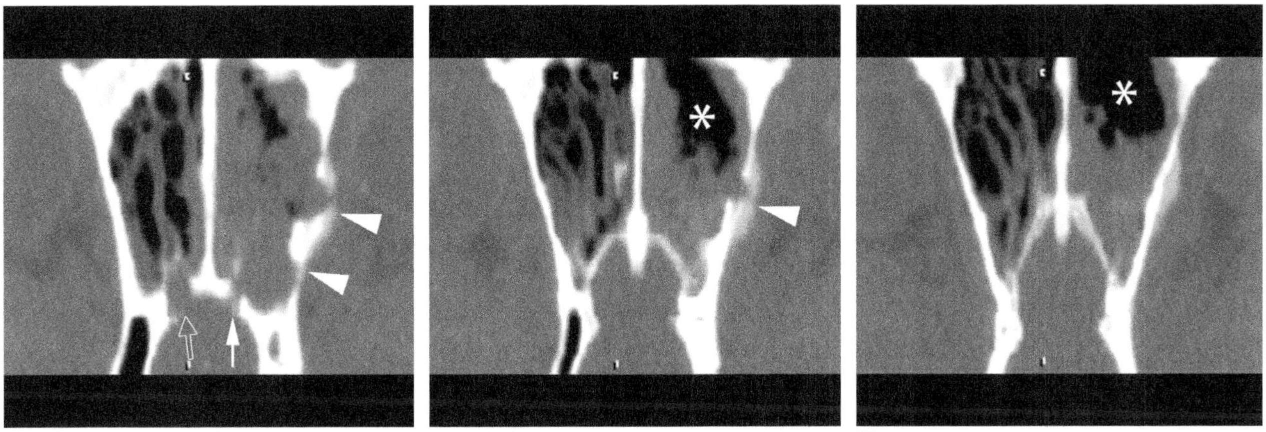

(d) CT, DP

(e) CT, DP

(f) CT, DP

11y MC Rottweiler with chronic left-sided mucopurulent and hemorrhagic nasal discharge. There is nasal turbinate atrophy with associated residual mucosal hypertrophy in the left nasal cavity (a,e,f: asterisk). The left frontal sinus contains a soft-tissue mass with entrapped fragmented gas (c: large arrow). A mixed pattern of frontal bone osteolysis and periosteal reactive productive response is also seen (b–e: arrowheads). A focal defect in the left dorsal cribriform plate is seen on both transverse and dorsal plane reformatted images (c,d: small arrow), and a second defect is suspected on the right side (d: open arrow), although there is no overt nasal disease adjacent to the cribriform plate on the right. Nasal biopsy confirmed a diagnosis of mycotic rhinosinusitis.

Figure 1.1.16 Mycotic Rhinosinusitis—Aspergillosis (Canine)   CT & MR

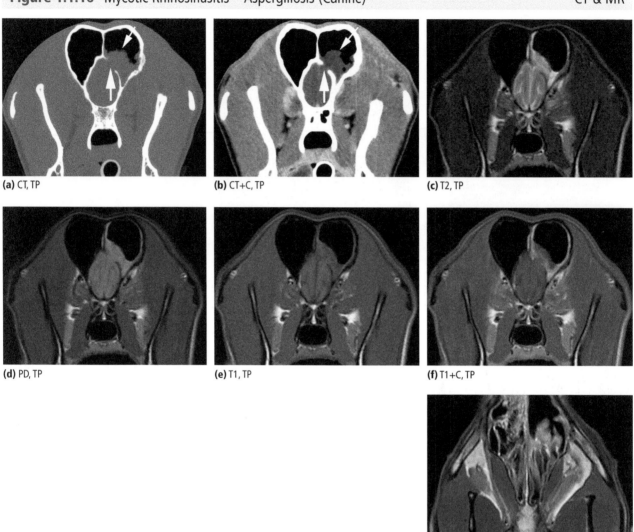

(a) CT, TP   **(b)** CT+C, TP   **(c)** T2, TP

(d) PD, TP   **(e)** T1, TP   **(f)** T1+C, TP

(g) T1+C, DP

14y MC Labrador Retriever with chronic left-sided nasal discharge. CT images were acquired at the time of initial evaluation. MR images were acquired approximately 2 months later. A large, focal defect is seen in the left frontal bone (**a**,**b**: large arrow). An adjacent irregularly margined soft-tissue mass is consistent with a fungus ball (**a**,**b**: small arrow). The bone defect is again seen on the subsequent MRI examination (**c–f**). Ill-defined contrast enhancement is seen within the defect, likely due to focal meningeal enhancement and possible left olfactory bulb invasion. A dorsal plane MR image shows a signal void within the left nasal cavity due to turbinate atrophy (**g**). Contrast-enhancing soft tissue in the caudal aspect of the nasal cavity likely represents hypertrophy of residual nasal mucosa. Nasal biopsy and fungal culture confirmed a diagnosis of mycotic rhinosinusitis due to *Aspergillus* species.

Figure 1.1.17 Cryptococcosis (Feline)

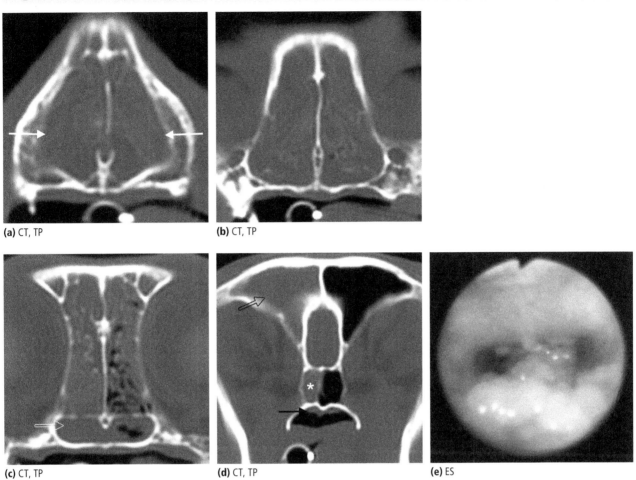

(a) CT, TP

(b) CT, TP

(c) CT, TP

(d) CT, TP

(e) ES

15y M Domestic Shorthair with stertor, sneezing, and progressive open-mouth breathing. The left and right nasal passages are completely opacified with soft tissue material, but bony turbinates are largely preserved (**a**: arrows). The left and right maxillary recesses, the nasopharynx (**c**: open arrow), and the left frontal (**d**: black open arrow) and sphenopalatine (**d**: asterisk) sinuses are also completely opacified with soft-tissue or fluid attenuating material. The dorsal wall of the nasopharynx appears irregular and thickened (**d**: black arrow), and the nasopharyngeal lumen is narrowed. Rhinoscopy revealed polypoid pharyngeal mucosal inflammation (**e**), and *Cryptococcus neoformans* was cultured from the tissue.

Figure 1.1.18 Nasal Lymphoma (Feline)

CT & MR

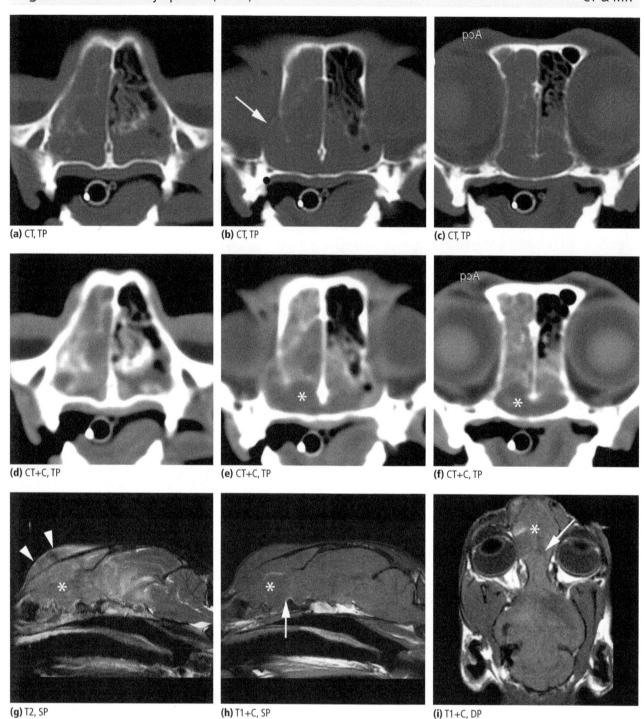

(a) CT, TP

(b) CT, TP

(c) CT, TP

(d) CT+C, TP

(e) CT+C, TP

(f) CT+C, TP

(g) T2, SP

(h) T1+C, SP

(i) T1+C, DP

12y MC Domestic Shorthair with chronic bilateral serosanguinous nasal discharge. Paired unenhanced (**a–c**) and contrast-enhanced (**d–f**) CT images progressing from rostral to caudal were acquired at the time of initial diagnosis. Soft-tissue opacity fills the nasal cavity, and there is underlying predominantly right-sided turbinate destruction. A poorly defined, contrast-enhancing mass is present in the ventral nasal cavity and extends into the nasopharynx (**e,f**: asterisk). There is lateral displacement of the frontal and/or palatine bone forming the deep part of the right orbit due to intranasal tumor expansion (**b**: arrow). The cat was treated with chemotherapy, and signs resolved for approximately 1 year. MR images (**g–i**) were acquired approximately 1 year following the CT examination after a recent onset of intracranial signs. There is a large, mildly contrast-enhancing soft-tissue mass within the nasal cavity, which extends caudally to involve the frontal sinuses (**g–i**: asterisk). Destruction of nasal and maxillary bones has occurred with dorsal extension of the neoplasm resulting in facial deformity (**g**: arrowheads). The mass also breaches the cribriform plate caudally (**h,i**: arrow) and extends into the rostral aspect of the cranial vault with associated forebrain edema (**g**).

Figure 1.1.19 Nasal Lymphoma (Canine)   CT

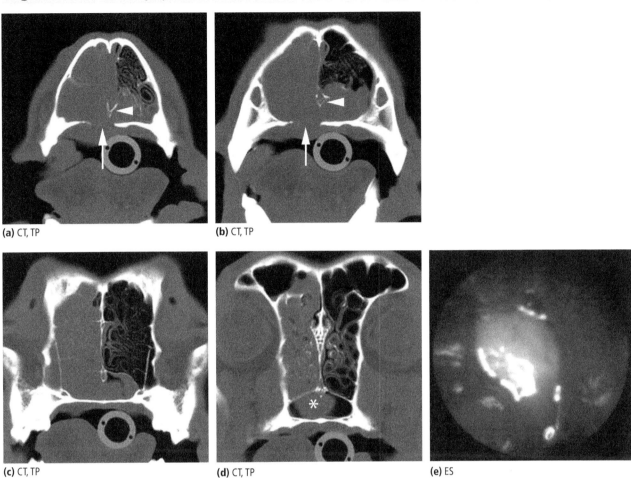

(a) CT, TP

(b) CT, TP

(c) CT, TP

(d) CT, TP

(e) ES

3y MC Rhodesian Ridgeback with a 3-month history of nasal discharge and stertor. There is a predominantly right-sided nasal mass that extends beyond midline to fill the ventral part of the left nasal cavity rostral to the maxillary sinuses. The mass extends caudally to the nasopharynx (**d**: asterisk). Nearly complete osteolysis of the right nasal ectoturbinates is evident (**a**,**b**), and there is destruction of the palatine portion of the maxilla and the palatine bone (**a**,**b**: arrow). Vomer bone destruction is also present where the mass extends across midline (**a**,**b**: arrowhead). Retrograde rhinoscopy revealed a nasopharyngeal mass (**e**).

Figure 1.1.20   Nasal Transitional Cell Carcinoma (Canine)   CT

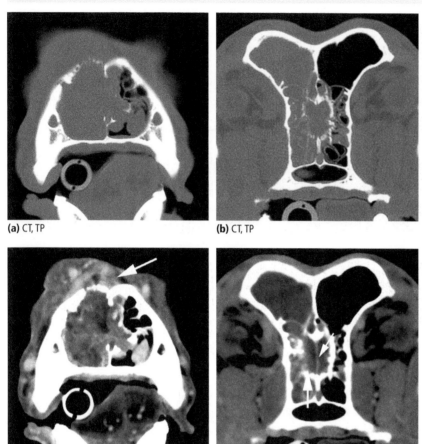

(a) CT, TP

(b) CT, TP

(c) CT+C, TP

(d) CT+C, TP

7y MC Golden Retriever cross with a 2-month history of right-sided epistaxis. A large soft-tissue mass fills the right nasal cavity and extends across midline (**a**). The right ectoturbinates are obliterated by the mass, and there is right maxillary and nasal septum destruction (**a**). Regional destruction of the right side of the cribriform plate is seen (**b**), and the right frontal sinus is filled with fluid-attenuating material. The nasal mass enhances heterogeneously and extends through the breach in the right maxillary bone (**c**: arrow). There is prominent meningeal enhancement adjacent to the right cribriform osteolytic region (**d**: large arrow) as well as an associated mild midline shift of the interolfactory longitudinal fissure (**d**: small arrow). Material within the right frontal sinus does not contrast enhance, confirming fluid and exudate entrapment from sinus obstruction. Nasal biopsy revealed transitional cell carcinoma.

Figure 1.1.21 Nasal Carcinoma (Canine)   MR

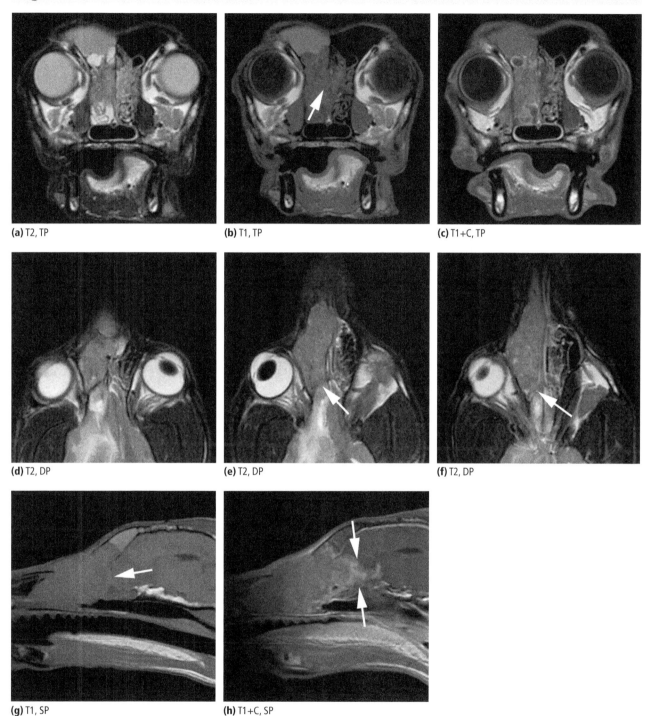

(a) T2, TP

(b) T1, TP

(c) T1+C, TP

(d) T2, DP

(e) T2, DP

(f) T2, DP

(g) T1, SP

(h) T1+C, SP

12y FS Australian Shepherd with progressive stertor. Transverse images (**a–c**) are at the same anatomic level at the rostral extent of the cribriform plate. Representative dorsal plane images (**d–e**) are ordered from dorsal to ventral. A large mass of mixed-signal intensity fills the right nasal cavity, obliterating the right ecto- and endoturbinates. Cribriform bone margins are ill-defined or absent and indicative of destruction (**b,e–g**: arrow). There is right olfactory and frontal lobe T2 hyperintensity associated with the breach of the cribriform plate and intracranial extension of the contrast-enhancing mass (**h**: arrows). Right frontal obstructive sinusitis is also present (**a–c,g**).

Figure 1.1.22 Nasal Anaplastic Adenocarcinoma (Canine)   CT

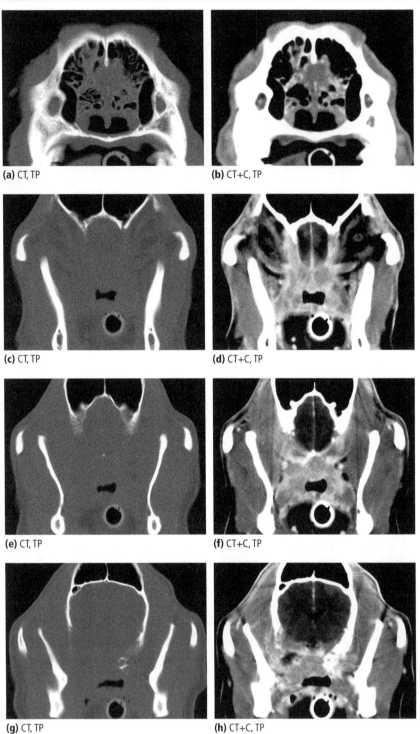

(a) CT, TP

(b) CT+C, TP

(c) CT, TP

(d) CT+C, TP

(e) CT, TP

(f) CT+C, TP

(g) CT, TP

(h) CT+C, TP

13y MC Schnauzer with trismus and temporal muscle atrophy. Representative CT images include unenhanced (**a,c,e,g**) and corresponding contrast-enhanced (**b,d,f,h**) images. A highly aggressive mass extends from the ethmoid bone to the retropharyngeal region. Mass margins are ill defined on the contrast-enhanced images with enhancement extending along fascial planes and invading temporal and pterygoid musculature. Marked destruction of ethmoid, frontal, palatine, pterygoid, and sphenoid bones is evident, and the mass extends into the cranial vault. Cytologic evaluation revealed aggressive, anaplastic adenocarcinoma.

Figure 1.1.23 Nasal Chondrosarcoma (Canine)   CT

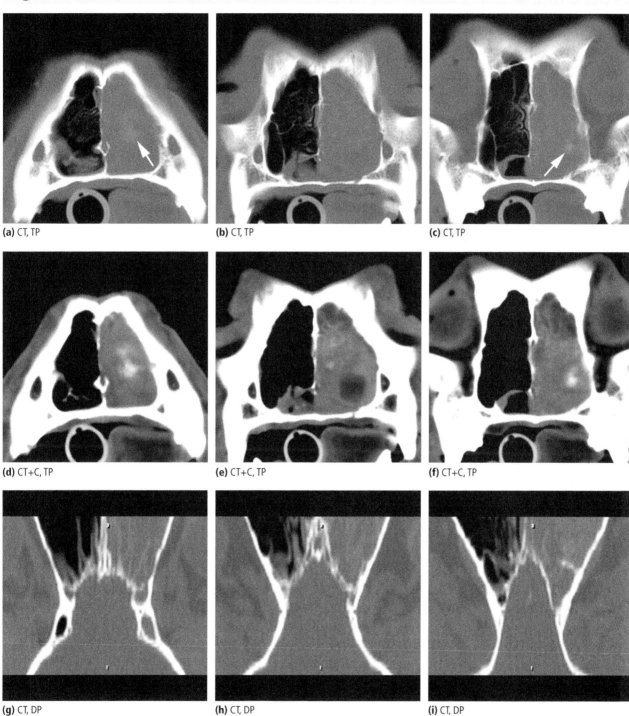

(a) CT, TP

(b) CT, TP

(c) CT, TP

(d) CT+C, TP

(e) CT+C, TP

(f) CT+C, TP

(g) CT, DP

(h) CT, DP

(i) CT, DP

6y FS Labrador Retriever cross with chronic epistaxis. Representative unenhanced (**a–c**) and corresponding contrast-enhanced (**d–f**) transverse images are ordered from rostral to caudal. Representative dorsal plane images are ordered from dorsal to ventral. A partially mineralized soft-tissue mass fills the left nasal cavity (**a–c**). Extensive turbinate destruction has occurred, but foci of amorphous intralesional mineralization are evident (**a,c**: arrow). The mass contrast enhances heterogeneously (**d–f**), and the mineralized foci are accentuated in the narrowly windowed enhanced images. The cribriform plate is intact (**g–i**). Nasal biopsy confirmed a diagnosis of chondrosarcoma.

Figure 1.1.24 Nasal Osteosarcoma (Canine)   CT

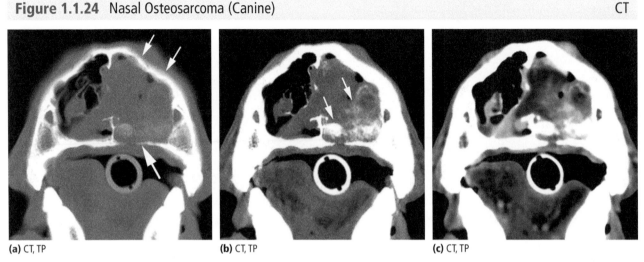

(a) CT, TP   (b) CT, TP   (c) CT, TP

11y FS Rottweiler with a 3-month history of sneezing and epistaxis. Representative transverse images are all at the same anatomic level in the midnasal cavity. Images **a** and **b** are the same image presented in a wide and a narrow window, respectively. A partially mineralized soft-tissue mass fills the left nasal cavity, with the extent of mineralization best seen in the narrowly windowed image (**b**: arrows). There is also associated destruction of the hard palate (**a**: large arrow) and productive reactivity of the maxilla (**a**: small arrows). The mass heterogeneously contrast enhances. A nasal biopsy confirmed a highly aggressive and infiltrative osteosarcoma.

Figure 1.1.25 Osteochondrosarcoma (Canine)   CT

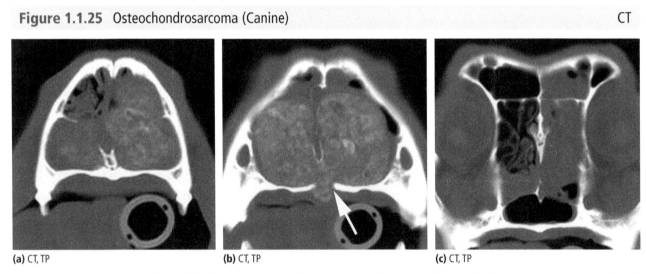

(a) CT, TP   (b) CT, TP   (c) CT, TP

5y MC Labrador Retriever with nasal discharge and stertor. There is a smoothly margined mineralized mass occupying the midnasal cavity. This mass extends ventrally through a bony defect at the rostral aspect of the palatine bone, and there is associated destruction of the nasal septum (**b**: arrow). Moderate fluid accumulation in the caudal nasal cavity and the left frontal sinus is also evident (**c**). This mass has the stippled, granular imaging features characteristic of multilobular osteochondrosarcoma. Although these neoplasms most commonly originate from flat bones comprising the calvarium, they have also been reported to arise from the hard palate.

Figure 1.1.26 Nasal Mast Cell Tumor (Canine)   CT & MR

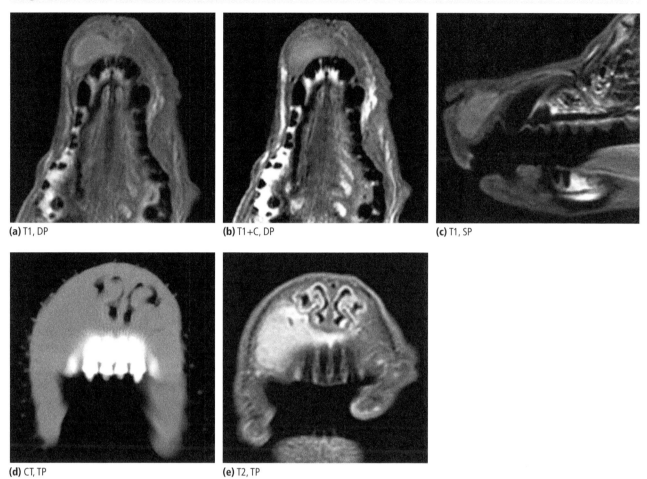

(a) T1, DP

(b) T1+C, DP

(c) T1, SP

(d) CT, TP

(e) T2, TP

8y FS Labrador Retriever with a rostral nasal mass. A well-defined ovoid mass is located adjacent to the right nares (**a–c**). The mass is soft-tissue attenuating on the CT image (**d**) and moderately T1 hyperintense (**b**) and markedly T2 hyperintense (**e**) on MR images. The T2 hyperintensity extends beyond the mass margins, indicating the presence of perilesional edema. The mass is only mildly contrast enhancing, which slightly diminishes lesion conspicuity because of the degree of enhancement of adjacent normal tissues (**b**). Biopsy revealed grade II–III mast cell tumor.

References

1. De Rycke LM, Saunders JH, Gielen IM, van Bree HJ, Simoens PJ. Magnetic resonance imaging, computed tomography, and cross-sectional views of the anatomy of normal nasal cavities and paranasal sinuses in mesaticephalic dogs. Am J Vet Res. 2003;64:1093–1098.
2. Losonsky JM, Abbott LC, Kuriashkin IV. Computed tomography of the normal feline nasal cavity and paranasal sinuses. Vet Radiol Ultrasound. 1997;38:251–258.
3. Noller C, Henninger W, Gronemeyer DH, Hirschberg RM, Budras KD. Computed tomography-anatomy of the normal feline nasolacrimal drainage system. Vet Radiol Ultrasound. 2006;47:53–60.
4. Hasegawa M, Kern EB. The human nasal cycle. Mayo Clin Proc. 1977;52:28–34.
5. Webber RL, Jeffcoat MK, Harman JT, Ruttimann UE. MR demonstration of the nasal cycle in the beagle dog. J Comput Assist Tomogr. 1987;11:869–871.
6. Schlueter C, Budras KD, Ludewig E, Mayrhofer E, Koenig HE, Walter A, et al. Brachycephalic feline noses: CT and anatomical study of the relationship between head conformation and the nasolacrimal drainage system. 2009;11:891–900.
7. Berent AC, Weisse C, Todd K, Rondeau MP, Reiter AM. Use of a balloon-expandable metallic stent for treatment of nasopharyngeal stenosis in dogs and cats: six cases (2005-2007). J Am Vet Med Assoc. 2008;233:1432–1440.
8. Saunders JH, van Bree H, Gielen I, de Rooster H. Diagnostic value of computed tomography in dogs with chronic nasal disease. Vet Radiol Ultrasound. 2003;44:409–413.
9. Lefebvre J, Kuehn NF, Wortinger A. Computed tomography as an aid in the diagnosis of chronic nasal disease in dogs. J Small Anim Pract. 2005;46:280–285.
10. Karnik K, Reichle JK, Fischetti AJ, Goggin JM. Computed tomographic findings of fungal rhinitis and sinusitis in cats. Vet Radiol Ultrasound. 2009;50:65–68.
11. Johnson LR, Drazenovich TL, Herrera MA, Wisner ER. Results of rhinoscopy alone or in conjunction with sinuscopy in dogs with

aspergillosis: 46 cases (2001–2004). J Am Vet Med Assoc. 2006; 228:738–742.

12. Johnson EG, Wisner ER. Advances in respiratory imaging. Vet Clin North Am Small Anim Pract. 2007;37:879–900.

13. Saunders JH, Clercx C, Snaps FR, Sullivan M, Duchateau L, van Bree HJ, et al. Radiographic, magnetic resonance imaging, computed tomographic, and rhinoscopic features of nasal aspergillosis in dogs. J Am Vet Med Assoc. 2004;225:1703–1712.

14. Saunders JH, van Bree H. Comparison of radiography and computed tomography for the diagnosis of canine nasal aspergillosis. Vet Radiol Ultrasound. 2003;44:414–419.

15. Saunders JH, Zonderland JL, Clercx C, Gielen I, Snaps FR, Sullivan M, et al. Computed tomographic findings in 35 dogs with nasal aspergillosis. Vet Radiol Ultrasound. 2002;43:5–9.

16. Whitney BL, Broussard J, Stefanacci JD. Four cats with fungal rhinitis. J Feline Med Surg. 2005;7:53–58.

17. Petite AF, Dennis R. Comparison of radiography and magnetic resonance imaging for evaluating the extent of nasal neoplasia in dogs. J Small Anim Pract. 2006;47:529–536.

18. Sako T, Shimoyama Y, Akihara Y, Ohmachi T, Yamashita K, Kadosawa T, et al. Neuroendocrine carcinoma in the nasal cavity of ten dogs. J Comp Pathol. 2005;133:155–163.

19. Schoenborn WC, Wisner ER, Kass PP, Dale M. Retrospective assessment of computed tomographic imaging of feline sinonasal disease in 62 cats. Vet Radiol Ultrasound. 2003;44:185–195.

20. Tromblee TC, Jones JC, Etue AE, Forrester SD. Association between clinical characteristics, computed tomography characteristics, and histologic diagnosis for cats with sinonasal disease. Vet Radiol Ultrasound. 2006;47:241–248.

21. Drees R, Forrest LJ, Chappell R. Comparison of computed tomography and magnetic resonance imaging for the evaluation of canine intranasal neoplasia. J Small Anim Pract. 2009;50:334–340.

1.2

Ear

Normal ear

The ear is divided into external, middle, and internal components. The external ear includes the pinna, the external ear canal, and external acoustic meatus. The middle ear includes the tympanic membrane, the osseous bulla, and the auditory ossicles. The inner ear, located within the temporal bone, includes the semicircular canals, vestibule, and cochlea. Together these structures define the labyrinth. CT and MR appearance of the normal ear have been previously reported (Figures 1.2.1, 1.2.2).[1,2]

Although the normal tympanic membrane can be seen on CT and MR images, it is usually obscured by the presence of adjacent horizontal canal or bulla effusion in patients with external and/or middle ear disease. The auditory ossicles and labyrinth are likewise visible on normal CT and MR images[3,4] but are typically more difficult to accurately identify in the presence of middle and inner ear disease. Thinly collimated CT images (1 mm or less) and 3D sequences to produce thin MR images are recommended to fully evaluate the labyrinth if subtle disease is suspected.

Inflammatory disorders

Otitis externa

Uncomplicated otitis externa is characterized by inflammation of the external ear canal. Hyperplastic thickening of the canal lining occurs as a response to chronic inflammation, causing ceruminous and aqueous exudates to fill the canal lumen. Exudates are generally hypoattenuating to adjacent canal epithelium on CT

images. Exudates are typically hyperintense on MR T2 images and of variable intensity on T1 images depending on the cellular and macromolecular content of the exudative fluid. Canal lining hyperplasia is strongly contrast enhancing on CT and MR images because of the high vascular density of the inflamed canal wall (Figure 1.2.3).

Inflammatory polyps

Inflammatory polyps may arise from the external ear canal epithelium in association with otitis externa. Polyps are typically vascular, resulting in moderate enhancement and increased conspicuity on contrast-enhanced CT and MR images (Figure 1.2.4).

Polyps may also arise from the epithelial lining of the tympanic membrane or within the auditory canal extending into the nasopharynx and most commonly occur in the cat (Figure 1.2.5). Polyps may not be readily distinguished from surrounding fluid on unenhanced CT and MR images but are easily detected on contrast-enhanced images. Neoplastic masses may also occasionally arise within or adjacent to the tympanic bulla and should be distinguished from inflammatory polyps.

Cellulitis, abscesses and fistulae

Pericanalicular cellulitis, abscesses, and fistulae may occur secondary to otitis externa when the canal wall is breached. Abscesses have a typical cavitary appearance with a fluid-filled center that appears hypoattenuating on CT, hyperintense on MR T2 images, and of variable intensity on T1 images, depending on the cellular and macromolecular content of the exudative fluid. Abscess walls and surrounding cellulitic tissue are highly contrast

Atlas of Small Animal CT and MRI, First Edition. Erik R. Wisner and Allison L. Zwingenberger.
© 2015 John Wiley & Sons, Inc. Published 2015 by John Wiley & Sons, Inc.

enhancing on both CT and MR images as a result of high vascular density and increased vascular permeability (Figure 1.2.6). Gravitational migration of inflammation may result in development of fistulae that may be tracked back to the external ear canal by conventional or CT fistulography.

Bulla effusion

While not necessarily inflammatory, bulla effusion must be differentiated from otitis media. Unilateral or bilateral sterile bulla effusion can occur secondary to obstruction of auditory canal flow (Figure 1.2.5). This entity has been described as a common sequela to either nasal disease, particularly in association with pharyngeal masses or pharyngitis, or to brachycephalic syndrome.[5–7] In affected dogs, the effusion is progressive but is not accompanied by clinical signs other than loss of hearing. Bulla fluid accumulates from bulla lining secretions and therefore contains macromolecules and cellular debris that appear fluid attenuating on CT images, hyperintense on T2 images, and of variable intensity on T1 images.

Otitis media

Bulla effusion may be the only abnormal imaging feature in early otitis media, although the disorder is often present concurrent with otitis externa and may involve the petrosal part of the temporal bone, depending on chronicity and severity. Exudative effusion appears soft-tissue attenuating on CT images, hyperintense on T2 images, and of intermediate intensity on T1 images (Figure 1.2.7). The bulla lining typically becomes thickened and irregular and markedly contrast enhances on both CT and MR images. With increasing chronicity, the bulla wall may become thickened and irregularly margined as a result of reactive osteitis, and the bulla cavity volume may increase, presumably because of the effect of hydrostatic pressure from the effusion (Figure 1.2.8). On CT images, one must use caution in assessing the thickness of the osseous bulla wall because replacement of air by fluid within the bulla cavity may artifactually increase apparent thickness. Thickening and/or expansion of the osseous bulla may also be present without other abnormal imaging findings in patients with previous otitis media that has resolved.

Otitis interna and intracranial extension

Osteitis of the petrous temporal bone is commonly associated with chronic otitis media, and progression to otitis interna is suggested by the presence of cranial nerve VII and VIII deficits. Infection may progress through the internal acoustic meatus or by direct extension through osteolysis of the petrous temporal bone. Some combination of osteosclerosis and osteolysis of the petrous temporal bone may be seen, and meningeal and cranial nerve VII/VIII enhancement is often present on contrast-enhanced images (Figures 1.2.9, 1.2.10, 1.2.11).[8]

Cholesteatoma

Aural cholesteatomas are epidermoid cysts that form expansile masses of keratin debris and keratinized squamous epithelium. They may be congenital or acquired; however, in dogs cholesteatomas appear to be acquired and are likely initiated by underlying otitis media. Cholesteatomas are most often unilateral, but bilateral lesions can occur. Imaging findings include a combination of bulla expansion, reactive osteoproliferation, and bulla osteolysis (Figure 1.2.12). A soft-tissue mass is present centrally in the region of the tympanic bulla, which usually contrast enhances heterogeneously or peripherally. In some patients, osteolysis of the petrous and squamous parts of the temporal bone may occur, with resulting intracranial extension of disease (Figure 1.2.13). In these cases, neurologic signs associated with cranial nerves VII and VIII may be evident, and regional meningeal contrast enhancement is sometimes present.[9] Sclerosis and osteoproliferation of the temporomandibular joint and paracondylar process can be seen.

Neoplasia

Neoplastic masses may arise within the external ear canal. The World Health Organization (WHO) recognizes both ceruminous gland adenomas and ceruminous gland adenocarcinomas in this category.

Ceruminous gland adenomas expand into and may occlude the external ear canal, leading to secondary otitis externa; however, the integrity of the external ear canal wall is typically maintained (Figure 1.2.14). Adenomas appear similar to inflammatory polyps. As with polyps, adenomas contrast enhance on both CT and MR images, increasing conspicuity.

Ceruminous adenocarcinomas are often well advanced by the time of imaging evaluation, and the specific site of origin may not be easily determined. These tumors are aggressive and highly invasive, typically obliterating the external ear canal and often extending to the middle and inner ear. Adenocarcinomas are also highly destructive, resulting in osteolysis of the osseous bulla and erosion of the petrous and squamous parts of the temporal bone (Figure 1.2.15). These tumors are highly but heterogeneously contrast enhancing on both CT and MR images. Depending on the size of the mass, adjacent structures, such as the pharynx, larynx, mandibular salivary gland, and temporal musculature, may be involved. Intracranial extension can occur with advanced disease, resulting in intracranial mass effect and meningeal contrast enhancement. The scan volume should always include the mandibular and medial retropharyngeal lymph nodes since reactive lymphadenopathy and regional metastasis are common.

The WHO recognizes squamous cell carcinoma of the tympanic bulla and tympanic adenocarcinoma as tumors arising from the middle and inner ear. As with ceruminous adenocarcinomas of the external ear, malignant tumors of the middle ear may be advanced by the time they are imaged, and the specific location of origin may be difficult or impossible to determine. Tympanic squamous cell carcinomas and adenocarcinomas appear similar to ceruminous gland carcinomas of the external ear on imaging studies, and differentiation is unlikely. These tumors are also highly invasive and bone destructive, typically involving the internal ear and often extending intracranially (Figures 1.2.16, 1.2.17). Malignant tumors are highly but heterogeneously contrast enhancing on both CT and MR images. Pharyngeal and cervical adnexa are also frequently affected, and regional lymphadenopathy is common.

Degenerative disorders

Cartilage mineralization

Mineralization of the supportive cartilage of the external ear canal may be seen as an incidental finding but is more often associated with chronic otitis externa. Mineralization appears primarily in the horizontal ear canal as linear or plaque-like mineral attenuation on CT (Figure 1.2.18) and may appear as an amorphous signal void in the region of the external ear on MRI.

Otolithiasis

Otolithiasis of the middle ear has been described in dogs with active or previous otitis media. Authors ascribed the otoliths to mineralization of necrotic debris in the osseous bulla, but otoliths sometimes appear to arise directly from the internal bulla margins and may well represent a proliferative osseous response. On CT images, otoliths appear within the tympanic bulla as solitary or multiple mineral densities of variable shape and size (Figure 1.2.19). Concurrent otitis media may also be seen.

Figure 1.2.1   Normal Ear (Canine)   CT

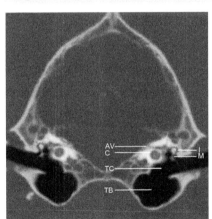

The normal canine ear on CT examination with thin collimation and bone algorithm. The vestibular aqueduct (AV) contains an extension of the membranous labyrinth and connects with the meninges of the brain. The cochlea is visible as a small, circular structure (C). The incus (I) and malleolus (M) are visible in the dorsal portion of the ear. The air-filled space of the ear is divided into the tympanic cavity (TC) and tympanic bulla (TB) by the tympanic septum (not shown).

(a) CT, TP

Figure 1.2.2   Normal Ear (Canine)   MR

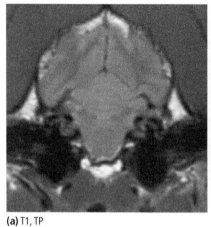

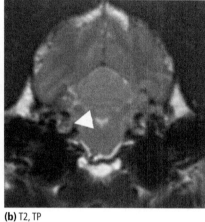

MR images of the normal canine ear. A transverse T1 image is shown on the left, T2 on the right. The cochlea is visible as a hyperintense structure on the T2 image (**b**: arrowhead).

(a) T1, TP   **(b)** T2, TP

Figure 1.2.3   Otitis Externa (Canine)   CT

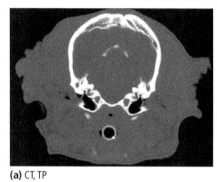

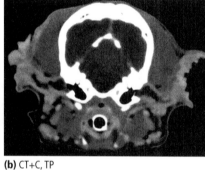

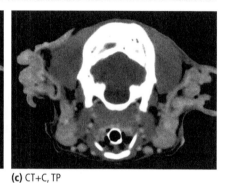

(a) CT, TP   **(b)** CT+C, TP   **(c)** CT+C, TP

1y MC Maltese with a history of chronic otitis externa. The external ear canals are occluded because of stenosis and exudates (**a**). Contrast-enhanced images show marked enhancement and redundancy of the external ear canal walls (**b,c**). Gas and fluid within the canal lumen can be distinguished from adjacent enhancing epithelium (**b**). Biopsy revealed severe diffuse chronic lymphoplasmacytic otitis externa with epithelial hyperplasia and ceruminous and sebaceous gland hyperplasia.

Figure 1.2.4   Inflammatory Polyp—External Ear (Feline)   CT

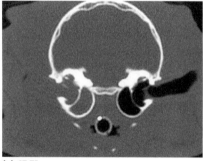

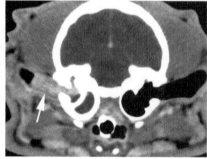

(a) CT, TP   **(b)** CT+C, TP

1y MC Domestic Shorthair with history of right-sided ear infections. Fluid/soft-tissue opacity within the right external ear canal and tympanic bulla is indicative of otitis externa and otitis media (**a**). On a contrast-enhanced image, a well-delineated contrast-enhancing mass is seen within the horizontal part of the right external ear canal and the bulla (**b**: arrow). The mass is distinguished from nonenhancing fluid in the bulla. An excisional biopsy revealed inflammatory polyp and suppurative otitis externa.

Figure 1.2.5 Obstructive Bulla Effusion—Nasopharyngeal Polyp (Feline)   CT

(a) CT, TP   **(b)** CT+C, TP   **(c)** CT+C, SP

3mo F Domestic Shorthair with a history of stertor and increased respiratory effort. Bilateral tympanic bulla effusion is seen, associated with mild bulla wall thickening (**a**). A large polyp completely occludes the nasopharyngeal lumen (**b,c**: arrow). The nasopharyngeal mass likely occludes the auditory canals, resulting in obstructive bulla effusion. The polyp was removed endoscopically using traction.

Figure 1.2.6 Otitis Externa and Media with Abscessation and Cellulitis (Canine)   CT

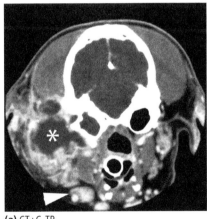

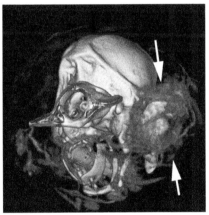

(a) CT+C, TP   **(b)** CT+C, 3D, OBL

3y MC Cocker Spaniel with a history of bilateral chronic otitis externa. A right-sided external ear canal ablation procedure was performed 2 years prior to the CT examination. A poorly marginated, fluid-filled mass is present adjacent to the right middle ear (**a**: asterisk). The mass is peripherally contrast enhancing, and enhancement extends along subcutaneous and interfascial planes. The right tympanic bulla is fluid filled, indicative of otitis media. The ipsilateral mandibular lymph nodes are enlarged (**a**: arrowhead). The 3D colorized rendering illustrates the prominent vascular density of the periphery of the lesion (**b**: arrows). Excisional biopsy revealed severe chronic granulomatous inflammation with intralesional ceruminous debris.

Figure 1.2.7   Otitis Media (Canine)   MR

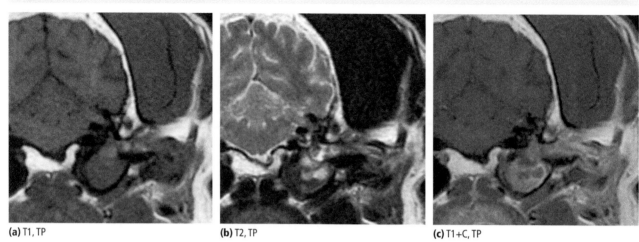

(a) T1, TP   **(b)** T2, TP   **(c)** T1+C, TP

10y M Golden Retriever with uncomplicated otitis media. The tympanic bulla contains material of mixed intensity on both the unen-hanced T1 image and the T2 image (**a,b**). The majority of the contents contrast enhance in the periphery of the bulla, indicating a pro-nounced thickening of the bulla lining (**c**). The nonenhancing regions represent entrapped fluid. The wall of the bulla is nonuniform in thickness and is irregularly margined because of reactive bulla osteitis (**c**). External ear canal stenosis, canal wall thickening, and marked contrast enhancement are indicative of concurrent otitis externa.

Figure 1.2.8   Otitis Media with Thickened Tympanic Bulla (Canine)   CT

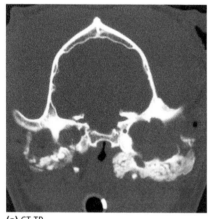

5y FS Labrador Retriever with a history of chronic bilateral otitis externa. Both external ear canals and tympanic bullae are filled with fluid-attenuating material. The left tympanic bulla cavity has expanded. There is a marked irregular proliferative bony response involving both bulla walls. The proliferative response is consistent with reactive osteitis associated with chronic otitis media.

(a) CT, TP

Figure 1.2.9   Otitis Media and Interna—Cranial Nerve VIII Involvement (Canine)   CT

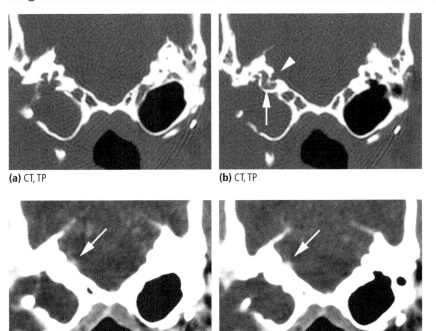

(a) CT, TP

(b) CT, TP

(c) CT+C, TP

(d) CT+C, TP

6y MC Cocker Spaniel with chronic ear infections. Bilateral ear canal ablations were performed 2 years previously, and the dog has recently developed right-sided peripheral vestibular signs. On sequential unenhanced images, the right tympanic bulla is filled with fluid-attenuating material, and there is partial osteolysis of the bulla wall laterally. The right internal acoustic meatus (**b**: arrowhead) and a portion of the cochlea (**b**: arrow) are seen. On contrast-enhanced images, there is enhancement of tissues surrounding the tympanic bulla consistent with a clinically confirmed abscess. There is also focal intracranial contrast enhancement in the location of the cochlear branch of the vestibulocochlear nerve (**c,d**: arrow), suggesting extension of disease through the internal acoustic meatus.

Figure 1.2.10   Otitis Media and Interna with Intracranial Extension (Canine)   MR

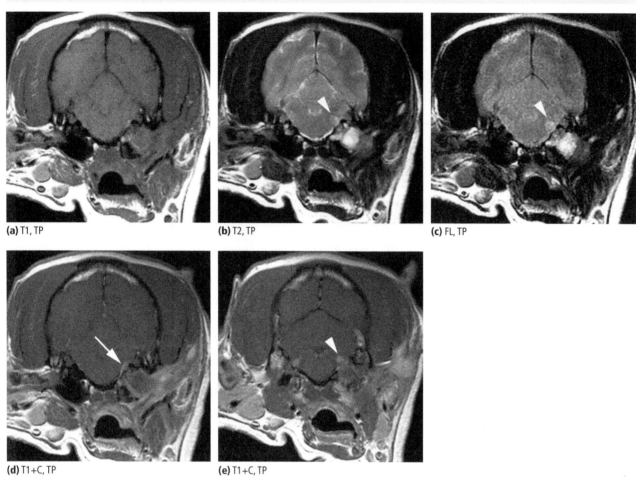

(a) T1, TP   **(b)** T2, TP   **(c)** FL, TP

(d) T1+C, TP   **(e)** T1+C, TP

13y West Highland White Terrier with a history of chronic otitis externa/media. A left-sided external ear canal ablation and bulla osteotomy were performed 18 months previously. The dog currently has peripheral vestibular signs. Images **a–d** are all at the same level. Image **e** is slightly more caudal. The residual bulla cavity is fluid and tissue filled. There is increased signal intensity of the left petrous temporal bone on all image sequences. There is also focal T2 hyperintensity of the left vestibulocochlear nerve (**b**: arrowhead), which is seen as increased signal intensity on the FLAIR sequence (**c**: arrowhead), suggesting cranial nerve VIII neuritis. Focal meningeal and petrosal contrast enhancement are present (**d**: arrow), indicative of meningitis. Enlargement of the left vestibulocochlear nerve is also seen on contrast-enhanced images (**e**: arrowhead).

Figure 1.2.11 Otitis Media and Interna—Meningeal Enhancement (Feline)   MR

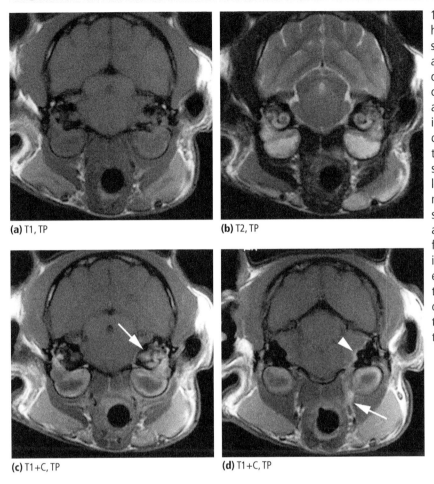

(a) T1, TP

(b) T2, TP

(c) T1+C, TP

(d) T1+C, TP

11y FS Domestic Shorthair with 1-week history of left-sided peripheral vestibular signs. Images **a–c** were acquired at the same anatomic level. Image **d** is slightly more caudal. The tympanic bullae contain material consistent with exudative fluid based on T1 and T2 signal characteristics. Marked thickening of the bulla epithelial lining is evident on contrast-enhanced images (**c,d**). In addition, there is enhancement of the soft-tissue structures encased within the left osseous labyrinth (**c**: arrow). Focal meningeal enhancement is also evident adjacent to the internal surface of the petrous temporal bone (**d**: arrowhead). This constellation of imaging features is consistent with otitis media, otitis interna, and regional meningitis. Contrast enhancement within fascial planes adjacent to the left tympanic bulla is indicative of cellulitis (**d**: arrow). Biopsy acquired at the time of bulla osteotomy revealed lymphohistiocytic and neutrophilic otitis media.

Figure 1.2.12 Cholesteatoma (Canine)   CT

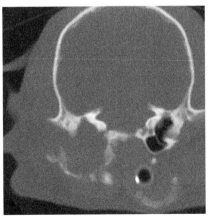

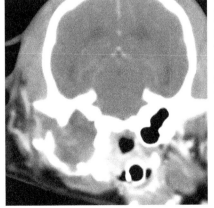

(a) CT, TP

(b) CT+C, TP

15y FS Miniature Poodle with a 6-month history of right-sided otitis externa. Marked expansion and osseous remodeling of the right tympanic bulla is seen. Soft-tissue attenuating material fills the bulla and the horizontal ear canal. Bulla contents and soft tissues adjacent to the bulla wall are mildly contrast enhancing. Histologic features of biopsy material were consistent with cholesteatoma.

Figure 1.2.13 Cholesteatoma with Otitis Interna (Canine) MR

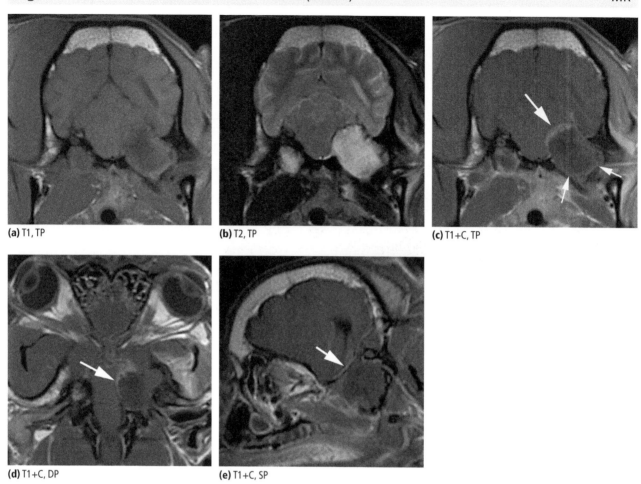

(a) T1, TP   **(b)** T2, TP   **(c)** T1+C, TP

(d) T1+C, DP   **(e)** T1+C, SP

7y FS French Bulldog with head tilt. There is a well-demarcated expansile mass emanating from the left tympanic bulla, which has eroded the petrous temporal bone and adjacent occipital bone, extends into the cranial vault, and has resulted in brainstem deformation. The mass is heterogeneous but T1 hypointense and moderately T2 hyperintense. There is irregular peripheral contrast enhancement (**c**: small arrows) and adjacent meningeal enhancement (**c–e**: large arrow). Similar signal changes are noted in the right tympanic bulla but are confined within the bulla cavity. Pronounced left-sided temporal, masseter, and pterygoid muscle atrophy is also evident. Biopsy revealed neutrophilic inflammatory response with abundant keratin-like debris consistent with cholesteatoma.

Figure 1.2.14 Ceruminous Adenoma—External Ear (Feline) CT

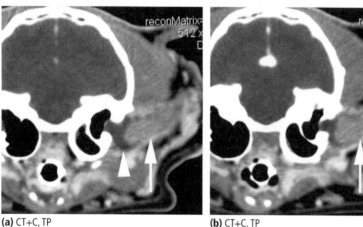

(a) CT+C, TP   **(b)** CT+C, TP

8y MC Domestic Shorthair with unilateral otitis externa. A well-delineated contrast-enhancing mass is seen within the horizontal part of the right external ear canal on contrast-enhanced images (**a,b**: arrow). Fluid is entrapped between the tympanic membrane and the mass in the proximal part of the canal (**a**: arrowhead). Thickening of the ipsilateral tympanic bulla and a small volume of exudate adherent to the bulla wall are suggestive of previous otitis media. Excisional biopsy revealed ceruminous adenoma of the external ear canal and chronic otitis externa.

Figure 1.2.15 Ceruminous Adenocarcinoma (Canine)   CT

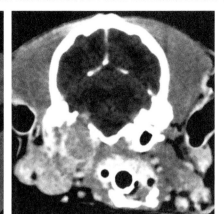

(a) CT, TP   **(b)** CT+C, TP

11y FS Lhasa Apso with a previously diagnosed right-sided ceruminous gland adenocarcinoma that was partially excised as part of an external ear canal ablation 1 year prior to the CT scan. Complete osteolysis of the tympanic bulla and partial osteolysis of the petrous temporal bone are evident on the unenhanced CT image (**a**). A large soft-tissue mass is present adjacent to the skull base, causing laryngeal displacement to the left of midline. Mass margins are ill defined, and normal fascial planes are obscured. The mass enhances on the contrast-enhanced image (**b**). Margins are moderately well defined, but there is intracranial extension of the mass through the petrous temporal bone defect.

Figure 1.2.16 Squamous Cell Carcinoma (Canine)   CT

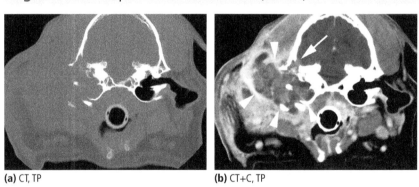

(a) CT, TP   **(b)** CT+C, TP

12y FS Golden Retriever with a mass associated with the right ear. A large, irregularly margined mass arises from the right middle ear (**a**). The external ear canal is not evident, and osteolysis of portions of the tympanic, petrosal, and squamous parts of the temporal bone is seen. The mass moderately and heterogeneously contrast enhances, and the bulk of the mass appears to be contained by the residual bulla and grossly distended external ear canal (**b**: arrowheads). There is also intracranial extension of the mass through a fenestration in the temporal bone (**b**: arrow). Ill-defined contrast enhancement is also present in peritumoral tissues. Biopsy of the mass revealed aural squamous cell carcinoma.

Figure 1.2.17   Squamous Cell Carcinoma (Canine)   MR

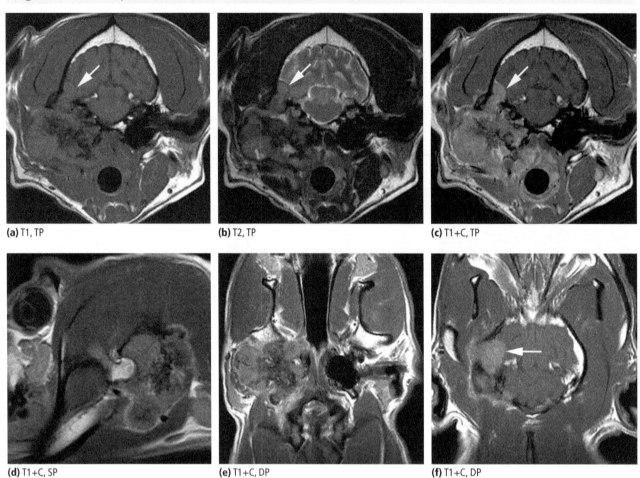

(a) T1, TP   **(b)** T2, TP   **(c)** T1+C, TP

(d) T1+C, SP   **(e)** T1+C, DP   **(f)** T1+C, DP

7y MC Labrador Retriever with a 1-month history of head tilt. There is a large, irregularly margined, and highly invasive mass of mixed-signal intensity arising from the region of the right middle ear (**a**,**b**). An amorphous signal void seen centrally within the mass on multiple sequences suggests partial mineralization. The right tympanic bulla is absent, and incomplete destruction of the petrosal and squamous parts of the right temporal bone is evident. The mass extends intracranially (**a**,**b**,**c**,**f**: arrow) and incorporates the right temporomandibular joint (**d**,**e**). Biopsy revealed squamous cell carcinoma.

Figure 1.2.18   Cartilage Mineralization (Canine)   CT

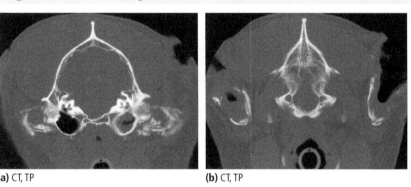

(a) CT, TP   **(b)** CT, TP

6y M German Shepherd Dog with longstanding history of bilateral otitis externa. Pronounced mineralization of the horizontal and vertical external ear canal walls is evident (**a**,**b**). External ear canals are occluded because of stenosis and exudates (**a**,**b**). Fluid-attenuating material is also present within the left tympanic bulla, indicative of concurrent otitis media (**a**). Biopsy of the canal wall revealed chronic neutrophilic otitis externa with osseous metaplasia.

Figure 1.2.19 Otitis Media with Otolith (Canine)   CT

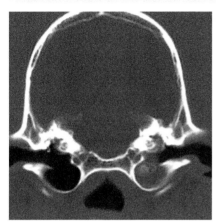

9y MC Australian Shepherd with chronic nasal discharge. The left tympanic bulla is fluid filled and contains multiple discrete mineral opacities. Biopsy acquired during bulla osteotomy yielded a histologic diagnosis of chronic otitis media with inspissated and mineralized debris.

(a) CT, TP

References

1. Allgoewer I, Lucas S, Schmitz SA. Magnetic resonance imaging of the normal and diseased feline middle ear. Vet Radiol Ultrasound. 2000;41:413–418.
2. Russo M, Covelli EM, Meomartino L, Lamb CR, Brunetti A. Computed tomographic anatomy of the canine inner and middle ear. Vet Radiol Ultrasound. 2002;43:22–26.
3. Garosi LS, Dennis R, Schwarz T. Review of diagnostic imaging of ear diseases in the dog and cat. Vet Radiol Ultrasound. 2003; 44:137–146.
4. Rohleder JJ, Jones JC, Duncan RB, Larson MM, Waldron DL, Tromblee T. Comparative performance of radiography and computed tomography in the diagnosis of middle ear disease in 31 dogs. Vet Radiol Ultrasound. 2006;47:45–52.
5. McGuinness SJ, Friend EJ, Knowler SP, Jeffery ND, Rusbridge C. Progression of otitis media with effusion in the Cavalier King Charles spaniel. Vet Rec. 2013;172:315.
6. Woodbridge NT, Baines EA, Baines SJ. Otitis media in five cats associated with soft palate abnormalities. Vet Rec. 2012;171:124.
7. Detweiler DA, Johnson LR, Kass PH, Wisner ER. Computed tomographic evidence of bulla effusion in cats with sinonasal disease: 2001-2004. J Vet Intern Med. 2006;20:1080–1084.
8. Sturges BK, Dickinson PJ, Kortz GD, Berry WL, Vernau KM, Wisner ER, et al. Clinical signs, magnetic resonance imaging features, and outcome after surgical and medical treatment of otogenic intracranial infection in 11 cats and 4 dogs. J Vet Intern Med. 2006;20:648–656.
9. Travetti O, Giudice C, Greci V, Lombardo R, Mortellaro CM, Di Giancamillo M. Computed tomography features of middle ear cholesteatoma in dogs. Vet Radiol Ultrasound. 2010;51:374–379.

1.3

Temporomandibular joint

Normal temporomandibular joint

The normal temporomandibular joint (TMJ) includes the articular surfaces of the condyloid process of the mandible and the mandibular fossa of the temporal bone, between which lies a cartilaginous articular disc. These structures are surrounded by a joint capsule and supported by a lateral ligament and adjacent muscles of mastication. High-resolution imaging protocols are necessary to visualize these structures.[1,2] Osseous structures are well visualized on CT images, although the intrinsic soft tissues of the joint are not clearly delineated (Figure 1.3.1). On MR images, the condyloid process and region of the mandibular fossa appear T1 and T2 hyperintense centrally, as a result of medullary fat, with a well to poorly defined signal void peripherally defining the subchondral bone margins. The articular disc is sometimes visible and has T1 iso- to hyperintensity and variable T2 intensity compared to muscle (Figure 1.3.2).[3]

Developmental disorders

Subchondral cysts

Subchondral bone cysts are occasionally seen in the condyloid process and are often clinically silent. Some cysts appear to be closed, while others may communicate with the joint space at the caudal aspect of the process. On CT images, cysts appear as spherical defects with well-demarcated dense bone margins (Figure 1.3.3). On MR images, cysts are typically T2 hyperintense and T1 hypointense centrally with a well-defined signal void peripherally because of the dense bone margin (Figure 1.3.4).

Temporomandibular dysplasia

Temporomandibular dysplasia has been reported in several canine breeds, including Dachshunds, Cocker Spaniels, Cavalier King Charles Spaniels, and Irish Setters.[4,5] The disorder is clinically characterized by temporomandibular joint laxity, resulting in subluxation or luxation, and an inability to close the mouth. CT imaging features include flattening of the condyloid process and mandibular fossa and hypoplasia of the retroarticular process (Figure 1.3.5). Although overt luxation is uncommon, the joint frequently appears incongruent or subluxated (Figure 1.3.6). As with other forms of dysplasia, the phenotypic expression of this disorder is variable, and imaging findings may be subtle in some patients.

Craniomandibular osteopathy

Craniomandibular osteopathy is an autosomal recessive developmental disease primarily affecting young West Highland White and other Terriers but also reported in a number of other breeds.[6–8] Clinical signs include swelling of the jaw due to bilaterally symmetrical new bone production, which can involve the mandibular body, ramus, and articular parts of the mandible. With severe manifestations, proliferative new bone encases the temporomandibular joints and extends to the temporal regions of the calvarium. Although radiographic evaluation usually suffices for diagnosis of the disorder, CT imaging may be useful to more accurately characterize the extent of temporomandibular joint involvement. CT imaging features include symmetrically distributed uniformly dense proliferative medullary and external

Atlas of Small Animal CT and MRI, First Edition. Erik R. Wisner and Allison L. Zwingenberger.
© 2015 John Wiley & Sons, Inc. Published 2015 by John Wiley & Sons, Inc.

woven bone formation involving the mandible and possibly the temporomandibular joints (Figure 1.3.7).

Trauma

Injury to the temporomandibular joint is a common sequela of head trauma. Although conventional radiographic imaging can be used to diagnose temporomandibular injury, it consistently underestimates the severity of trauma, particularly when complex fractures are present. Luxations and fractures are well delineated using CT imaging, with imaging features dependent on the specific trauma sustained (Figures 1.3.8, 1.3.9, 1.3.10, 1.3.11).[9]

Inflammatory disorders

Septic arthritis and osteomyelitis of the temporomandibular joint are occasionally encountered as a result of extension of otitis externa/media or a direct penetrating injury and may include articular cartilage and subchondral bone destruction, joint distension, and surrounding cellulitis (Figure 1.3.12).[10] General features of septic arthritis are described in Chapter 6.3.

Neoplasia

Although uncommon, neoplasia involving the temporomandibular joint may arise from intrinsic structures of the joint or from encroachment from adjacent neoplasms. Benign bone tumors, such as osteomas that arise from the mandible or temporal bone, may impinge on the temporomandibular joint and will typically appear as a dense, well-delineated mass on CT and as a low or no signal intensity mass on all MR sequences. CT features of sarcomas and carcinomas in this region may include osteolysis and soft-tissue mass with nonuniform contrast enhancement (Figure 1.3.13). MR features are similar and may also include replacement of T1 and T2

hyperintense medullary fat with lower intensity tumor (Figures 1.3.14, 1.3.15).

Degenerative disorders

Osteoarthrosis

Although commonly performed in people because of the high incidence of debilitating degenerative temporomandibular joint disorders, there are few reports on the use of high-resolution CT and MR imaging for diagnosis of this disorder in veterinary medicine. Although articular cartilage and the articular disc should be well visualized by MR using appropriate coils and pulse sequences, MR features of degenerative temporomandibular joint disease have not been fully described in dogs and cats. CT imaging features include narrowing of the joint space (best seen on sagittal plane reformatted images), condyloid process remodeling, subchondral bone sclerosis, and periarticular new bone formation (Figure 1.3.16). Similarly, MR imaging findings may include joint space narrowing and subchondral bone and periarticular new bone signal void.

Ankylosis

Occasionally, periarticular productive remodeling may be exuberant enough to restrict temporomandibular joint range of motion. This can be due either to primary temporomandibular degenerative joint disease or an adjacent proliferative response of the temporal bone associated with chronic otitis. True ankylosis is defined as bone fusion or synostosis. Most patients with reduced range of motion, in fact, have extracapsular or fibrous ankylosis. CT imaging findings consist of osteoarthrosis features in addition to more pronounced periarticular new bone formation (Figure 1.3.17). Comparable MR features would be expected in the form of ill-defined and nonuniform periarticular signal void on all sequences.

Figure 1.3.1 Normal Tempormandibular Joint (Canine) CT

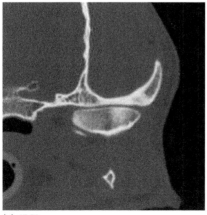 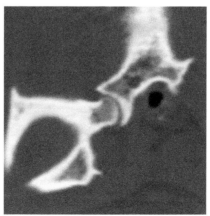

7y MC Australian Shepherd. Osseous structures are well visualized on CT images, although the intrinsic soft tissue structures of the joint are not clearly delineated.

(a) CT, TP   **(b)** CT, SP

Figure 1.3.2   Normal Temporomandibular Joint (Canine)   MR

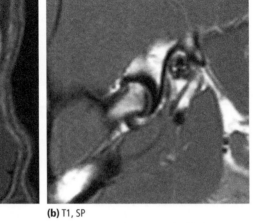

2y M Pit Bull Terrier. The condyloid process and region of the mandibular fossa appear T1 and T2 hyperintense centrally because of medullary fat, with a well to poorly defined signal void peripherally defining the subchondral bone margins. The apparent irregularity of the subchondral bone of the condyle on transverse images is due to partial volume averaging.

(a) T1, TP   **(b)** T1, SP

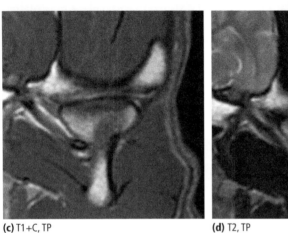

(c) T1+C, TP   **(d)** T2, TP

Figure 1.3.3   Subchondral Cyst of the Condylar Process (Canine)   CT

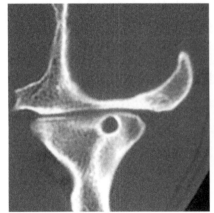

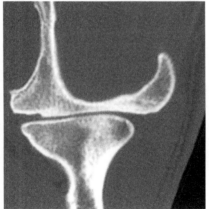

3y M Rottweiler. A CT scan of the head was performed as part of a diagnostic evaluation for chronic otitis. A well-delineated circular subchondral bone cyst is seen in the left mandibular condylar process (**a**). Contents are fluid-dense and surrounded by a thin rim of compact bone. The left condyle (**b**) is unremarkable and included in this figure in the same orientation for comparison. The cyst was clinically silent and identified as an incidental finding on this study.

(a) CT, TP   **(b)** CT, TP

Figure 1.3.4 Subchondral Cyst of the Condylar Process (Canine)   MR

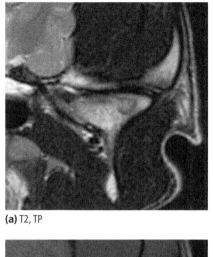

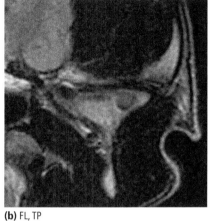

Adult MC Weimaraner. The MR study was part of a diagnostic evaluation of central neurologic signs. A well-delineated circular subchondral bone cyst is seen in the left mandibular condylar process. The center of the cyst has high water content, as suggested by the T2 hyperintensity and unenhanced T1 hypointensity. The low signal seen on the FLAIR image further suggests low cellular or macromolecular concentration, although the center does mildly contrast enhance.

(a) T2, TP   **(b)** FL, TP

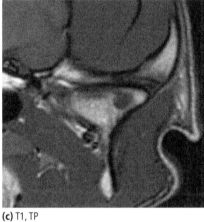

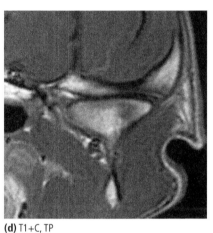

(c) T1, TP   **(d)** T1+C, TP

Figure 1.3.5 Mandibular Condylar Dysplasia (Canine)   CT

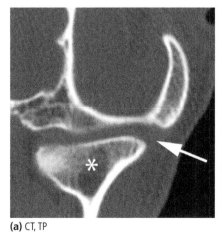

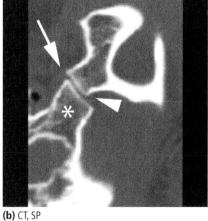

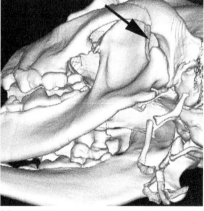

(a) CT, TP   **(b)** CT, SP   **(c)** CT, 3D, OBL

10mo MC Bassett Hound with a history of pain when opening the mouth and periodic episodes of inability to close the mouth. The sagittal reformatted image is oriented rostral to the left and caudal to the right. The left manibular condyle is misshapen (**a,b**: asterisk), and there is evidence of subluxation of the temporomandibular joint (**a–c**: arrow). The sagittal image reveals abnormal flattening of the articulating surfaces and striking hypoplasia of the retroarticular process resulting in ventral subluxation (**b**: arrowhead). Temporomandibular joint findings were bilaterally symmetrical in this dog.

Figure 1.3.6 Mandibular Condylar Dysplasia with Unilateral Luxation (Canine) CT

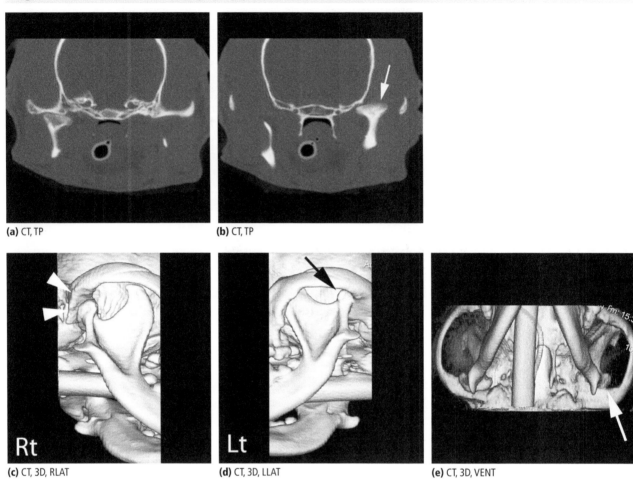

(a) CT, TP

(b) CT, TP

(c) CT, 3D, RLAT

(d) CT, 3D, LLAT

(e) CT, 3D, VENT

3y MC Lhasa Apso presented to the emergency service with temporomandibular luxation. The representative transverse images (**a,b**) are ordered from caudal to rostral. The left condyloid process is luxated rostrodorsally (**b,d,e**: arrow), and the right condyloid process is subluxated (**a,c**). The condyloid processes are misshapen, and the mandibular fossae are flattened with hypoplastic retroarticular processes (**c**: arrowheads).

Figure 1.3.7 Craniomandibular Osteopathy (Canine)   CT

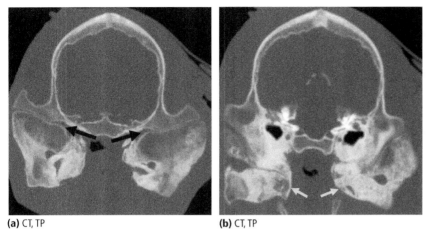

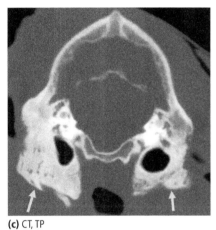
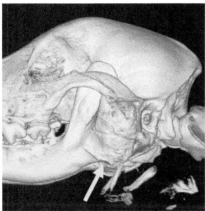

1y MC Golden Retriever with a history of mandibular swelling and pain. The representative transverse images (**a–c**) are ordered from rostral to caudal. There is marked, irregular, periosteal productive response that is symmetrically affecting the caudal mandible and temporomandibular joints. This productive response has extended to the temporomandibular joints (**a**: black arrows) and involves the temporal bones (**b–d**: arrows).

(a) CT, TP   **(b)** CT, TP

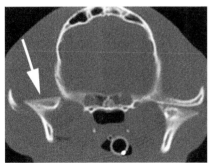
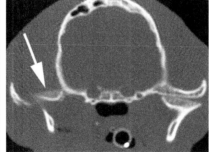

(c) CT, TP   **(d)** CT, 3D, LLAT

Figure 1.3.8 Unilateral Temporomandibular Joint Luxation (Feline)   CT

Mature MC Domestic Shorthair hit by a car within the past 24 hours. The representative transverse images are ordered from rostral to caudal. Images reveal a rostral and dorsal luxation of the right mandibular condylar process (**a,b**: arrow).

(a) CT, TP   **(b)** CT, TP

Figure 1.3.9 Temporomandibular Fracture–Luxation (Canine)   CT

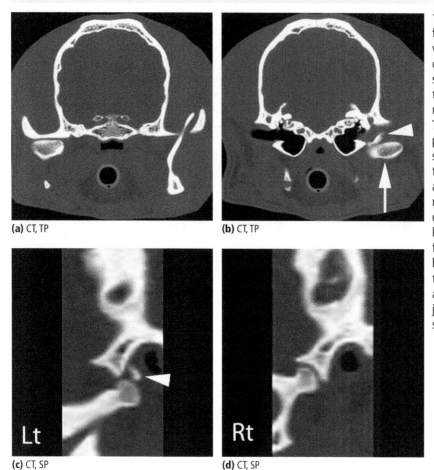

(a) CT, TP

(b) CT, TP

(c) CT, SP

(d) CT, SP

Lt

Rt

1y MC Lhasa Apso with a history of having fallen off a ledge. The representative transverse images are ordered from rostral to caudal. The two images reformatted in the sagittal plane are oriented in the same direction for easier comparison. In both images, rostral is to the left and caudal is to the right. There is caudal luxation of the left condyloid process. Although the head position is symmetrical, the left process is not seen on the rostral image (**a**) but comes into view on a more caudal image (**b**: arrow). The sagittal reformatted image of the left temporomandibular joint (**c**) clearly shows the caudal luxation as well as a caudally displaced fracture of the retroarticular process (**c**: arrowhead). The fracture fragment is also evident on the transverse images (**b**: arrowhead). The appearance of the right temporomandibular joint (**d**) is normal by comparison. Fluid is also seen within the left external ear canal (**b**).

Figure 1.3.10 Inflammatory Mandibular Mass with Temporomandibular Subluxation (Feline) CT

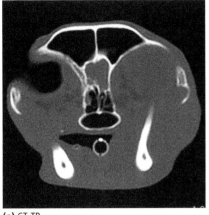

(a) CT, TP

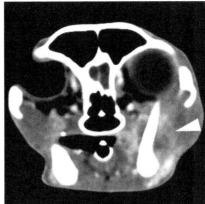

(b) CT+C, TP

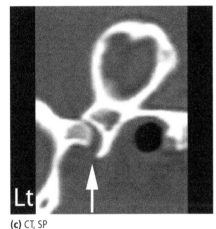

(c) CT, SP

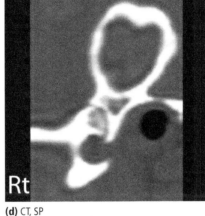

(d) CT, SP

12y FS Domestic Shorthair with iatrogenic open wound in the oropharyngeal region following a traumatic pill administration. Clinical signs included malocclusion, oral pain, and inability to close the mouth. The cat had a previous enucleation that is unrelated to the current presenting complaint. The transverse images are comparable unenhanced and contrast-enhanced images. The two images reformatted in the sagittal plane are oriented in the same direction for easier comparison. In both images, rostral is to the left and caudal is to the right. A heterogenously contrast-enhancing mass is evident surrounding the body of the mandible on the left (**b**: arrowhead). The left temporomandibular joint is subluxated as a result of extraarticular encroachment by the mass (**c**: arrow). The right temporomandibular joint is normal by comparison (**d**). Biopsy of the oropharyngeal region confirmed the presence of suppurative abscess and cellulitis.

Figure 1.3.11   Condylar Fossa Fracture (Canine)

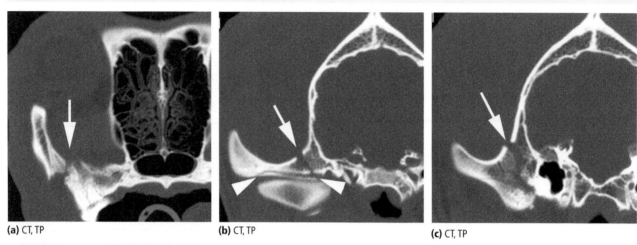

(a) CT, TP   **(b)** CT, TP   **(c)** CT, TP

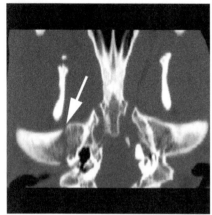

(d) CT, DP

1y German Shepherd Dog hit by a car 24 hours previously. The representative transverse images are ordered from rostral to caudal. A transverse fracture is seen in the rostral part of the right zygomatic bone near its articulation with the maxilla (**a**: arrow). A second, mildly displaced comminuted articular fracture is present near the origin of the zygomatic process of the right temporal bone (**b–d**: arrow). Another fracture line is evident coursing parallel to the subchondral bone margin of the fossa (**b**: arrowheads).

Figure 1.3.12 Temporomandibular Septic Arthritis (Canine)   MR

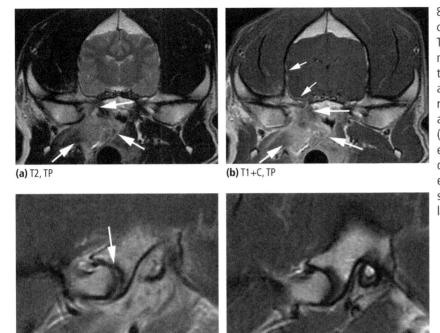

(a) T2, TP

(b) T1+C, TP

(c) T1+C, SP

(d) T1+C, SP

8y FS Rhodesian Ridgeback with regional cellulitis associated with otitis media/interna. T2 hyperintensity is seen adjacent to the medial margin of the right temporomandibular joint, the right lateral pterygoid muscle, and the dorsal aspect of the pharynx (**a**: arrows). The same region contrast enhances (**b**: large arrows), and additional meningeal enhancement is evident (**b**: small arrows). There is periarticular contrast enhancement involving the right temporomandibular joint, with associated intraarticular enhancement, and a diminished subchondral signal void (**c**: arrow). The left temporomandibular joint is normal by comparison (**d**).

Figure 1.3.13   Temporomandibular Fibrosarcoma (Canine)   CT

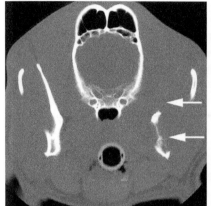

(a) CT, TP

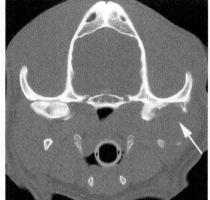

(b) CT, TP

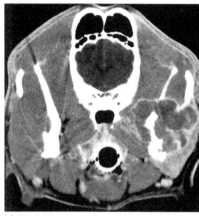

(c) CT+C, TP

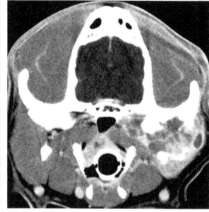

(d) CT+C, TP

6y M Golden Retriever with recent onset of oral pain. A large, aggressive bone-destructive mass is centered on the caudal aspect of the left side of the mandible. Osteolysis of the left mandibular ramus (**a**: arrows) and condyloid process (**b**: arrow) is evident. Bone destruction extends to and includes the subchondral bone of the process, implying an intraarticular component to the mass. On comparable contrast-enhanced images, the mass has a complex, lobular appearance (**c**,**d**). Aspiration biopsy revealed the mass to be a fibrosarcoma.

Figure 1.3.14 Temporal Bone Chondrosarcoma (Canine) MR

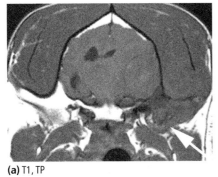

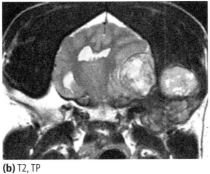

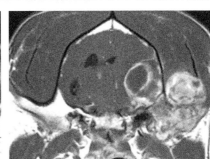

(a) T1, TP

(b) T2, TP

(c) T1+C, TP

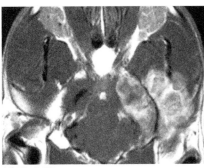

(d) T1+C, DP

8y FS German Shepherd Dog with neurologic signs relating to left cerebral and thalamic disease. A large, locally invasive complex mass arises from the temporal bone, with components extending intracranially and into the adjacent temporal musculature. Left temporal bone medullary signal intensity is reduced on unenhanced T1 images (**a**: arrow) as a result of marrow displacement by the mass, and cortical margins are attenuated. Multiple high intensity foci suggest the mass is multicameral and cystic (**b**). The mass is nonuniformly contrast enhancing (**c,d**). Biopsy revealed a highly anaplastic chondrosarcoma.

Figure 1.3.15 Temporomandibular Sarcoma (Canine) MR

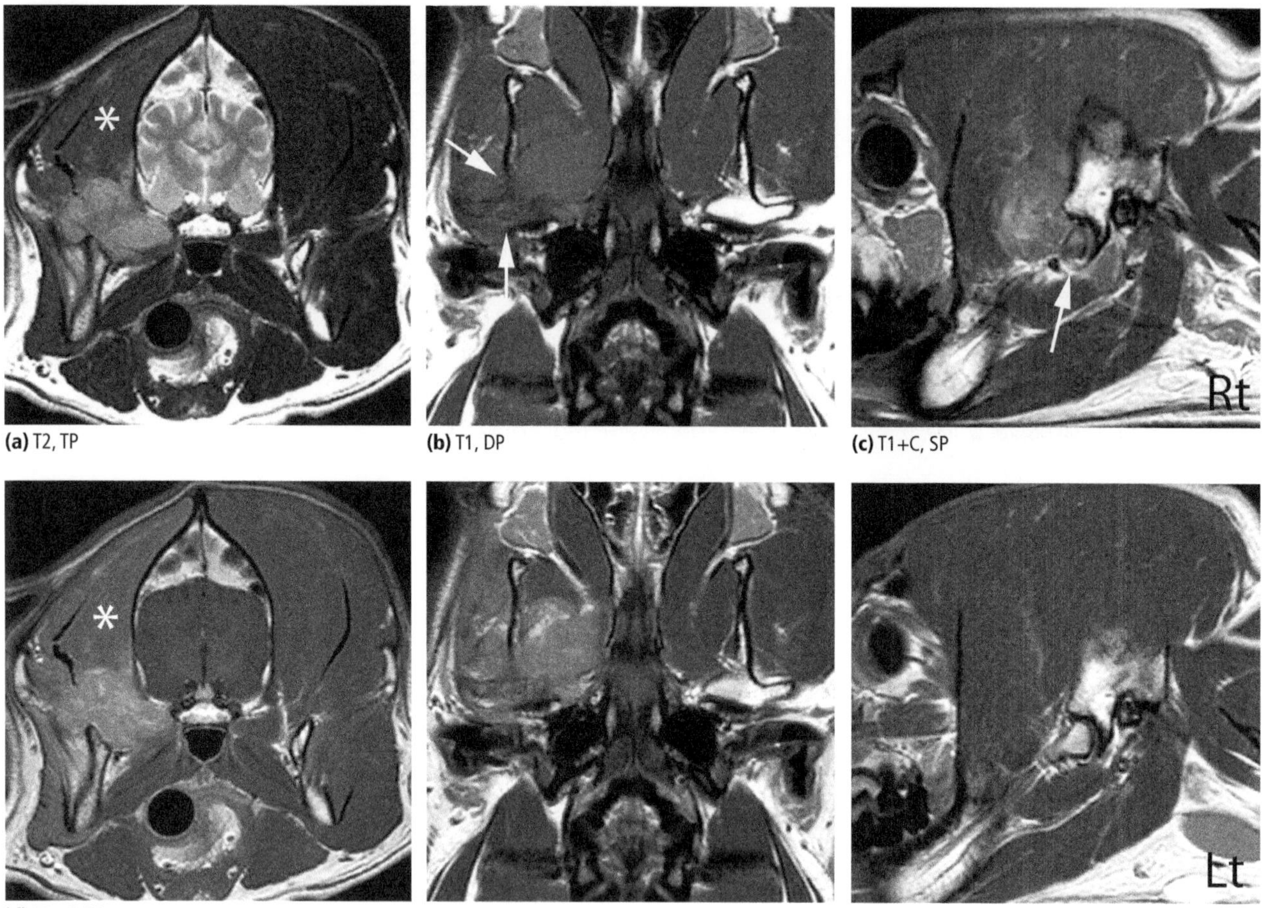

(a) T2, TP

(b) T1, DP

(c) T1+C, SP

(d) T1+C, TP

(e) T1+C, DP

(f) T1+C, SP

8y MC Rottweiler with progressive right temporal and masseter muscle atrophy and pain upon opening the mouth. A poorly margined lobular mass arises in the region of the right mandibular process, resulting in mandibular cortical bone destruction and diminished marrow signal intensity on the unenhanced T1 image (**b**: arrows). The mass is moderately and uniformly contrast enhancing (**c–e**). Replacement of the normal right condyloid process architecture by the mass with extension into the right temporomandibular joint space is best seen on the right sagittal image (**c**: arrow). The left temporomandibular joint is normal by comparison (**f**). Right temporal and masseter muscle atrophy is seen associated with increased T2 and T1 signal intensity (**a,d**: asterisk), consistent with dysfunction of the mandibular branch of the right trigeminal nerve. Aspiration biopsy of abnormal spindle cells was consistent with sarcoma.

Figure 1.3.16 Temporomandibular Osteoarthrosis (Canine)   CT

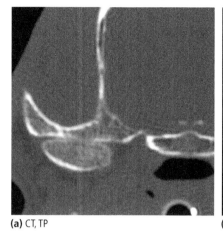
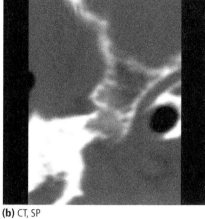

6y MC Miniature Schnauzer with a history of difficulty opening its mouth. Tests to assess for the presence of immune-mediated joint disease were negative. In the sagittal image, rostral is oriented to the left and caudal is to the right. Marked narrowing of the temporomandibular joint space is evident on both the transverse and sagittal images (a,b), implying a loss of articular cartilage and meniscal degeneration. Imaging findings are consistent with temporomandibular osteoarthrosis.

(a) CT, TP   **(b)** CT, SP

Figure 1.3.17 Temporomandibular Partial Ankylosis (Canine)   CT

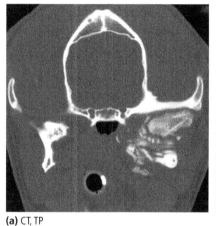
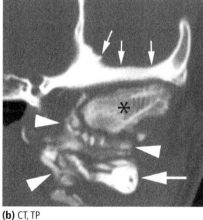

5y FS Labrador Retriever with a history of chronic otitis externa, a 1-year history of pain on opening the mouth, and more recent inability to open mouth. Image **b** represents a magnified view of the left temporomandibular joint from image **a**. In the sagittal image (**c**), rostral is oriented to the left and caudal is to the right. Subchondral bone remodeling of the left condylar process (**b,c**: asterisk) and marked periarticular bone proliferation surround the left temporomandibular joint. Reactive bone surrounds the medial and ventral aspect of the condylar process (**b**: arrowheads) and the angular process (**b,c**: large arrows). The left zygomatic process is thickened and sclerotic (**b**: small arrow). Milder changes to the right temporomandibular joint are also evident (**d**).

(a) CT, TP   **(b)** CT, TP

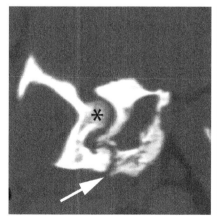
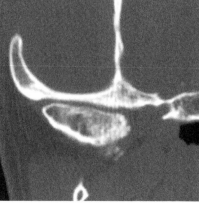

(c) CT, SP   **(d)** CT, TP

References

1. Gabler K, Bruhschwein A, Kiefer I, Loderstedt S, Oechtering G, Ludewig E. [Computed tomography imaging of the temporomandibular joint in dogs and cats. Effect of different scan parameters on image quality]. Tierarztl Prax K H. 2011;39:145–153.

2. Gabler K, Bruhschwein A, Loderstedt S, Oechtering G, Ludewig E. [Magnetic resonance imaging of the temporomandibular joint in dogs and cats. Effect of different coils on image quality]. Tierarztl Prax K H. 2011;39:79–88.

3. Macready DM, Hecht S, Craig LE, Conklin GA. Magnetic resonance imaging features of the temporomandibular joint in normal dogs. Vet Radiol Ultrasound. 2010;51:436–440.

4. Hoppe F, Svalastoga E. Temporomandibular dysplasia in American Cocker Spaniels. J Small Anim Pract. 1980;21:675–678.

5. Robins G, Grandage J. Temporomandibular joint dysplasia and open-mouth jaw locking in the dog. J Am Vet Med Assoc. 1977; 171:1072–1076.

6. Franch J, Cesari JR, Font J. Craniomandibular osteopathy in two Pyrenean mountain dogs. Vet Rec. 1998;142:455–459.

7. Padgett GA, Mostosky UV. The mode of inheritance of craniomandibular osteopathy in West Highland White terrier dogs. Am J Med Genet. 1986;25:9–13.

8. Ratterree WO, Glassman MM, Driskell EA, Havig ME. Craniomandibular osteopathy with a unique neurological manifestation in a young Akita. J Am Anim Hosp Assoc. 2011;47:e7–12.

9. Fricke J, Linn K, Anthony JM. Treatment for traumatic craniofacial deformation with restriction of the temporomandibular joint in a dog. J Vet Dent. 2008;25:246–248.

10. Seiler G, Rossi F, Vignoli M, Cianciolo R, Scanlon T, Giger U. Computed tomographic features of skull osteomyelitis in four young dogs. Vet Radiol Ultrasound. 2007;48:544–549.

1.4

Skull

Introduction

The skull is made up of many bones that fuse as the animal becomes skeletally mature. CT is an excellent modality to depict and study the complex anatomy of the skull using multi-planar 2D images as well as 3D renderings. The foramina of the skull, through which vasculature and the cranial nerves exit, have been described on CT and MR images.[1] CT imaging of the skull is prone to beam-hardening artifact because of the thickness of the bones, particularly the temporal bone region. Axial images tend to produce fewer artifacts than helical images, especially in cats and smaller dogs.

The skull is generally symmetric along the sagittal plane, which can be used for comparisons of paired structures during interpretation. However, variations of normal anatomy that cause asymmetry exist, especially in asymptomatic cats whose frontal and sphenoid sinuses are often unequally sized and whose nasal septum may be deviated.[2]

Developmental disorders

Occipitoatlantoaxial malformations

Congenital occipitoatlantoaxial malformations are rare in dogs; however, hypermotility or stenosis can cause severe neurologic compromise secondary to compression of the spinal cord. The occipital bone, foramen magnum, atlas, and ligamentous structures make up this region.[3] The spectrum of abnormalities includes hypoplasia of the occipital condyles, fusion of the atlas to the occiput, multiple separate centers of ossification, and malformation of the dens. The abnormally fused cranial segments may result in atlantoaxial instability or subluxation causing spinal cord compression. CT and MR imaging allow 3D visualization of the malformation itself as well as the effects on the spinal cord (Figure 1.4.1). Dogs should be positioned with care if instability is suspected.

Atlantooccipital overlapping

Atlantooccipital overlapping is rostral malposition of the atlas and axis resulting in compression of the cerebellum and kinking of the medulla oblongata. Since it is seen with other congenital anomalies, such as Chiari-like malformation (see Chapter 2.3) and dens hypoplasia resulting in atlantoaxial instability (see Chapter 3.1), it may be a consequence of other anomalies; however, it can also be seen as a sole abnormality.[4]

Syringomyelia, seen as a continuous or intermittent T2 hyperintense fluid collection in the spinal cord parenchyma, is associated with the chronic compression. Fibrous bands dorsal to the atlantoaxial or atlantooccipital junctions can also be seen with many of these disorders and contribute to the spinal cord compression.

Benign calvarial hyperostosis

Benign calvarial hyperostosis has been described in young Bull Mastiffs as a diffuse thickening of the bones of the calvarium, with some similarities to craniomandibular osteopathy. On MR images of one patient, the frontal bones were markedly thickened with hypointense T1 and T2 signal due to loss of normal marrow signal and T2 hyperintensity of the surrounding tissues.[5]

Atlas of Small Animal CT and MRI, First Edition. Erik R. Wisner and Allison L. Zwingenberger.
© 2015 John Wiley & Sons, Inc. Published 2015 by John Wiley & Sons, Inc.

T2* GRE images accentuated the signal from bone and provided good image quality for evaluating hyperostosis. Contrast-enhanced T1 images with fat saturation were recommended to reveal tissue enhancement.[5] CT imaging also demonstrates the increased bone attenuation in this syndrome (Figure 1.4.2).

Trauma

Skull fractures

Skull fractures due to trauma, such as vehicular trauma or fall from a height, are best appreciated on CT images. Radiographs cause superimposition of complex anatomy, and the asymmetry of the fractures and skull make interpretation difficult. Significantly more maxillofacial injuries were identified on CT images as compared to radiographs in cats and dogs.[6] Common regions of trauma to the calvarium include the sphenoid and pterygoid bones, the frontal bone, and the temporal bone (Figures 1.4.3, 1.4.4). Fractures of the temporomandibular joint and maxilla/mandible are discussed in Chapters 1.3 and 1.9. Gas may enter the calvarium as a result of open trauma to the skull and is identified as signal void on MR images and hypoattenuating regions on CT images. Associated hemorrhage may be seen in the dural tissues or brain (see Chapter 2.4). 3D reformations of CT images of the skull may be helpful in depicting the spatial location of fragments. However, small fractures are often best seen in the two-dimensional images.

Inflammatory disorders

Masticatory myositis

Masticatory myositis is an autoimmune inflammatory condition of the masseter, temporal, and pterygoid muscles in which autoantibodies are directed against myosin.[7] Affected dogs have pain opening the mouth and atrophy of the muscles of mastication. The atrophy can be seen on both CT and MR images. The affected muscles are hypoattenuating on CT on unenhanced images and have diffuse or peripheral enhancement on contrast-enhanced images (Figure 1.4.5).[8] Regions of myositis appear hyperintense on MR T2 sequences and, similar to CT, are contrast enhancing (Figure 1.4.6). Nonenhancing regions represent areas of necrosis (Figure 1.4.7).

Abscess

Abscesses can occur in the musculature of the head secondary to penetrating wounds from the skin, oral cavity, and pharynx or secondary to otitis media. Areas of abscessation appear hypoattenuating on CT and hyperintense on T2 MR images. On both modalities, contrast enhancement tends to be peripheral (Figure 1.4.8).

A contrast-enhancing tract may help to localize any foreign material or to trace the origin of the wound.

Osteomyelitis

Penetrating wounds to the head can result in intramuscular abscesses in the muscles of the head (Figure 1.4.9, Figure 2.7.6). Bite wounds and direct trauma can cause bacterial osteomyelitis of the skull to develop. CT features of osteomyelitis in the skull include soft tissue swelling, multifocal bone lysis with poorly defined cortical margins, regions of sclerosis, and irregular periosteal reaction.[9] Sequestra, identified as separate bone fragments in the affected region, can develop in chronic infections (Figure 1.4.9). The infection can extend to the meninges or brain if the full thickness of the skull is involved, appearing as contrast enhancement on CT and MR images (Figure 2.7.6).

Neoplasia

Osteomas are benign tumors of unknown etiology, comprised of compact or cancellous bone, that occasionally occur in the skull. Periosteal osteomas arise from the surface of the bone, while endosteal osteomas develop in the center of the bone.[10] These tumors have been reported in cats and dogs in the region of the skull. These may appear on CT images as primarily compact peripheral types, with uniform, hyperattenuating centers and smooth margins; or central cancellous types, with slightly lower attenuation and more irregular margins with invasion into adjacent bone (Figure 1.4.10).[10] These masses may affect the skull, oral cavity, or orbit.[11,12]

Osteosarcoma occurs most commonly in the maxilla and mandible in the axial skeleton and also occurs in the bones of the calvarium (Figure 1.4.11).[13] Chondrosarcoma occurs in the flat bones of the skull, most commonly in the nasal cavity. Imaging characteristics of primary bone tumors are similar on CT and MR images, with expansile irregular new bone production, cortical lysis, and associated soft-tissue masses with heterogeneous contrast enhancement (Figure 1.4.12). Other primary bone tumors, such as fibrosarcoma, hemangiosarcoma, as well as metastatic neoplasia, are infrequently encountered.

Multilobular osteochondrosarcoma occurs in the flat bones of the skull of dogs and occasionally in cats.[13] It is comprised of multiple lobules of bone or cartilage separated by fibrous septae, which give it a characteristic stippled appearance on CT images (Figure 1.4.13). These tumors tend to be round and well circumscribed to irregular in shape. They often expand into the calvarium or orbit, causing a significant mass effect. Brain edema can be seen as T2 hyperintensity, and obstructive hydrocephalus may result (Figure 1.4.14). On CT images, the masses are mildly contrast enhancing.[14] MR imaging characteristics of these masses include T1 and T2 hypointensity with regions of hyperintensity. Contrast enhancement is heterogeneous to uniform.[15]

Rarely, intracranial tumors, such as meningioma, can expand outside the calvarium.[16] Meningioma in cats can also cause hyperostosis of the adjacent calvarium,[17] and hyperostosis with bone lysis has been reported in the dog.[18] Tumors of the soft tissues surrounding the head, such as adenocarcinoma or squamous cell carcinoma, can also involve the bones of the skull (Figures 1.4.15, 1.4.16, 1.4.17). Lipomas or liposarcomas have a characteristic fat attenuation (–100 HU) within the musculature or soft tissues (Figure 1.4.18).

Cats with pituitary adenomas may develop acromegaly secondary to secretion of growth hormone and insulin-like growth factor. They tend to develop increased frontal bone thickness and excess soft tissue in the nasal cavity, sinuses, and pharynx, which can be seen on CT images.[1,19]

Figure 1.4.1 Occipitoatlantoaxial Dysplasia (Canine) CT

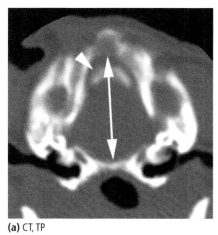 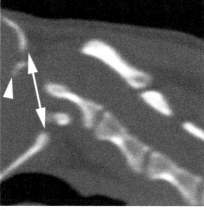 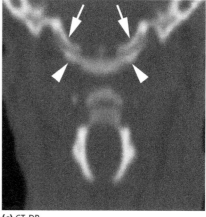

(a) CT, TP   (b) CT, SP   (c) CT, DP

8mo MC Yorkshire Terrier with atlantoaxial instability. An imaging diagnosis of occipital dysplasia was made as a component of a more complex anomaly of the atlantoaxial–occipital region. The transverse image is of the caudal aspect of the occipital bone at the level of the foramen magnum. The foramen magnum is larger than normal and elongated in the dorsal–ventral axis (**a**,**b**: two-headed arrow). The rostral margin of the dorsal arch of the atlas extends into the dorsal part of the foramen resulting in atlantooccipital overlapping (**a**,**b**: arrowhead). The occipital condyles (**c**: arrows) are hypoplastic but appear to articulate well with the articular fovea of the atlas (**c**: arrowheads). Marked rotational subluxation of the atlantoaxial joint is evident, and the odontoid process of the axis is hypoplastic (**b**).

Figure 1.4.2 Benign Calvarial Hyperostosis (Canine) CT

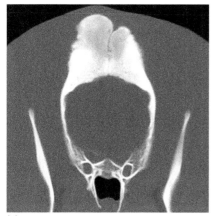

1y M Bernese Mountain Dog with prominent midline cranial mass. An irregular but well-defined osseous mass arises from the dorsal calvarium. The proliferative mass is dense and highly organized and has no appreciable overlying soft-tissue component. Bone biopsy revealed essentially normal bone tissue with considerable woven bone embedded in dense fibrous tissue overlying lamellar bone. This entity has previously been described in young Bull Mastiffs.

(a) CT, TP

Figure 1.4.3 Acute Skull Fracture (Canine)   CT

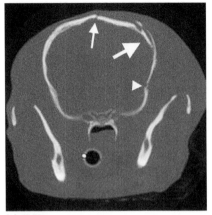

5y MC Pomeranian hit by a car earlier in the day. There is a depression fracture of the left side of the calvarium involving the interparietal suture (small arrow), the right parietal bone (large arrow), and the right parietotemporal suture (arrowhead). The dog also sustained multiple fractures involving the mandible, resulting in the asymmetry seen here. Additional CT or MR imaging is indicated to evaluate the extent of intracranial trauma.

(a) CT, TP

Figure 1.4.4 Skull Fractures (Feline)   CT

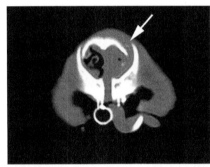
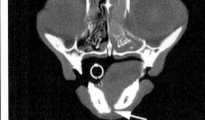
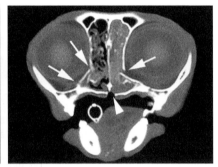

(a) CT, TP   **(b)** CT, TP   **(c)** CT, TP

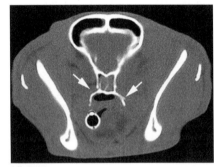
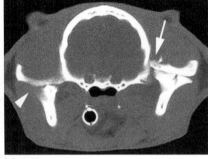

(d) CT, TP   **(e)** CT, TP

5y MC Domestic Shorthair that sustained trauma of unknown cause within the past 48 hours. This cat sustained a number of skull fractures commonly associated with high-impact trauma. Representative images are ordered from rostral to caudal. Injuries include a fracture–luxation involving the nasal and maxillary bones (a: arrow), mandibular symphyseal separation (b: arrow), fractures of the perpendicular processes of the palatine bones (c: arrows), separation of the palatine symphysis (c: arrowhead), fractures of the pterygoid bones (d: arrows), caudal luxation of the right condyloid process (e: arrowhead), and a fracture through the zygomatic process of the left temporal bone (e: arrow).

Figure 1.4.5 Masticatory Myositis (Canine)   CT

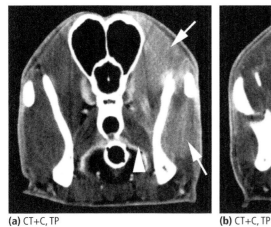
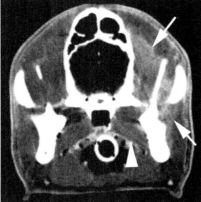

1.5y MC Rottweiler with rapidly progressive inability to open mouth. Representative CT images were acquired immediately following contrast medium administration. There is moderate, diffuse contrast enhancement of the left masseter and temporal muscles (**a**,**b**: arrows). Pterygoid muscles appear relatively unaffected (**a**,**b**: arrowhead). Muscle biopsy revealed diffuse, chronic, lymphoplasmacytic myositis with muscle atrophy and fibrosis.

(a) CT+C, TP   **(b)** CT+C, TP

Figure 1.4.6 Masticatory Myositis (Canine)   MR

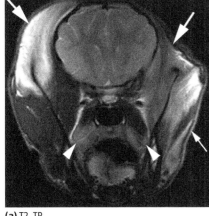
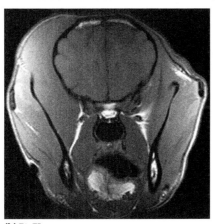
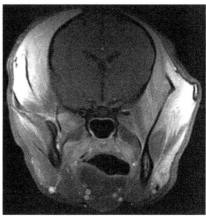

(a) T2, TP   **(b)** T1, TP   **(c)** T1+C, TP

9mo Miniature Pinscher with recent onset of left temporal muscle atrophy. The unenhanced T1 and T2 images are at the same anatomic level. The contrast-enhanced T1 image is more caudal. Marked atrophy of the left temporal muscle and moderate atrophy of the left masseter muscle are evident on all sequences. There is a pronounced increase in signal intensity of affected temporal (**a**: large arrows), masseter (**a**: small arrow), and pterygoid (**a**: arrowheads) muscles on the T2 image that corresponds to regions of mild hyperintensity present on the T1 image (**b**). The same regions markedly contrast enhance (**c**). Serum creatinine kinase was significantly elevated and an antibody test confirmed the diagnosis of masticatory myositis.

Figure 1.4.7 Masticatory Myositis (Canine)   MR

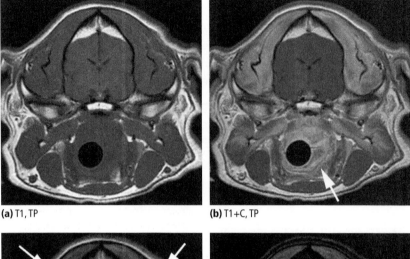

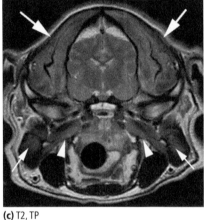

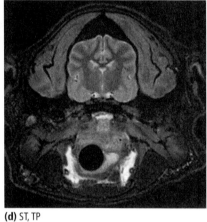

(a) T1, TP

(b) T1+C, TP

(c) T2, TP

(d) ST, TP

8y FS Golden Retriever with a 2-week history of weight loss, stridor, cranial nerve deficits, and temporal muscle atrophy. Bilaterally symmetrical temporal muscle atrophy is evident on all sequences. There is marked, diffuse, and symmetrical hyperintensity of temporal (c: large arrows), masseter (c: small arrows), and pterygoid (c: arrowheads) muscles on the T2 and STIR images corresponding to regional enhancement on the contrast-enhanced T1 image (b). A similar diffuse T2 hyperintensity and contrast enhancement pattern of the laryngeal tissues is evident (b: arrow). Necropsy revealed severe, bilateral, chronic, and diffuse lymphoplasmacytic myositis with myonecrosis and myodegeneration. This dog also had laryngeal cellulitis.

Figure 1.4.8 Temporal Muscle Abscess (Canine)   CT

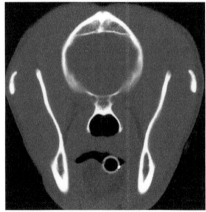

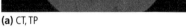

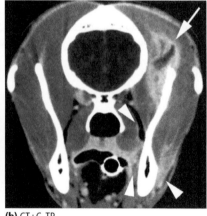

(a) CT, TP

(b) CT+C, TP

9y FS Chow with pain when opening mouth. A focal draining lesion was seen in the caudal oral cavity. The contrast-enhanced image shows a poorly delineated cavitary lesion within the left temporal muscle, consistent with an intramuscular abscess (b: arrow). Peripheral contrast enhancement extends to the medial surface of the coronoid process of the left mandible and to the external surface of the left parietal bone, but overt bone reactivity is not appreciated. Fascial and muscle contrast enhancement is also evident ventrally (b: arrowheads), indicative of more diffusely distributed cellulitis. Biopsy revealed chronic suppurative cellulitis.

Figure 1.4.9 Osteomyelitis (Canine)   CT

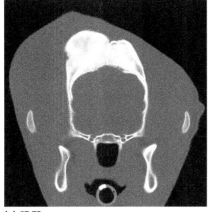

(a) CT, TP

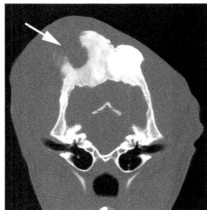

(b) CT, TP

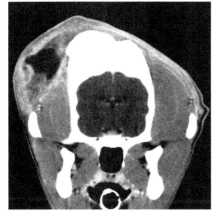

(c) CT+C, TP

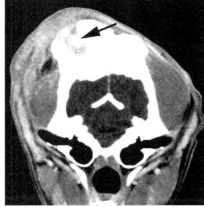

(d) CT+C, TP

1y Pit Bull Terrier with an 8-month history of progressive right-sided head and facial swelling. Representative images are unenhanced (**a**,**b**) and contrast enhanced (**c**,**d**) at comparable anatomic levels. Images are ordered from rostral to caudal. Marked asymmetry of the head is evident, and the underlying mass has both a soft tissue and an osseous component (**a**,**b**). A peripherally contrast-enhancing cavitary lesion is seen within the right temporal muscle, consistent with an abscess and surrounding cellulitis (**c**). Dense osteoproliferation is seen involving the right and left parietal bones (**a**,**b**). An involucrum is present toward the caudal aspect of the proliferative bone mass (**b**: arrow) and contains a focal mineral-dense body consistent with a sequestrum (**d**: arrow). Biopsy of bone and associated soft tissues revealed severe, chronic, suppurative, and necrotizing osteomyelitis with reactive new bone formation. The hyperostotic component of this lesion could represent underlying benign calvarial hyperostosis that became infected.

Figure 1.4.10   Osteoma (Canine)   CT & MR

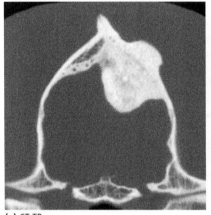
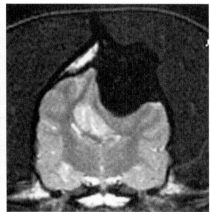

2y MC Golden Retriever with cranial mass. There is a smooth, dense production of bone centered on the parietal bone and expanding both intracranially and extracranially. The mass is hyperattenuating and uniform on CT images (**a**). On MR images, the mass effect is evident with compression of the brain and lateral ventricle next to the mass (**b**,**c**), as well as displacement of the falx cerebri to the right (**d**). There is T2 hyperintensity of the white matter next to the mass, (**b**) indicating edema.

(a) CT, TP   **(b)** T2, TP

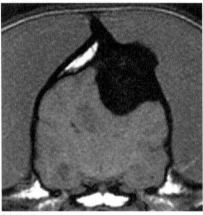
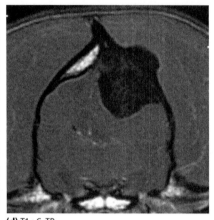

(c) T1, TP   **(d)** T1+C, TP

Figure 1.4.11   Osteosarcoma (Canine)

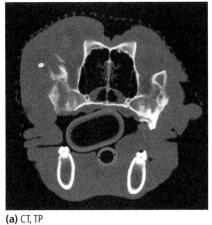

(a) CT, TP

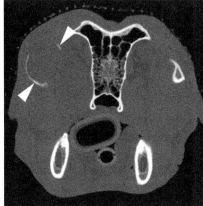

(b) CT, TP

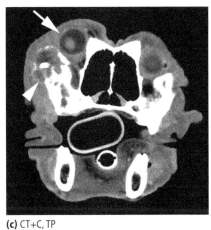

(c) CT+C, TP

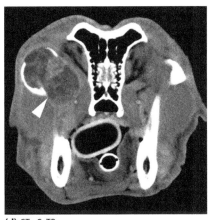

(d) CT+C, TP

4y F Bull Mastiff with a 2-month history of a right facial mass. Representative images are unenhanced (**a**,**b**) and contrast enhanced (**c**,**d**) at comparable anatomic levels. Images are ordered from rostral to caudal. A variably attenuating expansile mass appears to arise from within the right zygomatic bone (**a**,**b**) and is heterogeneously contrast enhancing (**c**,**d**: arrowhead). Cortical remnants of the zygomatic bone are still evident (**b**: arrowheads). The mass fills the orbital space, displacing the right globe dorsally (**c**: arrow). Biopsy revealed osteosarcoma with minimal osteoid, which reflects the predominantly destructive appearance of the mass on CT.

Figure 1.4.12   Chondrosarcoma (Canine)   CT

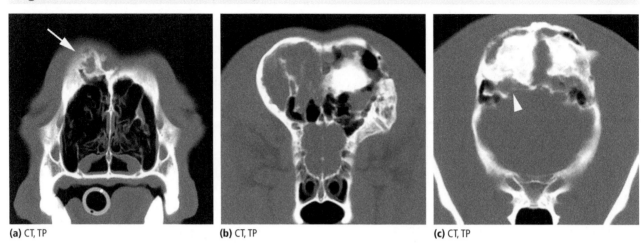

(a) CT, TP   **(b)** CT, TP   **(c)** CT, TP

8y MC Golden Retriever with a progressively enlarging rostral cranial mass. Representative CT images are ordered from rostral to caudal. Osteolysis and unorganized osteoproliferation of the caudal aspect of the right maxilla (**a**: arrow) and both frontal bones (**b,c**) is seen. The right frontal sinus is also filled with soft-tissue attenuating material that subsequently nonuniformly contrast enhances. There is also evidence of osteolysis of the internal margin of the right frontal bone (**c**: arrowhead). Slight meningeal enhancement at this site was noted on the contrast-enhanced images, but there was no evidence of further tumor extension. Biopsy revealed chondrosarcoma.

Figure 1.4.13   Multilobular Osteochondrosarcoma (Canine)   CT

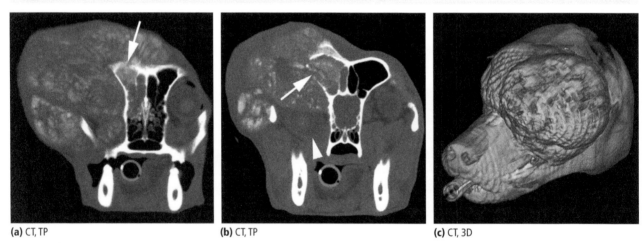

(a) CT, TP   **(b)** CT, TP   **(c)** CT, 3D

12y FS Dachshund Terrier cross with large craniofacial mass. Two representative images at the level of rostral extent (**a**) and middle (**b**) of the frontal sinus are included here. A partially and diffusely mineralized mass arises from the right frontal bone and extends around the right zygomatic arch. The mineralized component of the mass has a coarse, granular appearance characteristic of multilobular osteochondrosarcoma. The mass is osteodestructive (**a,b**: arrow) and displaces normal soft-tissue structures (**b**: arrowhead, right globe) but has virtually no soft-tissue component beyond the osseous margins. The 3D rendering reveals the full surface extent of the mass (**c**). Excisional biopsy confirmed multilobular osteochondrosarcoma.

Figure 1.4.14 Multilobular Osteochondrosarcoma (Canine)   CT & MR

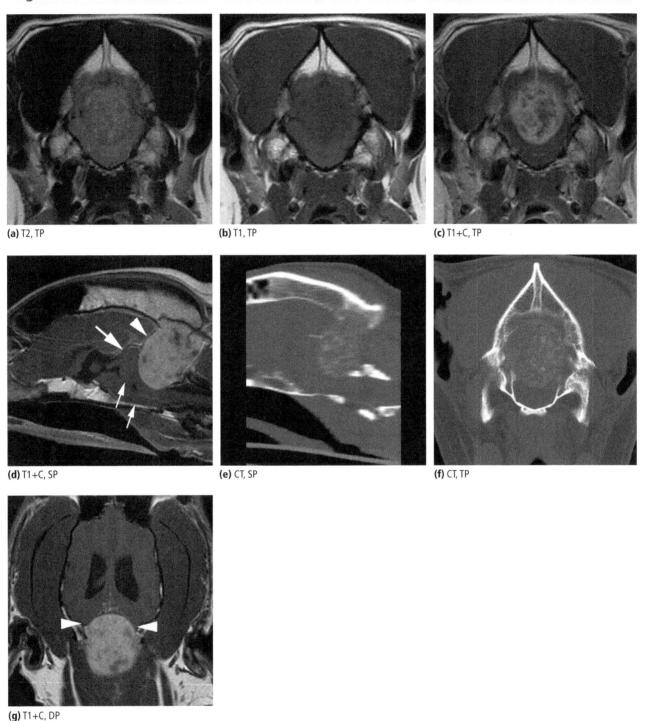

(a) T2, TP

(b) T1, TP

(c) T1+C, TP

(d) T1+C, SP

(e) CT, SP

(f) CT, TP

(g) T1+C, DP

7y FS Golden Retriever with a recent history of progressive incoordination. Neurologic examination localized neurologic deficits to the brainstem. A spherical mass arises from the occipital bone, causing extensive occipital osteolysis, and extends both intracranially and extracranially. The mass is hypointense on the unenhanced T1 image (**b**), has heterogeneous intensity and perilesional edema on the T2 image (**a**), and intensely and nonuniformly contrast enhances (**c,d,g**). The intracranial component of the mass is predominantly within the caudal fossa, causing rostral cerebellar displacement (**d**: large arrow), cerebellar and brainstem compression (**d**: small arrows), and obstructive hydrocephalus (**d,g**). The rostrodorsal aspect of the mass also encroaches on the caudal aspect of the rostral fossa, compressing the occipital lobes (**d,g**: arrowheads). Occipital osteolysis is also appreciated on the CT images (**e**). The coarse, granular, and diffuse mineralization (**e,f**) is characteristic of multilobular osteochondrosarcoma. Excisional biopsy confirmed the diagnosis of multilobular osteochondrosarcoma.

Figure 1.4.15 Adenocarcinoma (Feline)   CT

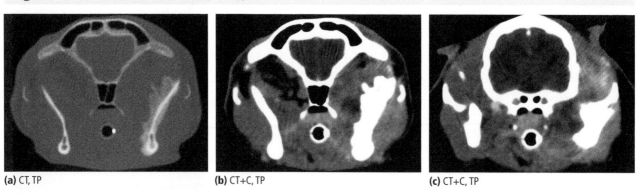

(a) CT, TP   (b) CT+C, TP   (c) CT+C, TP

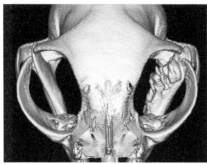

(d) CT, 3D

17y FS Domestic Shorthair with a 2-month history of pain on opening its mouth. Representative images include unenhanced and contrast-enhanced images at the level of the zygomatic process (a,b) of the frontal bone and a contrast-enhanced image near the level of the temporomandibular joint (c). A pronounced productive periosteal response is seen involving both the medial and lateral cortical surfaces of the left mandible. Contrast-enhanced images reveal a poorly defined, heterogeneously enhancing mass extending the length of the left mandible and extending into the left orbit. A biopsy of the mass was interpreted as adenocarcinoma of possible salivary origin.

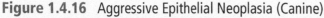

Figure 1.4.16 Aggressive Epithelial Neoplasia (Canine)   CT

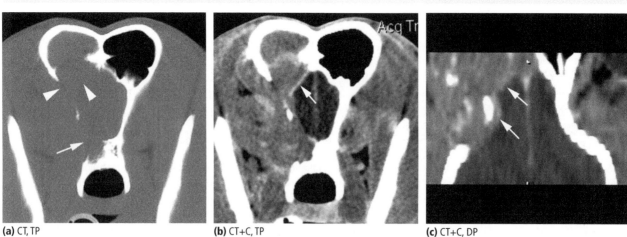

(a) CT, TP   (b) CT+C, TP   (c) CT+C, DP

11y Dalmatian with recent onset right-sided exophthalmia. A poorly defined right orbital mass is seen associated with aggressive osteolysis of the right frontal (a: arrowheads) and palatine (a: arrow) bones. The mass extends into the right frontal sinus and the rostral cranial vault and is in intimate contact with the contrast-enhancing meninges of the right olfactory bulb and frontal lobe (b,c: arrows). Fine-needle aspiration biopsy yielded a diagnosis of malignant epithelial neoplasia of possible basal cell origin.

Figure 1.4.17   Squamous Cell Carcinoma (Canine)

CT & MR

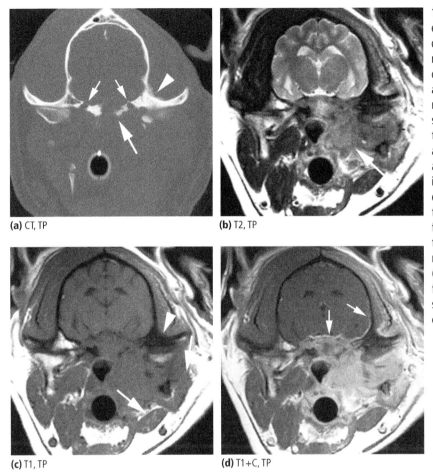

(a) CT, TP

(b) T2, TP

(c) T1, TP

(d) T1+C, TP

11y MC Shetland Sheepdog with left-sided epistaxis. There is a highly invasive and poorly defined soft-tissue mass centered on the left retropharyngeal region, causing profound osteolysis of the basisphenoid bone (**a**: large arrow) and obliterating the left pterygoid muscles (**b**: arrow). Periosteal reaction and sclerosis of the zygomatic process of the left temporal bone is also seen (**a,c**: arrowhead), and the left digastricus and masseter muscles are atrophied (**c**: arrows). Mass margins extend intracranially, and pronounced meningeal enhancement is evident ventrally and adjacent to the left temporal lobe (**d**: arrows). The oval foramina remain intact (**a**: small arrows), but the mandibular branch of the left trigeminal nerve cannot be delineated within the mass (**d**). The location and aggressive imaging features of this lesion are characteristic of squamous cell carcinoma. Biopsy of the mass confirmed squamous cell carcinoma.

Figure 1.4.18   Infiltrative Lipoma (Canine)

CT

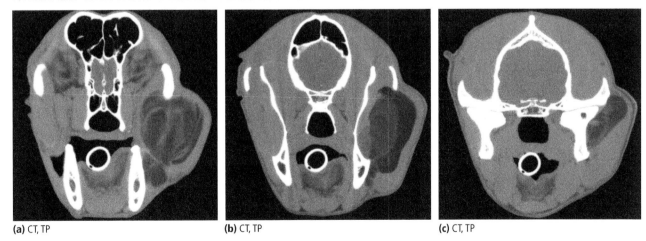

(a) CT, TP

(b) CT, TP

(c) CT, TP

8y FS Doberman Pinscher with a left-sided facial mass. Representative CT images are ordered from rostral to caudal. A well-defined fat-attenuating mass is present within the left masseter muscle. The striated pattern within the mass is due to adipose infiltration between muscle fasciculi A subchondral bone cyst is noted in the left condyloid process incidentally. Biopsy confirmed infiltrative lipoma.

References

1. Gomes E, Degueurce C, Ruel Y, Dennis R, Begon D. Anatomic study of cranial nerve emergence and associated skull foramina in cats using CT and MRI. Vet Radiol Ultrasound. 2009;50: 398–403.

2. Reetz JA, Maï W, Muravnick KB, Goldschmidt MH, Schwarz T. Computed tomographic evaluation of anatomic and pathologic variations in the feline nasal septum and paranasal sinuses. Vet Radiol Ultrasound. 2006;47:321–327.

3. Cerda-Gonzalez S, Dewey CW. Congenital diseases of the craniocervical junction in the dog. Vet Clin North Am Small Anim Pract. 2010;40:121–141.

4. Cerda-Gonzalez S, Dewey CW, Scrivani PV, Kline KL. Imaging features of atlanto-occipital overlapping in dogs. Vet Radiol Ultrasound. 2009;50:264–268.

5. McConnell JF, Hayes A, Platt SR, Smith KC. Calvarial hyperostosis syndrome in two bullmastiffs. Vet Radiol Ultrasound. 2006;47: 72–77.

6. Bar-Am Y, Pollard R, Kass P, Verstraete F. The diagnostic yield of conventional radiographs and computed tomography in dogs and cats with maxillofacial trauma. Vet Surg. 2008;37:294–299.

7. Neumann J, Bilzer T. Evidence for MHC I–restricted CD8+ T-cell-mediated immunopathology in canine masticatory muscle myositis and polymyositis. Muscle Nerve. 2006;33:215–224.

8. Reiter AM, Schwarz T. Computed tomographic appearance of masticatory myositis in dogs: 7 cases (1999–2006). J Am Vet Med Assoc. 2007;231:924–930.

9. Seiler G, Rossi F, Vignoli M, Cianciolo R, Scanlon T, Giger U. Computed tomographic features of skull osteomyelitis in four young dogs. Vet Radiol Ultrasound. 2007;48:544–549.

10. Fiani N, Arzi B, Johnson EG, Murphy B, Verstraete FJM. Osteoma of the oral and maxillofacial regions in cats: 7 cases (1999–2009). J Am Vet Med Assoc. 2011;238:1470–1475.

11. Grozdanic S, Riedesel EA, Ackermann MR. Successful medical treatment of an orbital osteoma in a dog. Vet Ophthalmol. 2013;16:135–139.

12. Fernandez M, Grau-Roma L, Roura X, Majó N. Lingual osteoma in a dog. J Small Anim Pract. 2012;53:480–482.

13. Ehrhart NP, Ryan SD, Fan TM. Tumors of the Skeletal System. In: Withrow SJ, MacEwen EG (eds): Withrow and MacEwen's Small Animal Clinical Oncology. 5th ed. Saunders Elsevier; 2013;463–503.

14. Hathcock JT, Newton JC. Computed tomographic characteristics of multilobular tumor of bone involving the cranium in 7 dogs and zygomatic arch in 2 dogs. Vet Radiol Ultrasound. 2000;41: 214–217.

15. Lipsitz D, Levitski RE, Berry WL. Magnetic resonance imaging features of multilobular osteochondrosarcoma in 3 dogs. Vet Radiol Ultrasound. 2001;42:14–19.

16. Karli P, Gorgas D, Oevermann A, Forterre F. Extracranial expansion of a feline meningioma. J Feline Med Surg. 2013;15: 749–753.

17. Troxel MT, Vite CH, Massicotte C, et al. Magnetic resonance imaging features of feline intracranial neoplasia: retrospective analysis of 46 cats. J Vet Intern Med. 2004;18:176–189.

18. Mercier M, Heller HLB, Bischoff MG, Looper J, Bacmeister CX. Imaging diagnosis – hyperostosis associated with meningioma in a dog. Vet Radiol Ultrasound. 2007;48:421–423.

19. Fischetti AJ, Gisselman K, Peterson ME. CT and MRI evaluation of skull bones and soft tissues in six cats with presumed acromegaly versus 12 unaffected cats. Vet Radiol Ultrasound. 2012;53:535–539.

1.5

Orbit

Introduction

The orbit is bounded by the frontal bones medially, the zygomatic arch caudolaterally, and the orbital ligament dorsally and contains the globe and associated vascular and glandular structures (Figures 1.5.1, 1.5.2). The zygomatic arch is curved and regular with a central suture. The orbital ligament spans the frontal process of the zygomatic bone and the zygomatic process of the frontal bone and is visible as a hyperattenuating structure on CT images and a hypointense structure on T1 and T2 images on MRI. In cats, the dorsal orbit is mainly bone as these processes are close together. Mineralization of the orbital ligament is common in dogs. Extrinsic ocular muscles, the zygomatic salivary gland (dogs), vasculature, the lacrimal gland and gland of the third eyelid, the globe, and the optic nerve fill the orbit. The ocular muscles enhance to a greater degree than surrounding musculature on MR images in normal dogs.[1] The nasolacrimal duct travels through the lacrimal canal in the lacrimal bone and maxilla to enter the nasal cavity rostrally and ventrally.[2,3] The optic nerve passes through the optic canal, formed by the pterygoid bone, to enter the calvarium.[4,5] It is best visualized on MR images in a dorsal oblique plane, parallel to the nerves. Several sequences may be used for visualization,[6,7] but 3D T1 weighted images with a 1–2 mm slice thickness are optimal.

Developmental disorders

Head conformation, particularly in brachycephalic breeds of cats, can alter the path of the normal nasolacrimal duct. The dorsal rotation of the facial bones and canine teeth causes the nasolacrimal duct to pass under the canine teeth and results in some obstruction to drainage.[8] Similar anatomic changes have been reported in brachycephalic dogs. CT is an excellent approach for performing dacryorhinocystography to evaluate the patency of the lacrimal duct and identify causes of obstruction (Figure 1.5.3). Dacryops, developmental cysts of the lacrimal system, can obstruct the lacrimal canal and deform the surrounding bones as they expand over time and can be imaged with CT or MR. They may contain sedimenting debris, best seen on T2 weighted MR images (Figure 1.5.4). The walls of such cysts exhibit mild contrast enhancement.

Trauma

Trauma to the skull often affects the orbit, either by fracturing the bones forming the orbital boundaries or by damaging the soft tissues within. Orbital fractures can be appreciated best on transverse images, but 3D images can also help to describe the displacement of the bones and alteration to orbital shape (Figure 1.5.5). Acute trauma results in sharply marginated fracture lines that may extend to the nasal cavity and calvarium. Chronic fractures may heal with malunion and deform the shape of the orbit by proliferative change or by areas of disruption of the skull (Figure 1.5.6). The globe may be acutely displaced from the orbit (Figure 1.5.7) or shrunken (phthisis bulbi) as a result of previous trauma.

Inflammatory disorders

Inflammation can affect the soft tissues within the orbit, often manifesting as exophthalmos or periorbital swelling. Penetrating trauma, foreign bodies, and infections

Atlas of Small Animal CT and MRI, First Edition. Erik R. Wisner and Allison L. Zwingenberger.
© 2015 John Wiley & Sons, Inc. Published 2015 by John Wiley & Sons, Inc.

of the eye may be initiating causes.[9] Cellulitis or myositis results in increased soft-tissue attenuating material or T2 hyperintensity of the orbital tissues. The volume of the tissues appears greater, and there is loss of definition of the normal fat and extraocular muscles (Figures 1.5.8, 1.5.9). The eyelids and surrounding tissues may also be affected. On contrast-enhanced images, there is diffuse enhancement of the tissues surrounding the globe. Abscesses may also form in the tissues of the orbit, resulting in fluid-attenuating, or T2 hyperintense and T1 hypointense, collections. These lesions are peripherally contrast enhancing (Figure 1.5.10). In addition to the extraocular muscles within the orbit, the pterygoid muscle is located medial to the zygomatic salivary gland and may also be affected by inflammatory disease (Figure 1.5.11). Rarely, the inflammation within the orbit may extend intracranially. MR imaging features of intracranial extension include T2, STIR, and FLAIR hyperintensity of the tissues in the skull foramina and orbital fissure, which do not extend into the brain or meninges.[10]

Zygomatic sialadenitis, often with sialocele formation, can be a cause of inflammation and exophthalmos in the orbit (see Chapter 1.7) (Figure 1.5.12).

Neoplasia

Neoplastic disease may arise from the soft tissues or osseous structures surrounding the orbit. On CT images, neoplasia usually has more clearly defined margins compared to inflammatory disease. Common tumors include carcinomas (adenocarcinoma, squamous cell carcinoma), sarcoma (fibrosarcoma, liposarcoma, rhabdomyosarcoma, osteosarcoma), round-cell neoplasia (lymphoma, mast cell tumor) and meningioma.[11-13] These tumors may primarily involve the tissues of the orbit, extend from the nasal cavity and maxilla (see Chapters 1.1, 1.4), or represent metastasis.[3,4,13] Imaging features include local bone destruction, irregular bone production, and increased soft-tissue mass within the orbit. Tumors are heterogeneously to intensely contrast enhancing (Figures 1.5.13, 1.5.14, 1.5.15, 1.5.16, 1.5.17, 1.5.18, 1.5.19). The surrounding structures should be evaluated to determine the involvement of bone, nasal cavity, optic nerve, and cranium.

Myxosarcoma has a predilection to the orbit in dogs, with CT and MR imaging characteristics of extensive, fluid-filled cavities within the orbit and surrounding fascial planes. They can extend to the temporomandibular joints and mimic a salivary mucocele.[14]

Osteoma and multilobular tumor of bone also occur in this location.[15] Osteoma has a characteristic smooth, uniform attenuation on CT images and may enlarge to affect adjacent structures by mass effect.

Restrictive orbital myofibroblastic sarcoma of cats, which was previously named idiopathic sclerosing orbital pseudotumor, is an invasive, low-grade neoplasm affecting the orbital tissues. CT and MR images show diffuse thickening of the orbital tissues, sclera, and eyelids with intense contrast enhancement.[16,17] The disease often affects both eyes and/or the oral cavity (Figure 1.5.20).

Figure1.5.1 Normal Orbit (Canine)

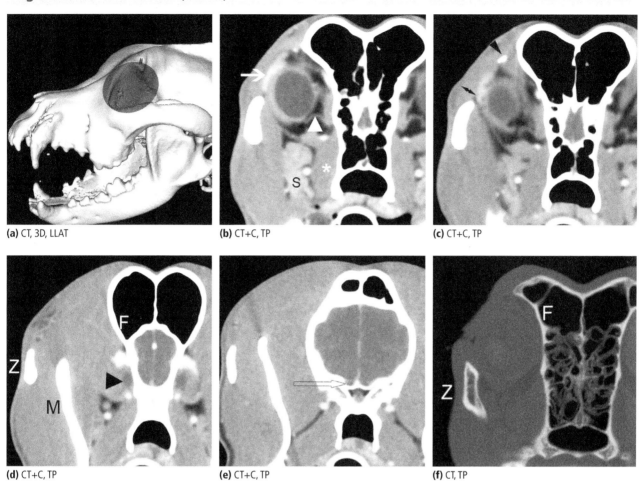

(a) CT, 3D, LLAT

(b) CT+C, TP

(c) CT+C, TP

(d) CT+C, TP

(e) CT+C, TP

(f) CT, TP

Images **b–e** are ordered from rostral to caudal. The orbit is represented by the shaded circle (**a**) and is mainly comprised of the frontal bone and zygomatic arch. The extraocular muscles (**b**: white arrowhead) are surrounded by fat. The zygomatic salivary gland is strongly contrast enhancing in the ventrolateral orbit. The pterygoid muscle (**b**: asterisk) lies medial to the gland. The orbital ligament (**c**: double-ended arrow) joins the zygomatic process of the frontal bone (**a**: #) to the zygomatic arch. Focal mineralization is common (**c**: small arrowhead). The lacrimal gland is ventral to the orbital ligament (**b**: thin white arrow) and is contrast enhancing. The ramus of the mandible is medial to the zygomatic arch. The optic nerve (**d**: black arrowhead) is hypoattenuating and travels toward the optic canal. The optic chiasm (**f**: open arrow) is visible within the calvarium. F (frontal sinus), M (mandible), S (zygomatic salivary gland), Z (zygomatic arch).

Figure 1.5.2 Normal Orbit (Canine)

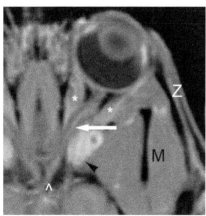

Dorsal reformatted image of the orbit. The zygomatic arch and mandible are visible as hypointense linear structures. The extrinsic ocular muscles are mildly hyperattenuating (asterisks) and are interleaved by fat. The optic nerve (arrow) travels in the center of the muscles toward the optic canal (caret). The ophthalmic venous plexus is strongly contrast enhancing (arrowhead). M (mandible), Z (zygomatic arch).

(a) T1+C, DP

Figure 1.5.3 Normal Nasolacrimal System (Canine)   CT

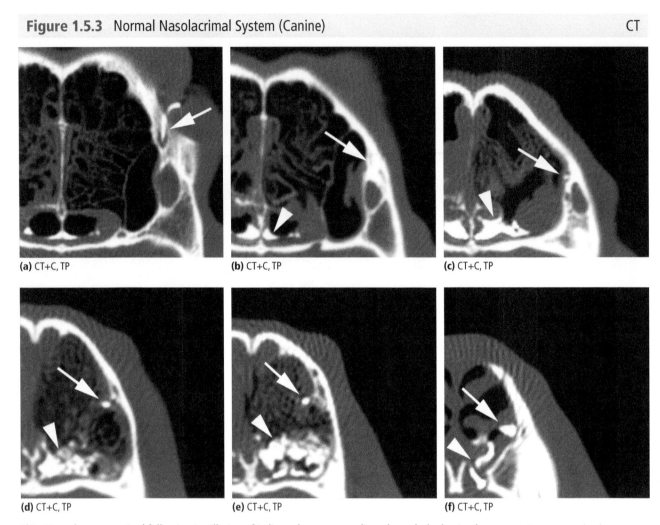

(a) CT+C, TP   **(b)** CT+C, TP   **(c)** CT+C, TP

(d) CT+C, TP   **(e)** CT+C, TP   **(f)** CT+C, TP

This CT study was acquired following instillation of iodinated contrast medium through the lacrimal punctum. Representative images are ordered from caudal to rostral, mimicking the order in which contrast medium flows through the duct. The normal nasolacrimal duct originates from the lacrimal sac, enters the lacrimal canal through the lacrimal bone (**a**: arrow), and continues rostrally within the maxillary bone (**b,c**: arrow). The duct exits the maxillary bone and continues to course rostrally (**d,e**: arrow), terminating in the nasal cavity (**f**: arrow). Contrast medium in the ventral aspect of the nasal cavity has exited the duct and is distributed in the dependent interstices of the turbinates (**b–f**: arrowhead).

Figure 1.5.4 Nasolacrimal Cyst (Canine)   CT & MR

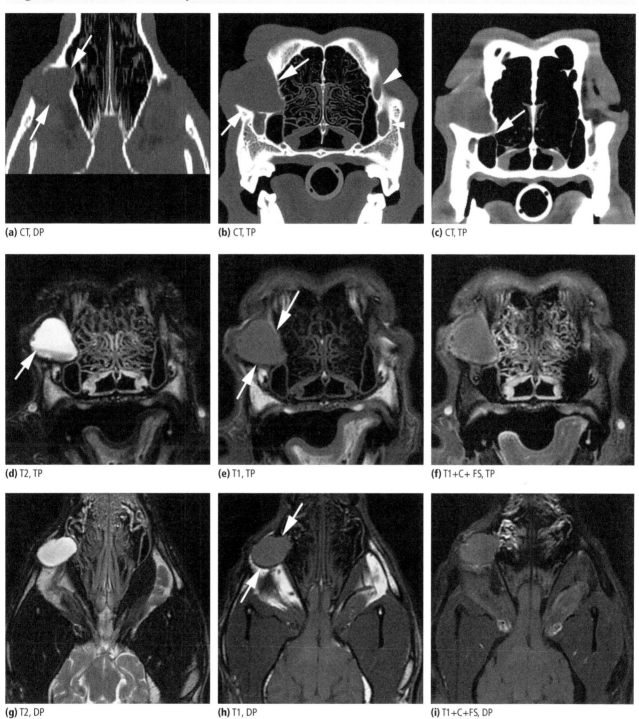

(a) CT, DP

(b) CT, TP

(c) CT, TP

(d) T2, TP

(e) T1, TP

(f) T1+C+ FS, TP

(g) T2, DP

(h) T1, DP

(i) T1+C+FS, DP

3y MC Golden Retriever with right-sided epiphora of 2-month duration. Images **b–f** are at approximately the same anatomic level near the proximal extent of the lacrimal canal. Similarly, images **a** and **g–i** are at the same anatomic level in the dorsal plane. A large expansile mass arises from the region of the lacrimal bone, causing resorptive deformation of the adjacent lacrimal, maxillary, and frontal bones (**a,b,e,h**: arrows). The mass also extends medially into the nasal cavity and causes deformation of the dorsal aspect of the maxillary sinus (**c**: arrow). Centrally, the mass is fluid attenuating on CT and is T2 hyperintense and T1 hypointense. A sedimentary layer is also appreciated on the transverse T2 image (**d**: arrow), further documenting a cystic character. The thin cystic wall minimally contrast enhances on both CT and MR studies (**c,f,i**). The normal appearance of the caudal extent of the contralateral lacrimal canal (**b**: large arrowhead) and the infraorbital canal (**b**: small arrowhead) is seen on the left. Excisional biopsy confirmed this to be a ductular cyst that arose near the proximal origin of the nasolacrimal duct.

Figure 1.5.5   Orbital Fracture (Feline)   CT

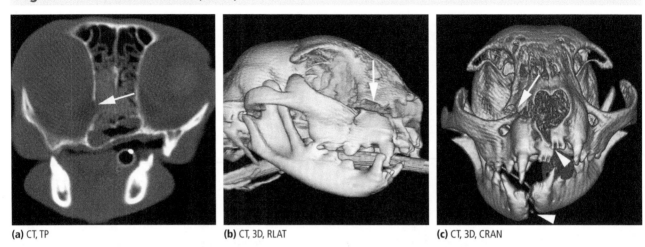

(a) CT, TP
(b) CT, 3D, RLAT
(c) CT, 3D, CRAN

2y MC Domestic Shorthair with acute head trauma of unknown cause. There is a moderately displaced fracture of the right ventromedial orbit (**a–c**: arrow). The fracture line is in the region of the convergence of the maxillary, lacrimal, and zygomatic bones. The cat also sustained a displaced fracture of the hard palate and separations of the incisive and mandibular symphyses (**c**: arrowheads).

Figure 1.5.6   Deformation of the Orbit—Chronic Trauma (Canine)   CT

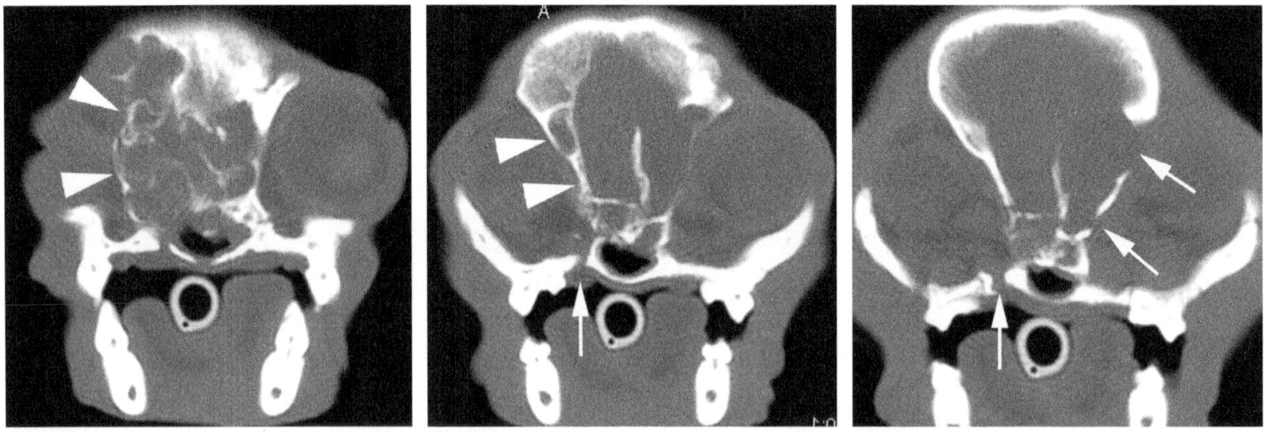

(a) CT, TP
(b) CT, TP
(c) CT, TP

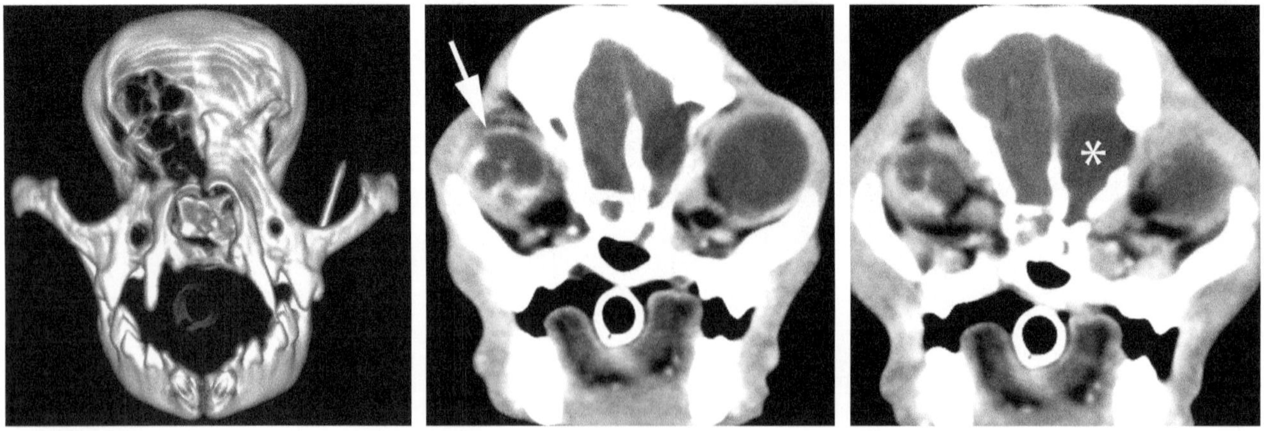

(d) CT, 3D, CRAN
(e) CT+C, TP
(f) CT+C, TP

16mo M Chihuahua bitten in the face 1 year prior. The representative transverse images **a–c** are ordered from rostral to caudal. Images **e** and **f** are contrast-enhanced images comparable to **b** and **c**, respectively. There is marked deformation of the right maxilla and frontal bone (**a,b**: arrowheads) and multiple fenestrations within the right maxilla and left frontal bone (**b,c**: arrows), causing both orbits to be misshapen. The 3D rendering (**d**) shows the extent of trauma and remodeling of the dorsal margin of the right orbit. Right-sided phthisis bulbi (**e**: arrow) and an intracranial cyst (**f**: asterisk) resulting from the previous trauma are also evident.

Figure 1.5.7   Globe Luxation (Canine)   CT

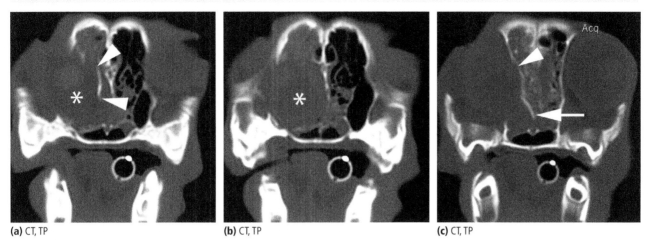

(a) CT, TP   **(b)** CT, TP   **(c)** CT, TP

4mo M Miniature Dachshund attacked by another dog 4 hours prior. Images are ordered from rostral to caudal. There are displaced fractures involving the right maxilla, frontal bone (**a,c**: arrowheads), and the perpendicular lamina of the palatine bone (**c**: arrow). There is obliteration of the right nasal turbinates and cranial luxation of the eye into the right nasal cavity (**a,b**: asterisk).

Figure 1.5.8   Retrobulbar Cellulitis (Canine)   MR

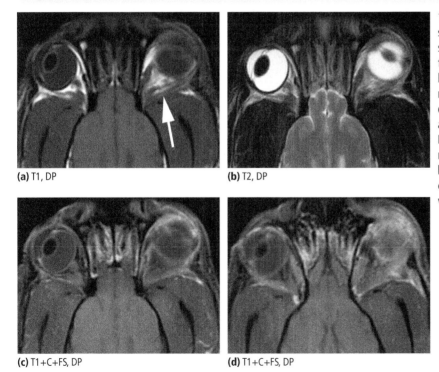

(a) T1, DP   **(b)** T2, DP

(c) T1+C+FS, DP   **(d)** T1+C+FS, DP

11y FS Pointer with 24-hour history of left-sided exophthalmos. Images **a–c** depict the same anatomy. Image **d** is slightly more ventral. There is a mild diffuse increase in extraocular musculature and adipose volume in the left retrobulbar space (**a**: arrow). There is also a loss of definition of muscle, scleral, conjunctival, and intraocular margins seen on all sequences. Diffuse retrobulbar and conjunctival enhancement is evident on the left (**c,d**). Conjunctival biopsy revealed neutrophilic and plasmocytic conjunctivitis. Clinical signs rapidly resolved with systemic and topical antibiotic therapy.

Figure 1.5.9 Extraocular Myositis (Canine)   MR

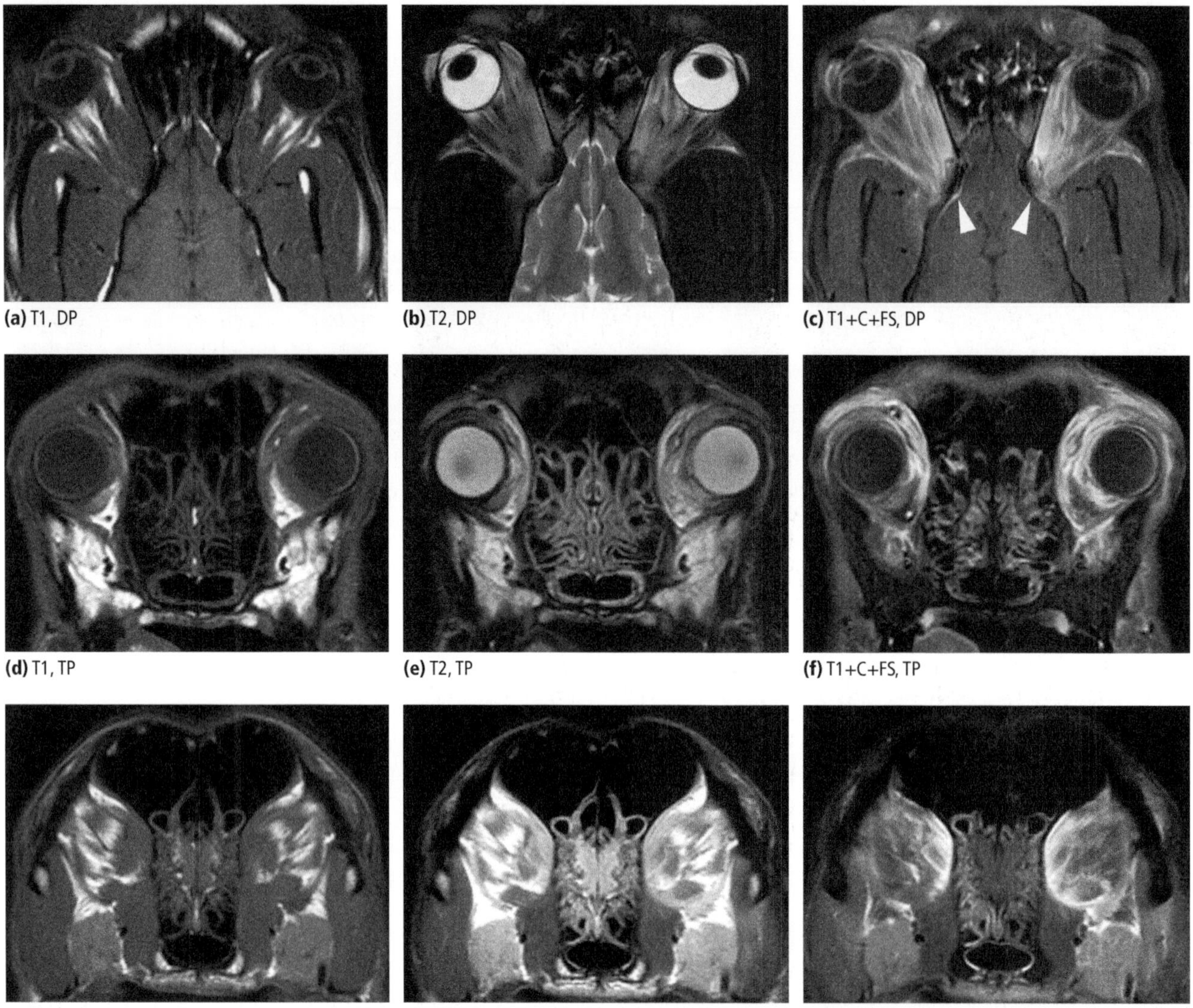

(a) T1, DP

(b) T2, DP

(c) T1+C+FS, DP

(d) T1, TP

(e) T2, TP

(f) T1+C+FS, TP

(g) T1, TP

(h) PD, TP

(i) T1+C+FS, TP

1y MC Labrador Retriever with bilateral blepharospasm and reduced response to retropulsion. Images **d–e** are at the level of the globe and images **g–i** are further caudal within the retrobulbar space. There is an increase in volume and loss of definition of the extraocular muscles (**a–c,g–i**). This is associated with an increase in extraocular muscle signal intensity on T2 images (**b,h**). There is diffuse contrast enhancement of the extraaxial muscles (**c,i**) and ocular adnexa (**f**), bilaterally. Focal meningeal enhancement is also present in the frontal lobar region bilaterally (**c**: arrowheads) and may represent an extension of the inflammatory response through the optic canal or orbital fissure. Extraocular muscle biopsy revealed chronic lymphohistiocytic myositis and myocyte atrophy, which is consistent with the microscopic description reported for extraocular myositis. Conjunctival biopsy revealed marked subacute fibrinosuppurative conjunctivitis.

Figure 1.5.10 Retrobulbar Abscess (Canine)   MR

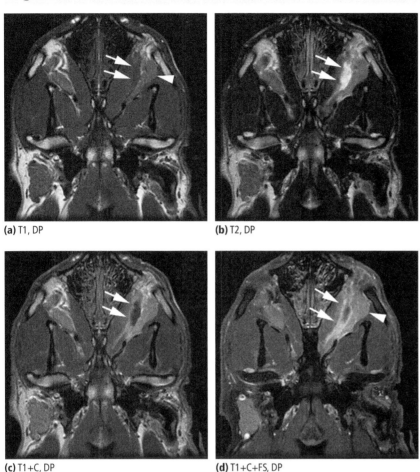

(a) T1, DP

(b) T2, DP

(c) T1+C, DP

(d) T1+C+FS, DP

10y MC Newfoundland with acute onset left-sided conjunctival hyperemia. Representative dorsal plane images all depict the same anatomy. These images are ventral to the globes and depict the ventral aspect of the orbits. A fusiform abscess that has T1 hypointensity and T2 hyperintensity (a–d: arrows) is evident centrally. The core does not contrast enhance, but the periphery intensely enhances (c,d). Distribution of contrast enhancement is best seen on the fat-suppressed contrast-enhanced T1 image (d). The left zygomatic salivary gland is also mildly enlarged and contrast enhances more than the contralateral gland as a result of secondary sialadenitis (a,d: arrowhead). Aspiration cytology revealed marked septic suppurative inflammation with a mixed bacterial population.

Figure 1.5.11 Pterygoid Abscess (Canine)   CT

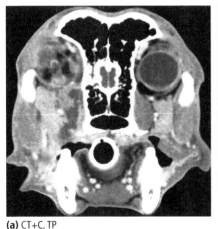

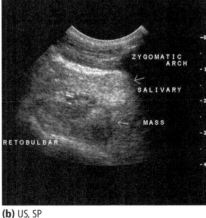

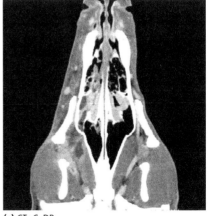

(a) CT+C, TP

(b) US, SP

(c) CT+C, DP

3y M Golden Retriever with right-sided buphthalmos and pain opening the mouth. There is an irregularly shaped, hypoattenuating region in the right pterygoid muscle (a,c). The pterygoid muscle is located medial to the hyperattenuating zygomatic salivary gland on the transverse images (a) and on ultrasound (b). The region of inflammation is hypoechoic and irregular on ultrasound images (b). There is additional soft-tissue opacity in the left nasal cavity indicating rhinitis. No migrating foreign bodies were observed, but this remains a primary differential as a cause of the abscess.

Figure 1.5.12 Zygomatic Sialoadenitis (Canine)   MR

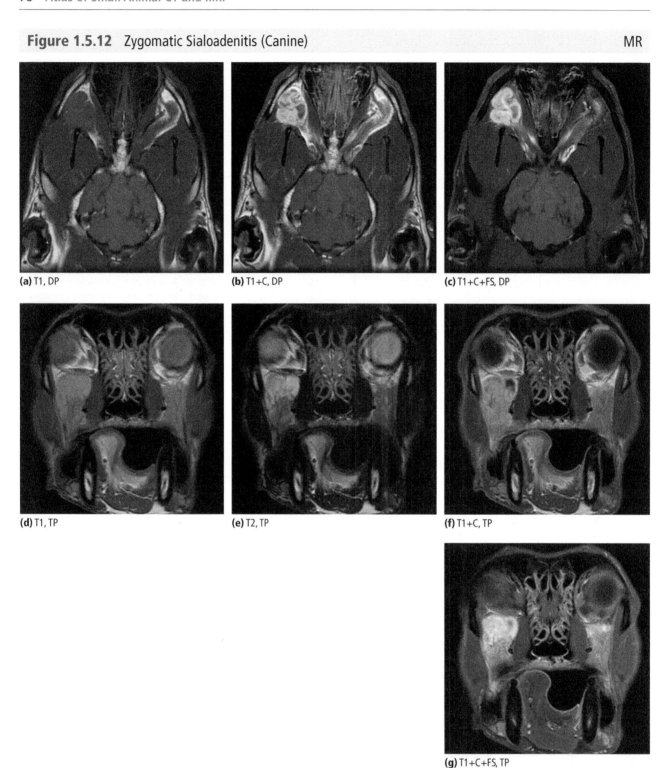

(a) T1, DP

(b) T1+C, DP

(c) T1+C+FS, DP

(d) T1, TP

(e) T2, TP

(f) T1+C, TP

(g) T1+C+FS, TP

8y MC German Shepherd cross with resistance to retropulsion of the right eye. Images **a–c** and **d–g** depict the same anatomy in dorsal and transverse planes, respectively. A well-demarcated lobular mass is seen in the ventral aspect of the right retrobulbar space (**a–g**). The mass is highly contrast enhancing and has a complex internal architecture consistent with salivary glandular tissue (**b,f,g**). Images **c** and **g** show the value of fat suppression for increasing conspicuity of contrast-enhancing lesions in the retrobulbar space. Aspiration biopsy of the mass revealed salivary tissue and chronic granulomatous inflammation.

Figure 1.5.13 Retrobulbar Lymphoma (Feline)

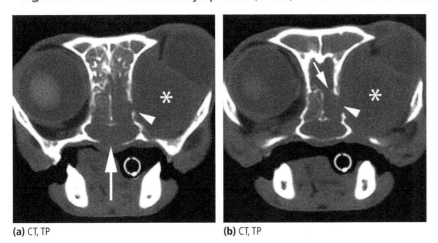

(a) CT, TP   **(b)** CT, TP

Mature cat of unknown age with left-sided exophthalmos. Representative transverse images are ordered from rostral to caudal. A large uniformly attenuating mass (**a,b**: asterisk) within the left retrobulbar space causes marked displacement of the globe. The mass has eroded through the perpendicular (**a,b**: arrowhead) and horizontal laminae of the palatine bone (**a**: large arrow) and fills the nasopharynx and the left sphenoidal sinus. The mass has also eroded through endoturbinates and the left ventral part of the cribriform plate (**b**: small arrow). Both frontal sinuses are fluid filled (**b**) as a result of obstructive sinusitis from the intranasal component of the mass (not seen). Aspiration biopsy confirmed lymphoma.

Figure 1.5.14 Retrobulbar Lymphoma (Canine)

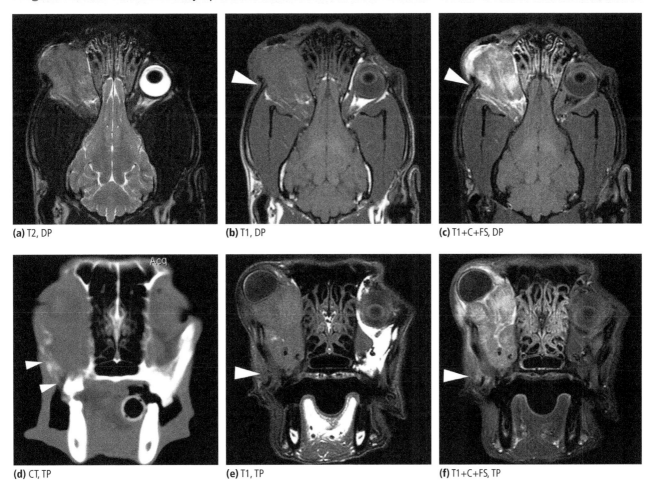

(a) T2, DP   **(b)** T1, DP   **(c)** T1+C+FS, DP

(d) CT, TP   **(e)** T1, TP   **(f)** T1+C+FS, TP

2y FS Golden Retriever with progressive right-sided exophthalmos. Images include dorsal and transverse MR images through the orbits as well as a comparable transverse CT image. There is a large, lobular retrobulbar mass involving the right orbit that compresses the globe and displaces it dorsally and laterally (**a–f**). Right zygomatic and maxillary bone destruction is evident on the MR images (**b,c,e,f**: arrowhead) but may be more easily recognized on the CT image (**d**: arrowheads). The mass heterogeneously contrast enhances (**c,f**), and there is associated conjunctival and adnexal enhancement as well. Tissue core biopsy revealed non-B-, non-T-cell lymphoma.

Figure 1.5.15   Metastatic Orbital Carcinoma (Feline)   CT

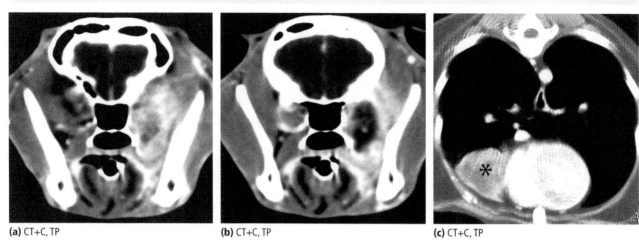

(a) CT+C, TP   **(b)** CT+C, TP   **(c)** CT+C, TP

17y FS Domestic Shorthair with swelling of the left side of the head and diminished retropulsion of the left eye. A right middle lung lobe mass was seen on thoracic radiographs. Representative transverse CT images are through the caudal aspect of the retrobulbar spaces and are ordered from rostral to caudal. An ill-defined, peripherally contrast-enhancing mass is present within the caudal extent of the left retrobulbar space (**b**). Contrast enhancement also extends to surrounding musculature and fascial planes (**a**). A large well-defined mass is present in the ventral part of the right middle lung lobe (**c**: asterisk). Tissue biopsies from necropsy revealed a primary bronchogenic carcinoma of the right middle lung lobe and an aggressive, highly invasive metastatic mass of the left retrobulbar space.

Figure 1.5.16   Orbital Melanoma (Canine)   CT

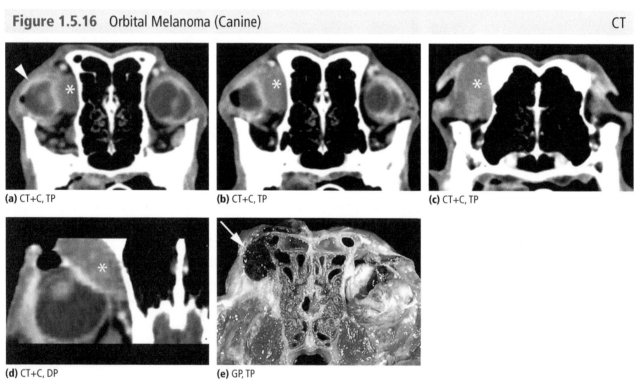

(a) CT+C, TP   **(b)** CT+C, TP   **(c)** CT+C, TP

(d) CT+C, DP   **(e)** GP, TP

13y FS Golden Retriever with right-sided exophthalmos. Representative transverse CT images (**a–c**) are ordered from rostral to caudal. The gross pathology image **e** is approximately comparable to CT image **a**. A well-delineated sessile soft-tissue mass is seen within the medial aspect of the right orbit (**a–d**: asterisk), causing compression and lateral displacement of the adjacent globe (**a**: arrowhead). The mass is only minimally contrast enhancing. Tissue biopsy revealed melanotic melanoma. A highly pigmented mass is seen in the dorsomedial aspect of the right orbit on the gross pathology image (**e**: arrow).

Figure 1.5.17 Orbital Fibrosarcoma (Canine)   CT

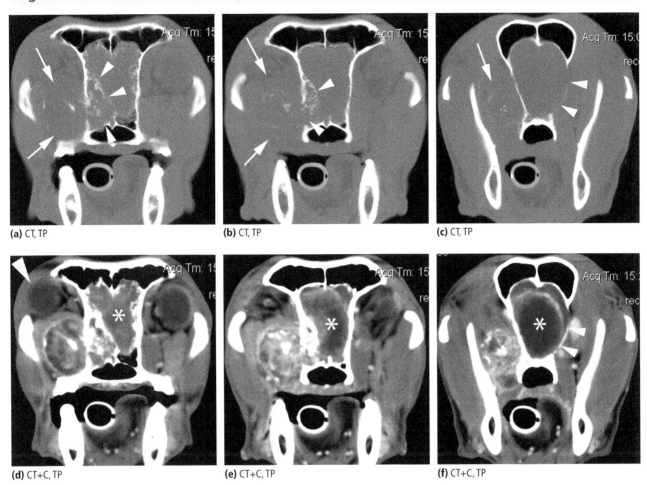

(a) CT, TP   **(b)** CT, TP   **(c)** CT, TP

(d) CT+C, TP   **(e)** CT+C, TP   **(f)** CT+C, TP

7y FS Retriever cross with right-sided exophthalmos and intracranial neurologic signs. Representative unenhanced (**a–c**) and comparable contrast-enhanced (**d–f**) images are ordered from rostral to caudal. An ill-defined partially mineralized soft-tissue mass is present in the right retrobulbar space (**a–c**: arrows), causing dorsal and rostral displacement of the right globe (**d**: arrowhead). There is osteolysis and medial displacement of the right frontal bone, perpendicular lamina of the right palatine bone, and ethmoturbinates (**a,b**: arrowheads). The mass extends into the olfactory and frontal regions of the cranial vault (**d–f**: asterisk). The expansile intracranial component of the mass also results in attenuation and lateral displacement of the left frontal and palatine bones (**c,f**: arrowheads). The mass has a heterogeneous contrast-enhancement pattern in the retrobulbar space (**d,e**) and a peripheral enhancement pattern intracranially (**f**: asterisk). Histologic diagnosis following necropsy was highly anaplastic sarcoma consistent with fibrosarcoma. The intracranial component was centrally necrotic, consistent with the pattern of contrast enhancement seen on CT images.

Figure 1.5.18   Orbital Rhabdomyosarcoma (Canine)   MR

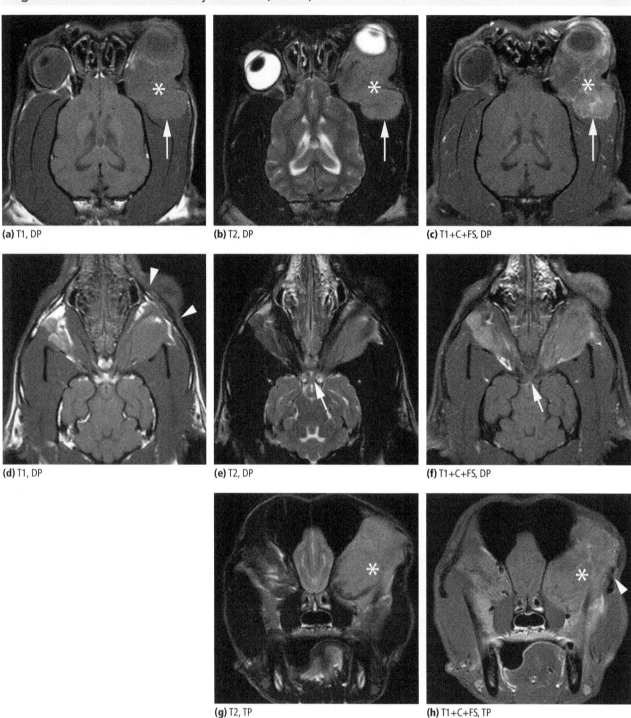

(a) T1, DP

(b) T2, DP

(c) T1+C+FS, DP

(d) T1, DP

(e) T2, DP

(f) T1+C+FS, DP

(g) T2, TP

(h) T1+C+FS, TP

3y MC Tibetan Terrier with a 2-week history of left-sided exophthalmos. Representative dorsal plane images are at (**a–c**) and ventral to (**d–f**) the level of the eyes. There is a large irregularly shaped mass within the retrobulbar space (**a–c,g,h**: asterisk), which is isointense to gray matter on both T1 and T2 images. The mass invades the left temporal muscle (**a–c**: arrow) and appears to cause osteolysis of the left zygomatic bone (**d,h**: arrowheads). The mass is nonuniformly contrast enhancing. Incidentally, the optic chiasm and origins of the optic nerves are particularly well seen in this study (**e,f**: arrow), and the origin of the left optic nerve does not appear to be involved. Histologic diagnosis following necropsy was rhabdomyosarcoma.

Figure 1.5.19 Orbital Meningioma (Canine)   MR

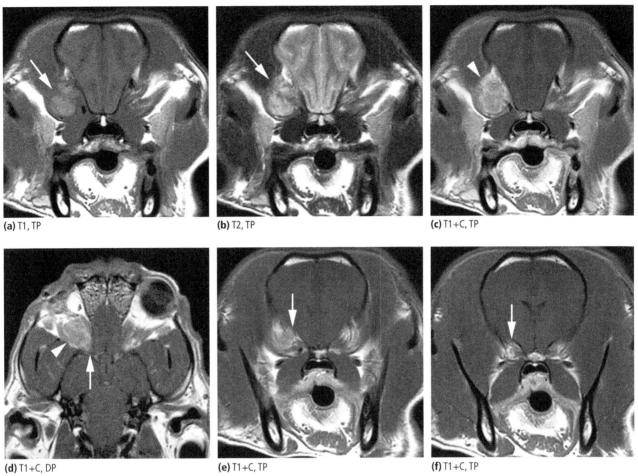

(a) T1, TP   **(b)** T2, TP   **(c)** T1+C, TP

(d) T1+C, DP   **(e)** T1+C, TP   **(f)** T1+C, TP

7y MC Cavalier King Charles Spaniel with a 4-month history of progressive right-sided exophthalmos. The first three images (**a–c**) depict the same anatomy and are at the level of the caudal aspect of the retrobulbar spaces. Images **e** and **f** are slightly more caudal and are ordered from rostral to caudal with image **f** at the caudal-most extent of the retrobulbar spaces. There is a well-defined mass in the caudal aspect of the right retrobulbar space that is hyperintense to gray matter on both T1 and T2 images (**a**,**b**: arrow). The mass is moderately and uniformly contrast enhancing (**c**,**d**: arrowhead). The caudal extent of the mass is adjacent to the region of the orbital fissure and optic canal (**d–e**,**f**: arrow). These structures are not clearly seen on the images, but the arrows indicate their approximate location. Upon surgical exploration, the mass was found to arise from the ophthalmic branch of the right trigeminal nerve (cranial nerve V) as it exited the orbital fissure. Excisional biopsy revealed meningioma. Although a specific preoperative diagnosis could not be made from MR images, the caudal and central location of the mass within the retrobulbar space and the uniform contrast-enhancement pattern is suggestive of a neoplasm arising from one of the nerves arising from the orbital fissure or optic canal.

Figure 1.5.20 Feline Restrictive Orbital Myofibroblastic Sarcoma (Feline)   MR

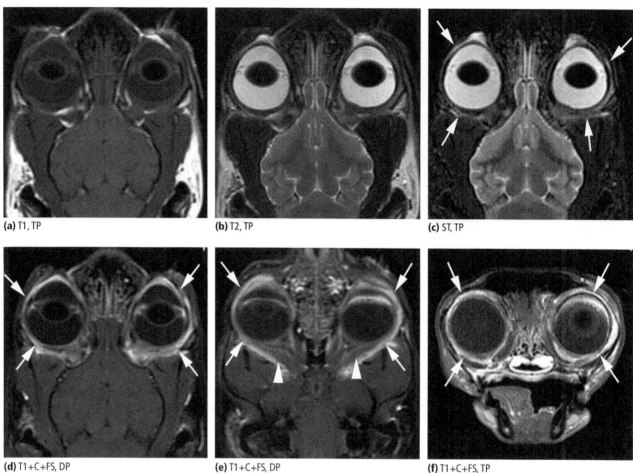

(a) T1, TP **(b)** T2, TP **(c)** ST, TP

(d) T1+C+FS, DP **(e)** T1+C+FS, DP **(f)** T1+C+FS, TP

16y FS Siamese with bilateral conjunctival and episcleral hyperemia, corneal ulcerations, and reduced extraocular muscle function. Images **a–d** are at the same anatomic level. Image **e** is somewhat more ventral and highlights the caudoventral recesses of the orbits. There is pronounced thickening of the sclera and episcleral tissues, which is best seen on the contrast-enhanced images (**d–f**: arrows). Periorbital edema is also evident on the STIR image (**c**: arrows). There is a loss of thickening of the extraocular muscles and loss of muscle margin definition associated with retrobulbar contrast enhancement (**e**: arrowheads). Biopsy confirmed a diagnosis of restrictive orbital myofibroblastic sarcoma involving both orbits. Thomasy et al (2013).[16] Reproduced with permission from Wiley.

References

1. Joslyn S, Richards S, Boroffka S, Mitchell M, Hammond G, Sullivan M. Magnetic resonance imaging contrast enhancement of extra-ocular muscles in dogs with no clinical evidence of orbital disease. Vet Radiol Ultrasound. 2013;55:63–67.

2. Noller C, Henninger W, Gronemeyer DH, Hirschberg RM, Budras KD. Computed tomography-anatomy of the normal feline nasolacrimal drainage system. Vet Radiol Ultrasound. 2006;47:53–60.

3. Nykamp SG, Scrivani PV, Pease AP. Computed tomography dacryocystography evaluation of the nasolacrimal apparatus. Vet Radiol Ultrasound. 2004;45:23–28.

4. Couturier L, Degueurce C, Ruel Y, Dennis R, Begon D. Anatomical study of cranial nerve emergence and skull foramina in the dog using magnetic resonance imaging and computed tomography. Vet Radiol Ultrasound. 2005;46:375–383.

5. Murphy CJ, Samuelson DA, Pollock RV. The Eye. *Miller's Anatomy of the Dog*: W.B. Saunders Company, 2012;746–785.

6. Boroffka SAEB, Görig C, Auriemma E, Passon-Vastenburg MHAC, Voorhout G, Barthez PY. Magnetic resonance imaging of the canine optic nerve. Vet Radiol Ultrasound. 2008;49:540–544.

7. Morgan RV, Daniel GB, Donnell RL. Magnetic resonance imaging of the normal eye and orbit of the dog and cat. Vet Radiol Ultrasound. 1994;35:102–108.

8. Schlueter C, Budras KD, Ludewig E, Mayrhofer E, Koenig HE, Walter A, et al. Brachycephalic feline noses: CT and anatomical study of the relationship between head conformation and the nasolacrimal drainage system. J Feline Med Surg. 2009;11: 891–900.

9. Hamilton HL, Whitley RD, McLaughlin SA. Exophthalmos secondary to aspergillosis in a cat. J Am Anim Hosp Assoc. 2000;36:343–347.

10. Kneissl S, Konar M, Fuchs-Baumgartinger A, Nell B. Magnetic resonance imaging features of orbital inflammation with intracranial extension in four dogs. Vet Radiol Ultrasound. 2007;48:403–408.

11. Boroffka SA, Verbruggen A-M, Grinwis GC, Voorhout G, Barthez PY. Assessment of ultrasonography and computed tomography for the evaluation of unilateral orbital disease in dogs. J Am Vet Med Assoc. 2007;230:671–680.
12. Headrick JF, Bentley E, Dubielzig RR. Canine lobular orbital adenoma: a report of 15 cases with distinctive features. Vet Ophthalmol. 2004;7:47–51.
13. Wiggans KT, Skorupski KA, Reilly CM. Presumed solitary intraocular or conjunctival lymphoma in dogs and cats: 9 cases (1985–2013). J Am Vet Med Assoc. 2014;244:460–470.
14. Dennis R. Imaging features of orbital myxosarcoma in dogs. Vet Radiol Ultrasound. 2008;49:256–263.
15. Fiani N, Arzi B, Johnson EG, Murphy B, Verstraete FJM. Osteoma of the oral and maxillofacial regions in cats: 7 cases (1999–2009). J Am Vet Med Assoc. 2011;238:1470–1475.
16. Bell CM, Schwarz T, Dubielzig RR. Diagnostic Features of Feline Restrictive Orbital Myofibroblastic Sarcoma. Vet Pathol. 2010;48:742–750.
17. Thomasy SM, Cissell DD, Arzi B, Vilches-Moure JG, Lo WY, Wisner ER, et al. Restrictive orbital myofibroblastic sarcoma in a cat – Cross-sectional imaging (MRI & CT) appearance, treatment, and outcome. Vet Ophthalmol. 2013;16:1–7.

1.6

Globe

Introduction

CT is often used to image the structures of the orbit and surrounding skull (see Chapter 1.5). It can also be used for imaging the major structures of the globe, including the anterior and vitreous chambers, as well as the lens (Figure 1.6.1). MRI is an excellent modality to image the structures of the globe and optic nerve. The cornea, anterior and posterior chambers, ciliary body, lens, vitreous chamber, and retina are visible on standard sequences (Figure 1.6.2).[1] The optic nerve can also be evaluated and followed to the optic chiasm, both in transverse images and when dorsal or sagittal plane sequences are oriented obliquely along the long axis of the nerve. The optic nerve is surrounded by cerebrospinal fluid (CSF), which appears hyperintense on T2 and hypointense on T1 images. Fat nullifying sequences, such as STIR, as well as thin collimation can help to suppress the bright fat signal and allow visualization of the CSF and nerve.[2] Disorders of the optic nerve are discussed in Chapter 2.10.

Trauma

Trauma to the eye commonly presents as proptosis, with the possibility of additional trauma to the surrounding bones and soft tissues of the orbit (Figure 1.6.3). Penetrating trauma to the eye is not commonly evaluated with CT or MRI, but hemorrhage, inflammation, and altered anatomic structures would be expected findings. Foreign bodies and associated inflammation in the sclera can be seen as a mass lesion that deforms the scleral shape with contrast enhancement.[3] Traumatic ruptures

of the lens and globe have been reported to be better seen on MR than on CT images.[4]

Inflammatory disorders

Optic neuritis can be seen on MR images as hyperintensity of one or both optic nerves in water-sensitive imaging sequences. The nerve may be hyperintense within the orbit and/or at the level of the optic chiasm.[5]

Granulomatous meningoencephalitis has been reported to involve the optic nerves. On MR images, it appears as isointense regions on T1 and T2 weighted images, with intense contrast enhancement (see Chapter 2.10).[6]

Anterior uveitis is defined as inflammation of the anterior chamber of the eye. On MR images, increased signal intensity can be seen on T1 images, and contrast enhancement may also be observed (Figure 1.6.4). Episcleritis involves inflammation of the tissues surrounding the sclera. The periocular tissues are thickened and T1 and T2 hyperintense and are intensely contrast enhancing (Figure 1.6.5).

Neoplasia

Melanoma arising from the uvea has been described on MR imaging in dogs. The mass was T1 hyperintense and T2 hypointense with contrast enhancement (Figure 1.6.6).[7] T1 hyperintensity is a property of melanin that has been described in other regions of the body. A case of melanoma arising from the choroid and surrounding the optic nerve was T1 and T2 hypointense.[8] On CT images, melanoma may appear hyperattenuating

---

Atlas of Small Animal CT and MRI, First Edition. Erik R. Wisner and Allison L. Zwingenberger.
© 2015 John Wiley & Sons, Inc. Published 2015 by John Wiley & Sons, Inc.

to the vitreous (Figure 1.6.7). Round cell neoplasia such as lymphoma can also primarily involve the eye (Figure 1.6.8). Metastatic disease due to other neoplasms can also occur. Neoplasia should be considered in patients with ocular hemorrhage where there is a clear fluid–fluid interface on MR images (Figure 1.6.9).

Degenerative disorders

Retinal detachment

Retinal detachment is uncommon in cats but may be caused by bullous or effusive mechanisms, a tear with vitreous filling the space between the retinal and choroid, or contraction of postinflammatory fibrous strands in the vitreous pulling the retina anteriorly.[9] The CT appearance of retinal detachment is a V-shaped linear structure (shaped like seagull wings) with the apex centered at the optic disc (Figure 1.6.10). Hyperattenuating material between the retina and the choroid may indicate proteinaceous fluid or hemorrhage.[10] Bullous retinal detachment due to fluid accumulation has been reported in cats with hypertension.[9] On MR images, the fluid external to the retina is hyperintense on T1 and T2 images (Figure 1.6.11).

Cataracts/lens luxation

Cataracts are a degenerative disease of the lens that results in increased density and opacification. On CT images, cataracts appear as hyperattenuating strands within the lens, which can progress to involve the entire lens (Figure 1.6.12). On MR images, the lens becomes decreased in signal intensity (Figure 1.6.13). The lens is normally hyperattenuating to the vitreous on CT images and hypointense on MR images. Deformation of the shape of the lens can also occur with cataract formation. Glaucoma can result in luxation of the lens into the vitreous chamber (Figure 1.6.13).

Prostheses

Some patients are fitted with ocular prostheses following enucleation. If CT or MR imaging is performed, characteristic artifacts may occur. Silicone-based prostheses may contain pigments to mimic brown or black eye color. In one study, the brown-pigmented prosthesis contained iron oxide or titanium dioxide, producing susceptibility artifact. A black prosthesis was pigmented with carbon black and did not produce ferromagnetic artifact, with no signal on any sequence (Figure 1.6.14).[11] On CT images, the prostheses tend to be hyperattenuating (Figure 1.6.15).

Figure 1.6.1   Normal Globe (Canine)   CT

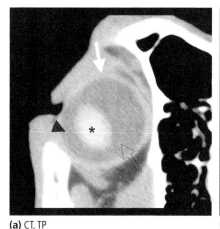
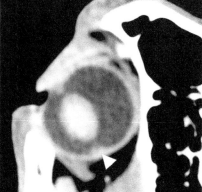

The lens is hyperattenuating (**a**: asterisk) and maintains its position through circumferential attachment to the ciliary body (**b**: white arrowhead). The anterior chamber (**a**: black arrowhead) and vitreous chamber (**a**: open arrow) are fluid attenuating. The sclera is hyperattenuating and surrounds the posterior portion of the eye (**a**: white arrow).

(a) CT, TP   (b) CT+C, TP

Figure 1.6.2 Normal Globe (Feline)   MR

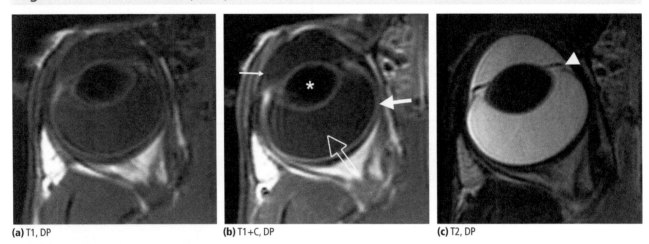

(a) T1, DP   (b) T1+C, DP   (c) T2, DP

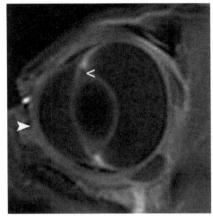

(d) T1+C+FS, SP

The lens is visible as a hypointense structure with a hyperintense capsule (**b**: asterisk). The ciliary body supports the lens (**c**: arrowhead) and is contrast enhancing (**d**). The anterior (**b**: small white arrow), posterior (**d**: <), and vitreous chambers (**b**: open arrow) are hypointense on T1 and hyperintense on T2 images. The cornea (**d**: arrowhead) is visible anteriorly. The enhancing retina (**b**: large solid white arrow) is present posterior to the vitreous.

Figure 1.6.3   Trauma with Proptosis (Canine)   CT

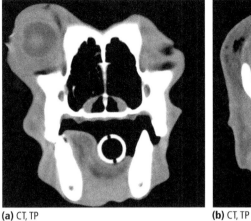

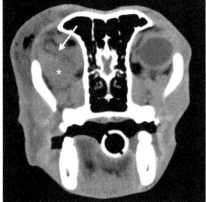

3y FS Brittany Spaniel with acute head trauma of unknown cause. Transverse images are ordered from rostral to caudal. The globe is located cranial and lateral to the orbit (a). There is soft-tissue swelling within the orbit (b: asterisk), likely due to hemorrhage and edema. The optic nerve appears enlarged and surrounded by hypoattenuating tissue as it crosses this region (b: arrow).

(a) CT, TP

(b) CT, TP

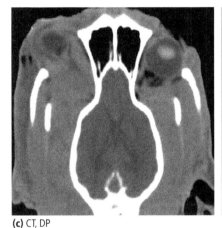

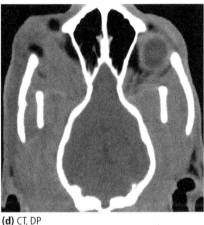

(c) CT, DP

(d) CT, DP

Figure 1.6.4   Anterior Uveitis (Canine)   MR

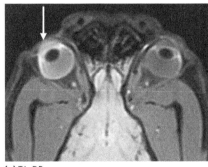

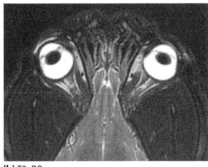

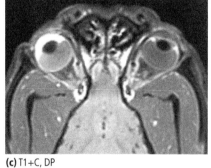

(a) T1, DP

(b) T2, DP

(c) T1+C, DP

1y M Labrador Retriever with progressive swelling and cloudiness of the right eye. Glaucoma and uveitis were diagnosed following a complete ophthalmic examination. There is increased signal intensity of the right anterior chamber on T1 images (a: arrow) compared to the normal eye. There is a similar but more subtle increase in vitreous attenuation in the same eye. On contrast-enhanced images, there is marked enhancement of the fluid in the anterior chamber (c). The eye was enucleated after a corneal rupture, and plant material was found within the lens capsule.

Figure 1.6.5   Scleritis/Episcleritis (Canine)   MR

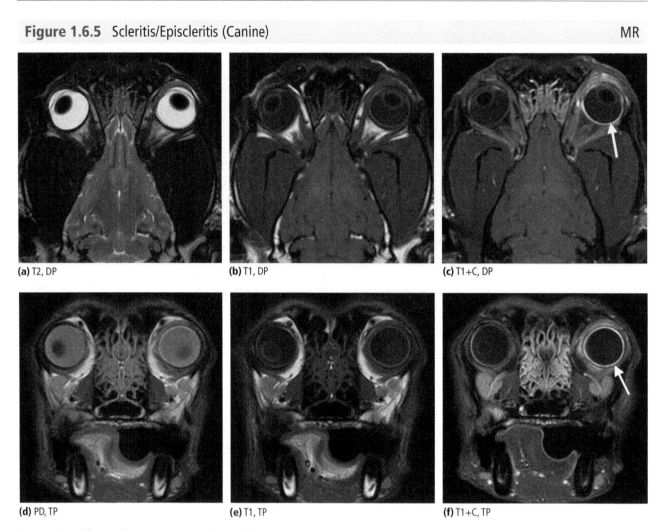

(a) T2, DP   **(b)** T1, DP   **(c)** T1+C, DP

(d) PD, TP   **(e)** T1, TP   **(f)** T1+C, TP

9y F Border Collie mix that was presented for eye infection. There is thickening of the tissues surrounding the eye as well as the sclera itself, best seen on contrast-enhanced images (**c**,**f**: arrow). The sclera is contrast enhancing and thickened compared to the normal eye (**b**,**c**,**f**).

Figure 1.6.6   Intraocular Melanoma (Canine)   MR

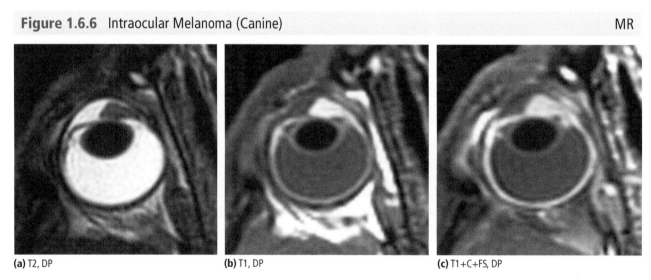

(a) T2, DP   **(b)** T1, DP   **(c)** T1+C+FS, DP

11y M Golden Retriever with red-eye of 3-week duration. This was a melanotic melanoma of the anterior uvea, explaining the pronounced T1 hyperintensity on the unenhanced image. The diagnosis was confirmed histologically following enucleation.

Figure 1.6.7 Intraocular Melanoma (Canine) CT

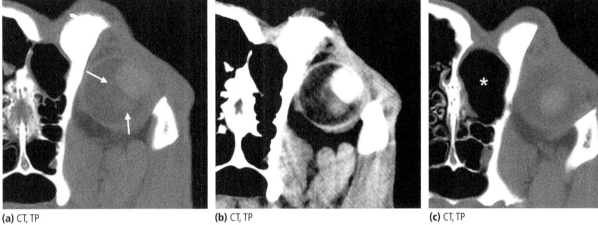

(a) CT, TP   **(b)** CT, TP   **(c)** CT, TP

11y MC German Shepherd Dog with aspergillosis and an incidentally discovered ocular mass. The mass (**a**: arrows) is visible as a lobular, soft-tissue attenuating structure caudal to the lens. There is interruption of the frontal bone and absent nasal turbinates (**c**: asterisk) due to previous rhinosinusitis. Vitreous humor aspirate revealed melanotic melanoma.

Figure 1.6.8   Intraocular Lymphoma (Feline)

MR

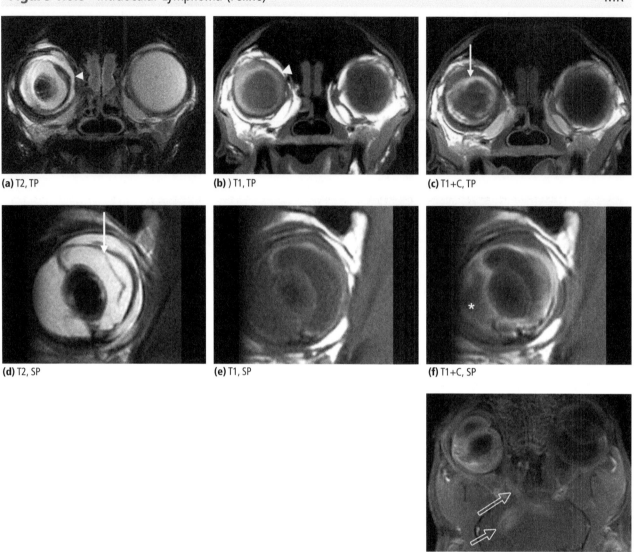

(a) T2, TP   **(b))** T1, TP   **(c)** T1+C, TP

(d) T2, SP   **(e)** T1, SP   **(f)** T1+C, SP

(g) T1+C, DP

12y MC Domestic Longhair who is FIV positive, with blindness and decreased mentation. There is nuclear sclerosis of the right lens (**a**). Retinal detachment is present (**d**: arrow) with thickening of the retinal tissue on contrast-enhanced images (**c**: arrow). The material posterior to the retina is T2 hyperintense and T1 hypointense (**a**,**b**: arrowhead). The anterior chamber is filled with contrast-enhancing material (**f**: asterisk). The optic nerve is enlarged and contrast enhancing, extending through the orbital fissure to a hyperintense, contrast-enhancing mass within the brain (**g**: open arrows). Lymphoma was diagnosed after enucleation of the eye.

Figure 1.6.9 Intraocular Hemorrhage, Retinal Separation and Panuveitis (Canine)   MR

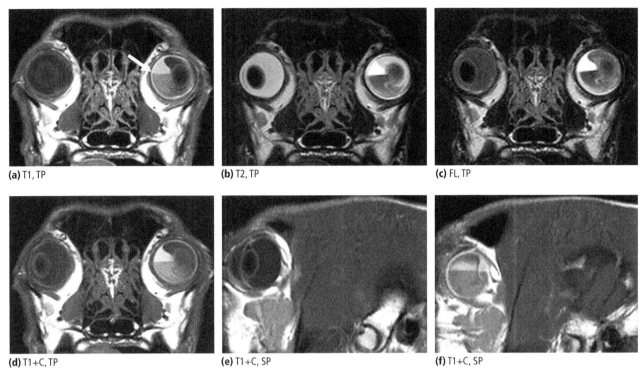

(a) T1, TP

(b) T2, TP

(c) FL, TP

(d) T1+C, TP

(e) T1+C, SP

(f) T1+C, SP

11y MC Border Collie with a history of ocular hemorrhage. There is increased intensity within the vitreous chamber of the left globe on T1 (**a**) and T2 (**b**) weighted sequences. The retina is poorly defined and appears detached. There is a clearly demarcated line (**a**: arrow) separating two different fluid signals in the vitreous chamber. Neither component nulls on the FLAIR image (**c**), and the lesion does not enhance on contrast-enhanced images (**d**). The normal right globe (**e**) can be compared with the abnormal globe (**f**) on sagittal images. A hemangiosarcoma metastasis was found in the iris on histopathology and was the source of intraocular hemorrhage, which was confirmed on postmortem examination. The partitioning was thought to be due to separation of serum and cellular components.

Figure 1.6.10 Bullous Retinal Detachment (Feline)   CT

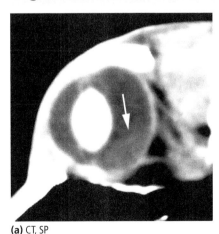

(a) CT, SP

8y MC Domestic Shorthair with hypertension, acute onset blindness, and obtundation. The CT study was performed on an emergent basis to evaluate for intracranial causes of obtundation. There is a broad-based, hyperattenuating structure (arrow) on the ventral aspect of the globe. The most caudal aspect of the structure is in the region of the optic disc. The hyperattenuation indicates hemorrhage or proteinaceous fluid. Nuclear sclerosis was also present. Imaging findings were confirmed by full ophthalmic examination.

Figure 1.6.11   Retinal Detachment (Feline)   MR

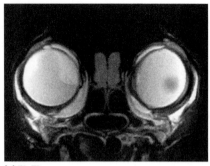 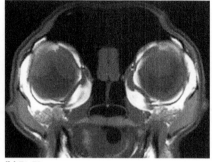 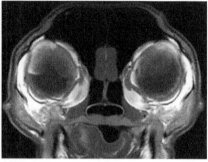

(a) T2, TP   **(b)** T1, TP   **(c)** T1+C, TP

18y MC Domestic Shorthair with progressive central nervous system disease, diabetes mellitus, and chronic renal failure. There is bilateral retinal detachment with a classic "V" shape centered at the optic disc. The material posterior to the retina is hyperintense on T2 images (**a**) and slightly hyperintense on T1 images (**b**) and represents retroretinal exudate. Bullous serous retinal detachment, confirmed by complete ophthalmic examination, was thought to be secondary to systemic hypertension.

Figure 1.6.12   Hypermature Cataract (Canine)   CT

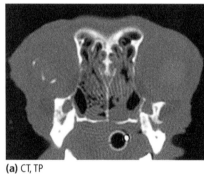 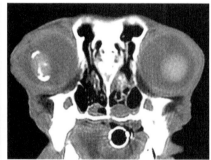

11y Poodle/Maltese cross. A cataract had been developing in the right eye for the previous 4 years. In the bone window (**a**) and soft-tissue window (**b**), mineral attenuating regions are visible in the peripheral and central regions of the right lens. The cataract was brunescent and resulted in loss of vision.

(a) CT, TP   **(b)** CT, TP

Figure 1.6.13 Luxated Lens, Hypermature Cataract, Retinal Detachment (Canine) MR

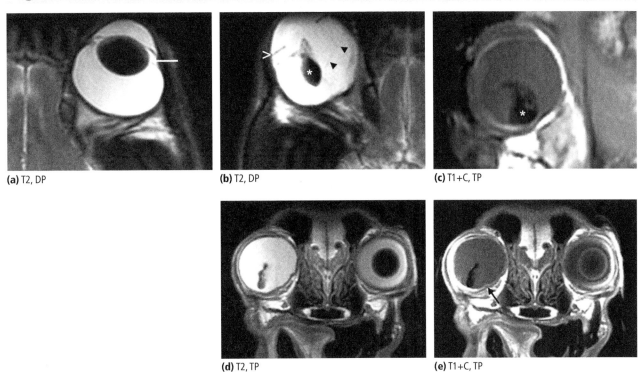

(a) T2, DP

(b) T2, DP

(c) T1+C, TP

(d) T2, TP

(e) T1+C, TP

The left lens is in a normal position caudal to the iris (**a**: white arrow). The right lens is misshapen and reduced in size as a result of a hypermature cataract (**b,c**: asterisk) and has been displaced caudal to the iris (**b**: >) into the vitreous (**b–e**). The sclera is slightly irregular in the right eye (**e**: black arrow), and the right globe is larger than the left (**d,e**). There is a thin hypointense linear structure (**b**: arrowheads) medial to the luxated lens that represents the detached retina. These findings, confirmed on postmortem examination, were attributed to glaucoma and to systemic hypertension.

Figure 1.6.14 Ocular Prosthesis (Canine)

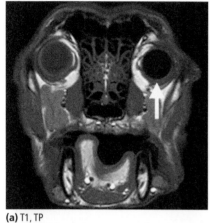

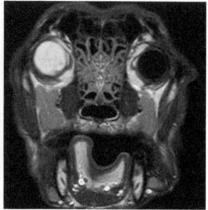

13y MC Golden Retriever with history of uveitis and prosthetic implantation in the left eye. The prosthesis (**a**: arrow) is hypointense to the normal right eye on all sequences (**a–d**).

(a) T1, TP   (b) T2, TP

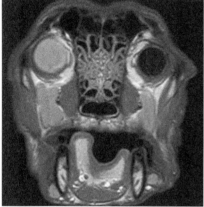

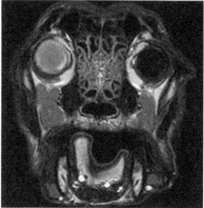

(c) PD, TP   (d) FL, TP

Figure 1.6.15 Ocular Prosthesis (Canine)

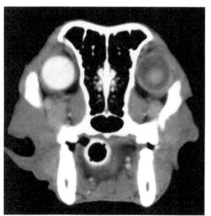

11y FS Golden Retriever presented for evaluation of a brainstem mass. The right globe is uniformly hyperattenuating, consistent with an ocular prosthesis.

(a) CT, TP

References

1. Morgan RV, Daniel GB, Donnell RL. Magnetic resonance imaging of the normal eye and orbit of the dog and cat. Vet Radiol Ultrasound. 1994;35:102–108.

2. Boroffka SAEB, Görig C, Auriemma E, Passon-Vastenburg MHAC, Voorhout G, Barthez PY. Magnetic resonance imaging of the canine optic nerve. Vet Radiol Ultrasound. 2008;49:540–544.

3. Welihozkiy A, Pirie CG, Pizzirani S. Scleral and suprachoroidal foreign body in a dog – a case report. Vet Ophthalmol. 2011; 14:345–351.

4. Krosigk von F, Steinmetz A, Ellenberger C, Oechtering G. [Magnetic resonance imaging and ultrasonography in dogs and cats with ocular and orbital diseases. Part 1: Ocular diseases]. Tierarztl Prax K H. 2012;40:7–15.

5. Armour MD, Broome M, Dell'Anna G, Blades NJ, Esson DW. A review of orbital and intracranial magnetic resonance imaging in 79 canine and 13 feline patients (2004–2010). Vet Ophthalmol. 2011;14:215–226.

6. Kitagawa M, Okada M, Watari T, Sato T, Kanayama K, Sakai T. Ocular granulomatous meningoencephalomyelitis in a dog: magnetic resonance images and clinical findings. J Vet Med Sci. 2009;71:233–237.

7. Kato K, Nishimura R, Sasaki N, et al. Magnetic resonance imaging of a canine eye with melanoma. J Vet Med Sci. 2005;67: 179–182.

8. Miwa Y, Matsunaga S, Kato K, et al. Choroidal melanoma in a dog. J Vet Med Sci. 2005;67:821–823.

9. Christmas R, Guthrie B. Bullous retinal detachment in a cat. Can Vet J. 1989;30:430–431.

10. LeBedis CA, Sakai O. Nontraumatic orbital conditions: diagnosis with CT and MR imaging in the emergent setting. Radiographics. 2008;28:1741–1753.

11. Dees DD, Knollinger AM, Simmons JP, Seshadri R, MacLaren NE. Magnetic resonance imaging susceptibility artifact due to pigmented intraorbital silicone prosthesis. Vet Ophthalmol. 2012;15:386–390.

1.7

Salivary glands

Introduction

The salivary glands include the mandibular, zygomatic, parotid, and lingual glands. The mandibular salivary gland is a large, oval, uniform structure located caudal to the mandible. On CT images it has a uniform texture (Figure 1.7.1). The parotid salivary gland is thin, elongated, and has a finely textured lobular structure. It is located lateral to the vertical ear canal and cranial and dorsal to the mandibular salivary gland. The parotid and mandibular salivary glands are moderately hyperintense to muscle on T1 images, but the mandibular salivary gland is hyperintense to the parotid on T2 images (Figure 1.7.2). The zygomatic salivary gland is variable in size and shape, and it is located in the orbit, lateral to the pterygoid muscles and ventral to the globe (Figure 1.7.3). Contrast enhancement on CT is slightly heterogeneous because of the glandular architecture. The major sublingual salivary gland is fused to the cranial capsule of the mandibular salivary gland. It appears triangular in shape in the sagittal plane (Figure 1.7.1) and may be more difficult to visualize on MR images. Glands are isointense to hyperintense to adjacent musculature on T1 and hyperintense on T2 images (Figure 1.7.4).[1] The salivary glands moderately to intensely contrast enhance on both CT and MR images.

Sialography of the salivary glands using CT has been performed in cadavers by placing a cannula and extension set in the oral salivary duct. Diluted nonionic contrast medium mixed with methylcellulose was used to fill the ducts. The parotid duct travels from the rostral and ventral border of the gland, lateral to the masseter muscle, to the level of the 4th premolar. The mandibular duct travels medial and parallel to the mandible and enters the oral cavity at the level of the sublingual caruncle. The zygomatic duct enters the oral cavity caudal to the parotid duct at the level of the first upper molar and often has several diverticula.[2]

Inflammatory disorders

Zygomatic sialadenitis is an inflammatory condition of the zygomatic salivary gland. The position of the gland in the ventrolateral orbit causes secondary exophthalmos when enlarged and inflamed. CT and MR imaging show an enlarged, hypoattenuating (CT) and T1 hypointense, T2 and FLAIR hyperintense (MR) gland with surrounding loss of detail due to inflammation (Figures 1.7.5, 1.7.6).[3] The disease is usually unilateral but can also be bilateral. Formation of fluid-attenuating or T2 hyperintense sialoceles is common. The mandibular and parotid salivary glands are occasionally affected by sialadenitis. This appears on CT images as enlargement of the gland lateral and ventral to the ear canal (Figure 1.7.7). Affected glands are intensely contrast enhancing and often retain their glandular structures, including ducts, despite the inflammatory change. The structure may become disrupted with sialocele or abscess formation (Figure 1.7.8).

Neoplasia

Tumors of the salivary glands are uncommon. These lesions produce mass effect in the regional tissues of the head and irregular enlargement of the gland of origin. Contrast enhancement may be strong to heterogeneous if there is fluid present or regions of necrosis. Tumors can be differentiated from sialadenitis by the disruption

---

Atlas of Small Animal CT and MRI, First Edition. Erik R. Wisner and Allison L. Zwingenberger.
© 2015 John Wiley & Sons, Inc. Published 2015 by John Wiley & Sons, Inc.

of the normal architecture of the gland. Examples include adenocarcinoma of the mandibular (Figure 1.7.9) and parotid (Figure 1.7.10) salivary glands, as well as zygomatic basal cell adenocarcinoma (Figure 1.7.11)

Sialolithiasis and sialocele

When the salivary ducts are blocked by mucus concretions or sialoliths, the production of saliva causes expansion of cavities within the salivary gland, which extend beyond the normal borders. These fluctuant masses tend to contain fluid in large thin-walled chambers in the ventral mandibular area, sublingual region, or orbit (see zygomatic sialadenitis earlier in this chapter). The communication with the salivary gland may be difficult to localize on CT and MR images. Other imaging characteristics include fluid that is hypoattenuating on CT (0 HU) with no contrast

enhancement (Figure 1.7.12), and MR hyperintensity on T2 images with hypointensity on T1 images (Figure 1.7.13). The fluid compartments may exhibit peripheral contrast enhancement on CT and MR images. The location of the fluid in relation to the salivary glands may suggest a gland of origin. For example, fluid in the sublingual region is likely associated with obstruction to the sublingual salivary duct (Figure 1.7.13). Sialoceles may also occur bilaterally, appearing as roughly symmetric fluid-filled masses on both sides of the mandible (Figure 1.7.14). If sialoliths are responsible for the ductal obstruction, they may be seen on CT images within the fluid of the mass, within the ipsilateral or contralateral gland, or within the duct itself (Figure 1.7.15). Sialoceles may also form in other salivary glands, including minor glands that are less commonly seen on imaging examinations.[4]

Figure 1.7.1 Normal Parotid and Mandibular Salivary Glands (Canine)   CT

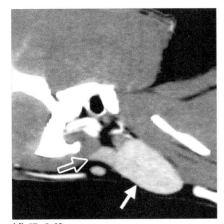

(a) CT+C, TP   **(b)** CT+C, TP   **(c)** CT+C, TP

(d) CT+C, SP

6y MC Boxer. Representative images were acquired immediately following contrast medium administration and are ordered from rostral to caudal. The normal mandibular salivary glands are characteristically oval in shape and smoothly margined (**a–d**: arrows). The normal parotid salivary glands are more elongated and have lobular margins (**a–c**: arrowheads). Both glands are highly and uniformly contrast enhancing. The major sublingual salivary gland is a small triangular structure fused to the cranial margin of the mandibular salivary gland (**d**: open arrow).

Figure 1.7.2 Normal Parotid and Mandibular Salivary Glands (Canine) MR

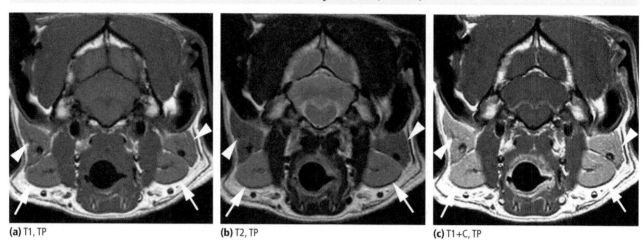

(a) T1, TP **(b)** T2, TP **(c)** T1+C, TP

4y MC Terrier. The normal mandibular salivary glands are characteristically oval in shape and smoothly margined (**a–c**: arrows). The normal parotid salivary glands are more elongated and have a mildly heterogeneous appearance (**a–c**: arrowheads). Although the glands have similar hyperintensity to muscle on unenhanced T1 images, the mandibular salivary glands are hyperintense compared to the parotid glands on T2 images. Both glands are intensely and uniformly contrast enhancing (**c**).

Figure 1.7.3 Normal Zygomatic Salivary Gland (Canine) CT

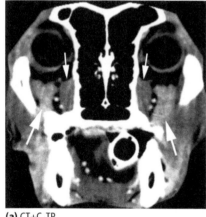

7y MC Weimaraner cross. Normal zygomatic salivary glands moderately contrast enhance (large arrows). The nonuniformity of enhancement is consistent with the glandular architecture. The medial pterygoid muscle is located adjacent and medial to the zygomatic salivary gland at this level (small arrows).

(a) CT+C, TP

Figure 1.7.4 Normal Zygomatic Salivary Gland (Canine) MR

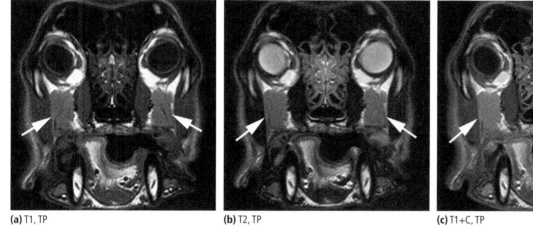

(a) T1, TP   **(b)** T2, TP   **(c)** T1+C, TP

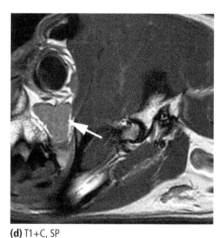

(d) T1+C, SP

5y MC Golden Retriever. Zygomatic salivary glands (**a–d**: arrows) are extremely variable in both size and shape. Glands are hyperintense to adjacent musculature on both T1 and T2 images (**a,b**) and are moderately and uniformly enhancing on contrast-enhanced T1 images (**c,d**).

Figure 1.7.5 Zygomatic Sialadenitis (Canine) CT

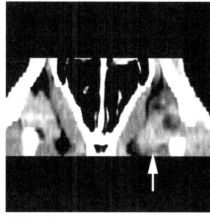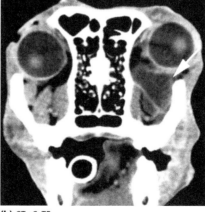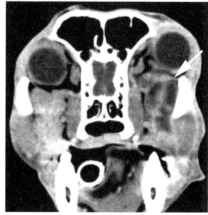

(a) CT+C, DP   **(b)** CT+C, TP   **(c)** CT+C, TP

2y MC Australian Shepherd with left-sided exophthalmos. A multicameral cystic mass arises from the left zygomatic salivary gland (**a–c**: arrow), causing dorsal displacement of the left globe. The right zygomatic salivary gland is normal in appearance. Aspiration cytology of the mass revealed neutrophilic inflammation consistent with zygomatic sialoadenitis.

Figure 1.7.6 Zygomatic Sialadenitis (Canine) MR

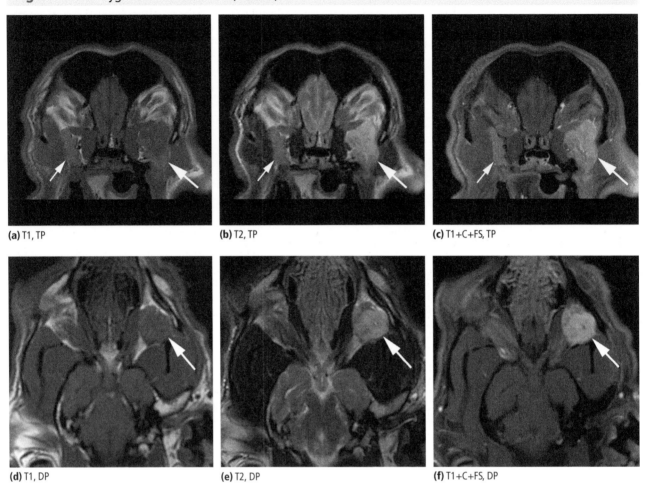

(a) T1, TP   **(b)** T2, TP   **(c)** T1+C+FS, TP

(d) T1, DP   **(e)** T2, DP   **(f)** T1+C+FS, DP

9y FS Cocker Spaniel with left-sided exophthalmos. The left zygomatic salivary gland (**a–f**: large arrow) is markedly enlarged and is T1 hypointense and T2 hyperintense to the contralateral gland (**a–c**: small arrow). The contrast-enhanced images reveal that the glandular architecture is retained, including the arborizing ductal pattern, suggesting diffuse inflammation rather than neoplasia. Clinical signs resolved with antibiotic and anti-inflammatory therapy.

Figure 1.7.7 Parotid Sialoadenitis (Canine) CT

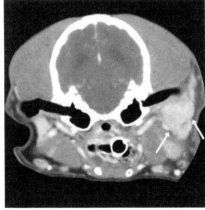

1y MC Pembroke Welsh Corgi with pain on palpation of left ear. The left parotid salivary gland, ventral and lateral to the ear canal, is enlarged and thickened compared to the right side. There is intense contrast enhancement on transverse images (**a**: arrows), which correlates with the contrast-enhanced gland on the 3D images (**b**: arrows).

(a) CT+C, T   **(b)** CT+C, 3D, VENT

Figure 1.7.8 Mandibular Salivary Gland Abscess (Canine)   CT

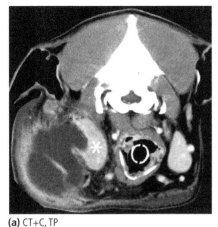
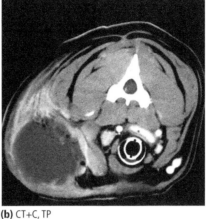

(a) CT+C, TP   **(b)** CT+C, TP

12y MC Rottweiler with a ventral cervical mass. Representative contrast-enhanced images are ordered from rostral to caudal. There is a large predominantly fluid attenuating cavitary mass contiguous with the lateral margin of the right mandibular salivary gland (a: asterisk). The lateral contour of the gland is altered, and the fluid center extends into the glandular parenchyma (a). The mass is thick walled, peripherally enhancing, and poorly margined. The center consists predominantly of fluid but also includes a small volume of fragmented gas (b). A mixed bacterial population was cultured from a fluid aspirate.

Figure 1.7.9 Mandibular Salivary Adenocarcinoma (Feline)   CT

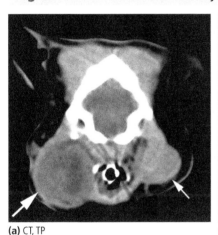
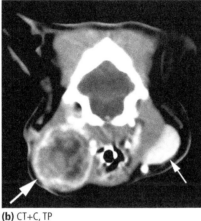

(a) CT, TP   **(b)** CT+C, TP

8y FS Siamese with a ventral cervical mass. Representative images are at the level of the mandibular salivary glands. There is a large, spherical, low-attenuation mandibular salivary mass in the right ventral cervical region (a,b: large arrow). The mass contrast enhances nonuniformly centrally and has a thin but prominent peripheral rim of enhancement (b). The normal left mandibular salivary gland is also evident (a,b: small arrow). Biopsy confirmed mandibular salivary adenocarcinoma.

Figure 1.7.10 Parotid Salivary Adenocarcinoma (Canine)   CT

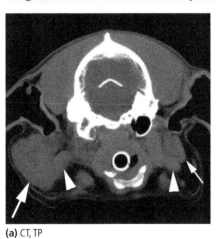
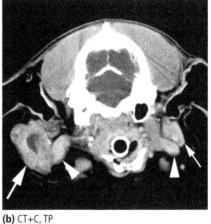
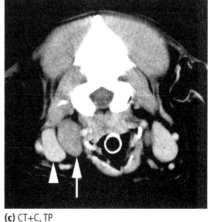

(a) CT, TP   **(b)** CT+C, TP   **(c)** CT+C, TP

13y MC Golden Retriever with a slowly enlarging mass. There is a large, irregularly margined mass arising from the right parotid salivary gland (a,b: large arrow). The normal left parotid gland is also seen (a,b: small arrow). The cranial poles of the mandibular salivary glands can also be seen medial to the parotid glands (a,b: arrowheads). An enlarged right mandibular lymph node is also present (a,b: adjacent to left arrowhead). The mass nonuniformly contrast enhances revealing a central cavitary component (b). Further caudally, a markedly enlarged right medial retropharyngeal lymph node is evident (c: arrow) adjacent to the mandibular gland (c: arrowhead). Biopsy of the mass and lymph nodes confirmed a diagnosis of parotid salivary adenocarcinoma with regional lymph node metastasis.

Figure 1.7.11   Zygomatic Salivary Gland Basal Cell Adenocarcinoma (Feline)   CT

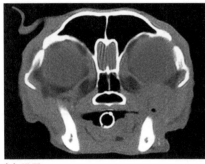 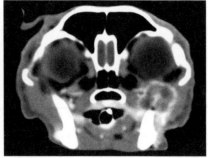

(a) CT, TP   **(b)** CT+C, TP

14y MC Japanese Bobtail with ulcerated oral lesion. A roughly spherical mass is seen immediately ventral to the left globe. The mass is nonuniformly contrast enhancing centrally and has a thin, prominent peripheral rim of enhancement. Contrast enhancement extends to the mandible, and mass margins are poorly delineated. A focal gas collection ventral to the mass is due to the associated oral ulcer. Biopsy revealed basal cell adenocarcinoma of the zygomatic salivary gland.

Figure 1.7.12   Mandibular Sialocele (Canine)   CT

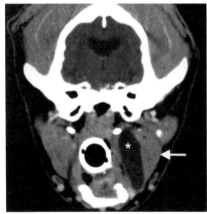

10y MC Afghan Hound. The CT study was performed as part of a diagnostic evaluation of suspected pituitary-dependent Cushing's syndrome. An oval fluid-dense mass (**a**: asterisk) is located medial to the left digastricus muscle (**a**: arrow). The attenuation of the fluid was 0 HU and was similar on unenhanced and contrast-enhanced images. The clinical diagnosis was sialocele arising from the mandibular salivary gland (not seen in this image).

(a) CT+C, TP

Figure 1.7.13 Sialocele (Canine)   MR

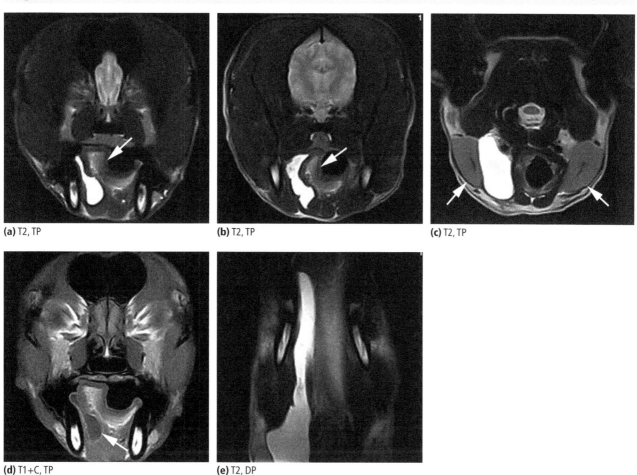

(a) T2, TP   **(b)** T2, TP   **(c)** T2, TP

(d) T1+C, TP   **(e)** T2, DP

5y M Samoyed with fluctuant sublingual mass. Images **a–c** are ordered from rostral to caudal. Image **d** is at approximately the same anatomic level as **a**. Compartmentalized fluid extends along the length of the oral cavity, terminating caudal to the larynx (**a–d**). The uniformly hyperintense T2 signal and the T1 hypointensity (**d**: arrow) verify the fluid composition of the mass. Fluid is distributed to the right of midline and is sublingual for much of its length. The tongue (**a,b**: arrows) is adjacent to the fluid compartment and distorts its medial margin. The right and left mandibular salivary glands are also seen (**c**: arrows). The characteristic sublingual location of the fluid collection and the normal appearance of the mandibular salivary gland suggest a sialocele arising from obstruction of the monostomatic sublingual salivary duct. Dr S.Cizinauskas, Animal Hospital Aisti, Finland, 2014. Reproduced with permission from S. Cizinauskas.

Figure 1.7.14 Parotid Duct Obstruction (Feline)   CT

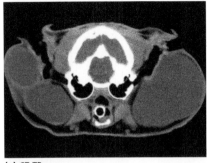

(a) CT, TP

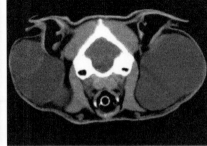

(b) CT, TP

16y Domestic Longhair with bilateral facial swelling. Representative unenhanced and comparable contrast-enhanced images are ordered from rostral to caudal. Bilateral well-circumscribed, thin-walled, fluid-attenuating masses are present ventrolaterally. Other images (not shown) documented these masses are tubular. Although the masses peripherally enhance, central attenuation remains unchanged, indicative of compartmentalized fluid. Aspiration cytology confirmed the fluid was saliva. Attempts to catheterize the parotid ducts were unsuccessful because of stenosis at the oral papilla.

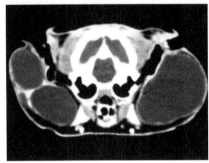

(c) CT+C, TP

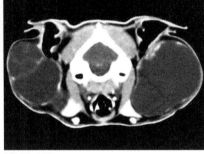

(d) CT+C, TP

Figure 1.7.15 Sialocele with Sialoliths (Canine)   CT

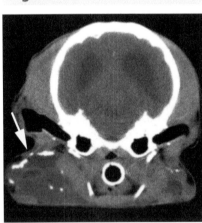

(a) CT, TP

10y MC Maltese with a fluctuant ventral cervical mass. The CT image is at a level just rostral to the mandibular salivary gland. An ill-defined and diffusely hypoattenuating mass (arrow) is present adjacent to the right external ear canal and tympanic bulla. Multiple focal mineral opacities are distributed within the mass. Smaller numbers are seen on the left side. The mass was thought to represent a sialocele containing multiple sialoliths.

References

1. Weidner S, Probst A, Kneissl S. MR anatomy of salivary glands in the dog. Anatom Histol Embryol. 2012;41:149–153.
2. Kneissl S, Weidner S, Probst A. CT sialography in the dog – a cadaver study. Anatom Histol Embryol. 2011;40:397–401.
3. Cannon MS, Paglia D, Zwingenberger AL, Boroffka SA, Hollingsworth SR, Wisner ER. Clinical and diagnostic imaging findings in dogs with zygomatic sialadenitis: 11 cases (1990–2009). J Am Vet Med Assoc. 2011 ed. 2011;239:1211–1218.
4. Watanabe K, Miyawaki S, Kanayama M, et al. First case of salivary mucocele originating from the minor salivary gland of the soft palate in a dog. J Vet Med Sci. 2012;74:71–74.

1.8

Lymph nodes

Introduction

The lymph nodes of the head include the facial, parotid, mandibular, and lateral and medial retropharyngeal lymph nodes. These lymph nodes drain the head and oral cavity, and the mandibular and medial retropharyngeal lymph nodes are routinely evaluated on CT and MRI scans for signs of abnormality. Lymph from the rostral lymph nodes passes through the lymph node chain sequentially and may mix and cross to the contralateral side before reaching the medial retropharyngeal lymph nodes.[1]

The mandibular lymph node group consists of three to four lymph nodes surrounding the facial vein on the ventral neck and are, in aggregate, 10–25 mm in length (Figures 1.8.1, 1.8.3). The parotid lymph nodes (one or two nodes) are located lateral to the temporomandibular joint, medial to the parotid salivary gland and are detected infrequently on CT and MR images. The medial retropharyngeal nodes are located between the mandibular salivary gland and common carotid artery and are 30–70 mm in length in dogs and average $20.7 \times 4.2 \times 13.1$ mm in cats (Figures 1.8.2, 1.8.4).[2,3] The lateral retropharyngeal lymph nodes are less frequently seen in normal animals.

Lymph nodes are isoattenuating to muscle on CT and strongly contrast enhance. They are hypointense to fat and isointense to muscle on T1 images and hypointense to fat and hyperintense to muscle on T2 images. Lymph nodes are isointense to fat on contrast-enhanced T1 images.[4] The lymph nodes of the head are generally less than 5 mm in width. In the caudal part of the neck, the superficial cervical lymph nodes are located lateral to the serratus ventralis and scalenus muscles.

Lymphography has been used in experimental studies to determine lymph flow from regions of the head to sentinel lymph nodes using CT and MR.[5,6] This may be a useful technique to trace potential routes of metastasis in head and neck cancer.

Inflammatory disorders

Lymph nodes affected by regional disease, such as abscesses, myositis, otitis externa, and other inflammatory disorders, undergo hyperplasia as part of the immune response. On CT and MR images, the lymph nodes appear mildly to moderately enlarged. On CT, reactive lymph nodes are normally iso attenuating to hypoattenuating on unenhanced images and moderately to strongly contrast enhancing with a uniform or central pattern (Figure 1.8.5).[7,8] Lymph nodes are similarly mildly to moderately enlarged on MR images with homogeneous to heterogeneous contrast enhancement.[9] The parotid and lateral retropharyngeal lymph nodes may be visible when enlarged. In severe cases, lymph nodes may become abscessed with central hypoattenuating regions and peripheral contrast enhancement (Figure 1.8.6). Reactivity may also cause poor margination and soft-tissue stranding in surrounding fat.

Neoplasia

Neoplasia of the head and oral cavity may metastasize to the regional lymph nodes. The mandibular and medial retropharyngeal lymph nodes should be evaluated for enlargement, heterogeneity, and change of shape to detect metastatic disease (Figures 1.8.7, 1.8.8, 1.8.9).

Atlas of Small Animal CT and MRI, First Edition. Erik R. Wisner and Allison L. Zwingenberger.
© 2015 John Wiley & Sons, Inc. Published 2015 by John Wiley & Sons, Inc.

Metastatic deposits tend to lodge in the lymphatic sinuses of affected nodes, and when macrometastases are present, filling defects can be identified on contrast-enhanced images. On CT images, these need to be distinguished from fat within the lymph node hilus, which can mimic a parenchymal filling defect. On MR images of dogs with mast cell tumors, affected lymph nodes were larger and more heterogeneous on T2 and contrast-enhanced images than normal lymph nodes.[10] Lymph nodes in cats with metastatic disease from squamous cell carcinoma were not significantly larger than normal lymph nodes.[11] Therefore, affected lymph nodes cannot always be detected on CT and MR images, and fine-needle aspiration cytology is necessary for diagnosis.

Lymphoma may also affect the lymph nodes of the head and neck. Diffuse large-cell B-cell lymphoma results in marked enlargement of the retropharyngeal and/or mandibular lymph node groups. The contrast enhancement in these lymph nodes is uniform with a slightly foamy appearance. Small lymph nodes that are not normally identified, such as the parotid lymph node, may become visible with increased size (Figure 1.8.10). T-cell lymphoma may affect a single lymph node in the head with similar imaging characteristics.

Figure 1.8.1 Normal Mandibular Lymph Nodes (Canine)   CT

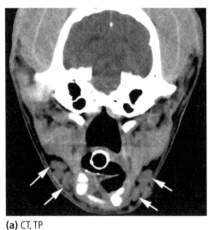

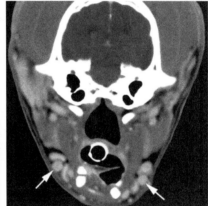

5y MC English Setter. Mandibular lymph node aggregates are seen ventrally (**a**: arrows). Normal mandibular nodes are variable in both size and number. Normal lymph nodes are highly and uniformly contrast enhancing (**b**). The facial vein (**b**: arrows) courses next to the lymph nodes and should be distinguished from them by viewing serial contiguous images (not shown).

(**a**) CT, TP   (**b**) CT+C, TP

Figure 1.8.2 Normal Mandibular Lymph Nodes (Canine)   MR

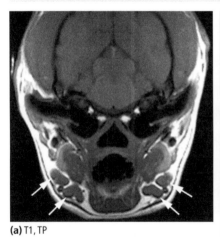

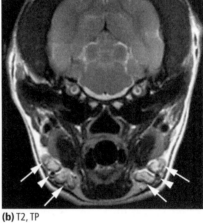

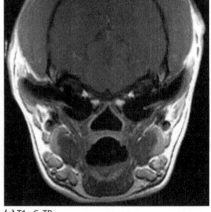

(**a**) T1, TP   (**b**) T2, TP   (**c**) T1+C, TP

1y M Shetland Sheepdog. Mandibular lymph node aggregates are seen ventrally, appearing isointense to muscle on T1 images (**a**: arrows) and hyperintense on T2 images (**b**: arrows). Normal mandibular lymph nodes are variable in both size and number. Normal lymph nodes are highly and uniformly contrast enhancing (**c**). The facial vein (**b**: arrowheads) courses next to the lymph nodes and can be distinguished from the lymph nodes on MR by the flow void artifact.

Figure 1.8.3 Normal Medial Retropharyngeal Lymph Nodes (Canine)   CT

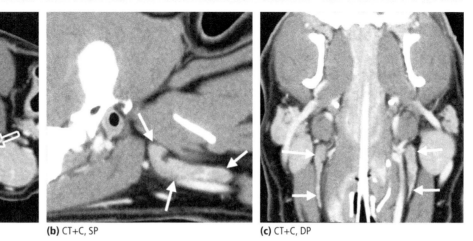

(a) CT+C, TP   **(b)** CT+C, SP   **(c)** CT+C, DP

8y MC Beagle with nasolacrimal duct obstruction. On transverse images (**a**), the medial retropharyngeal lymph nodes (**a**: arrow) appear as oval, isoattenuating structures medial to the mandibular salivary gland (**a**: M) and lateral to the carotid artery. A hypoattenuating linear structure representing fat in the hilus is visible in the rostral portion of the lymph node (**a**: open arrow). Sagittal and dorsal plane images (**b,c**) show the elongated, oval shape of the lymph node (**b,c**: arrows). Strong, mildly heterogeneous contrast enhancement is visible on all images.

Figure 1.8.4 Normal Medial Retropharyngeal Lymph Nodes   MR

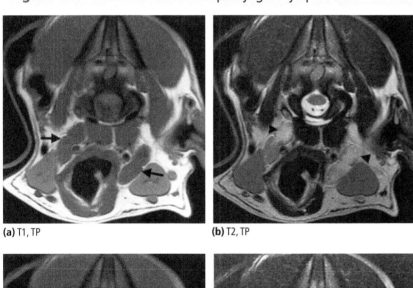

1y FS Border Collie with seizures. The medial retropharyngeal lymph nodes are larger and more heterogeneous than adult nodes in this young dog. There is isointense signal on T1 images (**a**: arrows) and heterogeneous hyperintense signal on T2 images (**b**: arrowheads). The signal is hyperintense with heterogeneity on T1 contrast-enhanced images (**c**) and uniform and isointense on FLAIR images (**d**).

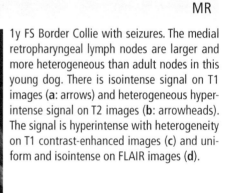

(a) T1, TP   **(b)** T2, TP

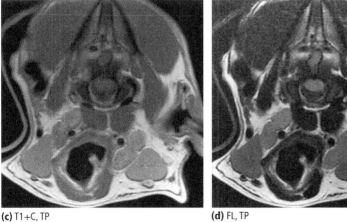

(c) T1+C, TP   **(d)** FL, TP

Figure 1.8.5 Reactive Lymphadenopathy (Canine)

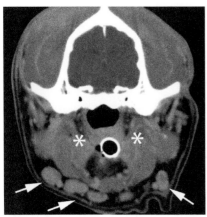

(a) CT+C, TP

12y MC Labrador Retriever with cervical necrotizing cellulitis and septicemia. The pharyngeal soft tissues are thickened and fascial margins are poorly delineated as a result of diffuse regional cellulitis (asterisks). Mandibular lymph nodes are variably enlarged and are somewhat more spherical than normal (arrows). Contrast enhancement is uniform. Low-density foci in some nodes are attributable to fat within the lymph node hilus. Microscopic evaluation of mandibular lymph nodes following euthanasia revealed marked diffuse plasmacytosis and lymphocytosis, consistent with node reactivity.

Figure 1.8.6 Pyogranulomatous Lymphadenopathy & Lymph Node Abscess (Canine)

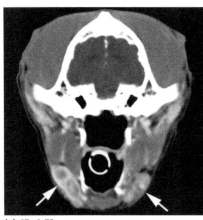   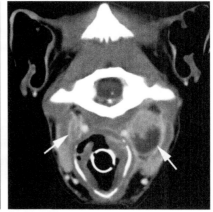

(a) CT+C, TP   **(b)** CT+C, TP

7y MC Weimaraner with recent-onset difficulty swallowing and pain on manipulation of the head and neck. Representative contrast-enhanced CT images are at the level of the mandibular (**a**) and retropharyngeal (**b**) lymph nodes. Mandibular lymph nodes are enlarged and have extensive nodal and ill-defined perinodal contrast enhancement (**a**: arrows). Similar findings are seen associated with the medial retropharyngeal lymph nodes (**b**: arrows). In addition, the left medial retropharyngeal lymph node is greatly enlarged and contains a fluid component ventrally consistent with frank abscessation. Aspiration cytology from the medial retropharyngeal lymph node confirmed suppurative inflammation and necrosis.

Figure 1.8.7 Regional Lymph Node Metastasis (Canine)

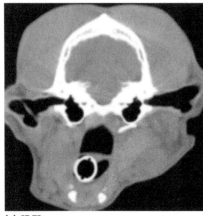   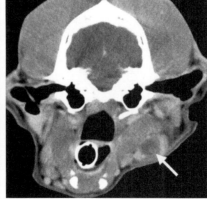

(a) CT, TP   **(b)** CT+C, TP

10mo F German Shepherd Dog with an undifferentiated oral sarcoma, present since 8 weeks of age. The left mandibular lymph node is markedly enlarged on the unenhanced image (**a**). Following contrast administration, there is peripheral enhancement of the mandibular lymph node with a central nonenhancing region representing metastasis (**b**: arrow). Fine-needle aspiration cytology confirmed nodal metastasis.

Figure 1.8.8   Regional Lymph Node Metastasis (Canine)   CT

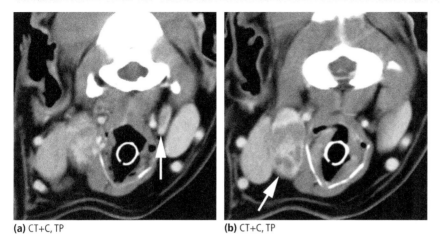

(a) CT+C, TP   **(b)** CT+C, TP

8y MC Labrador Retriever with previously excised right tonsillar squamous-cell carcinoma. Representative CT images are at the level of the medial retropharyngeal lymph nodes and are ordered from rostral to caudal. The left medial retropharyngeal lymph node (**a**: arrow) is normal in size, shape, and contrast enhancement. The central linear filling defect represents the normal fat-filled lymph node hilus. The right medial retropharyngeal lymph node is markedly enlarged and has irregular margins (**b**: arrow). Multiple parenchymal contrast filling defects are characteristic of lymph node metastatic deposits. Aspiration cytology of the right medial retropharyngeal node confirmed metastatic squamous cell carcinoma.

Figure 1.8.9   Regional Lymph Node Metastasis (Canine)   CT

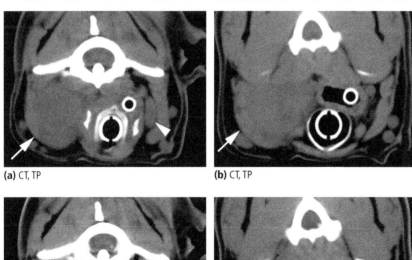

(a) CT, TP   **(b)** CT, TP

(c) CT+C, TP   **(d)** CT+C, TP

7y MC Springer Spaniel cross with previously excised right tonsillar squamous cell carcinoma. Representative unenhanced (**a,b**) and contrast-enhanced (**c,d**) images are at the level of the medial retropharyngeal lymph nodes and are ordered from rostral to caudal. The right medial retropharyngeal lymph node (**a–d**: arrow) is markedly enlarged and irregularly shaped, has mildly indistinct margins, and nonuniformly contrast enhances. Filling defects, most clearly seen in (**d**), are indicative of nodal metastasis. By comparison, the left medial retropharyngeal node (**a,c**: arrowhead) is normal in size, shape, and contrast enhancement characteristics. Aspiration cytology of the right medial retropharyngeal node confirmed metastasis of the tonsillar squamous cell carcinoma as well as moderate plasmacytic and lymphocytic reactivity.

Figure 1.8.10   Lymphoma (Canine)   CT

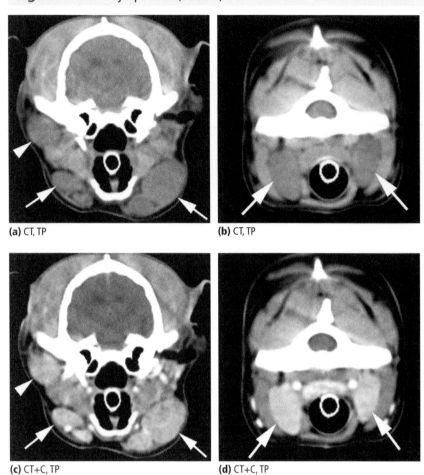

(a) CT, TP

(b) CT, TP

(c) CT+C, TP

(d) CT+C, TP

9y M Fox Terrier. CT was performed for lymphoma staging. Representative unenhanced (**a,b**) and contrast-enhanced (**c,d**) images are at the level of the mandibular (**a,c**: arrows) and medial retropharyngeal (**b,d**: arrows) lymph nodes. The lymph nodes are markedly enlarged but retain an oval shape and smooth contours. Contrast enhancement is characteristically uniform with a slightly foamy appearance. The right parotid lymph node, often not easily recognized on CT in normal dogs, is prominent in this patient (**a,c**: arrowheads). Mandibular lymph node biopsy documented T-cell lymphoma.

References

1. Belz GT, Heath TJ. Lymph pathways of the medial retropharyngeal lymph node in dogs. J Anat. 1995;186:517–526.
2. Kneissl S, Probst A. Comparison of computed tomographic images of normal cranial and upper cervical lymph nodes with corresponding E12 plastinated-embedded sections in the dog. Vet J. 2007;174:435–438.
3. Nemanic S, Nelson NC. Ultrasonography and noncontrast computed tomography of medial retropharyngeal lymph nodes in healthy cats. Am J Vet Res. 2012;73:1377–1385.
4. Kneissl S, Probst A. Magnetic resonance imaging features of presumed normal head and neck lymph nodes in dogs. Vet Radiol Ultrasound. 2006;47:538–541.
5. Wisner ER, Katzberg RW, Griffey SM, Drake CM, Haley PJ, Vessey AR. Indirect computed tomography lymphography using iodinated nanoparticles: time and dose response in normal canine lymph nodes. Acad Radiol. 1995;2:985–993.
6. Mayer MN, Kraft SL, Bucy DS, Waldner CL, Elliot KM, Wiebe S. Indirect magnetic resonance lymphography of the head and neck of dogs using Gadofluorine M and a conventional gadolinium contrast agent: A pilot study. Can Vet J. 2012;53:1085.
7. Reiter AM, Schwarz T. Computed tomographic appearance of masticatory myositis in dogs: 7 cases (1999–2006). J Am Vet Med Assoc. 2007;231:924–930.
8. Hardie EM, Linder KE, Pease AP. Aural cholesteatoma in twenty dogs. Vet Surg. 2008;37:763–770.
9. Cannon MS, Paglia D, Zwingenberger AL, Boroffka SA, Hollingsworth SR, Wisner ER. Clinical and diagnostic imaging findings in dogs with zygomatic sialadenitis: 11 cases (1990–2009). J Am Vet Med Assoc. 2011;239:1211–1218.
10. Pokorny E, Hecht S, Sura PA, et al. Magnetic resonance imaging of canine mast cell tumors. Vet Radiol Ultrasound. 2012;53:167–173.
11. Gendler A, Lewis JR, Reetz JA, Schwarz T. Computed tomographic features of oral squamous cell carcinoma in cats: 18 cases (2002–2008). J Am Vet Med Assoc. 2010;236:319–325.

1.9

Oral cavity

Introduction

CT is an excellent imaging modality to investigate the oral cavity because of the prevalence of high-attenuation structures. CT provides excellent contrast and spatial resolution within the oral cavity. The extent of lesion invasion has been shown to be improved with MR imaging compared to CT in a small number of cases.[1] Thin-collimation CT images in bone and soft-tissue algorithms are ideal for evaluation of both dense structures and soft tissues of the mouth. Contrast medium is employed when soft tissues are suspected of being abnormal, and 3D images may be useful for surgical planning. The normal structures of the tooth are visible as layers of differing attenuation on thinly collimated images (Figure 1.9.1).

Developmental disorders

Congenital anomalies of the teeth are occasionally seen on CT images. Supernumerary teeth appear as complete dental structures adjacent to the normal tooth at an abnormal angulation because of displacement (Figure 1.9.2). These have been reported to occur with high frequency in Greyhounds at the level of maxillary P1.[2] The maxillary second premolar and the maxillary first molar frequently have fused roots in cats and are occasionally absent.[3]

Brachycephalic syndrome has been assessed using CT, with increased thickness of the soft palate being the main associated finding in severely affected animals.[4]

Trauma

The oral cavity is often affected by trauma in dogs and cats, such as injury by other animals or vehicular trauma. Structures such as the mandible, maxilla, and teeth may be fractured or displaced by the traumatic event. CT is used to increase the diagnostic yield of such injuries compared to radiographs, especially for the purpose of surgical planning.[5] Multiplanar reformatted images and 3D images can add information to the transverse 2D images by displaying the affected structures in relationship to each other. Developing teeth may be damaged in traumatic events, which causes altered development of the tooth and occasionally of the adjacent structures (Figures 1.9.3, 1.9.4).

Inflammatory disorders

Dental disease can result in abscess formation around affected tooth roots and may be observed on CT images as contoured or rounded regions of alveolar bone osteolysis surrounding the tooth roots (Figure 1.9.5). Occasionally, the medial wall of the alveolus will be eroded by the infectious process and cause regional rhinitis (Figure 1.9.6). Dental disease may also progress to frank osteomyelitis, producing regional osteolysis and irregular to smooth periosteal reaction surrounding the affected bone (Figure 1.9.7).

Soft tissues of the oral cavity, such as the tongue, can be affected by inflammation and abscessation due to trauma or penetrating foreign bodies. On CT and MR images, abscessation appears as an encapsulated lesion

---

Atlas of Small Animal CT and MRI, First Edition. Erik R. Wisner and Allison L. Zwingenberger.
© 2015 John Wiley & Sons, Inc. Published 2015 by John Wiley & Sons, Inc.

with central fluid intensity or attenuation and circumferential contrast enhancement. Oral infection can spread to other neighboring tissues of the head, such as the pharynx and brain (Figure 1.9.8).

Odontogenic neoplasia

Odontogenic neoplasia is challenging to classify, and recent reports indicate that further study is required to accurately diagnose these tumors.[6] There are several categories that can be used to group the dental tumors, based on the WHO classification scheme.[7,8]

Cysts

Dentigerous cysts are rare and form from squamous epithelium surrounding tooth remnants (Figure 1.9.2). Radicular cysts are lined with squamous epithelium and occur adjacent to the tooth root (Figure 1.9.9). These lesions cause expansile bone destruction surrounding the tooth of origin and an associated fluid-attenuating mass.

Tumors of the periodontal ligament

Fibromatous epulis is a common lesion of soft-tissue proliferation in the oral cavity, some of which undergo mineralization (Figure 1.9.10). Fibromatous epulides and ossifying fibromatous epulides are subdivided histologically into focal fibrous hyperplasia, which is inflammatory and benign, and peripheral odontogenic fibroma, having dental epithelium and a neoplastic behavior.[9] CT imaging features of these lesions have not been described.

Tumors of odontogenic epithelium without odontogenic mesenchyme

Canine acanthomatous ameloblastoma (acanthomatous epulis) is an aggressive tumor that can affect the underlying bone of the maxilla or mandible. This lesion occurs mainly in medium to large-breed dogs of middle age, most frequently in the rostral mandible. The majority of dogs had osteolysis of the apical border of the alveolus with an expansile pattern (Figure 1.9.11).[10] The soft-tissue component of the mass shows intense, uniform contrast enhancement. Amyloid-producing odontogenic tumors are benign, mineralizing masses without encapsulation and are relatively rare (Figure 1.9.12).

Tumors of odontogenic epithelium with odontogenic mesenchyme

Ameloblastic fibroma is a rare tumor that has a benign behavior and does not recur after excision.[11] Imaging characteristics of a single case include an expansile soft-tissue mass with expansion of the surrounding mandible (Figure 1.9.13). Ameloblastic fibro-odontoma is similar to ameloblastic fibroma with the addition of enamel and dentin. Feline inductive odontogenic tumor is unique to cats and is rare, with no imaging features described.[12]

Complex odontoma is comprised of dental tissue that does not form recognizable tooth-like structures (Figure 1.9.14). These masses are disorganized and highly attenuating with expansion of the surrounding bone. Compound odontoma is a malformation of dental tissues that are not organized into a normal tooth structure.

Oral cavity neoplasia

The most common types of neoplasia encountered in the oral cavity are squamous cell carcinoma, melanoma, and fibrosarcoma. More rarely encountered tumors, such as liposarcoma, may arise as a soft-tissue attenuating mass in the fatty tissues of the tongue (Figure 1.9.15) with intense contrast enhancement.

Squamous cell carcinoma is an aggressive tumor affecting cats and dogs. In cats, it may cause a mass effect in the soft palate, sublingual or lingual region, lip, buccal mucosa, maxilla, or mandible.[13] When adjacent to bone, squamous cell carcinoma frequently results in osteolysis, with a primarily lytic appearance and peripheral expansion of mineralized tissue with heterogeneous contrast enhancement (Figure 1.9.16). When the soft palate is thickened in cats, adjacent otitis media or bulla effusion may occur concurrently (Figure 1.9.17).[14] Metastasis to the mandibular and retropharyngeal lymph nodes is common and results in lymph node enlargement with heterogeneous enhancement or well-defined parenchymal filling defects.

Oral melanoma may also affect the soft tissues of the mouth and can cause osteolysis of adjacent bone. The soft tissue portion of the mass is expansile and heterogeneously contrast enhancing (Figures 1.9.18, 1.9.19). Metastasis to local lymph nodes is also common, causing enlargement and peripheral contrast enhancement with central nonenhancing regions (Figure 1.9.20).

Fibrosarcoma is the third most common oral tumor in dogs and is generally locally destructive with osteolytic lesions (Figure 1.9.21). CT scanning can improve outcomes by defining the tumor margins for surgical planning.[15]

Primary bone tumors, including osteosarcoma, also occur in the oral cavity. They form destructive and productive lesions centered on the bone of origin and expand peripherally (Figure 1.9.22).

Figure 1.9.1 Normal Tooth Anatomy (Canine) — CT

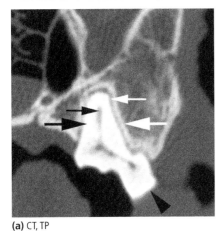

Normal left maxillary first molar. The central lucent pulp cavity (small black arrow) is surrounded by a dense cementum layer (large black arrow). The thin lucent layer of the periodontal ligament (small white arrow) is in turn surrounded by the dense lamina dura of the alveolus (large white arrow). The outer layers of the crown (black arrowhead) are composed of dense enamel and dentin.

(a) CT, TP

Figure 1.9.2 Supernumerary Teeth and Dentigerous Cyst (Canine) — CT

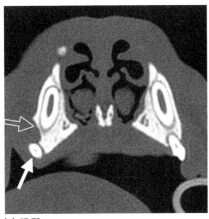 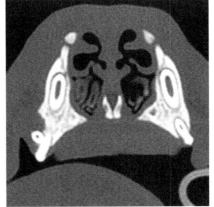

9mo F Boxer with dental abnormalities. There is a partially erupted supernumerary right maxillary P1 adjacent to the normal P1 tooth (a: solid arrow). A concave erosion of the mandibular surface indicates the presence of a dentigerous cyst associated with the tooth root (a: open arrow).

(a) CT, TP   (b) CT, TP

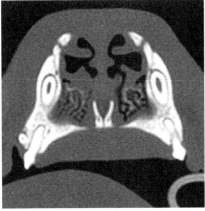 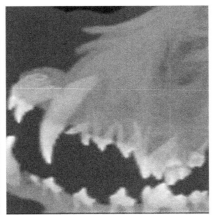

(c) CT, TP   (d) CT, SP, MIP

Figure 1.9.3 Trauma (Canine)

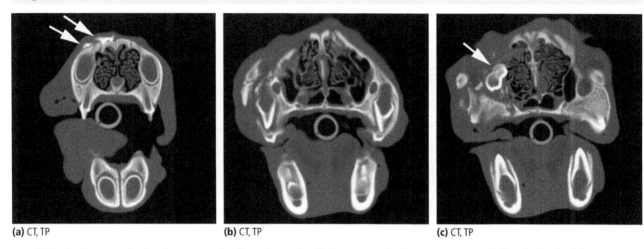

(a) CT, TP **(b)** CT, TP **(c)** CT, TP

4mo M Husky bitten on the face by another dog 2 weeks previously. Representative images were acquired at the level of the unerupted canine tooth roots (**a**), the third maxillary premolars (**b**), and the maxillary recess (**c**). A comminuted fracture of the right maxilla is present, associated with dental fractures and tooth fragment migration. Mineralized dental fragments are seen subcutaneously (**a**: arrows), and the unerupted left first molar is lodged within the left maxillary recess (**c**: arrow).

Figure 1.9.4 Trauma (Canine)

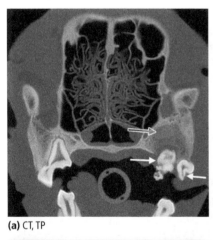 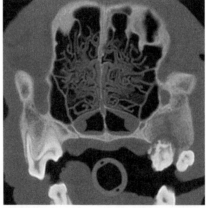

1y MC Great Dane with unilateral nasolacrimal duct obstruction and a history of being bitten in the face as a puppy. There is disorganization of the left maxillary fourth premolar with altered structure and two unequally sized fragments (**a**: solid arrows). The maxillary bone surrounding the tooth roots is expansile with a lytic component (**a**: open arrow). The frontal sinuses are asymmetric, and the zygomatic and maxillary bones are malformed. This has affected formation of the nasolacrimal duct on the left side, compared to the normal duct on the right (**d**: arrowheads).

(a) CT, TP **(b)** CT, TP

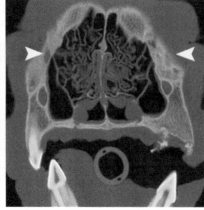

(c) CT, TP **(d)** CT, TP

Figure 1.9.5 Periapical Abscess (Canine)

CT

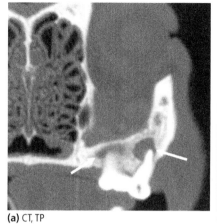 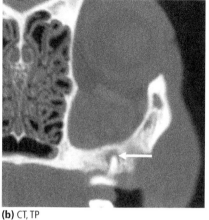

11y FS Australian Cattle Dog. The CT scan was performed for an unrelated disorder. Representative sequential images acquired at the level of the fourth maxillary premolar are shown and ordered from rostral to caudal. There is focal destruction of periapical alveolar bone of the rostral (**a**: arrows) and caudal (**b**: arrow) roots, and of the left maxillary fourth premolar. Imaging findings are characteristic of periapical abscess.

(a) CT, TP

(b) CT, TP

Figure 1.9.6 Abscess and Rhinitis (Feline)

CT

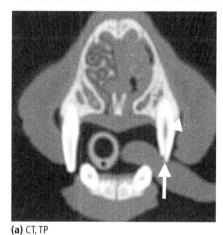 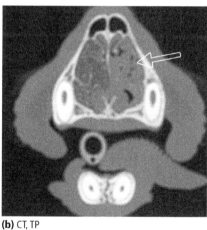 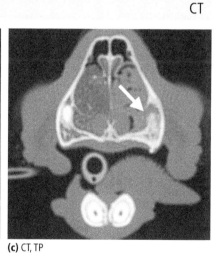

(a) CT, TP

(b) CT, TP

(c) CT, TP

The left maxillary canine tooth is fractured at the tip (**a**: arrow), and the pulp chamber is widened compared to the right side (**a**: arrowhead). The adjacent nasal cavity is filled with soft-tissue opacity material (**b**: open arrow). The alveolus is lytic and open to the adjacent nasal cavity (**c**: arrow).

Figure 1.9.7 Mandibular Osteomyelitis and Osteonecrosis (Canine)

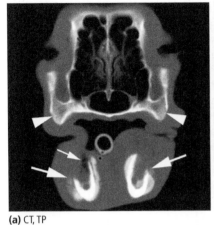

(a) CT, TP

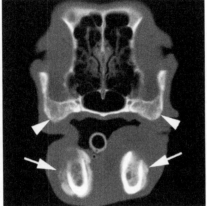

(b) CT, TP

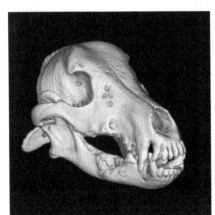

(c) CT, 3D, OBL

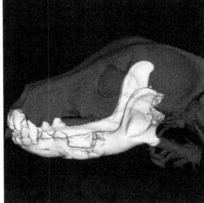

(d) CT, 3D, LLAT

4y M Scottish Terrier with history of suppurative, ulcerative stomatitis. The dog has had numerous tooth extractions performed previously. The molars and caudal premolars are missing. Representative sequential images acquired at the level of the first maxillary molar are shown and ordered from rostral to caudal (**a**,**b**). The alveolar processes in the maxilla are blunted, and the alveolar cavities have filled with organized bone (**a**,**b**: arrowheads). Large post-extraction defects remain in the mandible, accompanied by alveolar bone destruction and adjacent reactive periosteal production (**a**,**b**: large arrows). A focal gas collection is also evident within the right mandibular alveolar cavity (**a**: small arrow). The 3D renderings reveal the full extent of mandibular periodontal osteolysis and adjacent reactive periosteal remodeling.

Figure 1.9.8 Sublingual Abscess with Extension to Pharynx and Meninges (Canine)   MR

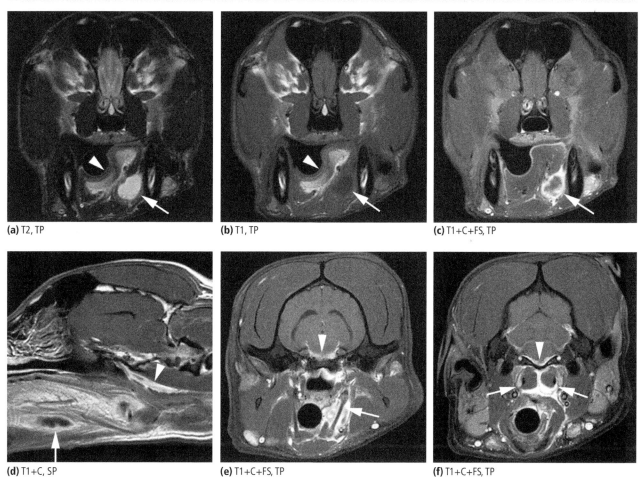

(a) T2, TP   **(b)** T1, TP   **(c)** T1+C+FS, TP

(d) T1+C, SP   **(e)** T1+C+FS, TP   **(f)** T1+C+FS, TP

6y MC Labrador Retriever with lethargy and difficulty prehending food. Images **a–c** are at the same anatomic level near the base of the tongue. Images **e** and **f** are further caudal and are ordered from rostral to caudal. A fluid-filled, cavitary sublingual mass is seen that is T1 hypointense, T2 hyperintense, and peripherally contrast enhancing (**a–d**: arrow). The tongue is otherwise normal in appearance, having a T1 and T2 hyperintense center of intrinsic musculature and adipose tissue surrounded by a low-intensity peripheral layer (**a,b**: arrowhead). Diffuse contrast enhancement is present surrounding the oropharynx, the left epihyoid bone (**e**: arrow), and the longus capitus muscles (**f**: arrows). Marked meningeal enhancement is also evident ventral to the brainstem (**d–f**: arrowhead), indicating intracranial extension, presumably through one of the foramina of the skull base. Lingual biopsy revealed severe neutrophilic and necrotizing glossitis with abscessation, likely due to a migrating plant awn foreign body. Cerebrospinal fluid cytology revealed marked suppurative inflammation.

Figure 1.9.9 Radicular Cyst (Canine)   CT

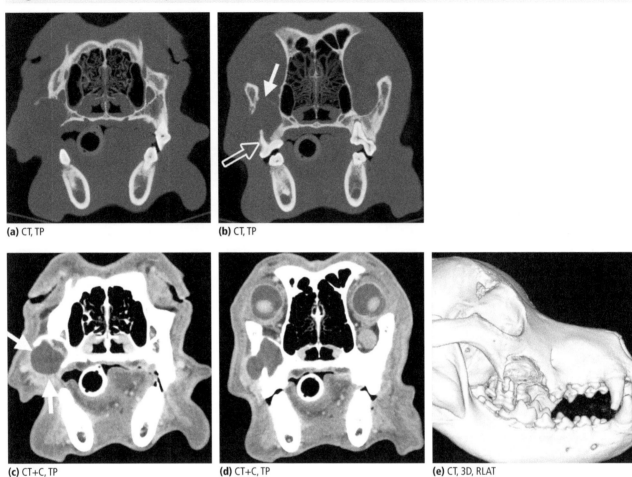

(a) CT, TP   (b) CT, TP

(c) CT+C, TP   (d) CT+C, TP   (e) CT, 3D, RLAT

10y MC Labrador Retriever with a facial mass. The right maxillary fourth premolar was previously removed on suspicion of tooth root abscess. Unenhanced (**a,b**) and comparable contrast-enhanced transverse images (**c,d**) are ordered from rostral to caudal. On bone windowed images, a cystic expansile lesion is present in the right maxilla (**b**: solid arrow), extending from the third premolar to the right mandibular first molar tooth roots (**b**: open arrow) and into the orbit. There is peripheral enhancement of the lesion on contrast-enhanced images (**c**: arrows), and fluid-attenuating material is present centrally. The circular-shaped mandibular lysis can be seen on the 3D image (**e**). The fourth maxillary premolar is absent. Exisional biopsy confirmed the mass to be a radicular cyst.

Figure 1.9.10 Ossifying Fibromatous Epulis (Canine)   CT

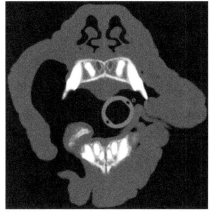

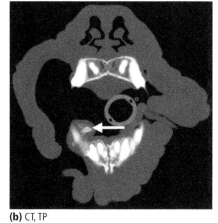

4y MC Great Dane with rapidly enlarging oral mass. There is a sessile, mineralized mass at the rostral aspect of the right mandibular canine tooth (**b**: arrow). On enhanced images, the mass is uniformly and intensely contrast enhancing (**d**). Excisional biopsy confirmed ossifying fibromatous epulis.

(a) CT, TP

(b) CT, TP

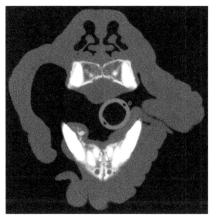

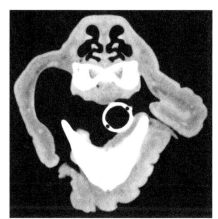

(c) CT, TP

(d) CT+C, TP

Figure 1.9.11   Acanthomatous Ameloblastoma (Canine)   CT

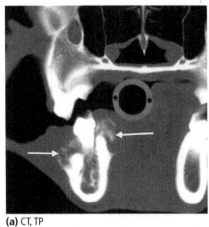

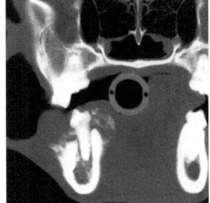

(a) CT, TP   **(b)** CT, TP

10y MC Border Collie presenting with an oral mass. There is a combined destructive and productive osseous lesion involving the body of the right mandible surrounding the first and second molars (**a**: arrows). Intensely contrast-enhancing lobular soft tissue is also present dorsal to the osseous component of the mass (**c,d**). Excisional biopsy confirmed the mass to be an acanthomatous ameloblastoma.

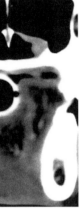

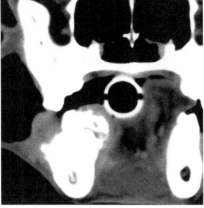

(c) CT+C, TP   **(d)** CT+C, TP

Figure 1.9.12 Amyloid Producing Odontogenic Tumor (Canine)   CT

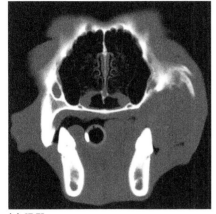

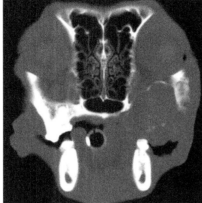

(a) CT, TP

(b) CT, TP

8y M Terrier mix with orbital swelling. There is an expansile productive and destructive bone lesion involving the rostral aspect of the left zygomatic arch and left caudal maxilla (**a**,**b**). After intravenous administration of iodinated contrast medium, the soft-tissue component of the lesion has a multicameral appearance with hypoattenuating loculated regions and good enhancement of interspersed soft tissues and septae (**c**: arrows). Contrast enhancement demonstrates extension of the mass proximally from the level of the second premolars caudally into the ventral orbit (**d**). The left fourth maxillary premolar and left maxillary molars are not present. Biopsy confirmed the mass to be an amyloid-producing odontogenic tumor.

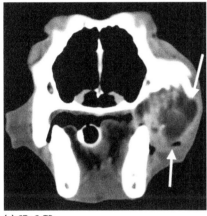

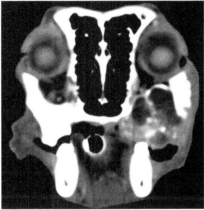

(c) CT+C, TP

(d) CT+C, TP

Figure 1.9.13   Ameloblastic Fibroma (Canine)   CT

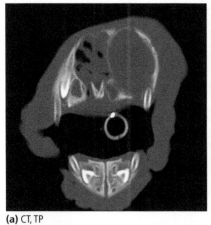

(a) CT, TP

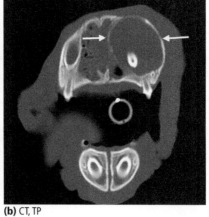

(b) CT, TP

4mo FS Labrador Retriever with facial swelling. Images are ordered from rostral to caudal (**a–c**). The left maxillary canine (**c**: open arrow) is displaced into the left nasal cavity and is surrounded by fluid-attenuating material. The maxilla surrounding the tooth root is expanded and displaced into the nasal cavity with deviation of the nasal septum (**b,c**: arrows). The mass was surgically excised along with the canine tooth and was confirmed to be an ameloblastic fibroma (**d**).

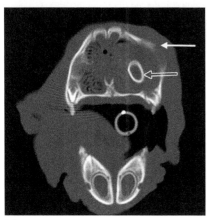

(c) CT, TP

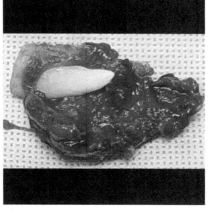

(d) GP

Figure 1.9.14   Compound Odontoma (Canine)   CT

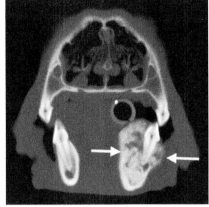

(a) CT, TP

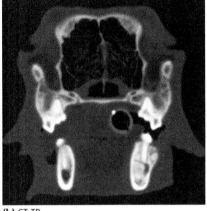

(b) CT, TP

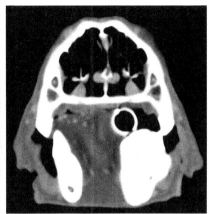

(c) CT+C, TP

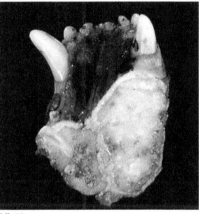

(d) GP

3y MC Golden Retriever with an oral mass. There is an expansile, primarily productive mass in the left mandible on the lingual and buccal sides of the teeth (a: arrows). There is cortical lysis, but the margin of the mass is smooth and regular. No soft-tissue component is present on contrast-enhanced images (c). A diagnosis of compound odontoma was confirmed with excisional biopsy (d).

Figure 1.9.15   Lingual Liposarcoma (Canine)   CT

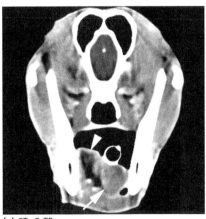

(a) CT+C, TP

12y MC Fox Terrier with a left-sided lingual mass. A well-circumscribed, moderately contrast-enhancing mass (arrow) arises from the left side of the tongue (arrowhead) and is displaced ventrally by the overlying endotracheal catheter. The tongue is otherwise normal in appearance, having a relatively low-density center of intrinsic musculature and adipose tissue surrounded by a soft-tissue dense peripheral layer. Biopsy of the mass revealed it to be a moderately well-differentiated liposarcoma.

Figure 1.9.16 Squamous Cell Carcinoma (Canine) CT

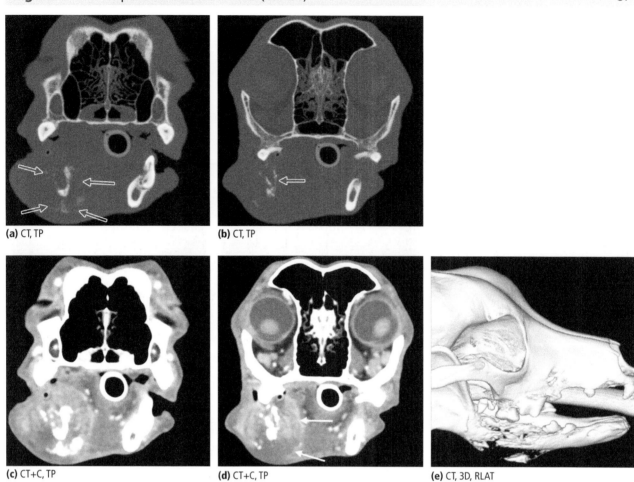

(a) CT, TP

(b) CT, TP

(c) CT+C, TP

(d) CT+C, TP

(e) CT, 3D, RLAT

8y FS Border Collie with possible infected tooth. There is marked osteolysis and irregular bone production surrounding the caudal left mandible (**a,b**: open arrows). Multiple teeth are absent. There is a large soft-tissue mass associated with the osseous lesion, which is intensely, heterogeneously contrast enhancing (**d**: arrows). The 3D image shows the extent of the osseous component of mandibular lesion (**e**). Biopsy confirmed squamous cell carcinoma.

Figure 1.9.17 Squamous Cell Carcinoma with Metastasis (Feline) CT

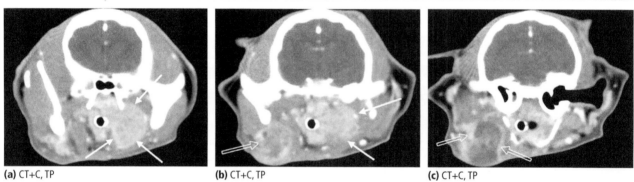

(a) CT+C, TP

(b) CT+C, TP

(c) CT+C, TP

9y FS Domestic Shorthair with a neck mass. On contrast-enhanced images of the head, there is a large, intensely enhancing mass in the left soft palate and tonsillar region (**a,b**: arrows). The contralateral mandibular lymph node is markedly enlarged and heterogeneously contrast enhancing (**b,c**: open arrows). Fluid is visible in the tympanic bulla secondary to the soft palate thickening (**c**). Postmortem examination confirmed primary squamous cell carcinoma with regional lymph node metastasis.

Figure 1.9.18 Melanotic Melanoma (Canine)   CT

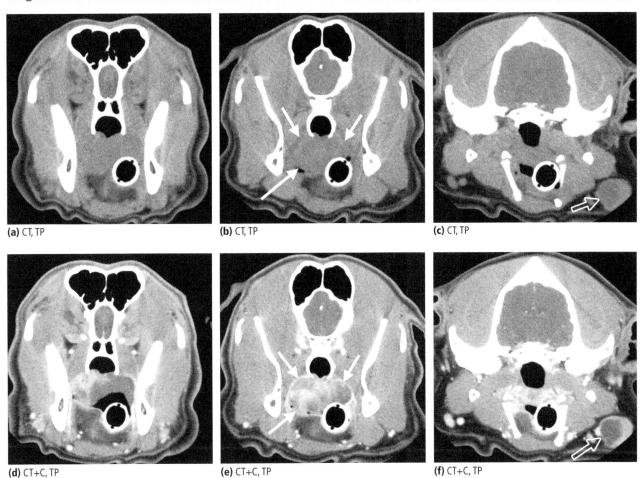

(a) CT, TP

(b) CT, TP

(c) CT, TP

(d) CT+C, TP

(e) CT+C, TP

(f) CT+C, TP

10y MC Labrador Retriever with difficulty eating. There is a mass in the region of the soft palate and tonsils that is multilobular in shape (**b**: arrows). On contrast-enhanced images, the mass is peripherally and heterogeneously enhancing (**e**: arrows). The left mandibular lymph node is enlarged with a central, hypoattenuating, nonenhancing region (**c,f**: open arrow) and peripheral contrast enhancement. Primary melanotic melanoma with regional lymph node metastasis was confirmed by excisional biopsy.

Figure 1.9.19   Amelanotic Melanoma (Canine)   CT

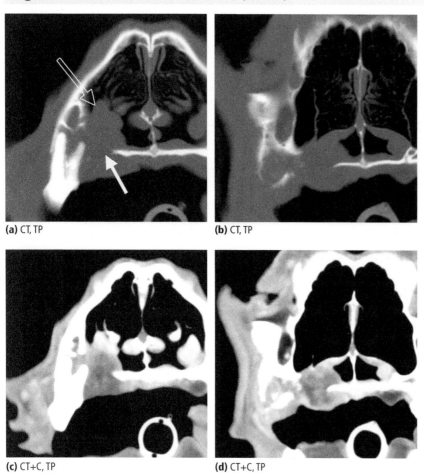

(a) CT, TP

(b) CT, TP

(c) CT+C, TP

(d) CT+C, TP

10y MC Labrador Retriever with a history of an ulcerated maxillary oral mass. There is lysis of the hard palate (**a**: arrow) and the medial aspect of the maxilla surrounding the right fourth maxillary premolar tooth. The mass extends into the right nasal cavity (**a**: open arrow) and the oral cavity. On contrast-enhanced images, the mass is centrally poorly enhancing and peripherally strongly enhancing. A diagnosis of amelanotic melanoma was confirmed with excisional biopsy.

Figure 1.9.20   Lingual Melanoma with Regional Metastasis (Canine)   CT

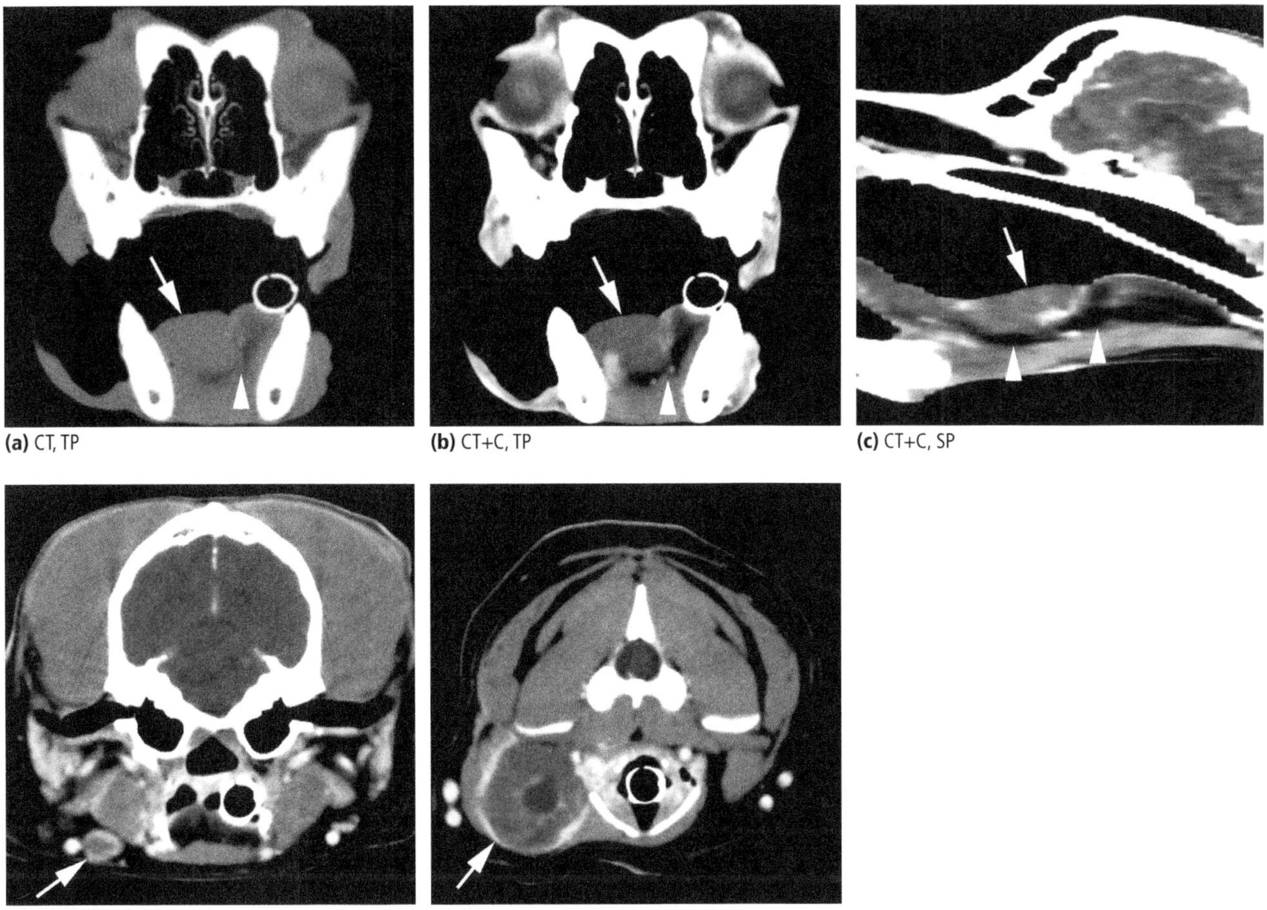

(a) CT, TP

(b) CT+C, TP

(c) CT+C, SP

(d) CT+C, TP

(e) CT+C, TP

9y FS Terrier cross with a tongue mass. Images **a** and **b** are at the same anatomic level. Images **d** and **e** are further caudal and are ordered from rostral to caudal. A smoothly margined ovoid lingual mass (**a–c**: arrow) compresses and displaces adjacent normal tongue parenchyma (**a–c**: arrowheads). The right mandibular (**d**: arrow) and medial retropharyngeal (**e**: arrow) lymph nodes are markedly enlarged, and contrast enhancement is nonuniform and reduced centrally, consistent with regional metastasis. Lingual biopsy revealed melanoma, and lymph node aspirates confirmed regional metastasis.

Figure 1.9.21   Maxillary Fibrosarcoma (Canine)   CT

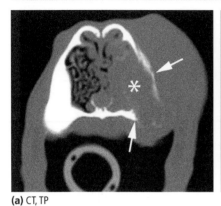

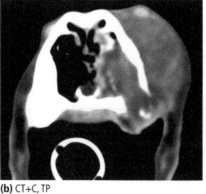

(a) CT, TP   **(b)** CT+C, TP

11y Standard Poodle with enlarging left maxillary mass. Representative CT images are at the level of the maxillary canine teeth. There is a left-sided soft-tissue mass with an intranasal component, the latter of which has resulted in adjacent ectoturbinate destruction (**a**: asterisk). The left maxillary canine tooth is missing, and osteolysis of the alveolus and lateral maxillary cortex is evident (**a**: arrows). The mass moderately and heterogeneously contrast enhances (**b**). Biopsy revealed fibrosarcoma.

Figure 1.9.22   Maxillary Osteosarcoma (Canine)   CT

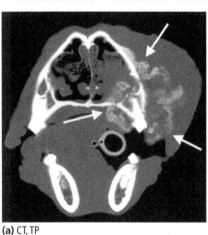

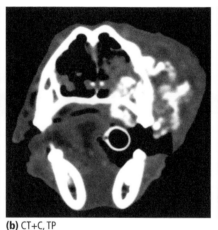

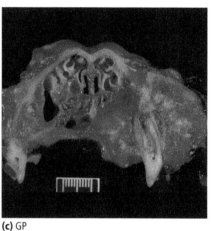

(a) CT, TP   **(b)** CT+C, TP   **(c)** GP

12y MC Miniature Schnauzer with left-sided facial swelling and an infraorbital draining tract. There is a mixed productive and destructive mass originating from the left maxilla (**a**: arrows). The mass extends into the nasal cavity, obliterating the ventral nasal turbinates. The mass is mildly enhancing on contrast-enhanced images. Biopsy confirmed osteosarcoma.

References

1. Kafka UCM, Carstens A, Steenkamp G, Symington H. Diagnostic value of magnetic resonance imaging and computed tomography for oral masses in dogs. J S Afr Vet Assoc. 2004;75:163–168.

2. Dole RS, Spurgeon TL. Frequency of supernumerary teeth in a dolichocephalic canine breed, the greyhound. Am J Vet Res. 1998;59:16–17.

3. Verstraete FJ, Terpak CH. Anatomical variations in the dentition of the domestic cat. J Vet Dent. 1997;14:137–140.

4. Grand J-GR, Bureau S. Structural characteristics of the soft palate and meatus nasopharyngeus in brachycephalic and non-brachycephalic dogs analysed by CT. J Small Anim Pract. 2011;52:232–239.

5. Bar-Am Y, Pollard RE, Kass PH, Verstraete FJM. The diagnostic yield of conventional radiographs and computed tomography in dogs and cats with maxillofacial trauma. Vet Surg. 2008;37:294–299.

6. Boehm B, Breuer W, Hermanns W. [Odontogenic tumours in the dog and cat]. Tierarztl Prax K H. 2011;39:305–312.

7. Head KW, Cullen JM, Dubielzig RR, et al. Histological classification of tumors of the alimentary system of domestic animals [Internet]. Head KW, Cullen JM, Dubielzig RR (eds): Washington, D.C.: WHO, Armed Forces Institute of Pathology; 2007. Available from: http://www.ncbi.nlm.nih.gov/books/NBK9565/#ch8.r71

8. Baba AI, Câtoi C, editors. Tumors of the alimentary system. Comparative Oncology [Internet]. Bucharest: The Publishing

House of the Romanian Academy; 2007. Available from: http://www.ncbi.nlm.nih.gov/books/NBK9565/

9. Fiani N, Verstraete FJM, Kass PH, Cox DP. Clinicopathologic characterization of odontogenic tumors and focal fibrous hyperplasia in dogs: 152 cases (1995–2005). J Am Vet Med Assoc. 2011; 238:495–500.

10. Schmidt A, Kessler M, Tassani-Prell M. [Computed tomographic characteristics of canine acanthomatous ameloblastoma – a retrospective study in 52 dogs]. Tierarztl Prax K H. 2012;40:155–160.

11. Miles CR, Bell CM, Pinkerton ME, Soukup JW. Maxillary ameloblastic fibroma in a dog. Vet Pathol. 2011;48:823–826.

12. Gardner DG, Dubielzig RR. Feline inductive odontogenic tumor (inductive fibroameloblastoma) – a tumor unique to cats. J Oral Pathol Med. 1995;24:185–190.

13. Gendler A, Lewis JR, Reetz JA, Schwarz T. Computed tomographic features of oral squamous cell carcinoma in cats: 18 cases (2002–2008). J Am Vet Med Assoc. 2010;236:319–325.

14. Woodbridge NT, Baines EA, Baines SJ. Otitis media in five cats associated with soft palate abnormalities. Vet Rec. 2012;171:124.

15. Frazier SA, Johns SM, Ortega J, et al. Outcome in dogs with surgically resected oral fibrosarcoma (1997–2008). Vet Comp Oncol. 2012;10:33–43.

1.10

Larynx, pharynx, and neck

Introduction

The soft tissues of the larynx, pharynx, and neck are investigated using both CT and MR imaging.[1] Both modalities have excellent sensitivity for evaluation of inflammatory and neoplastic lesions when contrast medium is used. CT has lower inherent soft-tissue contrast than MR, and sensitivity and interpretation confidence can be increased when the animal is scanned in the open-mouth position, using air as additional contrast.[2]

Developmental disorders

A laryngeal cyst causing upper airway obstruction has been reported in a dog. CT imaging characteristics were a fluid-attenuating mass with a thin rim of contrast enhancement that did not communicate with the laryngeal lumen.[3]

Trauma

Trauma due to bite wounds or other direct insult to the neck and laryngeal region may cause disruption of the hyoid apparatus at its attachment to the skull or its intrinsic joints. Symmetry of the hyoid apparatus is helpful in determining whether disruption has occurred, both on transverse and 3D images (Figures 1.10.1, 1.10.2). Trauma may also result in hematoma formation that causes a mass effect with characteristics of blood or proteinaceous fluid on MR images (Figure 1.10.3).

Inflammatory disorders

Nasopharyngeal polyps

Nasopharyngeal polyps arise from the tympanic bulla or auditory tube, are inflammatory in origin, and are most often seen in cats. On CT images, they have poorly defined margins and are hypoattenuating on unenhanced images. Following contrast administration, masses remain centrally hypoattenuating with an intensely contrast-enhancing margin (Figure 1.10.4). In most cats, a stalk connecting the polyp to the widened auditory tube can be seen.[4] Ipsilateral or bilateral otitis media is usually present as soft-tissue or fluid attenuating material within the bulla, which may be thickened, expanded, and occasionally lytic. Imaging features of otitis media are described in Chapter 1.2.

Foreign bodies

Inflammation of the pharyngeal region often occurs secondary to foreign bodies within the nasopharynx or penetrating foreign bodies from the skin or pharynx that localize in the neck or retropharyngeal region. Unless they are of sufficient size, plant material foreign bodies are often not directly visualized on CT or MR images. Larger foreign bodies, such as sticks, may have a definite shape and exhibit internal architecture.[5,6] On MR images, the foreign bodies may be isointense on T1 and hypointense or hyperintense on T2 images. On CT images, the foreign material may be hyperattenuating. There is surrounding tissue and edema that is

Atlas of Small Animal CT and MRI, First Edition. Erik R. Wisner and Allison L. Zwingenberger.
© 2015 John Wiley & Sons, Inc. Published 2015 by John Wiley & Sons, Inc.

hypoattenuating on CT or hyperintense on T2 on MR, with strong peripheral contrast enhancement (Figures 1.10.5, 1.10.6).[7] Fistulography may be considered to define any draining tracts and to attempt to outline the foreign body.

Neoplasia

Ectopic thyroid neoplasia has been recognized to occur in the laryngeal region, with possible invasion of the laryngeal lumen or ventral musculature.[8] Masses are oval or bilobed and are centered on the basihyoid bone with osteolysis (Figure 1.10.7), and normal thyroid glands are present. Metastasis to local lymph nodes or the lungs may occur. Primary thyroid neoplasia is discussed in Chapter 1.11.

The musculature of the larynx may also give rise to neoplasia, such as rhabdomyoma or rhabdomyosarcoma (Figure 1.10.8).[9] Neuroendocrine tumors, such as carotid body tumors, also occur in the region of the larynx and may be mistaken for thyroid carcinoma (Figure 1.10.9).[10]

The larynx, tonsils, and pharynx may be affected by oral tumors, such as fibrosarcoma or squamous cell carcinoma involving the soft palate or tongue (see Chapter 1.9, Figure 1.9.17 and Figure 1.10.10).[11] Round cell neoplasia may also arise in these soft tissues and cause nasopharyngeal obstruction and local lymph node enlargement (Figures 1.10.11, 1.10.12).

Idiopathic and other disorders

Upper airway obstruction may occur secondary to laryngeal paralysis or laryngeal collapse. On CT images, the imaging findings of laryngeal paralysis include failure to abduct the arytenoid cartilages, air-filled lateral ventricles, and a narrowed rima glottis. Everted laryngeal saccules, collapse of the cuneiform and corniculate processes, and narrowed rima glottis were seen in sedated dogs with laryngeal collapse.[12] These features may be difficult to assess in animals that are intubated under general anesthesia.

Figure 1.10.1 Hyoid Trauma (Canine)  CT

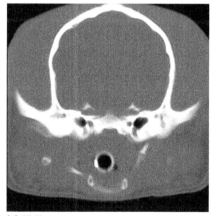 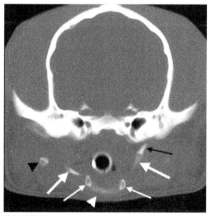

(a) CT, TP   **(b)** CT, TP

5y FS Jack Russell Terrier with a 3-month history of coughing, gagging, and nasal discharge. Images **a** and **b** are the same image with and without annotation. These are 5 mm collimated transverse images that include the basihyoid bone (**b**: arrowhead), caudal ends of the ceratohyoid bones (**b**: small arrows), portions of the epihyoid bones (**b**: large arrows), and the distal end of the left stylohyoid bone (**b**: black arrow). The caudal end of the angular process of the right mandible is also seen (**b**: black arrowhead). The right epihyoid bone is displaced laterally, indicative of trauma.

Figure 1.10.2   Hyoid Trauma (Feline)   CT

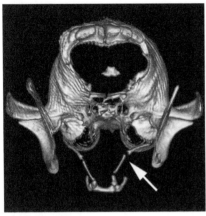

9y MC Domestic Shorthair with acute head and neck trauma of unknown cause. The cat also had difficulty swallowing on physical examination. There is asymmetry of the hyoid apparatus with medial displacement of the left epihyoid and stylohyoid bones (arrow). Swallowing function improved following 3 days of supportive care.

(a) CT, 3D, CAUD

Figure 1.10.3   Hematoma (Canine)   MR

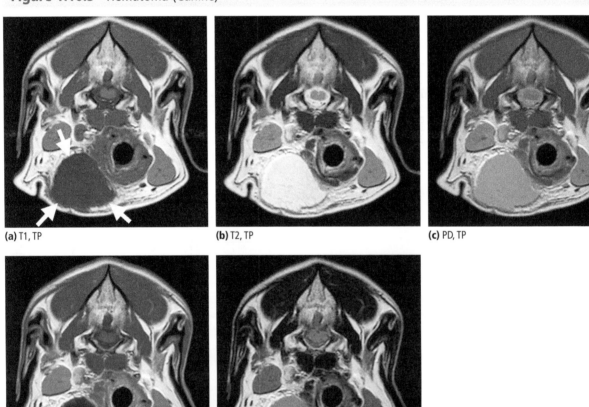

(a) T1, TP   **(b)** T2, TP   **(c)** PD, TP

(d) T1+C, TP   **(e)** FL, TP

8y MC Golden Retriever. Previous endoscopy (1 week prior) with laryngeal biopsy resulted in a hematoma. A large, well-circumscribed mass that is hypointense to muscle on T1 sequences and hyperintense to muscle on T2, PD, and FLAIR sequences is present in the right cranioventral cervical region adjacent to the larynx (**a**: arrows). There is a thin, peripheral rim of enhancement on contrast-enhanced images (**d**: arrowhead). The mass partially suppresses on the FLAIR image (**e**).

Figure 1.10.4 Nasopharyngeal Polyp (Feline)   CT

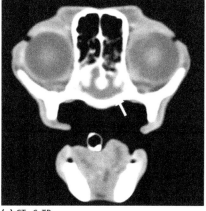

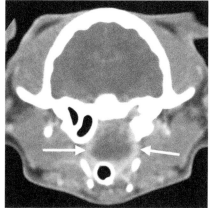

4y FS Domestic Shorthair with upper respiratory noise and open-mouth breathing. There is soft-tissue attenuating material filling the nasopharynx and choana on transverse images (**a**,**b**: arrows). The mass is well circumscribed and peripherally contrast enhancing (**c**: arrowhead). The left tympanic bulla is filled with a combination of mineral and soft-tissue attenuating material (**d**: open arrow).

(a) CT+C, TP

(b) CT+C, TP

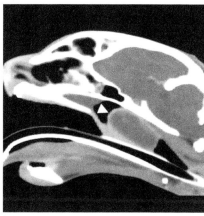

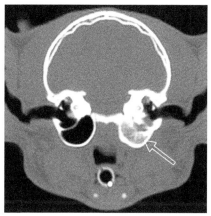

(c) CT+C, SP

(d) CT, TP

Figure 1.10.5   Retropharyngeal Cellulitis (Canine)   CT

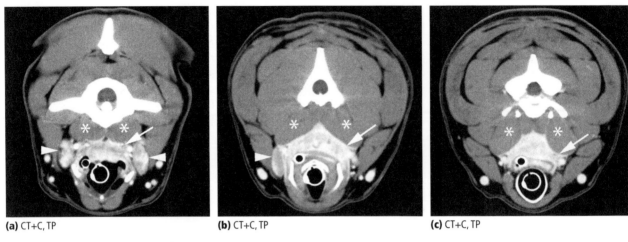

(a) CT+C, TP   **(b)** CT+C, TP   **(c)** CT+C, TP

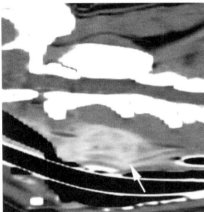

(d) CT+C, SP

4y FS Pit Bull Terrier with progressive dyspnea. Representative contrast-enhanced images are at the cranial cervical level and are ordered from cranial to caudal. A contrast-enhancing perilaryngeal and retropharyngeal mass (**a–d**: arrow) is evident, bounded by the longus capitus muscles dorsally (**a–c**: asterisks). The medial retropharyngeal lymph nodes (**a**,**b**: arrowheads) are moderately enlarged and have a nonuniform contrast-enhancement pattern. Biopsy of retropharyngeal tissue confirmed chronic neutrophilic and plasmacytic cellulitis with extensive fibrosis.

Figure 1.10.6   Pyogranulomatous Inflammation (Canine)   CT

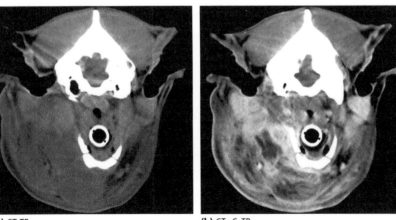

2y F German Shepherd with ventral cervical swelling. Marked, diffuse ventral cervical swelling is present, associated with loss of fascial plane definition (**a**) and heterogeneous and ill-defined contrast enhancement (**b**). Biopsy revealed pyogranulomatous cellulitis and myositis, likely due to migrating plant awn foreign body.

(a) CT, TP   **(b)** CT+C, TP

Figure 1.10.7 Hyoid Neoplasia (Canine) CT

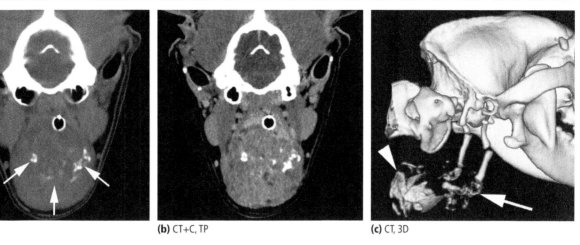

(a) CT, TP   **(b)** CT+C, TP   **(c)** CT, 3D

11y FS Labrador Retriever with a diagnosed thyroid carcinoma. A large ventral mass incorporates the hyoid apparatus, obliterating the basihyoid, thyrohyoid, and ceratohyoid bones (**a,c**). Remnants of these hyoid components are present within the mass (**a,c**: arrows). The mass moderately and heterogeneously contrast enhances (**b**). The thyroid and cricoid cartilages are uninvolved and appear intact (**c**: arrowhead). Aspiration cytology confirmed ectopic thyroid carcinoma.

Figure 1.10.8 Laryngeal Rhabdomyosarcoma (Canine) CT

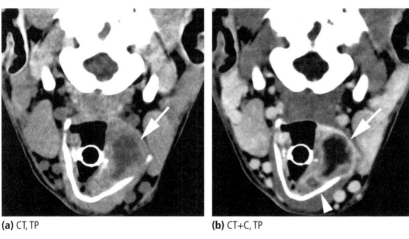

(a) CT, TP   **(b)** CT+C, TP

11y MC English Setter with a left-sided laryngeal mass. Images **a** and **b** are at the level of the larynx. Images **c** and **d** are at the level of the mandibular and medial retropharyngeal lymph nodes, respectively. There is a centrally hypoattenuating left laryngeal mass (**a,b**: arrow) that peripherally contrast enhances and causes rotational displacement of the cranial border thyroid cartilage (**b**: arrowhead). Ipsilateral mandibular (**c**: arrows) and medial retropharyngeal (**d**: arrow) lymph nodes appear normal. Biopsy revealed granular cell rhabdomyosarcoma. The dog was alive, and there was no evidence of mass recurrence 4 years following mass excision and permanent tracheostomy.

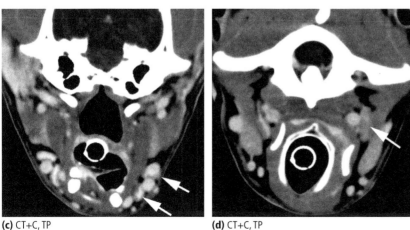

(c) CT+C, TP   **(d)** CT+C, TP

Figure 1.10.9 Neuroendocrine Tumor (Canine)

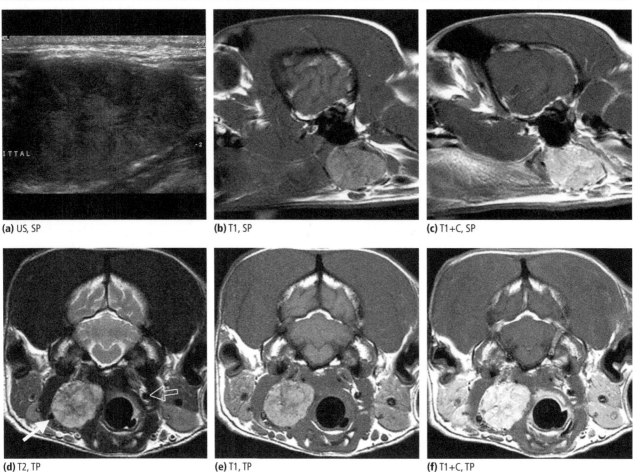

(a) US, SP

(b) T1, SP

(c) T1+C, SP

(d) T2, TP

(e) T1, TP

(f) T1+C, TP

14y FS Golden Retriever cross with a right ventral cervical mass. Images **d–f** are at the level of the larynx. An irregularly margined, ovoid mass is seen adjacent to the larynx in the region of the right retropharyngeal lymph node. The mass has a solid but heterogeneous center (**a–f**) and markedly contrast enhances (**c,f**). The right carotid artery is displaced laterally (**d**: arrow) compared to the left carotid artery (**d**: open arrow). Both thyroid lobes were identified and appeared normal (not shown). Biopsy revealed the mass to be a neuroendocrine tumor of indeterminate origin.

Figure 1.10.10 Neuroendocrine Tumor (Feline)

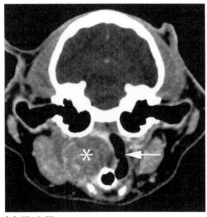

10y FS Siamese with intermittent dyspnea of 1-month duration. A large, predominantly right-sided contrast-enhancing mass (**a,b**: asterisk) arises from the right laryngeal wall, displacing and partially occluding the intralaryngeal ostium and caudal nasopharynx (**a**: arrow). Aspiration cytology revealed this mass to be a malignant neuroendocrine tumor.

(a) CT+C, TP

(b) CT+C, SP

Figure 1.10.11 Nasopharyngeal Undifferentiated Round Cell Tumor (Canine)

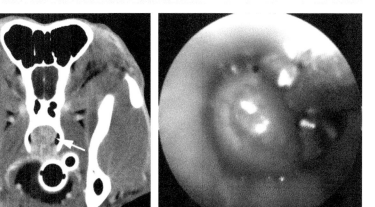

(a) CT+C, TP   **(b)** CT+C, TP   **(b)** ES

2y MC Labrador Retriever with progressive dyspnea. A well-defined, uniformly contrast-enhancing mass arises from the dorsal nasopharyngeal wall and nearly completely obstructs the nasopharyngeal lumen (**a,b**: arrow). Endoscopically acquired biopsy (**c**) revealed the mass to be a primitive undifferentiated round-cell tumor.

Figure 1.10.12 Laryngeal Lymphoma (Feline)

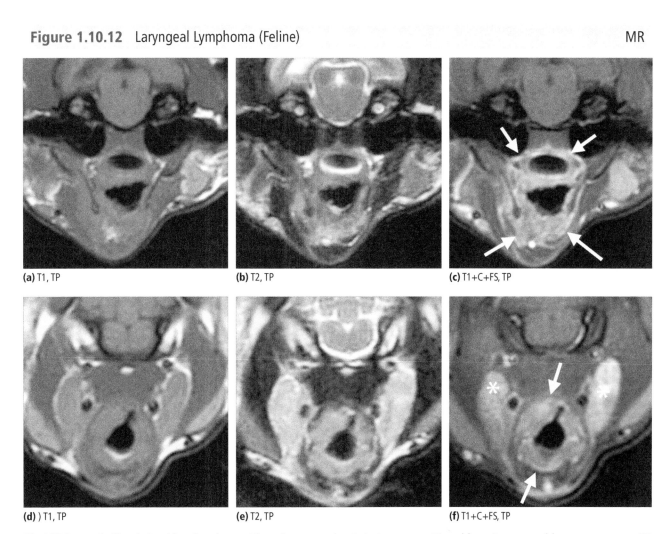

(a) T1, TP   **(b)** T2, TP   **(c)** T1+C+FS, TP

(d)) T1, TP   **(e)** T2, TP   **(f)** T1+C+FS, TP

11y MC Domestic Shorthair with voice change. There is a mass that is isointense on T1 and hyperintense and heterogeneous on T2 surrounding the pharynx and larynx. On contrast-enhanced T1 images, the mass is intensely enhancing (**c,f**: arrows). The retropharyngeal lymph nodes (**f**: asterisks) are moderately enlarged. The lymphoma was a large-cell T-cell type.

References

1. Vazquez JM, Arencibia A, Gil F, et al. Magnetic resonance imaging of the normal canine larynx. Anat Histol Embryol. 1998;27: 263–270.

2. Laurenson MP, Zwingenberger AL, Cissell DD, et al. Computed tomography of the pharynx in a closed vs. open mouth position. Vet Radiol Ultrasound. 2011;52:357–361.

3. Cuddy LC, Bacon NJ, Coomer AR, Jeyapaul CJ, Sheppard BJ, Winter MD. Excision of a congenital laryngeal cyst in a five-month-old dog via a lateral extraluminal approach. J Am Vet Med Assoc. 2010;236:1328–1333.

4. Oliveira CR, O'Brien RT, Matheson JS, Carrera I. Computed tomographic features of feline nasopharyngeal polyps. Vet Radiol Ultrasound. 2012;53:406–411.

5. Jones JC, Ober CP. Computed tomographic diagnosis of nongastrointestinal foreign bodies in dogs. J Am Anim Hosp Assoc. 2007;43:99–111.

6. Potanas CP, Armbrust LJ, Klocke EE, Lister SA, Jiménez DA, Saltysiak KA. Ultrasonographic and magnetic resonance imaging diagnosis of an oropharyngeal wood penetrating injury in a dog. J Am Anim Hosp Assoc. 2011;47:e1–e6.

7. Young B, Klopp L, Albrecht M, Kraft S. Imaging diagnosis: magnetic resonance imaging of a cervical wooden foreign body in a dog. Vet Radiol Ultrasound. 2004;45:538–541.

8. Rossi F, Caleri E, Bacci B, et al. Computed tomographic features of basihyoid ectopic thyroid carcinoma in dogs. Vet Radiol Ultrasound. 2013;54:575–581.

9. Dunbar MD, Ginn P, Winter M, Miller KB, Craft W. Laryngeal rhabdomyoma in a dog. Vet Clin Pathol. 2012;41:590–593.

10. Taeymans O, Penninck DG, Peters RM. Comparison between clinical, ultrasound, CT, MRI, and pathology findings in dogs presented for suspected thyroid carcinoma. Vet Radiol Ultrasound. 2013;54:61–70.

11. Gendler A, Lewis JR, Reetz JA, Schwarz T. Computed tomographic features of oral squamous cell carcinoma in cats: 18 cases (2002–2008). J Am Vet Med Assoc. 2010;236:319–325.

12. Stadler K, Hartman S, Matheson J, O'Brien R. Computed tomographic imaging of dogs with primary laryngeal or tracheal airway obstruction. Vet Radiol Ultrasound. 2011;52:377–384.

1.11

Thyroid and parathyroid

Normal thyroid and parathyroid

The normal thyroid gland is composed of two flattened ellipsoid lobes that lie adjacent and dorsolateral to the cranial segment of the cervical trachea. In dogs the right lobe is located slightly cranial to the left lobe. Canine thyroid gland size is variable and may be conjoined by an isthmus.[1] Feline thyroid lobes are approximately 2 cm in length by 0.5 cm in maximum width.[2] The thyroid gland is supplied by the cranial and caudal thyroid arteries and is highly perfused. Parathyroid glands average four in number, although there is individual variability. These glands are ovoid and less than 5 mm in longest diameter. Parathyroid glands are located toward the cranial and caudal poles of each thyroid lobe, with cranial glands tending to be located superficially and caudal glands embedded in thyroid parenchyma.

On transverse CT images, thyroid lobes are usually easily detected as small oval or triangular paratracheal structures that are denser than surrounding tissues as a result of the presence of iodine within the gland parenchyma (Figure 1.11.1**a**). On long-axis reformatted CT images, thyroid lobes have a characteristic elongated ovoid shape (Figure 1.11.1**b**). Unenhanced attenuation of canine and feline thyroid tissue is approximately 110 HU and 125 HU, respectively, and glands uniformly contrast enhance.[1,3]

On MR images, thyroid glands may have a homogeneous or heterogeneous appearance and are T1 isointense or mildly hyperintense and T2 hyperintense compared to adjacent cervical muscle (Figure 1.11.2). Normal thyroid glands are markedly and uniformly contrast enhancing.[4]

Normal parathyroid glands are not routinely recognized on either CT or MR images, although larger-diameter glands may appear as focal hyperintensities in T2-weighted MR images.

Because high-resolution ultrasound and scintigraphy studies are highly effective for evaluation of primary thyroid and parathyroid disorders, CT and MRI may be best employed as adjunct imaging techniques to assess extent and operability of aggressive thyroid neoplasia or for detection of ectopic thyroid and parathyroid masses.[5]

Hypothyroidism

Approximately half of dogs with functional hypothyroidism have lymphocytic thyroiditis, while the majority of the remainder suffer from idiopathic thyroid atrophy. Although descriptions of CT and MR features of hypothyroidism are lacking in the veterinary literature, those patients with thyroiditis would be expected to have thyroid enlargement, whereas idiopathic thyroid atrophy would result in reduced thyroid size (Figure 1.11.3). Thyroid glands of people with thyroiditis have reduced density on CT images as a result of diminished iodine concentration thought to be the result of follicular cell destruction.[6] Thyroiditis in people is also associated with increased T2 hyperintensity on MR imaging.[6]

Atlas of Small Animal CT and MRI, First Edition. Erik R. Wisner and Allison L. Zwingenberger.

Thyroid neoplasia

Feline functional thyroid nodular hyperplasia and adenoma

Functional benign adenomatous neoplasms and hyperplastic masses are common in the older cat. Because these are usually adequately characterized using other methods, descriptions of the CT and MR appearance of these lesions may have little clinical utility.

On both imaging modalities, thyroid glands are unilaterally or bilaterally enlarged and may include discrete mass lesions or diffuse lobar enlargement. Affected thyroid glands may have irregular margins and cystic components that appear hypoattenuating on CT images and hypointense and hyperintense on T1 and T2 MR images, respectively (Figure 1.11.4).[7] The thyroid glands of affected cats are moderately to markedly contrast enhancing and may be nonuniform in appearance.

Thyroid adenocarcinoma

Canine thyroid carcinomas are most commonly unilateral, are usually poorly encapsulated, and aggressively invade adjacent tissues and vessels. A tentative diagnosis is often made before CT or MR imaging is performed, and these studies are most useful for confirming thyroid origin, determining operability, and for specific surgical planning.[5]

On both CT and MR imaging, thyroid carcinomas are often large and may displace or invade adjacent cervical musculature, blood vessels, trachea, larynx, and esophagus (Figures 1.11.5, 1.11.6, 1.11.7, 1.11.8, 1.11.9). Some tumors appear to be well encapsulated, but others are unconstrained and highly invasive to adjacent tissues. Malignant tumors are typically highly vascular, and the parenchyma often appears heterogeneous and may have cystic and mineralized components. Regional lymph node metastasis is common.

On CT images, thyroid adenocarcinomas are generally isoattenuating to adjacent ventral cervical musculature on unenhanced images, with hypoattenuating and hyperattenuating regions within the parenchyma corresponding to cavitary lesions or mineralization, respectively, when present. Malignant neoplasms are markedly and nonuniformly contrast enhancing, and tumor thrombi may be evident in neoplasms with vascular invasion.[5]

On MR images, tumors are generally T1 hyperintense on unenhanced images and of mixed hyperintensity on T2 images. Contrast enhancement on MR images parallels that seen on CT, with tumor parenchyma markedly and heterogeneously contrast enhancing.[5]

Ectopic thyroid tumors may occasionally be encountered in the ventral cervical region (Figure 1.11.10) or cranial mediastinum (Figure 1.11.11). Ectopic thyroid tumors involving the hyoid apparatus are discussed in Chapter 1.10. CT and MR appearances of ectopic thyroid carcinomas are the same as described for in situ masses.

Other ventral cervical masses that can mimic the imaging appearance of thyroid carcinomas include carotid body tumors (Figure 1.11.12), hemangiosarcoma, undifferentiated carcinoma, granulomatous lymphadenitis, and paraesophageal abscess.

Parathyroid nodules

Disorders of the parathyroid glands resulting in hypercalcemia are categorized as primary or secondary hyperparathyroidism. Primary hyperparathyroidism is usually due to the presence of a solitary autonomously functional parathyroid adenoma or carcinoma, while secondary hyperparathyroidism is caused by hypocalcemia that leads to parathyroid hyperplasia of multiple glands. Both entities lead to parathyroid gland enlargement; however, neoplastic glands tend to be solitary and, on average, are larger than hyperplastic glands, although there is considerable overlap.

Little has been reported on the CT and MR imaging appearance of functional parathyroid nodules and masses in veterinary or human patients, presumably because they are easily detected and adequately characterized using diagnostic ultrasound.[8] CT would be expected to be an insensitive modality for detecting parathyroid lesions because of the relatively small size of parathyroid nodules and similarity in density to surrounding thyroid tissue.

On MR images parathyroid nodules may appear as well delineated T1 hypointense and T2 hyperintense lesions within or adjacent to thyroid parenchyma (Figure 1.11.13).[8]

Figure 1.11.1   Normal Thyroid Glands (Canine)

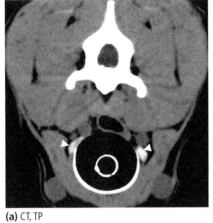 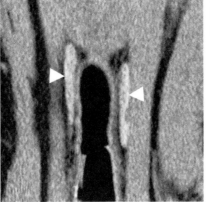

On unenhanced CT images, normal thyroid lobes are typically hyperattenuating as a result of iodine content (**a**,**b**: arrowheads).

(a) CT, TP

(b) CT, DP

Figure 1.11.2   Normal Thyroid Glands (Canine)

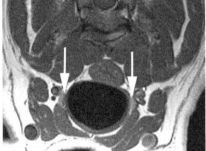 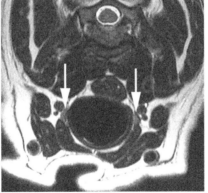

Left and right thyroid lobes are seen as small, roughly triangular structures on transverse T1 and T2 images (**a**,**b**: arrows) located adjacent to the tracheal wall and ventromedial to the common carotid arteries. Right (**c**: arrow) and left (**d**: arrow) thyroid lobes are well delineated on dorsal plane T1 3D-SPGR images, seen medial to the common carotid arteries (**c**,**d**: arrowhead), which course obliquely through this imaging plane.

(a) T1, TP

(b) T2, TP

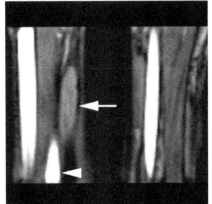 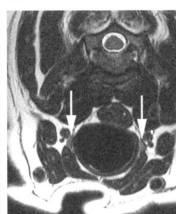 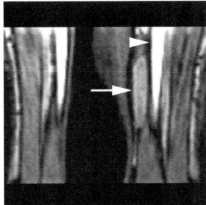

(c) T1, SPGR, DP

(d) T1, SPGR, DP

Figure 1.11.3 Hypothyroidism (Canine)   CT

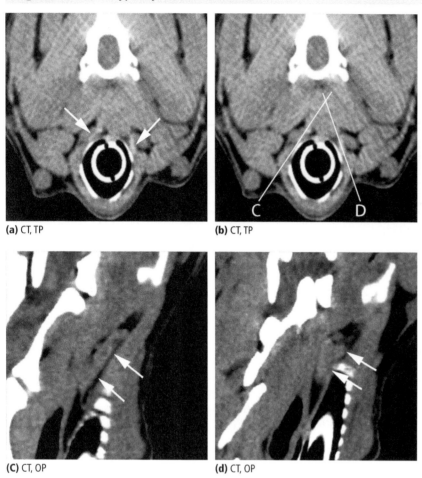

(a) CT, TP   **(b)** CT, TP

12y FS Weimaraner with documented hypothyroidism. Image **b** is the same image as **a** with line overlays showing the long-axis oblique planes depicted in **c** and **d**. The thyroid lobes are smaller than expected and are marginally hyperattenuating than adjacent soft tissues (**a**: arrows). The right (**c**: arrows) and left (**d**: arrows) thyroid lobes are easily delineated on the oblique images. Both lobes are small, and margins are abnormally lobular. Thyroid lobes viewed in long axis are distinguished from the medial retropharyngeal lymph nodes which can appear similar but are more cranial and located lateral to the neurovascular bundle.

(C) CT, OP   **(d)** CT, OP

Figure 1.11.4 Thyroid Adenoma (Feline)   CT

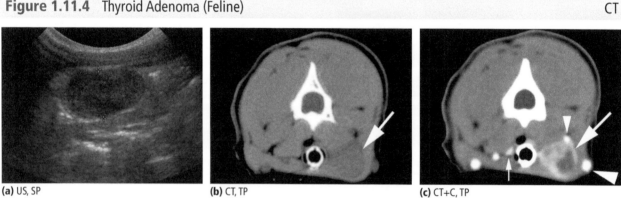

(a) US, SP   **(b)** CT, TP   **(c)** CT+C, TP

7y Himalayan with recent history of dysphagia and anorexia. An ovoid hypoattenuating mass is present in the left ventral cervical region on ultrasound examination (a). On CT images, the mass has attenuation less than adjacent soft tissues but significantly more than fat (b: arrow). The mass contrast enhances nonuniformly and margins are well defined (c: large arrow). The left common carotid artery is displaced dorsally (c: small arrowhead), and the left jugular vein is displaced laterally (c: large arrowhead). The right thyroid gland appears normal (c: small arrow). Excisional biopsy confirmed a diagnosis of thyroid adenoma.

Figure 1.11.5   Thyroid Carcinoma (Canine)

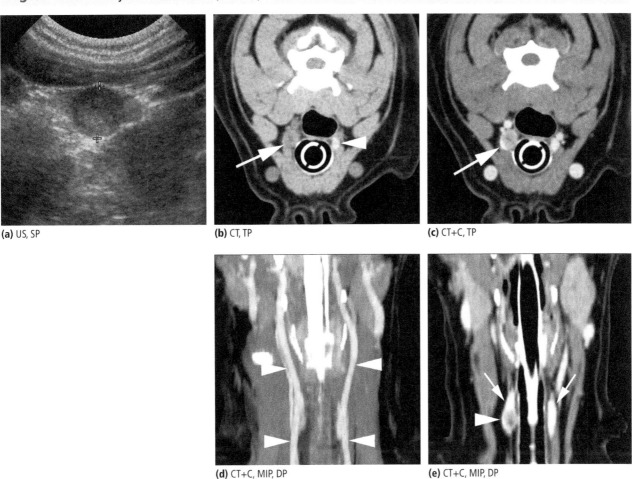

(a) US, SP

(b) CT, TP

(c) CT+C, TP

(d) CT+C, MIP, DP

(e) CT+C, MIP, DP

12y FS Labrador Retriever with previously diagnosed pulmonary and cervical masses. A spherical hypoechoic nodule is seen in the body of the right thyroid lobe on ultrasound examination (a). The mass is mildly hypoattenuating on an unenhanced CT image (b: arrow). The left thyroid lobe appears normal in size and is hyperattenuating (b: arrowhead). The mass moderately contrast enhances but less so than surrounding normal thyroid tissue (c: arrow) and the contralateral thyroid lobe. On dorsal plane maximum-intensity projections (MIP) of contrast-enhanced imaging data, a thick-slab MIP reveals the course of the two common carotid arteries dorsal to the thyroid lobes (d: arrowheads). A thinner-slab MIP excluding the carotid arteries reveals the thyroid lobes (e: arrows) and the specific location of the mass within the right lobe (e: arrowhead). Excisional biopsy revealed solid and follicular thyroid carcinoma with vascular and capsular invasion.

Figure 1.11.6 Thyroid Carcinoma and Thyroid Adenoma (Canine)

CT

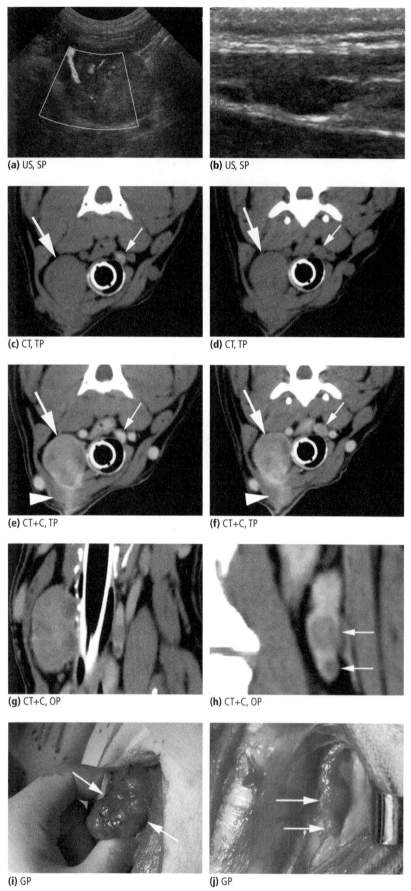

(a) US, SP

(b) US, SP

(c) CT, TP

(d) CT, TP

(e) CT+C, TP

(f) CT+C, TP

(g) CT+C, OP

(h) CT+C, OP

(i) GP

(j) GP

12y FS Australian Shepherd with a right-sided ventral cervical mass. Ultrasound examination revealed a large, solid vascular mass in the region of the right thyroid lobe (**a**). A smaller hypoechoic mass was seen within the body of the left thyroid lobe (**b**). Unenhanced and contrast-enhanced transverse CT images (**c–f**) are paired and ordered from cranial to caudal. A large right-sided, uniformly contrast-enhancing mass is present (**c–f**: large arrow). The mass margin is poorly defined ventrally, and there appears to be extracapsular extension of the mass and diffuse enhancement of adjacent tissues (**e,f**: arrowhead). A normal-appearing left thyroid lobe is seen on the more cranial CT image (**c,e**: small arrow). On the more caudal image, the left thyroid lobe is larger and has lower attenuation characteristics than expected, suggesting the presence of a second smaller left thyroid mass (**d,f**: small arrow). CT imaging findings are further documented on long-axis oblique axis reformatted CT images, and now two small nodules are seen in the left thyroid lobe (**h**: small arrows). Imaging findings were corroborated at the time of surgical excision (**i,j**: arrows). Excisional biopsy revealed right-sided thyroid carcinoma with extracapsular invasion and left-sided thyroid adenoma.

Figure 1.11.7   Thyroid Carcinoma (Canine)

CT

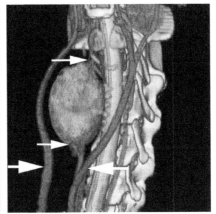

(a) CT+C, TP

(b) CT+C, 3D, OP

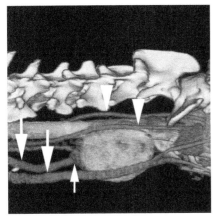

(c) CT+C, 3D, RLAT

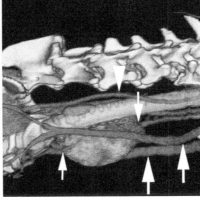

(d) CT+C, 3D, LLAT

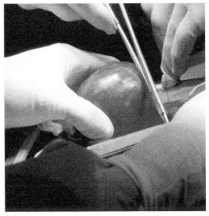

(e) GP

10y MC Rottweiler with a 4-month history of a ventral cervical mass. A large well-margined ovoid mass is seen in the right ventral cervical region. The mass is moderately and uniformly contrast enhancing (**a**: asterisk). The left thyroid lobe appears normal in size, location, and density (**a**: arrowhead), but a normal thyroid lobe was not identified on this study. 3D renderings reveal the specific location of the mass in relation to the jugular veins (**b–d**: large arrows) and common carotid arteries (**c**,**d**: arrowheads). Vascular supply to the mass from the cranial and caudal thyroid vessels can also be seen (**b–d**: small arrows). A well-encapsulated mass was excised (**e**). Excisional biopsy confirmed a diagnosis of thyroid carcinoma.

Figure 1.11.8 Invasive Thyroid Carcinoma (Canine)   CT

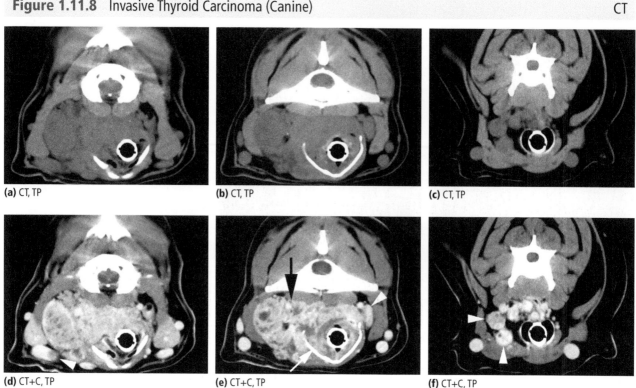

(a) CT, TP   **(b)** CT, TP   **(c)** CT, TP

(d) CT+C, TP   **(e)** CT+C, TP   **(f)** CT+C, TP

10y MC Labrador cross with a 3-month history of dysphagia and ventral cervical mass. Representative CT images are paired unenhanced (**a–c**) and contrast-enhanced (**d–f**) images ordered from cranial to caudal. An extensive soft-tissue mass with heterogeneous attenuation is seen in the right cervical region, extending from the hyoid apparatus rostrally to the mid-cervical region caudally. The mass displaces the larynx to the left, crosses midline, and extends into the dorsal and left lateral laryngeal and retropharyngeal regions. The mass is highly and heterogeneously contrast enhancing. The mass displaces the larynx to the left, invades the laryngeal soft tissues (**e**: small arrow), and incorporates the carotid artery and internal jugular vein on the right (**e**: black arrow). There are filling defects and distension of these vessels caudally (**f**: arrowheads) and of the right facial vein (**d**: arrowhead), indicating tumor invasion and the presence of tumor thrombus. The left retropharyngeal lymph nodes are enlarged and have a heterogeneous pattern of enhancement (**e**: arrowhead), suggesting contralateral regional lymph node metastasis. Postmortem examination confirmed a diagnosis of thyroid carcinoma involving both thyroid lobes with extensive infiltration into the adjacent soft tissues and metastasis to regional lymph nodes and lung. The mass extended into and expanded the oropharyngeal wall with marked compression of the pharynx and laryngeal opening.

Figure 1.11.9 Invasive Thyroid Carcinoma (Canine)   CT

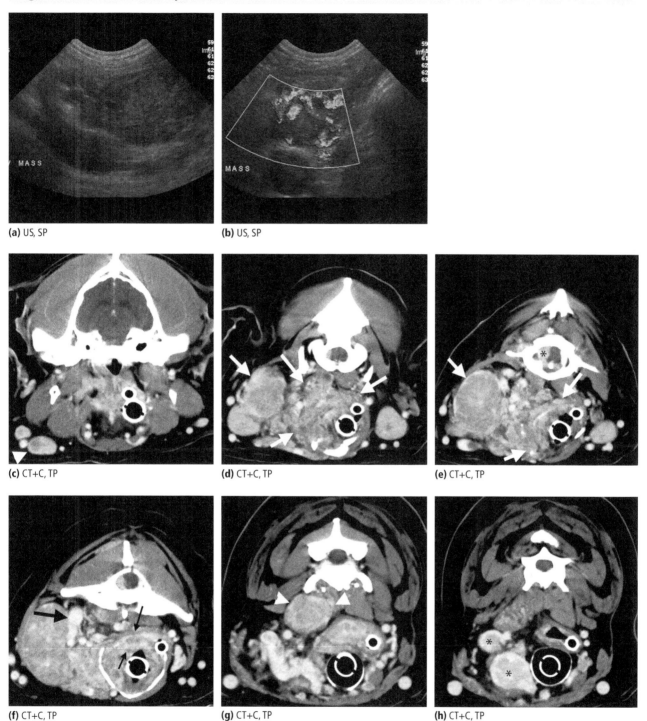

(a) US, SP

(b) US, SP

(c) CT+C, TP

(d) CT+C, TP

(e) CT+C, TP

(f) CT+C, TP

(g) CT+C, TP

(h) CT+C, TP

6y MC Old English Sheepdog with anorexia and right-sided laryngeal paralysis. On ultrasound images, the mass is hypoechoic and highly vascular (**a,b**). The mandibular lymph nodes are enlarged with nonenhancing central nodules, suggestive of metastatic disease (**c**: arrowhead). The diffuse, contrast-enhancing neoplastic tissue invades the larynx and cervical musculature (**d,e**: arrows). There is also a mass effect in the spinal canal associated with cord displacement and compression (**e**: asterisk). This either represents vascular invasion of tumor into the internal venous plexus or venous obstruction. There is esophageal invasion (**f**: small arrows) and tortuous vasculature surrounding the mass (**f**: large arrow). There is invasion of the subvertebral musculature caudally (**g**: arrowheads). Unidentified tumor vessels are enlarged and filled with tumor thrombus (**h**: asterisks).

Figure 1.11.10   Ectopic Thyroid Carcinoma (Canine)   MR

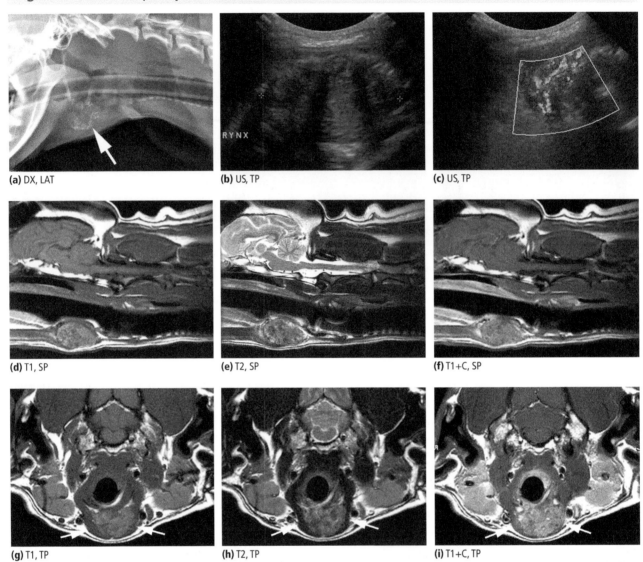

(a) DX, LAT   **(b)** US, TP   **(c)** US, TP

(d) T1, SP   **(e)** T2, SP   **(f)** T1+C, SP

(g) T1, TP   **(h)** T2, TP   **(i)** T1+C, TP

8y MC Labrador Retriever with recent weight loss and elevated T4 level. A partially mineralized mass is seen ventral to the hyoid apparatus and appears to involve the basihyoid bone (**a**: arrow). The mass appears solid and highly vascular on ultrasound images (**b,c**), and partial mineralization is again noted (**b**: shadowing). Marked uptake of technetium pertechnetate on a thyroid scintigraphic examination (not shown) confirmed thyroid origin of the mass. The mass is of mixed intensity on unenhanced T1 and T2 images (**d,e,g,h**) and moderately contrast enhances (**f,i**). Mass margins are poorly defined on the transverse images, suggesting invasion of the adjacent geniohyoideus and mylohyoideus muscles (**g–i**: small arrows). The mass also incorporated the basihyoid bone, which could not be seen on any images. Surgical excision was incomplete because of extensive laryngeal involvement.

Figure 1.11.11   Ectopic Thyroid Carcinoma (Canine)   CT

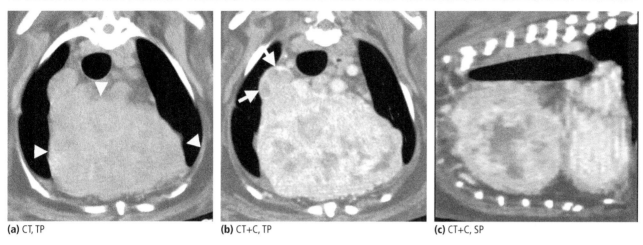

(a) CT, TP   **(b)** CT+C, TP   **(c)** CT+C, SP

10y F Shetland Sheepdog with swelling of the face and neck. There is a large, heterogeneous mass in the cranial mediastinum (**a**: arrowheads). The mass is causing dorsal displacement of the trachea (**a,b**) and caudal displacement of the heart (**c**). On contrast-enhanced images (**b,c**), there is heterogeneous enhancement and filling defects representing tumor thrombus within the cranial vena cava (**b**: arrows). Histologic diagnosis and anatomic distribution were confirmed on postmortem examination.

Figure 1.11.12   Malignant Carotid Body Tumor (Canine)   CT

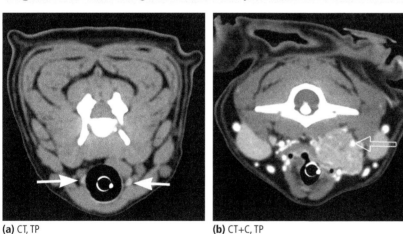

(a) CT, TP   **(b)** CT+C, TP

9y FS Boston terrier with a cervical mass. Carotid body tumors (Chemodectoma) are similar in location to thyroid masses. However, the normal, high-attenuating thyroid lobes are easily identified adjacent to the tracheal wall on the unenhanced image in this patient (**a**: arrows). The carotid body tumor is highly vascular and intensely contrast enhancing. In comparison to thyroid tumors where the carotid artery is usually displaced laterally, the carotid artery is contained within the mass (**b**: open arrow). Regional lymph node metastasis (not shown) was also confirmed from surgical excisional biopsy.

Figure 1.11.13 Parathyroid Carcinoma (Canine)   MR

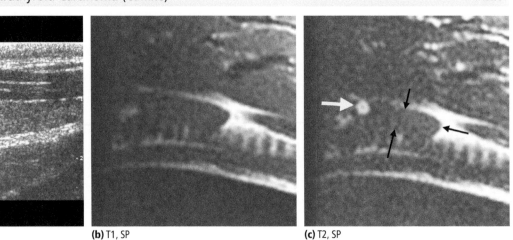

(a) US, SP   **(b)** T1, SP   **(c)** T2, SP

12y M Golden Retriever with hypercalcemia. There is a hypoechoic nodule seen in the cranial pole of the left thyroid lobe on ultrasound (a: calipers). On MR imaging, the mass is isointense on T1 images and hyperintense on T2 images (c: white arrow) within the thyroid gland (c: black arrows). The histologic diagnosis was documented on postmortem examination.

References

1. Taeymans O, Schwarz T, Duchateau L, Barberet V, Gielen I, Haskins M, et al. Computed tomographic features of the normal canine thyroid gland. Vet Radiol Ultrasound. 2008;49:13–19.
2. Drost WT, Mattoon JS, Weisbrode SE. Use of helical computed tomography for measurement of thyroid glands in clinically normal cats. Am J Vet Res. 2006;67:467–471.
3. Drost WT, Mattoon JS, Samii VF, Weisbrode SE, Hoshaw-Woodard SL. Computed tomographic densitometry of normal feline thyroid glands. Vet Radiol Ultrasound. 2004;45:112–116.
4. Taeymans O, Dennis R, Saunders JH. Magnetic resonance imaging of the normal canine thyroid gland. Vet Radiol Ultrasound. 2008;49:238–242.
5. Taeymans O, Penninck DG, Peters RM. Comparison between clinical, ultrasound, CT, MRI, and pathology findings in dogs presented for suspected thyroid carcinoma. Vet Radiol Ultrasound. 2012;54:61–70.
6. Jhaveri K, Shroff MM, Fatterpekar GM, Som PM. CT and MR imaging findings associated with subacute thyroiditis. AJNR Am J Neuroradiol. 2003;24:143–146.
7. Hofmeister E, Kippenes H, Mealey KL, Cantor GH, Lohr CV. Functional cystic thyroid adenoma in a cat. J Am Vet Med Assoc. 2001;219:190–193.
8. Cakal E, Cakir E, Dilli A, Colak N, Unsal I, Aslan MS, et al. Parathyroid adenoma screening efficacies of different imaging tools and factors affecting the success rates. Clin Imaging. 2012;36:688–694.

Section 2
Brain

2.1

Ventricular system and hydrocephalus

Normal ventricular system

The normal ventricular system consists of the third, fourth, and lateral ventricles. The third ventricle communicates with the lateral ventricles via the interventricular foramina, and the mesencephalic aqueduct connects the third and fourth ventricles (Figures 2.1.1, 2.1.2). Caudally, the fourth ventricle communicates with the central canal. Cerebrospinal fluid (CSF) is produced by the choroid plexus, located on the floor of the lateral ventricles and on the dorsal margins of the third and fourth ventricles. CSF circulates throughout the ventricular system and exits into the subarachnoid space through the lateral apertures of the fourth ventricle. CSF is resorbed primarily through arachnoid villi that extend into the dural venous sinuses and secondarily through lymphatic drainage of the meningeal sheaths surrounding nerve roots.[1] The ventricular system also includes a number of anatomic recesses that may appear more prominent in the presence of hydrocephalus.

Hydrocephalus

Hydrocephalus is defined as an abnormal distension of all or part of the ventricular system with CSF. Ventricular distension is typically caused by constant or intermittent increased hydrostatic pressure. The term hydrocephalus denotes the anatomic status of the ventricular system rather than an underlying cause. Hydrocephalus can be developmental or acquired and can result from obstruction of CSF drainage, from impaired CSF resorption, or from CSF overproduction.[2,3] The latter two forms are referred to as communicating or nonobstructive hydrocephalus. Use of a related term, ventriculomegaly, may

be more appropriate when passive ventricular enlargement occurs as a result of diminished brain parenchyma volume (also known as hydrocephalus *ex vacuo*) (Figure 2.1.3). Normal CSF has a density near that of pure water and will therefore have a HU value of close to 0 on unenhanced CT images and will be hypoattenuating to surrounding brain parenchyma. On unenhanced MR images, normal CSF will appear T1 hypointense and T2 hyperintense to brain parenchyma and will have no or low signal on water-nulling sequences, such as FLAIR. In patients with abnormal CSF due to hemorrhage, inflammation, or neoplasia, signal intensity may be significantly increased on T1 and pure water-nulling sequences depending on cellular and macromolecular content (Figure 2.1.4).

Congenital hydrocephalus

Congenital hydrocephalus occurs predominantly in brachycephalic and toy breeds (Figure 2.1.5). In some instances, mechanical obstruction from such entities as mesencephalic duct stenosis or Chiari malformation explains the presence of hydrocephalus; in other cases, no underlying cause is recognized.[4-6]

Obstructive hydrocephalus

Obstructive hydrocephalus may be due to intraluminal or extraluminal masses or other lesions that impair CSF flow within the ventricular system. The underlying causes of obstructive hydrocephalus vary widely, as do the imaging features of the ventricular system. Depending on the source and location of obstruction, hydrocephalus may be uniform or regional. Obstruction

Atlas of Small Animal CT and MRI, First Edition. Erik R. Wisner and Allison L. Zwingenberger.
© 2015 John Wiley & Sons, Inc. Published 2015 by John Wiley & Sons, Inc.

originating in or caudal to the fourth ventricle will tend to produce uniform ventricular distension, whereas obstruction in the third or lateral ventricles or in the interventricular foramina may produce asymmetrical, regional, or focal ventricular distension (Figures 2.1.6, 2.1.7).[2,6–10]

Communicating (nonobstructive) hydrocephalus

Impaired CSF resorption

Impaired CSF resorption is thought to occur with diminished resorptive capacity of the arachnoid villi.

Postulated causes include intraventricular hemorrhage and ventriculitis with cells or debris causing obstruction of the valvular flow mechanism of individual villi. Chronic hydrocephalus also appears to diminish resorptive function of the villi.[11]

Hydrocephalus from CSF overproduction

Hydrocephalus from overproduction of CSF is thought to occasionally occur in some patients with functional choroid plexus tumors in which the abnormally high rate of CSF production exceeds the rate of resorption (Figure 2.1.8).[12]

Figure 2.1.1 Normal Ventricles (Canine)   CT

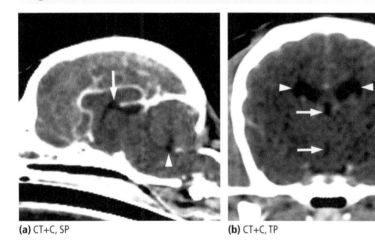

(a) CT+C, SP   (b) CT+C, TP

7y F Toy Poodle. Sagittal (a) and transverse (b) contrast-enhanced images of the brain. The normal appearance of the third ventricle surrounding the interthalamic adhesion (a,b: arrows), the lateral ventricles (b: arrowheads), and the fourth ventricle (a: arrowhead). The mesencephalic duct is also seen as a thin, curvilinear, hypoattenuating communication between the third and fourth ventricles (a).

Figure 2.1.2   Normal Ventricles (Canine)   MR

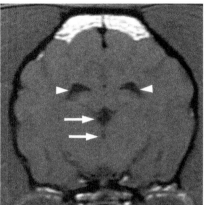

7y FS French Bulldog. The normal T1 hypointense appearance of the third ventricle surrounding the interthalamic adhesion (**a,b**: arrows), the lateral ventricles (**b**: arrowheads), and the fourth ventricle (**a**: arrowhead). The mesencephalic duct is also seen as a thin, curvilinear, hypointense communication between the third and fourth ventricles (**a**). Normal cerebrospinal fluid appears hyperintense on T2 images (**c**) and profoundly hypointense on FLAIR images (**d**).

(**a**) T1, SP   (**b**) T1, TP

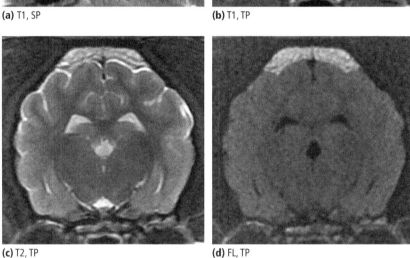

(**c**) T2, TP   (**d**) FL, TP

Figure 2.1.3   *Ex vacuo* Hydrocephalus (Canine)   CT & MR

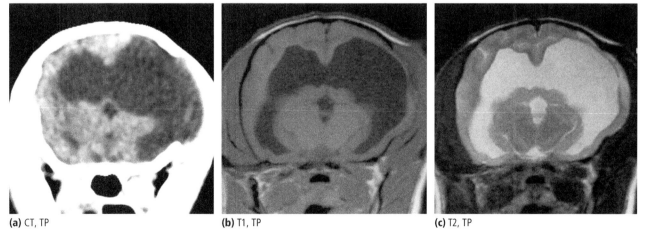

(**a**) CT, TP   (**b**) T1, TP   (**c**) T2, TP

4y MC Maltese recovering from a penetrating head injury (dog bite) 6 months previously. Posttraumatic cortical atrophy of the left cerebral hemisphere results in passive expansion of the left lateral ventricle to fill the potential space. This dog also has evidence of more generalized ventriculomegaly. Discontinuity of the overlying parietal bone from previous fracture is evident on both the CT and MR images.

Figure 2.1.4   Hydrocephalus with Abnormal Cerebrospinal Fluid (Feline)   MR

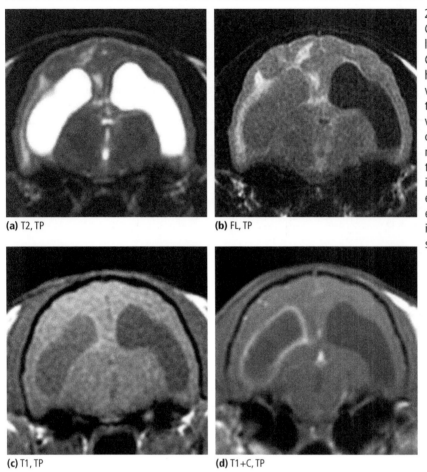

(a) T2, TP

(b) FL, TP

(c) T1, TP

(d) T1+C, TP

2y MC Domestic Shorthair with signs of a C1–C5 myelopathy. Bilateral lateral ventriculomegaly is seen on all MR sequences. Cerebrospinal fluid (CSF) is uniformly T2 hyperintense (**a**), but CSF in the right lateral ventricle is moderately intense compared to the low-intensity signal within the left lateral ventricle on FLAIR (**b**) and T1 (**c**) images, indicating compartmentalization and cells or macromolecules contaminating the CSF in the right lateral ventricle. Thickening and intense enhancement of the right lateral ependymal lining is evident on the contrast-enhanced T1 image (**d**). A diagnosis of feline infectious peritonitis was based on cerebrospinal fluid cytology and coronavirus titers.

Figure 2.1.5   Congenital Hydrocephalus (Canine)   MR

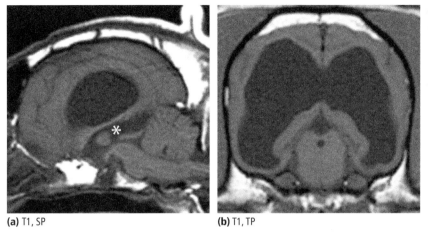

4y MC English Bulldog with intermittent seizures. Marked generalized hydrocephalus is
seen on all image sequences. Although
enlargement of the lateral ventricles is most
striking, third ventricular dilation is also evident,
which is best appreciated on the sagittal T1
image (**a**: asterisk). Ventriculomegaly was
thought to be breed related.

(a) T1, SP

(b) T1, TP

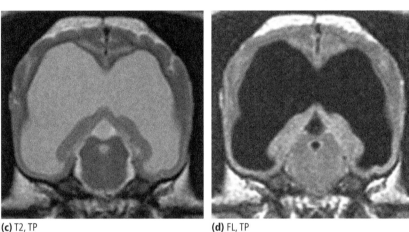

(c) T2, TP

(d) FL, TP

Figure 2.1.6   Obstructive Hydrocephalus (Feline)   MR

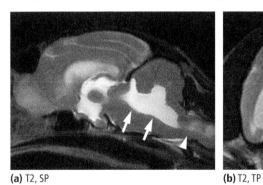 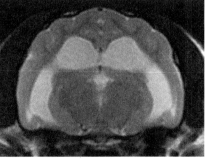 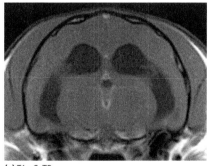

(a) T2, SP

(b) T2, TP

(c) T1+C, TP

7mo MC Domestic Shorthair with multifocal central nervous system signs. An obstructive mass was detected in the caudal brainstem and
in the spinal cord at the level of C1 (**a**: arrowhead). Marked generalized ventriculomegaly is evident on all images, and distension of the
fourth ventricle and mesencephalic duct is particularly prominent (**a**: arrows). A diagnosis of feline infectious peritonitis was based on
cerebrospinal fluid cytology and coronavirus titers.

Figure 2.1.7 Obstructive Hydrocephalus (Canine)

MR

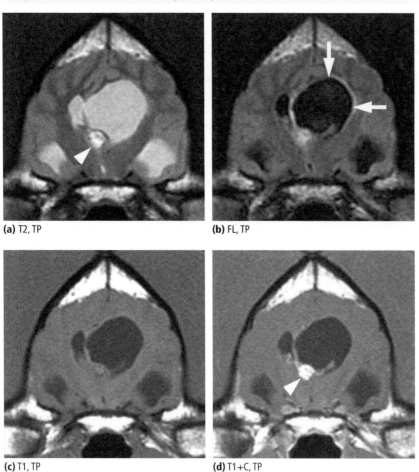

(a) T2, TP

(b) FL, TP

(c) T1, TP

(d) T1+C, TP

5y MC Labrador Retriever with hydrocephalus affecting the left lateral ventricle. A small contrast-enhancing mass is present on the ventral margin of the left lateral ventricle (**a**,**d**: arrowhead). The left lateral ventricle is markedly distended, and there is a thin rim of hyperintensity, best seen on the FLAIR image (**b**: arrows), thought to represent transependymal interstitial edema. A choroid plexus carcinoma involving the floor of the left lateral ventricle and causing partial foraminal obstruction was confirmed on postmortem examination.

Figure 2.1.8   Presumptive Overproduction Hydrocephalus (Canine)   MR

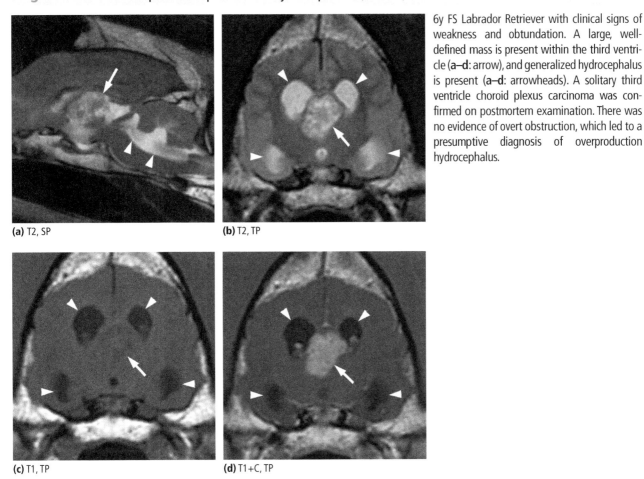

(a) T2, SP

(b) T2, TP

(c) T1, TP

(d) T1+C, TP

6y FS Labrador Retriever with clinical signs of weakness and obtundation. A large, well-defined mass is present within the third ventricle (**a–d**: arrow), and generalized hydrocephalus is present (**a–d**: arrowheads). A solitary third ventricle choroid plexus carcinoma was confirmed on postmortem examination. There was no evidence of overt obstruction, which led to a presumptive diagnosis of overproduction hydrocephalus.

References

1. Evans HE. Miller's Anatomy of the Dog. St. Louis: Elsevier Saunders, 2013.
2. de Stefani A, de Risio L, Platt SR, Matiasek L, Lujan-Feliu-Pascual A, Garosi LS. Surgical technique, postoperative complications and outcome in 14 dogs treated for hydrocephalus by ventriculoperitoneal shunting. Vet Surg. 2011;40:183–191.
3. Harrington ML, Bagley RS, Moore MP. Hydrocephalus. Vet Clin North Am Small Anim Pract. 1996;26:843–856.
4. Johnson RP, Neer TM, Partington BP, Cho DY, Partington CR. Familial cerebellar ataxia with hydrocephalus in bull mastiffs. Vet Radiol Ultrasound. 2001;42:246–249.
5. MacKillop E. Magnetic resonance imaging of intracranial malformations in dogs and cats. Vet Radiol Ultrasound. 2011;52: S42–51.
6. Thomas WB. Hydrocephalus in dogs and cats. Vet Clin North Am Small Anim Pract. 2010;40:143–159.
7. Lovett MC, Fenner WR, Watson AT, Hostutler RA. Imaging diagnosis – MRI characteristics of a fourth ventricular cholesterol granuloma in a dog. Vet Radiol Ultrasound. 2012;53:650–654.
8. Tani K, Taga A, Itamoto K, Iwanaga T, Une S, Nakaichi M, et al. Hydrocephalus and syringomyelia in a cat. J Vet Med Sci. 2001;63:1331–1334.
9. Targett MP, McInnes E, Dennis R. Magnetic resonance imaging of a medullary dermoid cyst with secondary hydrocephalus in a dog. Vet Radiol Ultrasound. 1999;40:23–26.
10. Vullo T, Manzo R, Gomez DG, Deck MD, Cahill PT. A canine model of acute hydrocephalus with MR correlation. AJNR Am J Neuroradiol. 1998;19:1123–1125.
11. Zhao K, Sun H, Shan Y, Mao BY, Zhang H. Cerebrospinal fluid absorption disorder of arachnoid villi in a canine model of hydrocephalus. Neurol India. 2010;58:371–376.
12. Fujimoto Y, Matsushita H, Plese JP, Marino R, Jr. Hydrocephalus due to diffuse villous hyperplasia of the choroid plexus. Case report and review of the literature. Pediatr Neurosurg. 2004;40:32–36.

2.2

Brain edema

Introduction

Brain edema may result from a wide array of causes, which can be divided into the four principal forms listed in Table 2.2.1.[1-3] Clinically, multiple forms of brain edema can occur simultaneously, and often the predominating form depends on the inciting cause as well as the time course of the disease. Whether intracellular or extracellular, edema appears mildly to moderately hypoattenuating to normal brain parenchyma on CT images and T1 hypointense and T2 hyperintense on MR images. Because edema fluid is distributed within a microenvironment of cells and macromolecules, it will also appear hyperintense on FLAIR and other pure water-nulling sequences.

Cytotoxic edema

Cytotoxic edema occurs as a result of ischemia resulting in cell membrane Na/K pump dysfunction, increased intracellular fluid volume, and cell swelling. Because of the underlying cause and the intracellular nature of this form of edema, white and gray matter may both be affected, and the distribution of edema roughly conforms to the geographic distribution of ischemia (Figure 2.2.1).[3] In most instances, cytotoxic edema occurs in combination with vasogenic edema. Diffusion-weighted imaging has been used to discriminate between the two forms following acute episodes of ischemia, with reduced apparent diffusion coefficient (ADC) intensity reflecting predominantly cytotoxic edema.[4]

Vasogenic edema

Vasogenic edema occurs because of a disruption of the tight junctions of the blood–brain barrier, resulting in extravasation of high-protein fluid into the brain. Vasogenic edema is extracellular, so it tends to preferentially accumulate in white matter, which has a sparser cellular density and therefore more potential space for fluid distribution compared to highly cellular gray matter.[3] Depending on the initiating cause and volume of fluid, edema can distribute widely (Figures 2.2.2, 2.2.3).

Interstitial or hydrocephalic edema

Interstitial edema most often occurs in association with obstructive hydrocephalus when intraventricular pressure increases, causing transependymal CSF migration into adjacent brain parenchyma. As a result, hydrostatic edema preferentially occurs within periventricular parenchyma and is extracellular (Figure 2.2.4). Unlike vasogenic edema, interstitial edema fluid is a transudate containing little in the way of cells or macromolecules.[3]

Osmotic edema

Osmotic edema occurs rarely and is caused by reduced plasma osmolality resulting from water intoxication, hemodialysis, or metabolic disorders that reduce plasma sodium or glucose concentration. The imbalance in brain extracellular fluid osmolality and plasma osmolality results in a fluid shift to the brain leading to formation of extracellular edema.[3]

Atlas of Small Animal CT and MRI, First Edition. Erik R. Wisner and Allison L. Zwingenberger.
© 2015 John Wiley & Sons, Inc. Published 2015 by John Wiley & Sons, Inc.

Table 2.2.1 Distribution and causes of brain edema.

	Cytotoxic	Vasogenic	Interstitial	Osmotic
Distribution	Intracellular gray and white matter	Extracellular predominately white matter	Extracellular periventricular	Extracellular
Cause	Cell membrane Na/K pump dysfunction due to cell hypoxia from ischemia	Disruption of blood–brain barrier resulting in extravasation of high-protein fluid	Increased intraventricular pressure. Usually from obstructive hydrocephalus	Systemic plasma hypo-osmolality

Figure 2.2.1 Cytotoxic Edema (Canine)   MR

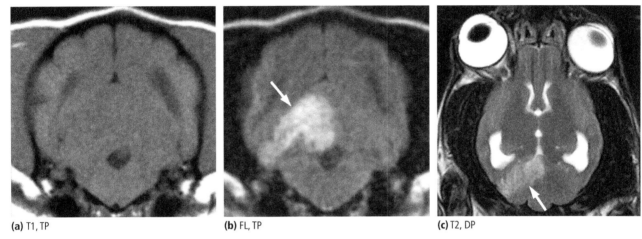

(a) T1, TP   (b) FL, TP   (c) T2, DP

3y FS Dachshund with right-sided cerebellar infarction. There is a well-circumscribed geographic region of FLAIR and T2 hyperintensity involving the right cerebellum (b,c: arrow). The T2 hyperintensity is due, in part, to intracellular cytotoxic edema resulting from cell hypoxia. The lesion distribution coincides with the tissue volume normally perfused by the right rostral cerebellar artery.

Figure 2.2.2 Vasogenic Edema (Canine)   CT

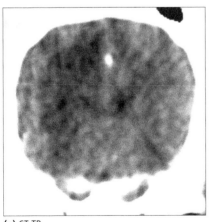

3y MC Basset Hound with aspergillosis involving the frontal sinus and forebrain. This unenhanced CT image is caudal to the primary lesion. Marked, diffuse hypoattenuation is evident involving the white matter of the right cerebral hemisphere because of the presence of vasogenic edema. Although edema is recognized on CT images, it may be less conspicuous than on corresponding MR images.

(a) CT, TP

Figure 2.2.3 Vasogenic Edema (Canine)   MR

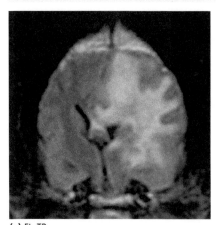

Adult dog of unknown age and gender with a large left frontal lobe meningioma. This image is at a level caudal to the mass. Marked, diffuse hyperintensity is evident involving the white matter of the left cerebral hemisphere, representing vasogenic edema. There is also diffuse volume expansion of the white matter associated with prominent right-sided midline shift.

(a) FL, TP

Figure 2.2.4 Interstitial Edema (Canine)   MR

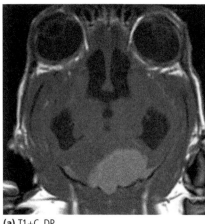 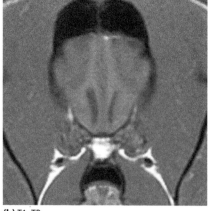 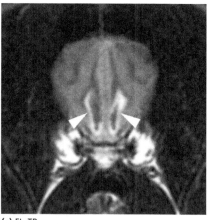

(a) T1+C, DP   **(b)** T1, TP   **(c)** FL, TP

6y FS Toy Poodle with a caudal fossa meningioma causing obstruction of the ventricular system (**a**). Images **b** and **c** are at the level of the rostral horns of the lateral ventricles. The thin, hyperintense rim surrounding the rostral horns of the lateral ventricles on the FLAIR image (**c**: arrowheads) represents transependymal migration of cerebrospinal fluid to the periventricular extracellular fluid space due to increased intraventricular hydrostatic pressure.

References

1. Betz AL, Iannotti F, Hoff JT. Brain edema: a classification based on blood–brain barrier integrity. Cerebrovasc Brain Metab Rev. 1989;1:133–154.
2. Iencean SM. Brain edema – a new classification. Med Hypotheses. 2003;61:106–109.
3. Nag S, Manias JL, Stewart DJ. Pathology and new players in the pathogenesis of brain edema. Acta Neuropathol. 2009;118: 197–217.
4. Loubinoux I, Volk A, Borredon J, Guirimand S, Tiffon B, Seylaz J, et al. Spreading of vasogenic edema and cytotoxic edema assessed by quantitative diffusion and T2 magnetic resonance imaging. Stroke. 1997;28:419–426; discussion 426–417.

2.3

Developmental disorders

Anomalous development of the brain

Brain malformation in the dog and cat can be induced by trauma, toxins, inflammatory disorders, serendipitous *in utero* aberrations, and genetic defects. Brain development can be broadly divided into five progressive stages of dorsal induction—ventral induction, neuronal proliferation, differentiation and histogenesis, neuronal migration, and myelination.[1] Anomalies can arise during any one of these stages, and the type of anomaly will reflect the predominant development activity at the time.

Most significant anomalies are rarely imaged with CT or MRI since many patients die or are euthanized early in life. Although classification schemes for developmental brain anomalies vary widely, we have chosen to organize this section into hindbrain herniations and malformations, diverticulation and cleavage disorders, malformations of cortical development, and nonneoplastic cysts.[2]

Hindbrain herniations and malformations

Chiari-like malformation

Chiari-like malformation is due to reduced volume of the caudal cranial fossa, resulting in cerebellar to caudal cranial fossa volume mismatch.[3-7] The disorder occurs primarily in Cavalier King Charles Spaniels, but other small and toy breed dogs can be affected.[3,4,8] The reduced caudal fossa volume results in crowding and repositioning of the cerebellum, which may sometimes encroach on or herniate through the foramen magnum. Cerebellar crowding also causes extramural compression of the fourth ventricle and central canal, which leads to obstructive hydrocephalus and syringohydromyelia.[3,9]

Clinical signs include pain, positional pain, hyperesthesia, and neurologic deficits, but severity of clinical signs correlate poorly to imaging findings.[10]

On CT images, the caudal fossa will appear smaller than normal, which may be best appreciated on sagittally reformatted images. Obstructive hydrocephalus and syringohydromyelia may also be seen.[3,6] Similar features will be seen on MR images, and a sagittal T2 sequence is often best for detecting ventricular and central canal distension and for recognizing cerebellar displacement and foraminal herniation (Figures 2.3.1, 2.3.2).[9-11]

Cerebellar hypoplasia

Cerebellar hypoplasia has been reported in cats as a sequela to *in utero* parvovirus infection.[12-14] The disorder has also been reported in dogs, but a distinction between cerebellar hypoplasia and cerebellar atrophy from degeneration may be challenging antemortem.[15-18] On MR images in people, the cerebellum is small and may appear to float in an expanded subarachnoid space. The number of folia may also be reduced.[19] Similar gross features have been reported in domestic animals (Figure 2.3.3).

Cerebellar vermian hypoplasia

Cerebellar vermian hypoplasia is a rare disorder in which the cerebellar vermis is hypoplastic or absent. In some patients, the cerebellar hemispheres and flocculus may also be involved and the caudal cranial fossa can be enlarged.[20] The anomaly is analogous to Dandy–Walker syndrome in people.

On unenhanced CT images, the cerebellar vermis is hypoplastic or absent, leaving a potential space filled by

Atlas of Small Animal CT and MRI, First Edition. Erik R. Wisner and Allison L. Zwingenberger.
© 2015 John Wiley & Sons, Inc. Published 2015 by John Wiley & Sons, Inc.

an expanded fourth ventricle, which is hypoattenuating compared to adjacent brain parenchyma.[21] Unenhanced MR imaging features are reported to be similar, with enlargement of the fourth ventricle appearing T1 hypointense and T2 hyperintense (Figure 2.3.4). Concurrent hydrocephalus has been reported in one dog.[22]

Diverticulation and cleavage disorders

Diverticulation and cleavage disorders include complex anomalies, such as holoprosencephaly and septo-optic dysplasia, that occur early in development and involve not only the brain but may affect the face, cranial nerves, and pituitary gland as well. Such anomalies are not well described in domestic animals since most affected animals likely die early in life. On both CT and MR images, these disorders will vary depending on the nature and severity of the anomaly.[2]

Malformations of cortical development

Malformations of cortical development represent a diverse group of developmental anomalies, including microencephaly, pachygyria–polymicrogyria, lissencephaly, and schizencephaly. These anomalies may feature variable and often reduced brain volume, cortical convolution anomalies, and cortical clefts. On both CT and MR images, the appearance of these disorders will vary depending on the nature and severity of the anomaly, although disruption of the normal contours of the cortex is a consistent feature (Figures 2.3.5, 2.3.6).[2]

Nonneoplastic cysts

Arachnoid cysts

Intracranial arachnoid cysts arise from the arachnoid membrane surrounding the brain, do not communicate with the ventricular system, and are thought to be primarily developmental (although acquired cysts are suspected to also occur). Young, small-breed brachycephalic dogs are most frequently affected, although cysts have also been reported in other canine breeds and in cats.[23–26] Arachnoid cysts most commonly arise from the quadrigeminal cistern but will occasionally occur in other locations.[24–26] Uncomplicated arachnoid cysts have a thin unicameral membrane, contain cerebrospinal fluid, and conform to the margins of adjacent structures.[23,24,26] Although many quadrigeminal arachnoid cysts are clinically silent, large cysts can produce cerebellar and occipital lobe compression leading to development of neurologic clinical signs.[24,27–29] The presence of intracystic hematomas has been reported and may lend credence to the thought that some arachnoid cysts are traumatic in origin, as described in people.[30]

On unenhanced CT images, uncomplicated intracranial arachnoid cysts have well-defined margins, contain fluid isoattenuating to cerebrospinal fluid, and do not contrast enhance (Figure 2.3.7). On MR images, cysts are clearly extraaxial, contain fluid isointense with CSF, and do not contrast enhance (Figures 2.3.8, 2.3.9).[24,26] Arachnoid cysts containing blood or organizing hematomas may have variable attenuation on CT and variable T1 and T2 signal intensity on MRI.[30]

Epidermoid and dermoid cysts

Epidermoid and dermoid cysts are rare and result from aberrant ectodermal cell migration and entrapment during neural tube closure. The most common locations are the fourth ventricle and cerebellopontine angle. Clinical signs may result from obstructive hydrocephalus.

Epidermoid cysts consist primarily of desquamated skin cells. These masses appear hypoattenuating to adjacent brain on unenhanced CT images and are T1 hypointense and T2 hyperintense on unenhanced MR images.[31,32] Epidermoid cysts would not be expected to enhance unless ruptured, producing a peripheral inflammatory response (Figure 2.3.10).

Dermoid cysts are more complex, containing hair follicles and sebaceous material that appear hypoattenuating on unenhanced CT images and T1 and T2 hyperintense on unenhanced MR images because of the lipid content. Fat-suppressed T1 sequences may be used to null the lipid signal to better characterize the lesion.[33,34] Similar to epidermoid cysts, dermoid cysts would not be expected to enhance unless ruptured, producing a peripheral inflammatory response.[33]

Figure 2.3.1 Chiari-like Malformation (Canine)

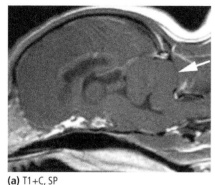

(a) T1+C, SP

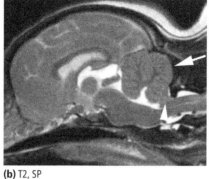

(b) T2, SP

5y F Cavalier King Charles Spaniel with intermittent neck pain and C1–C5 myelopathy. Image **c** is a magnification of image **b**. Malformation of the occipital bone (**a,b**: arrow) results in reduced caudal cranial fossa volume. Mild enlargement of the third and fourth ventricles (**a**) and sacculated cervical syringohydromyelia (**d**) are evident. Herniation of the cerebellum through the foramen magnum is best seen on sagittal T2 images (**b,c**: arrowhead).

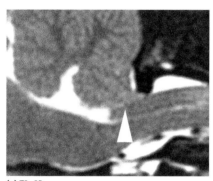

(c) T2, SP

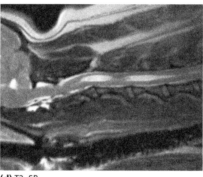

(d) T2, SP

Figure 2.3.2 Chiari-like Malformation (Canine)

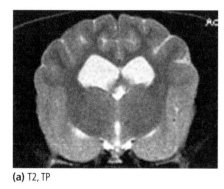

(a) T2, TP

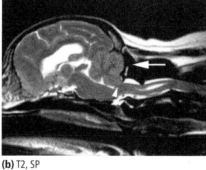

(b) T2, SP

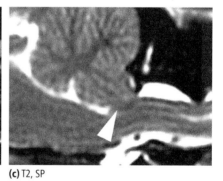

(c) T2, SP

6y MC Cavalier King Charles Spaniel with intermittent neck pain. Image **c** is a magnification of image **b**. Malformation of the occipital bone (**b**: arrow) results in reduced caudal cranial fossa volume. Ventriculomegaly and cervical syringohydromyelia are evident (**a,b**). Herniation of the cerebellum through the foramen magnum is best seen on sagittal T2 images (**b,c**: arrowhead).

Figure 2.3.3 Small Cerebellum – Probable Cerebellar Hypoplasia (Canine)   MR

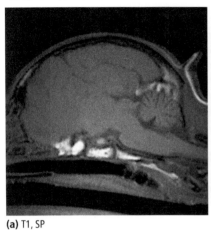

(a) T1, SP

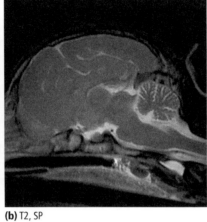

(b) T2, SP

3.5mo M Cocker Spaniel cross with neurologic signs referable to the cerebellum. The cerebellum is small, and the surface contours appear unusually well defined because of increased cerebrospinal fluid volume surrounding the cerebellar folia. The fourth ventricle and cerebellomedullary cistern are also larger than expected. This diagnosis was not confirmed by biopsy or postmortem examination.

Figure 2.3.4 Presumptive Cerebellar Vermian Hypoplasia (Canine)   MR

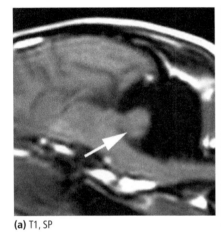

(a) T1, SP

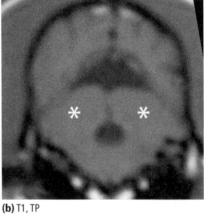

(b) T1, TP

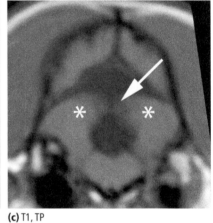

(c) T1, TP

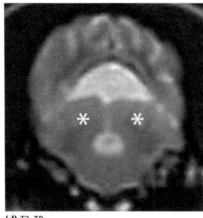

(d) T2, TP

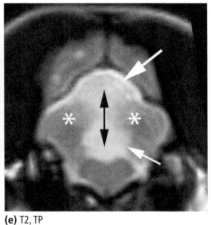

(e) T2, TP

Adult dog of unknown age and unknown clinical signs. The representative transverse images are at the level of the rostral (**b,d**) and caudal (**c,e**) cerebellum. The volume of the caudal fossa is larger than expected, and the cerebellum is markedly reduced in size (**a**: arrow). The fluid surrounding the cerebellum within the caudal fossa is likely compartmentalized cerebrospinal fluid within a grossly distended cerebellopontine cistern. Both cerebellar hemispheres are hypoplastic (**b–e**: asterisks), and the central cleft (**c**: arrow) is indicative of aplasia of the caudal aspect of the cerebellar vermis. There is free communication (**e**: black double-headed arrow) of the fourth ventricle (**e**: small arrow) with a markedly enlarged cerebellomedullary cistern (**e**: large arrow). Although not confirmed by postmortem exam, the constellation of imaging findings is characteristic of Dandy–Walker syndrome with cerebellar vermal hypoplasia/aplasia described in people.

Figure 2.3.5 Lissencephaly (Canine)   MR

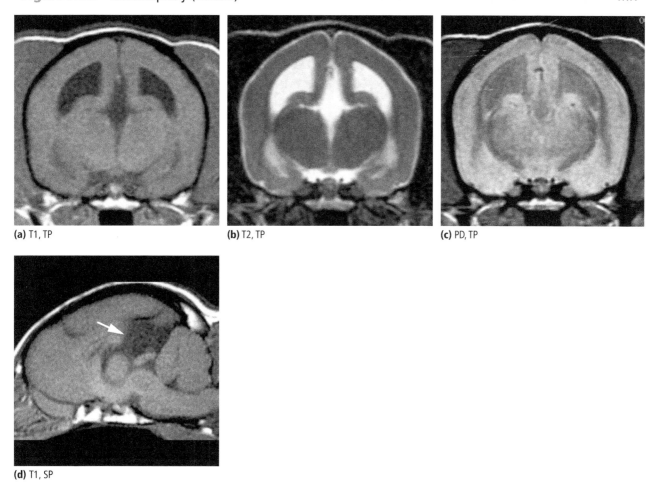

(a) T1, TP

(b) T2, TP

(c) PD, TP

(d) T1, SP

Lhasa Apso of unknown age. The normally complex surface convolutions of the cortical gyri and sulci are absent and mild, generalized hydrocephalus is present (**a–d**). In addition, there is a striking lack of white-matter architectural detail (**c**). This dog also has a quadrigeminal arachnoid cyst (**d**: arrow).

Figure 2.3.6 Complex Cortical Developmental Anomaly (Feline)   MR

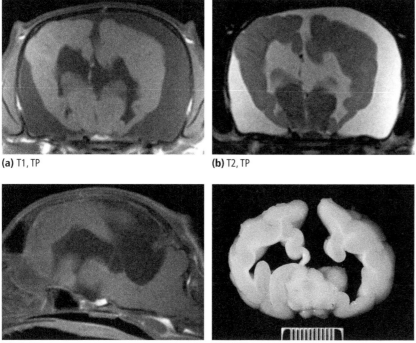

(a) T1, TP

(b) T2, TP

(c) T1, SP

(d) GP, TP

4mo F Domestic Shorthair with obtundation and rotary nystagmus. Representative transverse and parasagittal images reveal a complex brain anomaly that includes profound hydrocephalus and abnormal cortical and corpus callosum development (**a–c**). Postmortem examination documented hydrocephalus, hypoplasia of the corpus callosum, cortical gyral malformation, and pachygyria (**d**).

Figure 2.3.7 Arachnoid Cyst (Canine)   CT

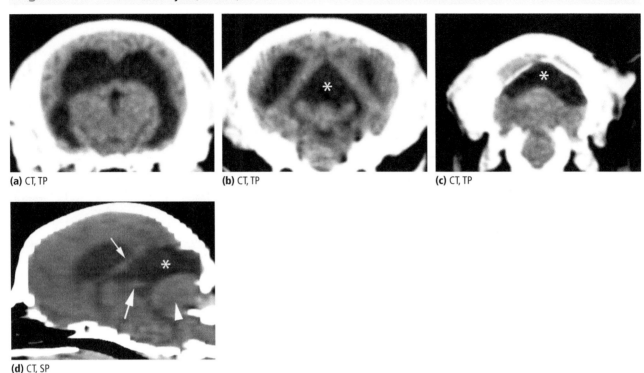

(a) CT, TP   **(b)** CT, TP   **(c)** CT, TP

(d) CT, SP

2y FS Maltese with unlocalized pain without neurologic deficits. Images **a–c** are representative transverse images of the brain at the level of the parietal lobes (**a**), occipital lobes (**b**), and cerebellum (**c**). Moderate, symmetrical lateral ventriculomegaly is present (**a**). A large, fluid-attenuating arachnoid cyst (**b–d**: asterisk) arises from the quadrigeminal cistern and is bounded ventrally by the tectum (**d**: large arrow) and cerebellum (**d**: arrowhead), rostrally by the corpus callosum (**d**: small arrow), and dorsally by the tentorium cerebelli (not seen). The cyst is predominantly subtentorial, and it displaces and compresses the cerebellum ventrally.

Figure 2.3.8 Arachnoid Cyst (Canine)   MR

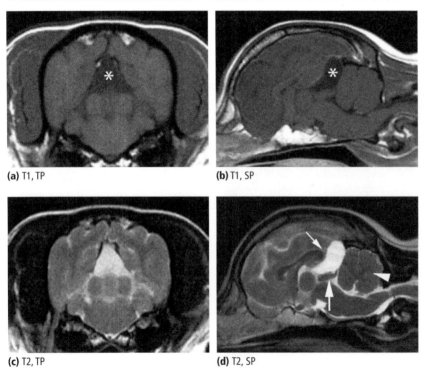

(a) T1, TP   **(b)** T1, SP

(c) T2, TP   **(d)** T2, SP

3y MC Shih Tzu with tetraparesis. The MR examination was performed to fully evaluate a diagnosed occipitoatlantoaxial malformation. Transverse images (**a,c**) are at the same level at the occipital lobes. A well-defined arachnoid cyst with pure-water signal characteristics arises from the quadrigeminal cistern (**a,b**: asterisk) and is bounded ventrally by the tectum (**d**: large arrow) and cerebellum (**d**: arrowhead), and rostrally by the corpus callosum (**d**: small arrow). Focal spinal cord narrowing and parenchymal T2 hyperintensity are also evident on image **d**, associated with the occipitoatlantoaxial malformation.

Figure 2.3.9   Arachnoid Cyst (Canine)

MR

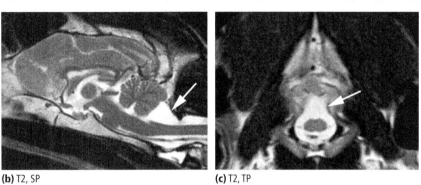

(a) T1+C, SP   **(b)** T2, SP   **(c)** T2, TP

4y M Belgian Tervuren with unclassified seizure-like activity of recent onset. Image **c** is at a level immediately rostral to the foramen magnum. A focal fluid dilation arises from the cerebellomedullary cistern (cisterna magna), ventral and caudal to the cerebellum, consistent with an arachnoid cyst (**a–c**: arrow). The location of the cyst, in combination with the elevation of the cerebellum and prominence of the third ventricle, mesencephalic duct, and fourth ventricle, suggests partial obstruction of the ventricular system.

Figure 2.3.10   Epidermoid Cyst (Canine)

MR

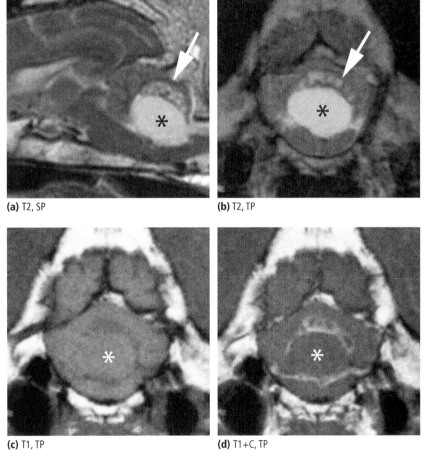

(a) T2, SP   **(b)** T2, TP

(c) T1, TP   **(d)** T1+C, TP

11y M Newfoundland with progressive neurologic deficits of 1-year duration. A large, ovoid, T2 hyperintense, T1 isointense mass is present in the caudal cranial fossa, causing rostrodorsal displacement and compression of the cerebellum and dorsal compression of the brainstem (**a–d**: asterisk). There is a complex, sessile mixed-intensity "cap" on the dorsal margin of the mass, best seen on T2 images (**a,b**: arrow). The mass nonuniformly and peripherally contrast enhances (**d**). The mass was confirmed to be an epidermoid cyst at the time of necropsy. The mass had ruptured, resulting in lipogranulomatous encephalitis surrounding the cyst, which was likely the cause for peripheral contrast enhancement on the MR examination.

References

1. Grossman RI, D.M. Y. Neuroradiology: The Requisites. Philadelphia, PA: Elsevier Inc., 2003.

2. Osborn AG. Diagnostic Imaging: Brain. Salt Lake City, UT: Amirsys Inc., 2005.

3. Cerda-Gonzalez S, Olby NJ, McCullough S, Pease AP, Broadstone R, Osborne JA. Morphology of the caudal fossa in Cavalier King Charles Spaniels. Vet Radiol Ultrasound. 2009;50:37–46.

4. Cross HR, Cappello R, Rusbridge C. Comparison of cerebral cranium volumes between cavalier King Charles spaniels with Chiari-like malformation, small breed dogs and Labradors. J Small Anim Pract. 2009;50:399–405.

5. Schmidt MJ, Kramer M, Ondreka N. Comparison of the relative occipital bone volume between Cavalier King Charles spaniels with and without syringohydromyelia and French bulldogs. Vet Radiol Ultrasound. 2012;53:540–544.

6. Schmidt MJ, Neumann AC, Amort KH, Failing K, Kramer M. Cephalometric measurements and determination of general skull type of Cavalier King Charles Spaniels. Vet Radiol Ultrasound. 2011;52:436–440.

7. Shaw TA, McGonnell IM, Driver CJ, Rusbridge C, Volk HA. Increase in cerebellar volume in Cavalier King Charles Spaniels with Chiari-like malformation and its role in the development of syringomyelia. PLoS One. 2012;7:e33660.

8. Rusbridge C, Knowler SP, Pieterse L, McFadyen AK. Chiari-like malformation in the Griffon Bruxellois. J Small Anim Pract. 2009;50:386–393.

9. Driver CJ, Rusbridge C, Cross HR, McGonnell I, Volk HA. Relationship of brain parenchyma within the caudal cranial fossa and ventricle size to syringomyelia in cavalier King Charles spaniels. J Small Anim Pract. 2010;51:382–386.

10. Lu D, Lamb CR, Pfeiffer DU, Targett MP. Neurological signs and results of magnetic resonance imaging in 40 cavalier King Charles spaniels with Chiari type 1-like malformations. Vet Rec. 2003;153:260–263.

11. Couturier J, Rault D, Cauzinille L. Chiari-like malformation and syringomyelia in normal cavalier King Charles spaniels: a multiple diagnostic imaging approach. J Small Anim Pract. 2008;49:438–443.

12. Aeffner F, Ulrich R, Schulze-Ruckamp L, Beineke A. Cerebellar hypoplasia in three sibling cats after intrauterine or early postnatal parvovirus infection. Dtsch Tierarztl Wochenschr. 2006;113:403–406.

13. Kilham L, Margolis G, Colby ED. Congenital infections of cats and ferrets by feline panleukopenia virus manifested by cerebellar hypoplasia. Lab Invest. 1967;17:465–480.

14. Sharp NJ, Davis BJ, Guy JS, Cullen JM, Steingold SF, Kornegay JN. Hydranencephaly and cerebellar hypoplasia in two kittens attributed to intrauterine parvovirus infection. J Comp Pathol. 1999;121:39–53.

15. Flegel T, Matiasek K, Henke D, Grevel V. Cerebellar cortical degeneration with selective granule cell loss in Bavarian mountain dogs. J Small Anim Pract. 2007;48:462–465.

16. Gandini G, Botteron C, Brini E, Fatzer R, Diana A, Jaggy A. Cerebellar cortical degeneration in three English bulldogs: clinical and neuropathological findings. J Small Anim Pract. 2005;46:291–294.

17. Speciale J, de Lahunta A. Cerebellar degeneration in a mature Staffordshire terrier. J Am Anim Hosp Assoc. 2003;39:459–462.

18. van der Merwe LL, Lane E. Diagnosis of cerebellar cortical degeneration in a Scottish terrier using magnetic resonance imaging. J Small Anim Pract. 2001;42:409–412.

19. Uhl M, Pawlik H, Laubenberger J, Darge K, Baborie A, Korinthenberg R, et al. MR findings in pontocerebellar hypoplasia. Pediatr Radiol. 1998;28:547–551.

20. Kornegay JN. Cerebellar vermian hypoplasia in dogs. Vet Pathol. 1986;23:374–379.

21. Lim JH, Kim DY, Yoon JH, Kim WH, Kweon OK. Cerebellar vermian hypoplasia in a Cocker Spaniel. J Vet Sci. 2008;9:215–217.

22. Schmidt MJ, Jawinski S, Wigger A, Kramer M. Imaging diagnosis – Dandy Walker malformation. Vet Radiol Ultrasound. 2008;49:264–266.

23. Kitagawa M, Kanayama K, Sakai T. Quadrigeminal cisterna arachnoid cyst diagnosed by MRI in five dogs. Aust Vet J. 2003;81:340–343.

24. Matiasek LA, Platt SR, Shaw S, Dennis R. Clinical and magnetic resonance imaging characteristics of quadrigeminal cysts in dogs. J Vet Intern Med. 2007;21:1021–1026.

25. Reed S, Cho DY, Paulsen D. Quadrigeminal arachnoid cysts in a kitten and a dog. J Vet Diagn Invest. 2009;21:707–710.

26. Vernau KM, Kortz GD, Koblik PD, LeCouteur RA, Bailey CS, Pedroia V. Magnetic resonance imaging and computed tomography characteristics of intracranial intra-arachnoid cysts in 6 dogs. Vet Radiol Ultrasound. 1997;38:171–176.

27. Dewey CW, Krotscheck U, Bailey KS, Marino DJ. Craniotomy with cystoperitoneal shunting for treatment of intracranial arachnoid cysts in dogs. Vet Surg. 2007;36:416–422.

28. Gallicchio B, Notari L. Animal behavior case of the month. Aggression in a dog caused by an arachnoid cyst. J Am Vet Med Assoc. 2010;236:1073–1075.

29. Kim JW, Jung DI, Kang BT, Kang MH, Park HM. Unilateral facial paresis secondary to a suspected brainstem arachnoid cyst in a Maltese dog. J Vet Med Sci. 2011;73:459–462.

30. Vernau KM, LeCouteur RA, Sturges BK, Samii V, Higgins RJ, Koblik PD, et al. Intracranial intra-arachnoid cyst with intracystic hemorrhage in two dogs. Vet Radiol Ultrasound. 2002;43:449–454.

31. De Decker S, Davies E, Benigni L, Wilson H, Pelligand L, Rayner EL, et al. Surgical treatment of an intracranial epidermoid cyst in a dog. Vet Surg. 2012;41:766–771.

32. Steinberg T, Matiasek K, Bruhschwein A, Fischer A. Imaging diagnosis – intracranial epidermoid cyst in a Doberman Pinscher. Vet Radiol Ultrasound. 2007;48:250–253.

33. Beard PM, Munro E, Gow AG. A quadrigeminal dermoid cyst with concurrent necrotizing granulomatous leukoencephalomyelitis in a Yorkshire Terrier dog. J Vet Diagn Invest. 2011;23:1075–1078.

34. Targett MP, McInnes E, Dennis R. Magnetic resonance imaging of a medullary dermoid cyst with secondary hydrocephalus in a dog. Vet Radiol Ultrasound. 1999;40:23–26.

2.4

Trauma, hemorrhage, and vascular disorders

Head trauma

Common causes of acute head trauma include high-impact automobile collisions, violent blunt-force and missile penetrating (gunshot) injury, bite wounds, and lower-impact injury from falls and collisions.

Skull fractures can be nondisplaced or displaced, and the latter may lead to higher brain morbidity when depressed (Figure 2.4.1). Fractures are variable in appearance and depend on both the source of trauma and the impact site. Because the neurocranium forms a rigid box, comminuted fractures are common, particularly in skeletally mature animals whose sutures have fused.

Computed tomography is generally the imaging modality of choice for initial evaluation of head injury in people because it can be rapidly performed and accurately detects skull fractures and intracranial hemorrhage. Magnetic resonance imaging is preferred when clinical signs are not explained by CT findings or in patients with subacute to chronic brain trauma.[1] Experience suggests that a similar approach should be used in veterinary patients (Figure 2.4.2).

Staging hemorrhage

Much emphasis has been placed on the importance of staging intraaxial intracranial hemorrhage in human medicine using MRI. In our experience, while it is an interesting intellectual exercise, staging of intraaxial hemorrhage in our veterinary patients is often less rewarding, as it seldom alters imaging diagnosis or patient management. In addition, while guidelines for staging intracranial hemorrhage in people are based on

accurate retrospective determination of the acute onset of a single bleeding episode, veterinary patients often have multiple sequential bleeds from a primary lesion, confounding the accuracy of staging. The information in Table 2.4.1 is extracted from the human MRI literature, but it should approximate hemorrhage-staging patterns in veterinary patients using unenhanced spin-echo T1 and T2 intensities (Figures 2.4.3, 2.4.4, 2.4.5).[2-5] In addition, T2* gradient echo sequences can be used to detect signal void from susceptibility of blood degradation products at most stages, though the susceptibility "bloom" sometimes overstates the actual hemorrhage volume. Because hematoma density is greater than that of normal brain parenchyma, acute to subacute hemorrhage is hyperattenuating compared to brain parenchyma on unenhanced CT images. Density gradually reduces to become isoattenuating with brain parenchyma over many days to weeks.[2-5]

Extraaxial hemorrhage

Extraaxial hemorrhage is classified as epidural, subdural, or subarachnoid, although in our experience subarachnoid hemorrhage is less frequently recognized.

Epidural hematoma

Epidural hematomas are most often traumatic in origin, arise in the potential space between the cranium and the dura mater, and typically occur from meningeal arterial hemorrhage. Epidural hematomas are described as having a characteristic biconvex or lenticular shape on cross-sectional images (Figure 2.4.6). Acute epidural

Atlas of Small Animal CT and MRI, First Edition. Erik R. Wisner and Allison L. Zwingenberger.
© 2015 John Wiley & Sons, Inc. Published 2015 by John Wiley & Sons, Inc.

hematomas appear hyperattenuating to brain paren-chyma on unenhanced CT images and will have variable unenhanced T1 and T2 intensity on MR images, depend-ing on the age of the hematoma.[6,7]

Subdural hematoma

Subdural hematomas are usually traumatic in origin, arise in the potential space between the dura mater and the arachnoid membrane, and typically occur as the result of venous sinus hemorrhage. Subdural hematomas are cres-cent shaped, conforming to the convex surface of the brain (Figure 2.4.7). Acute subdural hematomas will appear hyperattenuating to brain parenchyma on unenhanced CT images with a gradual reduction in density over time. They will have variable unenhanced T1 and T2 intensity on MR images, depending on the age of the hematoma.[6–8]

Subarchnoid hemorrhage

Head trauma may cause bleeding into the subarachnoid space. Acute subarachnoid hemorrhage will appear hyperattenuating and will generally conform to the convolutions of the cerebral cortex and the cisterns on unenhanced CT images. Acute subarachnoid hemor-rhage will appear T1 isointense and T2 and FLAIR hyperintense on MR images with a distribution similar to that seen on CT. Intensity patterns will change with chronicity (Figure 2.4.8).

Brain contusion and hemorrhage

Imaging features of brain contusion depend on the combination of edema and hemorrhage in the affected brain parenchyma. Edematous regions will appear hypoattenuating (Figure 2.4.1) and focal areas of hemor-rhage will appear hyperattenuating on unenhanced CT images (Figure 2.4.7). Edema will appear T1 hypointense and T2 hyperintense on MR images with hemorrhagic regions having a T2* signal void and an otherwise variable appearance depending on duration since trauma.[9,10] Edema and hemorrhage will increase brain parenchymal volume, which can lead to midline shift, ventricular compression, sulcal and gyral effacement, and brain herniation. Magnetic resonance angiography, diffusion and perfusion weighted imaging, and diffusion tensor imaging can all be used to further characterize the extent of injury.[1,11,12]

Vascular disorders

Primary intracranial vascular disease is uncommon in cats and dogs, as compared to stroke disorders in people. Stroke occurs when blood flow to the brain is disrupted, causing ischemia and eventual brain cell death. Stroke is caused by either spontaneous vascular disruption, leading to hematoma formation, or from vascular occlusion, resulting in hemorrhagic or nonhemorrhagic infarction. Vascular occlusion (ischemic infarction) may be due to either *in situ* thrombus formation or obstructing emboli originating elsewhere. Hemorrhagic ischemic infarction occurs when the mural integrity of an occluded vessel is disrupted, secondarily leading to extravasation. It may be impossible to distinguish between hemorrhagic ischemic infarction and hematoma resulting from vascular disrup-tion, as both will have similar imaging features. Most infarctions are arterial in origin, and although stroke from venous thrombosis is described in people, there are few comparable reports in veterinary medicine. The rostral and middle cerebral and the striate and rostral cerebellar arteries are the most commonly involved, and infarcts involving the cerebrum, thalamus/midbrain, and cerebel-lum have been reported.[13–17] Infarcts are described as ter-ritorial when they involve a major intracranial vessel and lacunar when smaller penetrating vessels are obstructed. Underlying causes for stroke include atherosclerosis, hypertension, and diabetes in people, although these have not been confirmed as predisposing factors in veterinary patients.[18]

Hematoma from vascular disruption

Hematomas from vascular disruption may occur as the result of vascular trauma or from spontaneous hemorrhage, as may occur with rupture of an intracra-nial vascular malformation. Imaging characteristics will vary depending on the size, location, and chronicity of the hematoma. Hematomas will generally appear as a hyperattenuating mass on unenhanced CT images, and there may be evidence of contrast enhancement if active bleeding (acute) or neovascularization (chronic) is present. MR imaging features will generally follow the scheme outlined in Table 2.4.1, although age can be ambiguous when multiple bleeding episodes occur over time. Secondary features of mass effect may include sur-rounding edema, midline shift, ventricular displacement and compression, and sulcus and gyrus effacement on both modalities (Figure 2.4.9).

Hemorrhagic infarction

Hemorrhagic infarctions may not be distinguishable from hematoma caused by vascular disruption (Figure 2.4.10). Imaging features of hematoma described above are also applicable to hemorrhagic infarction.

Nonhemorrhagic Infarction

CT imaging features of nonhemorrhagic infarction may be subtle and include focal or regional hypoattenuation from edema and variable, but often minimal, mass effect.[19]

Nonhemorrhagic infarction may appear mildly T1 hypointense and T2 hyperintense with variable mass effect involving both gray and white matter on unenhanced MR images (Figure 2.4.11). Due to restricted water diffusion, ischemic regions of the brain will appear hyperintense on diffusion-weighted images and hypointense on corresponding apparent diffusion coefficient (ADC) maps.[14] Perfusion images may define specific regions of perfusion deficit, and magnetic resonance angiographic (MRA) images can reveal relative or absolute flow deficits in affected vessels.[14,17,20] Gradient echo T2* images will display relatively little or no susceptibility effect.

Table 2.4.1   MR staging of intracranial hemorrhage.

Phase	Time	Compartment	Hemoglobin product	T1	T2
Hyperacute	<24 hours	Intracellular	Oxyhemoglobin	isointense	hyperintense
Acute	1–3 days	Intracellular	Deoxyhemoglobin	iso- to hypointense	hypointense
Early subacute	>3 days	Intracellular	Methemoglobin	hyperintense	hypointense
Late subacute	>7 days	Extracellular	Methemoglobin	hyperintense	hyperintense
Chronic	>14 days	Extracellular	Hemosiderin	hypointense	hypointense

Figure 2.4.1   Depression Fracture of Skull (Canine)   CT

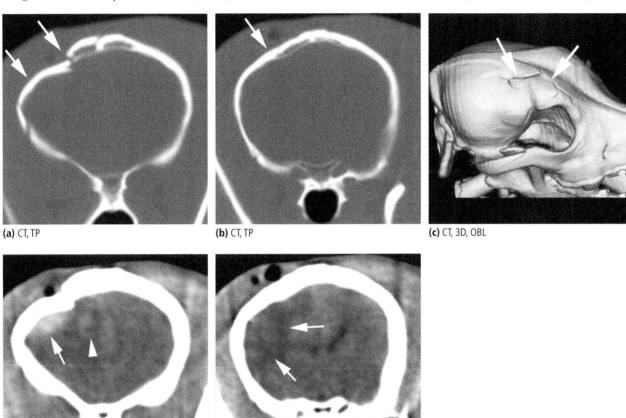

(a) CT, TP   (b) CT, TP   (c) CT, 3D, OBL

(d) CT, TP   (e) CT, TP

12y MC Jack Russell Terrier with acute head trauma following a kick to the head by a horse. The CT images were acquired approximately 8 hours after the incident. An open, comminuted depression fracture of the right frontal bone is evident on unenhanced, wide-windowed images (a–c: arrows). A focal hyperattenuating epidural hemorrhage is evident on the same unenhanced images (narrow window) adjacent to the internal surface of the largest fracture fragment (d: arrow). A smaller hyperattenuating lesion is present within the right frontal lobe, consistent with acute intraparenchymal hemorrhage (d: arrowhead). Regional hypoattenuation in the right frontal lobe is consistent with parenchymal edema (e: arrows). Decompressive craniotomy confirmed the epidural hematoma.

Figure 2.4.2   Acute Intracranial Hemorrhage (Canine)

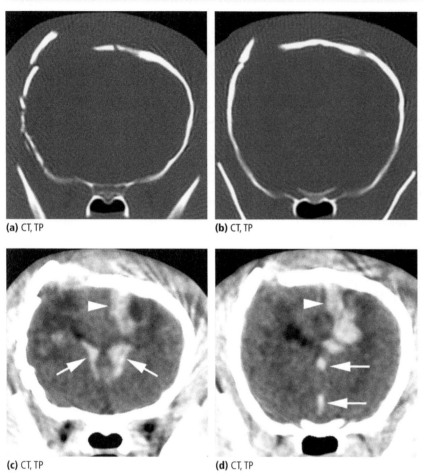

(a) CT, TP

(b) CT, TP

(c) CT, TP

(d) CT, TP

3y MC Chihuahua with acute head trauma of unknown cause. CT images were acquired approximately 36 hours after the injury. Displaced comminuted fractures of the right parietal and temporal bones are evident on unenhanced, wide-windowed images (**a,b**). The same images displayed using a soft-tissue algorithm and a narrow window reveal hyper-attenuating hemorrhage (65 HU) in the lateral (**c**: arrows) and third (**d**: arrows) ventricles. Additional hyperattenuating parenchymal hemorrhage and associated hypoattenuating edema are seen in the right and left parietal lobes (**c,d**: arrowhead).

Figure 2.4.3 Acute Intracranial Hemorrhage (Canine)

MR

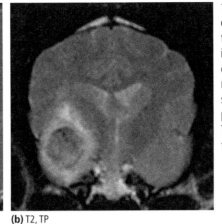

(a) T1, TP

(b) T2, TP

13y FS Corgi with a 1-day history of tonic/clonic seizures and a 2-year history of systemic hypertension. A well-delineated, T1 isointense (**a**), T2 hypointense (**b**) intraaxial cerebral mass is present in the region of the right piriform lobe. There is moderate edema surrounding the mass (**b**) as well as a thin peripheral rim of contrast enhancement (**c**). There is uniform susceptibility effect within the lesion (**d**).

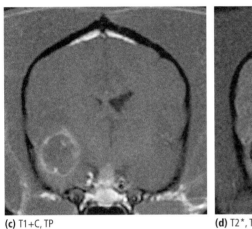

(c) T1+C, TP

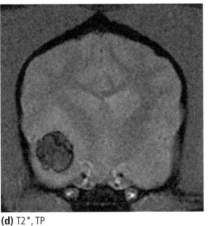

(d) T2*, TP

Figure 2.4.4 Subacute Intracranial Hemorrhage (Canine)

MR

(a) T1, TP

(b) T2, TP

(c) FL, TP

7y MC Greyhound with central nervous system deficits associated with an anesthetic recovery complication following routine dental prophylaxis performed 5 days previously. There is marked T1 hyperintensity (**a**) and mixed T2 intensity (**b**) involving the left cerebral hemisphere. The lesion involves primarily the cerebral cortex based on distribution on the T1 image, but more extensive edema involving gray and white matter is appreciated on T2 and FLAIR images (**b,c**), resulting in a midline shift. The 5-day history of intracranial signs and imaging characteristics are consistent with subacute hemorrhage.

Figure 2.4.5 Chronic Intracranial Hemorrhage (Canine)   MR

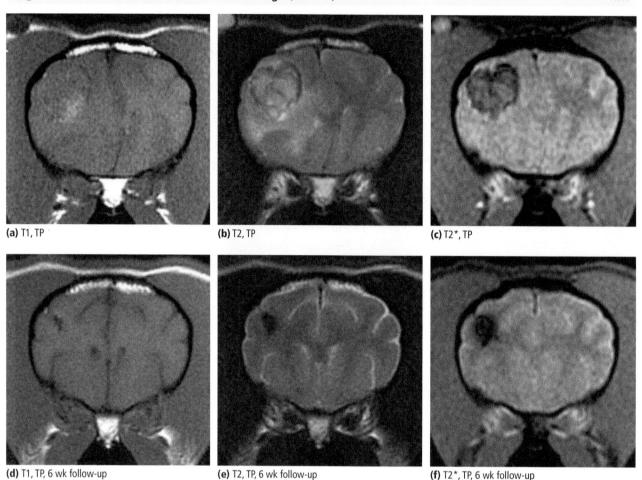

(a) T1, TP

(b) T2, TP

(c) T2*, TP

(d) T1, TP, 6 wk follow-up

(e) T2, TP, 6 wk follow-up

(f) T2*, TP, 6 wk follow-up

12y FS Poodle with 5-day history of right forebrain deficits. The initial MR examination (**a–c**) was acquired 5 days following the onset of clinical signs. The follow-up MR examination (**d–f**) was acquired approximately 6 weeks later, at which time the dog had clinically improved. On the initial examination, there is a large mass within the right frontal lobe that is T1 iso- to hyperintense (**a**) and of mixed T2 intensity (**b**). A prominent susceptibility effect is present on the T2* image (**c**). This constellation of imaging features is consistent with an acute to subacute intracranial hemorrhage, supported by the 5-day duration of clinical signs. The marked reduction in lesion volume and the uniform hypointensity evident on all imaging sequences on the second examination acquired 6 weeks later are consistent with a resolving chronic hematoma (**d–f**). A postmortem examination performed 1 year later for an unrelated cause of death revealed extensive neuropil loss and other chronic degenerative changes of the right frontal lobe consistent with residual effects of a healed infarct.

Figure 2.4.6 Acute Epidural Hemorrhage (Canine)   CT

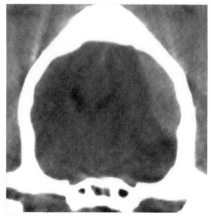

10y FS Labrador Retriever with lymphoplasmacytic encephalitis. The CT image was acquired immediately following CT-guided brain biopsy. Epidural hemorrhage is evident involving the left parietal region. The biconvex shape is consistent with an epidural hemorrhage. Although acute hemorrhage is hyperattenuating on unenhanced CT images, the increased attenuation in this patient is due, in part, to enhancement following intravenous contrast medium administration.

(a) CT+C, TP

Figure 2.4.7   Subacute Subdural Hemorrhage (Canine)

MR

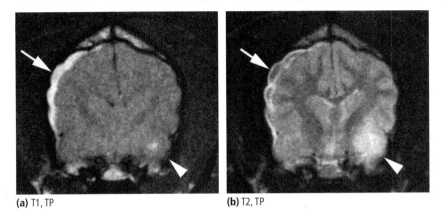

(a) T1, TP

(b) T2, TP

5y MC Mixed Breed with head trauma 4 days previously. A crescent-shaped, T1 hyperintense, right-sided subdural hematoma is present (a: arrow). The hemorrhage has central hypointensity and peripheral hyperintensity on the T2 image (b: arrow), consistent with subacute hemorrhage and the 4-day history of head trauma. A focal, nonenhancing, T1 hyperintense lesion is also present in the left pyriform lobe (a,b: arrowhead), associated with regional edema and consistent with subacute parenchymal hemorrhage. Given the location of this second lesion in relation to the subdural hematoma, it is thought to represent a contrecoup brain contusion. Necropsy confirmed both the subdural hematoma and the brain hemorrhage.

Figure 2.4.8   Multiple Compartment Intracranial Hemorrhage (Canine)

MR

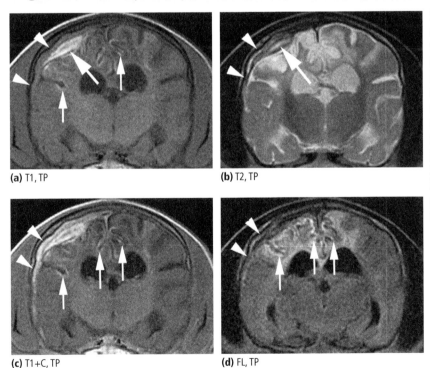

(a) T1, TP

(b) T2, TP

(c) T1+C, TP

(d) FL, TP

3mo FS Golden Retriever with acute blindness and seizures following head trauma 11 days prior to the MR examination. Signs of epidural, subdural, and subarachnoid hemorrhage are evident. Epidural hemorrhage is seen as a T1 isointense and T2 hyperintense contrast-enhancing crescent dissecting between the right hemispheric dura and parietal bone (a–d: arrowheads). Focal subdural hemorrhage is seen in the right dorsal parietal region and is T1 hyperintense and of mixed T2 intensity (a,b: large arrow). There is T1 hyperintensity and prominence of the sulci margins (a,c,d: small arrows), indicative of subarachnoid hemorrhage.

Figure 2.4.9   Intracranial Hemorrhage from Vascular Disruption or Hemorrhagic Infarction. (Canine)   CT & MR

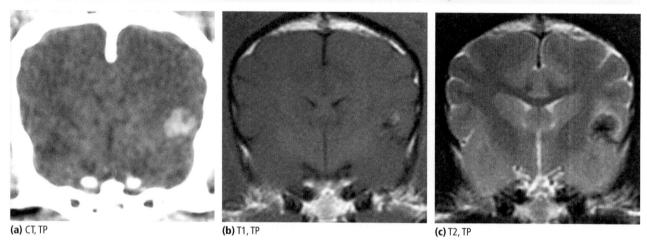

(a) CT, TP   **(b)** T1, TP   **(c)** T2, TP

12y Scottish Terrier with seizures occurring 2.5 weeks prior to the initial CT (**a**) and MR (**b,c**) examinations, which were acquired on the same day. A focal hyperattenuating subcortical lesion (65 HU) with a small hypoattenuating center is present in the left parieto-temporal region on the unenhanced CT image (**a**), consistent with acute to late subacute hemorrhage. The mixed T1 signal intensity and T2 hypointensity on the MR images are consistent with late subacute to early chronic hemorrhage and consistent with the 2.5-week delay from the onset of clinical signs. Although density of blood on CT diminishes with time, the hyperattenuation seen in this patient is also consistent with the 2.5-week staging of the hemorrhage. The lesion was thought to be a hemorrhagic infarction or spontaneous intracranial hemorrhage.

Figure 2.4.10 Hypertensive Infarction (Canine)

MR

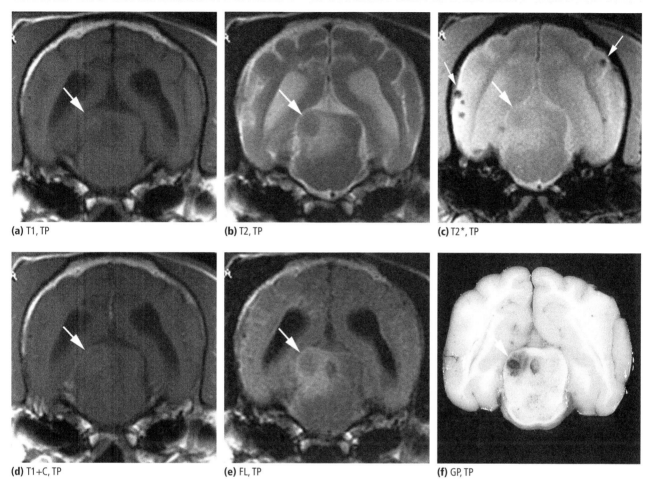

(a) T1, TP

(b) T2, TP

(c) T2*, TP

(d) T1+C, TP

(e) FL, TP

(f) GP, TP

13y FS Silky Terrier with previous diagnosis of hypertension and secondary hypertrophic cardiomyopathy. Nonambulatory for past 3 days with head tilt and hypertonic limbs. There is a T1 hyperintense, T2 isointense, minimally contrast-enhancing lesion of the right caudal colliculus with moderate surrounding edema (**a–f**: large arrow). The lesion produces minimal susceptibility artifact on the T2* gradient echo image (**c**). Additional T1, T2, and GE hypointense pinpoint lesions are evident in the cerebral cortex (**c**: small arrows). The caudal colliculus lesion is consistent with an acute to early subacute hemorrhagic infarct and is also consistent with the current 3–4-day clinical history. The hypointense cortical lesions represent resolved chronic infarcts. Both the acute and chronic vascular lesions were confirmed on postmortem examination. An acute arterial thrombus was documented at the caudal colliculus lesion site, and arterial mural hypertrophy supported systemic hypertension as the cause for the multiple intracranial infarcts.

Figure 2.4.11 Nonhemorrhagic Cerebellar Infarction (Canine) MR

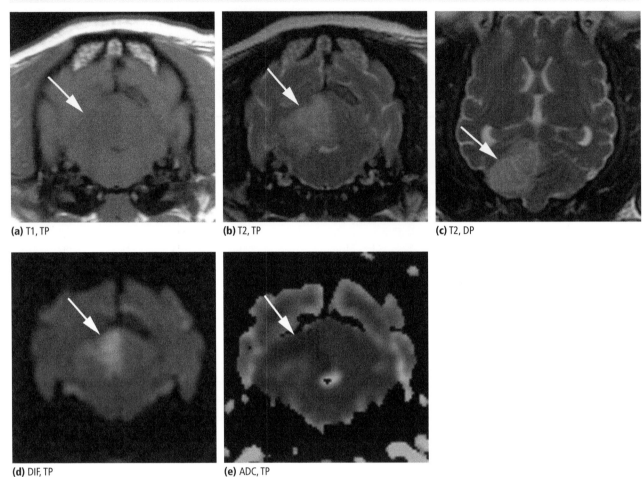

(a) T1, TP   **(b)** T2, TP   **(c)** T2, DP

(d) DIF, TP   **(e)** ADC, TP

13y FS Pug with central vestibular signs of 2-day duration. There is a well-delineated region of T1 hypointensity (**a**: arrow) and T2 hyperintensity (**b,c**: arrow) involving the right side of the cerebellum. The lesion has minimal mass effect and is not associated with other intracranial lesions. The focal area of hyperintensity on the B_{1000} diffusion image (**d**: arrow) and the corresponding region of hypointensity on the apparent diffusion coefficient map (**e**: arrow) are attributable to diffusion restriction in the ischemic tissue. MR findings and clinical signs are consistent with nonhemorrhagic cerebellar infarction caused by right rostral cerebellar artery thrombosis.

References

1. Le TH, Gean AD. Neuroimaging of traumatic brain injury. Mt Sinai J Med. 2009;76:145–162.
2. Anzalone N, Scotti R, Riva R. Neuroradiologic differential diagnosis of cerebral intraparenchymal hemorrhage. Neurol Sci. 2004;25 Suppl 1:S3–5.
3. Bradley WG, Jr. MR appearance of hemorrhage in the brain. Radiology. 1993;189:15–26.
4. Caceres JA, Goldstein JN. Intracranial hemorrhage. Emerg Med Clin North Am. 2012;30:771–794.
5. Freeman WD, Aguilar MI. Intracranial hemorrhage: diagnosis and management. Neurol Clin. 2012;30:211–240.
6. Provenzale J. CT and MR imaging of acute cranial trauma. Emerg Radiol. 2007;14:1–12.
7. Zee CS, Go JL. CT of head trauma. Neuroimaging Clin N Am. 1998;8:525–539.
8. Grundy SA, Liu SM, Davidson AP. Intracranial trauma in a dog due to being "swung" at birth. Top Companion Anim Med. 2009;24:100–103.
9. Kitagawa M, Okada M, Kanayama K, Sakai T. Traumatic intracerebral hematoma in a dog: MR images and clinical findings. J Vet Med Sci. 2005;67:843–846.
10. Tamura S, Tamura Y, Tsuka T, Uchida K. Sequential magnetic resonance imaging of an intracranial hematoma in a dog. Vet Radiol Ultrasound. 2006;47:142–144.
11. Duckworth JL, Stevens RD. Imaging brain trauma. Curr Opin Crit Care. 2010;16:92–97.
12. Kubal WS. Updated imaging of traumatic brain injury. Radiol Clin North Am. 2012;50:15–41.
13. Berg JM, Joseph RJ. Cerebellar infarcts in two dogs diagnosed with magnetic resonance imaging. J Am Anim Hosp Assoc. 2003;39:203–207.

14. Garosi L, McConnell JF, Platt SR, Barone G, Baron JC, de Lahunta A, et al. Clinical and topographic magnetic resonance characteristics of suspected brain infarction in 40 dogs. J Vet Intern Med. 2006;20:311–321.

15. Goncalves R, Carrera I, Garosi L, Smith PM, Fraser McConnell J, Penderis J. Clinical and topographic magnetic resonance imaging characteristics of suspected thalamic infarcts in 16 dogs. Vet J. 2011;188:39–43.

16. Major AC, Caine A, Rodriguez SB, Cherubini GB. Imaging diagnosis – magnetic resonance imaging findings in a dog with sequential brain infarction. Vet Radiol Ultrasound. 2012; 53:576–580.

17. McConnell JF, Garosi L, Platt SR. Magnetic resonance imaging findings of presumed cerebellar cerebrovascular accident in twelve dogs. Vet Radiol Ultrasound. 2005;46:1–10.

18. Garosi L, McConnell JE, Platt SR, Barone G, Baron JC, de Lahunta A, et al. Results of diagnostic investigations and long-term outcome of 33 dogs with brain infarction (2000–2004). J Vet Intern Med. 2005;19:725–731.

19. Paul AE, Lenard Z, Mansfield CS. Computed tomography diagnosis of eight dogs with brain infarction. Aust Vet J. 2010;88:374–380.

20. Tidwell AS, Robertson ID. Magnetic resonance imaging of normal and abnormal brain perfusion. Vet Radiol Ultrasound. 2011;52:S62–71.

2.5

Metabolic, toxic, and degenerative disorders

Inherited metabolic disorders

Lysosomal storage disorders

Lysosomal storage disorders are a group of more than 50 rare inherited diseases characterized by failure of lysosomes to metabolize lipids or glycoproteins. Most are autosomal recessive disorders that cause a single enzyme deficiency. Although the clinical presentations associated with this spectrum of diseases vary depending on the specific defect, most include central nervous system pathology and consequent neurologic clinical signs. Comprehensive coverage of these disorders is beyond the scope of this text, but we will highlight two representative examples.

Neuronal ceroid lipofuscinosis

Neuronal ceroid lipofuscinosis has been reported in many canine breeds, including Cocker Spaniels, Border Collies, American Bulldogs, Chihuahuas, Schnauzers, English Setters, Tibetan Terriers, and Polish Lowland Sheepdogs.[1–9] The underlying pathology includes generalized neuronal loss with diffuse astrogliosis. Remaining neurons contain an intracytoplasmic accumulation of yellow lipopigments.[7,8,10] Retinal cells can be similarly affected, and other organ involvement can occur. In a single case report of CT features of ceroid lipofuscinosis in a Border Collie, there was generalized cortical atrophy and ventricular dilation.[11] MR descriptions also include cortical atrophy and ventriculomegaly.[6,7,12] One citation describes intense enhancement of thickened meninges in a group of affected Chihuahuas, but this has not been reported elsewhere.[7] In our experience, there is also a loss of definition of the gray–white matter interface on proton density images and possible cerebellar atrophy (Figure 2.5.1).

Galactosialidosis

Galactosialidosis is caused by a cathepsin A mutation that results in β-galactosidase and neuraminidase deficiency. The disorder has three clinical variants and affects multiple organs, but the central nervous system is consistently involved. In people, neuropathologic features include atrophy of the optic nerve, thalamus, globus pallidus, lateral geniculate bodies, brainstem, and cerebellum.[13] Microscopic findings include neuronal loss, gliosis, and abnormal lysosomal storage in remaining neurons. A lysosomal storage disorder similar to galactosialidosis has been reported in a 5-year-old Schipperke dog with progressive cerebellar and central vestibular signs.[14] Enlarged and vacuolated neurons were seen on postmortem examination, which were documented to be due to the presence of glycolipid-laden intracytoplasmic lysosomes.

Imaging reports in people are lacking, but the MR features of the canine patient in Figure 2.5.2 with a presumptive diagnosis of galactosialidosis include cerebellar atrophy and ventriculomegaly. There was diffuse cerebellar purkinje cell and granular cell loss and extensive neuronal cytoplasmic lysosomal storage in the cerebellum and hippocampus on postmortem microscopic examination.

Acquired metabolic disorders

Thiamine deficiency

Thiamine deficiency is rare and usually results from animals being fed commercial or noncommercial diets deficient in thiamine.[15] The disorder has also been

Atlas of Small Animal CT and MRI, First Edition. Erik R. Wisner and Allison L. Zwingenberger.
© 2015 John Wiley & Sons, Inc. Published 2015 by John Wiley & Sons, Inc.

documented in dogs and cats fed commercial pet food formulations containing sulfur dioxide as a preservative.[16,17] Certain species of fish contain high levels of thiaminase, and some drugs can also induce thiamine deficiency. Clinical manifestations include neurologic, ocular, gastrointestinal, and cardiac signs.[15] As with other metabolic/toxic central nervous system disorders, specific regions of the brain are vulnerable, leading to symmetrical multifocal lesions on imaging studies. The lateral geniculate, dorsal cochlear, oculomotor, mammillary, and red nuclei and the caudal colliculi are most often involved. The cerebral cortex, cerebellar vermis, basal ganglia, and hippocampus can also be variably affected.[18,19] Microscopic pathology includes neuronal degeneration and necrosis, myelin degeneration, and secondary vascular changes.[20]

Lesions are usually well defined and bilaterally symmetric, have minimal mass-effect, appear T2 and FLAIR hyperintense, are variably T1 hypointense, and do not typically contrast enhance (Figure 2.5.3).[15,21,22] Not all vulnerable regions are affected in every patient.

Hepatic encephalopathy

MR features of the brains of dogs and cats with portosystemic shunts include T1 hyperintensity of the lentiform nuclei. These lesions are T2 isointense, do not contrast enhance, and subside following correction of portosystemic shunt (Figure 2.5.4).[23] Comparable MR lesions are described in people with chronic hepatic encephalopathy and are thought to be due to a focal accumulation of manganese, which has also been documented in dogs with the same condition.[24]

More fulminant clinical signs and MR imaging features occur with acute hepatic encephalopathy. MR findings in people include diffusion restriction, diffuse cortical T2 and FLAIR hyperintensity, and focal T2 and FLAIR hyperintensity of thalamic nuclei without contrast enhancement.[25–27] Intensity changes are due primarily to cytotoxic edema, but cortical laminar necrosis has also been described.[26,28] Similar MR features have been described in a dog with fulminant hepatic encephalopathy.[29]

Osmotic demyelination syndrome

Myelinolysis due to hypernatremia and from aggressive correction of hyponatremia has been reported in people.[30–39] Myelinolysis occurs due to a high gradient between intracellular and extracellular osmolarity, which injures cells as a result of abnormal transmembrane water transit. The general term osmotic demyelination syndrome defines the underlying pathology in both clinical conditions. In people, osmotic demyelination from rapid correction of hyponatremia occurs primarily in the central pontine region, but other sites have also been reported.[30,34,36,38] Hypernatremic osmotic demyelination, however, occurs both in the pons and in extrapontine locations, including white matter, corpus callosum, basal ganglia, hippocampus, cerebellum, and cortex.[33] Clinical signs vary depending on the vulnerable tissues affected but include neurocognitive changes and motor dysfunction. MR features of acute disease include focal or multifocal, T1 hypointense and T2 and FLAIR hyperintense lesions in the anatomic locations listed above and diffusion restriction on diffusion-weighted imaging. Lesions typically do not enhance.[28] Demyelination similar to that seen in people has been described in both the dog and cat (Figure 2.5.5).[40,41]

Peri-ictal encephalopathy

In people, MR imaging performed within a few days of generalized seizures reveals transient diffusion restriction, swelling, and T2 hyperintensity of cortical gray matter, subcortical white matter, and hippocampus. These changes are ascribed to seizure-induced transient vasogenic and cytotoxic edema.[42] MR features of peri-ictal encephalopathy in dogs have also been reported.[43] MR imaging features within 14 days of seizuring included variable T1 hypointensity and T2 hyperintensity of the piriform and temporal lobes (Figure 2.5.6). Contrast enhancement of the lesions occurred in only one dog, and lesions resolved within 10–16 weeks after the initial MR examinations. Microscopic features included edema, neovascularization, reactive astrocytosis, and acute neuronal necrosis and were similar to those reported in people. In our experience, lesion distribution may extend beyond the piriform and temporal lobes.

Toxic disorders

Radiation-induced brain injury

Neurotoxic effects of brain irradiation can be divided into an acute response, characterized by reversible vasogenic edema; an early delayed response (1–4 months following irradiation), involving edema and demyelination; and a late delayed response that includes irreversible vascular changes and necrotizing leukoencephalopathy.[44–46] Focal, multifocal, or diffuse T1 hypointensity and T2 hyperintensity may be seen associated with vasogenic edema or necrotizing leukoencephalopathy depending on the timing, irradiation target, and severity of radiation-induced injury. Necrotic regions may nonuniformly contrast enhance (Figure 2.5.7).[28] Late-phase responses can also include multifocal T2* susceptibility effects from lacunar infarction (Figure 2.5.8).[46]

Exogenous toxins

Neurotoxicity can occur from consumption of recognized toxins or from adverse effects of pharmaceuticals. The list of neurotoxins that affect the brain is extensive, and many do not produce pathology detectable with neuroimaging techniques. Clinically, exposure to a neurotoxin may not be recognized; therefore, diagnoses are often speculative and rarely confirmed. Comprehensive coverage of neurotoxicity is beyond the scope of this text, but we will highlight one representative example.

Metronidazole toxicity

Metronidazole has been documented to induce neurotoxicity in both dogs and cats.[47–49] Although clinical signs in the dog are referable primarily to the cerebellum, neurologic signs in the cat seem to be less specific.[47–49] MR imaging features of metronidazole toxicity in people include focal T2 and FLAIR hyperintensity, primarily in the dentate and other cerebellar nuclei, although similar lesions have been described in other regions of the brain. Lesions do not contrast enhance and resolve after discontinuation of the drug.[50,51] Although imaging findings of metronidazole toxicity have not been well described for dogs or cats, our limited experience suggests MR features are similar to those in people (Figure 2.5.9).

Degenerative disorders

Age-related degeneration

Gross changes in the brain that occur from age-related degeneration include cortical and hippocampal atrophy and ventricular enlargement.[52–55] The frontal lobes are particularly vulnerable, decreasing in volume disproportionately more than other parts of the cerebrum.[54,55] Underlying pathology includes neuronal loss due to accumulation of toxic proteins, oxidative damage, and cerebrovascular pathology.[53] CT and MR features include enlargement of the ventricular system and prominence of the brain cortical margins and sulci on T1 and T2 images due to expansion of subarachnoid space volume (Figure 2.5.10).[56]

Other degenerative disorders

Neurodegenerative disorders of the brain often have a known underlying cause, such as an inborn error of metabolism (lysosomal storage disorders) or an acquired metabolic, inflammatory, or toxic source, and the degenerative pathology represents an end stage of disease. Although each neurodegenerative disorder has specific pathologic characteristics, common features include neuronal loss with associated volume reduction, demyelination, and cavitation from tissue necrosis. Examples of reported neurodegenerative disorders in dogs and cats include neuroaxonal dystrophy,[57–59] leukoencephalomyelopathy,[60–65] and Alaskan Husky encephalopathy[66–68] (Figure 2.5.11).

Figure 2.5.1 Ceroid Lipofuscinosis (Canine)

MR

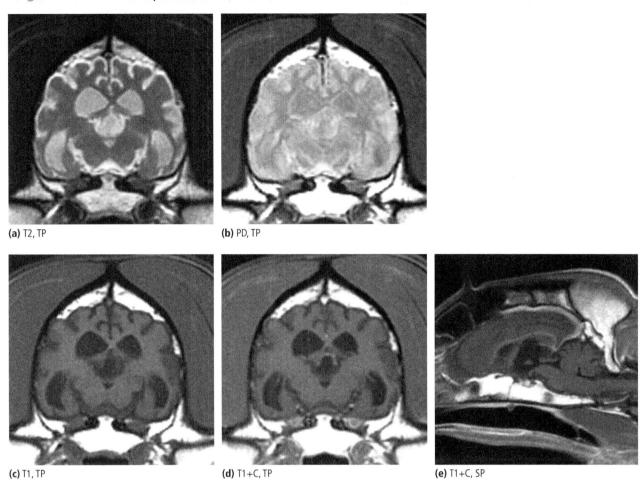

(a) T2, TP

(b) PD, TP

(c) T1, TP

(d) T1+C, TP

(e) T1+C, SP

2y MC Border Collie cross with 4-month history of progressive behavior changes, ataxia, and incoordination. There is generalized reduction in cerebral and cerebellar volume with concomitant generalized ventriculomegaly and prominence of the subarachnoid space due to gyral atrophy and sulcal widening (a,c–e). There is also loss of white and gray matter definition on the proton density image (b). Postmortem examination revealed neuronal accumulation of eosinophilic granular intracytoplasmic material. The material was autofluorescent and stained positive with PAS, LFB, and Sudan black B, all of which supported the diagnosis of neuronal ceroid lipofuscinosis.

Figure 2.5.2 Presumptive Galactosialidosis (Canine)

MR

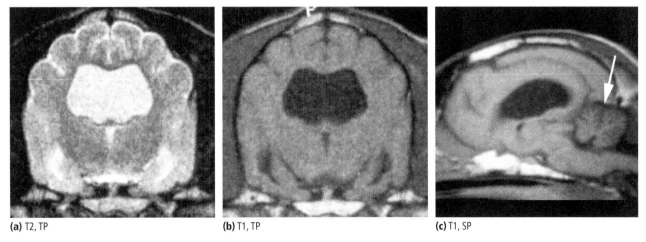

(a) T2, TP

(b) T1, TP

(c) T1, SP

3y MC Schipperke with 2-year history of progressive ataxia and intermittent seizures. There is marked symmetrical ventriculomegaly (a–c). The cerebellum is smaller than expected with greater definition of the folia due to atrophy and consequent expansion of the surrounding CSF volume (c: arrow). Postmortem examination revealed cerebellar atrophy associated with marked Purkinje and granular cell loss. There was also extensive neuronal lysosomal storage, noted in both the cerebellum and cerebrum. Although the diagnosis was not further documented, pathologic features in this patient were similar to those previously reported in another Schipperke with documented galactosialidosis.[14]

Figure 2.5.3 Presumptive Thiamine Deficiency (Feline)   MR

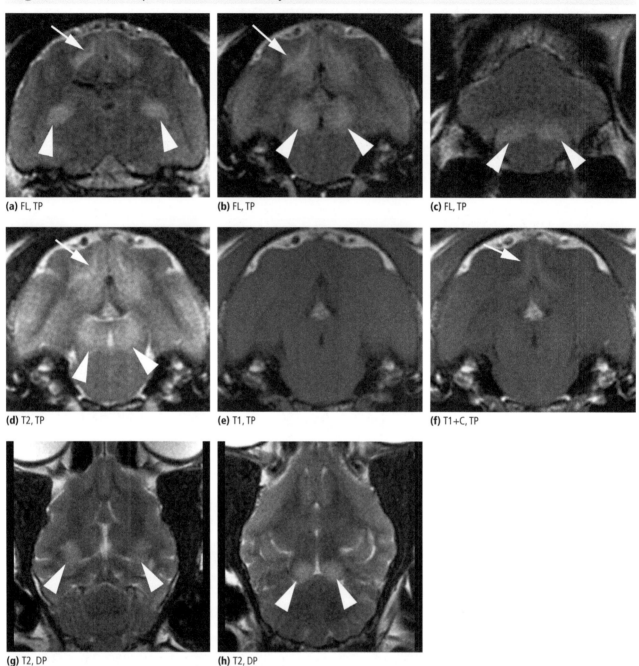

(a) FL, TP   **(b)** FL, TP   **(c)** FL, TP

(d) T2, TP   **(e)** T1, TP   **(f)** T1+C, TP

(g) T2, DP   **(h)** T2, DP

14y MC Domestic Shorthair with 2-day history of inappetence, vomiting, and ataxia. Neurologic examination revealed multifocal neurological deficits involving the cerebellum, brainstem, and cerebrum. There are focal regions of T2 and FLAIR hyperintensity involving the lateral geniculate nuclei (**a,g**: arrowheads), the caudal colliculi (**b,d,h**: arrowheads), and vestibular nuclei (**c**: arrowheads). Other thalamic nuclei were similarly affected (not shown). There is also ill-defined T2 and FLAIR hyperintensity of the axial regions of the parietal and occipital cortex (**a,b,d**: arrow), which enhance following contrast administration (**f**: arrow). These MR features are characteristic of multifocal polioencephalopathy due to thiamine deficiency. Further questioning of the owner revealed the cat had been fed an almost exclusively meat diet. Clinical signs resolved with dietary change and thiamine supplementation.

Figure 2.5.4 Chronic Hepatic Insufficiency from Portosystemic Shunt (Canine)   MR

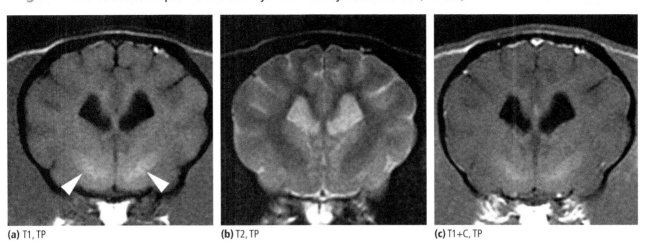

(a) T1, TP   **(b)** T2, TP   **(c)** T1+C, TP

6mo FS Shih Tzu with a single extrahepatic portosystemic shunt. Has infrequent seizures but is otherwise neurologically normal. Ill-defined bilateral T1 hyperintensity in the lentiform nuclei is seen (a: arrowheads). There is no corresponding change on T2 images (b) and no evidence of enhancement following contrast administration (c). These lesions are consistent with those described in dogs with liver insufficiency due to portosystemic shunting. The T1 hyperintensity is due to manganese accumulation.

Figure 2.5.5 Presumptive Osmotic Demyelination (Canine)   MR

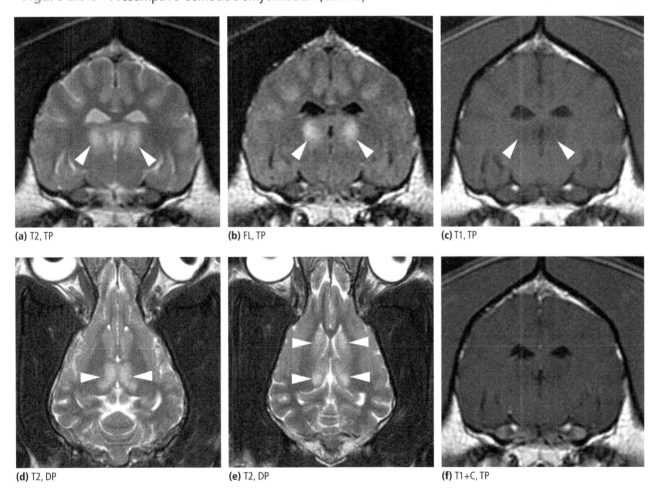

(a) T2, TP   **(b)** FL, TP   **(c)** T1, TP

(d) T2, DP   **(e)** T2, DP   **(f)** T1+C, TP

6y MC Golden Retriever with a recent history of consuming a large quantity of ocean water with subsequent progressive lethargy, ataxia, and seizures. Serum sodium at the time of admission was 191 mmol/l (normal range is 145–154 mmol/l). There are well-defined, focal, and symmetrical T2 and FLAIR hyperintense and T1 hypointense lesions involving the basal ganglia and thalamus (a–e: arrowheads). Diffuse, nonuniformly distributed, bihemispheric T2 and FLAIR hyperintensity and T1 hypointensity is seen in the cerebral cortex (a–c). Lesions do not enhance following contrast administration. The dog gradually responded to therapy. Although MR lesions were not confirmed, they are consistent with MR features described in people with hypernatremic osmotic demyelination.

Figure 2.5.6   Peri-ictal Encephalopathy (Canine)   MR

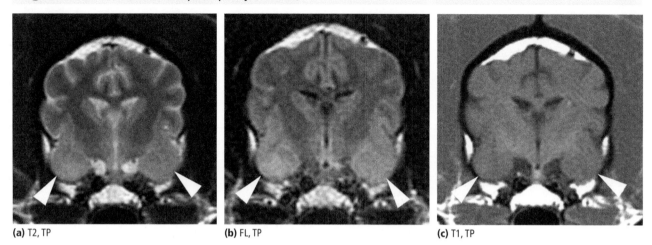

(a) T2, TP   **(b)** FL, TP   **(c)** T1, TP

7y MC crossbreed with frequent generalized seizures for the past 48 hours. There is moderate ill-defined T2 and FLAIR hyperintensity and T1 hypointensity involving both piriform lobes (**a–c**: arrowheads). No other abnormalities were seen on this examination, and the dog responded to medical management of seizures.

Figure 2.5.7   Early-delayed and Late-delayed Radiation Effects (Canine)   MR

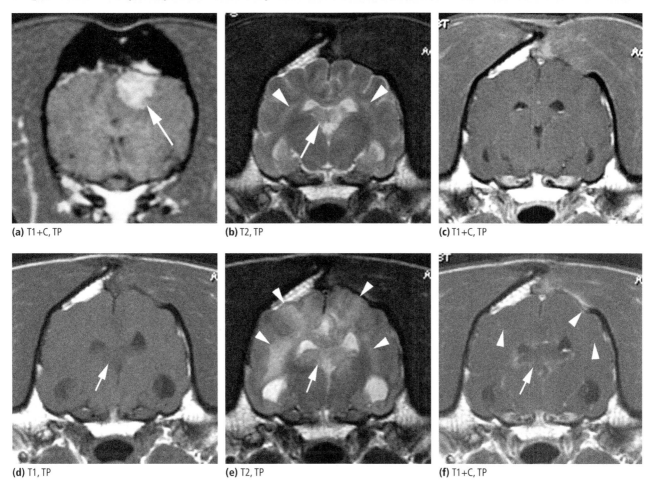

(a) T1+C, TP

(b) T2, TP

(c) T1+C, TP

(d) T1, TP

(e) T2, TP

(f) T1+C, TP

10y FS Border Collie with a frontal lobe meningioma that was incompletely surgically excised. A well-defined, uniformly contrast-enhancing extraaxial mass is seen in the region of the left frontal lobe on a preoperative MR examination (**a**: arrow). On an MR examination acquired 14 weeks following completion of a course of postoperative radiation therapy (**b,c**), there is evidence of T2 hyperintensity due to white matter edema in both cerebral hemispheres (**b**: arrowheads) and in the corpus callosum (**b**: arrow) with no evidence of contrast enhancement (**c**). On a second postoperative MR examination acquired 21 weeks following completion of radiation therapy (**d–f**), cerebral T2 hyperintensity has increased and involves both white and gray matter (**e**: arrowheads). The corpus callosum is T2 hyperintense and T1 hypointense (**d,e**: arrow) and appears larger than in the previous examination. There is irregular enhancement in this region (**f**: arrow) and in the meninges (**f**: arrowheads) following contrast administration. Postmortem examination findings were consistent with delayed radiation effects, including severe encephalomalacia, primarily affecting the white matter, but also extending into the adjacent gray matter, and lymphocytic perivascular encephalitis located within the cerebrum surrounding the ventricular system. White matter was necrotic with a neutrophilic inflammatory response. Vessels within the region had fibrinonecrosis of their walls with some vasculitis and numerous fibrin thrombi.

Figure 2.5.8 Late-delayed Radiation Effects (Canine)   MR

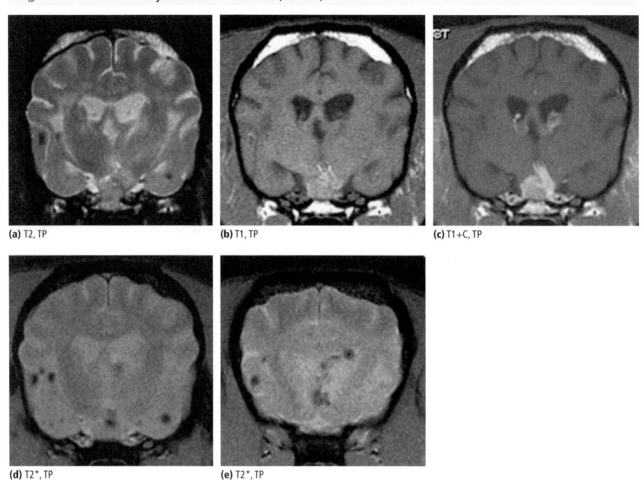

(a) T2, TP   **(b)** T1, TP   **(c)** T1+C, TP

(d) T2*, TP   **(e)** T2*, TP

10y MC Boston Terrier who underwent radiation therapy for a pituitary tumor 18 months previously. There is ill-defined, bihemispheric, white-matter T2 hyperintensity and T1 hypointensity (**a,b**). There are multiple focal signal voids in the deep gray matter and at the cerebral cortical gray–white matter interface, best seen on T2* images (**d,e**). The residual pituitary tumor is best seen on the contrast-enhanced T1 image (**c**). The signal voids represent susceptibility effect from multiple lacunar infarcts from the vascular effects of irradiation. The white matter T2 hyperintensity is consistent with necrotizing leukoencephalopathy.

Figure 2.5.9   Presumptive Metronidazole Toxicity (Canine)   MR

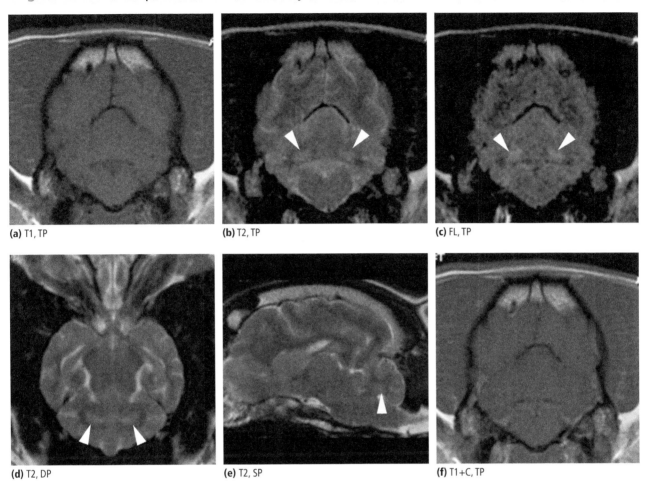

(a) T1, TP

(b) T2, TP

(c) FL, TP

(d) T2, DP

(e) T2, SP

(f) T1+C, TP

11y FS Poodle with a history of inflammatory bowel disease being treated long-term with metronidazole. Current neurologic signs include nystagmus and rolling. Symmetrical T2 and FLAIR hyperintensity of the dentate nuclei is present (**b–e**: arrowheads). There is no visible abnormality on the unenhanced T1 image (**a**) and no evidence of contrast enhancement (**f**). MR features are consistent with metronidazole neurotoxicity, and both serum and cerebrospinal fluid were positive for metronidazole on liquid chromatography/mass spectrometry analysis.

Figure 2.5.10   Age-related Degeneration (Canine)   MR

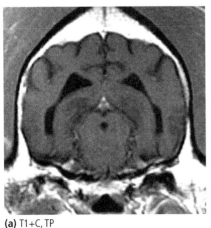

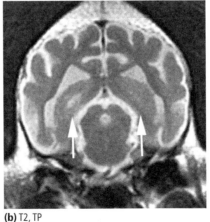

(a) T1+C, TP

(b) T2, TP

12y MC Shiba Inu with left-sided vestibular signs. There is prominence of the subarachnoid space and lateral ventricles due to cortical atrophy (**a,b**). The cortical mantle is thin, and gyri are smaller than expected. The hippocampus also appears small with central foci of increased T2 intensity (**b**: arrows). No other abnormalities were detected on the MR examination, and clinical signs resolved after approximately 2 weeks.

Figure 2.5.11 Alaskan Husky Encephalopathy (Canine)   MR

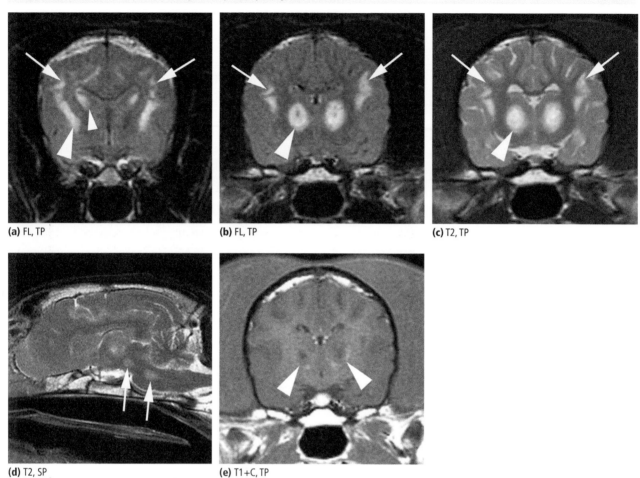

(a) FL, TP   **(b)** FL, TP   **(c)** T2, TP

(d) T2, SP   **(e)** T1+C, TP

9mo MC Alaskan Husky with ataxia, tetraparesis, and absent postural reactions. There are multiple focal T2 and FLAIR hyperintense lesions in the caudate nucleus (**a**: small arrowhead), putamen (**a**: large arrowhead), thalamus (**b,c**: arrowhead), red nucleus, and medulla (**d**: arrows). There are also ill-defined regions of T2 and FLAIR hyperintensity at the gray–white matter interface of the cerebrum (**a–c**: arrows). Thalamic lesions minimally and peripherally contrast enhance (**e**: arrowheads). Postmortem examination revealed severe bilaterally symmetrical encephalomalacia involving basal nuclei, thalamus, midbrain, pons, cerebral cortex, and cerebellar vermis gray matter, consistent with Alaskan Husky encephalopathy.

References

1. Evans J, Katz ML, Levesque D, Shelton GD, de Lahunta A, O'Brien D. A variant form of neuronal ceroid lipofuscinosis in American bulldogs. J Vet Intern Med. 2005;19:44–51.

2. Jolly RD, Hartley WJ, Jones BR, Johnstone AC, Palmer AC, Blakemore WF. Generalised ceroid-lipofuscinosis and brown bowel syndrome in Cocker spaniel dogs. N Z Vet J. 1994;42:236–239.

3. Jolly RD, Sutton RH, Smith RI, Palmer DN. Ceroid-lipofuscinosis in miniature Schnauzer dogs. Aust Vet J. 1997;75:67.

4. Katz ML, Khan S, Awano T, Shahid SA, Siakotos AN, Johnson GS. A mutation in the CLN8 gene in English Setter dogs with neuronal ceroid-lipofuscinosis. Biochem Biophys Res Commun. 2005; 327:541–547.

5. Katz ML, Narfstrom K, Johnson GS, O'Brien DP. Assessment of retinal function and characterization of lysosomal storage body accumulation in the retinas and brains of Tibetan Terriers with ceroid-lipofuscinosis. Am J Vet Res. 2005;66:67–76.

6. Koie H, Shibuya H, Sato T, Sato A, Nawa K, Nawa Y, et al. Magnetic resonance imaging of neuronal ceroid lipofuscinosis in a border collie. J Vet Med Sci. 2004;66:1453–1456.

7. Nakamoto Y, Yamato O, Uchida K, Nibe K, Tamura S, Ozawa T, et al. Neuronal ceroid-lipofuscinosis in longhaired Chihuahuas: clinical, pathologic, and MRI findings. J Am Anim Hosp Assoc. 2011;47:e64–70.

8. Narfstrom K, Wrigstad A, Ekesten B, Berg AL. Neuronal ceroid lipofuscinosis: clinical and morphologic findings in nine affected Polish Owczarek Nizinny (PON) dogs. Vet Ophthalmol. 2007; 10:111–120.

9. O'Brien DP, Katz ML. Neuronal ceroid lipofuscinosis in 3 Australian shepherd littermates. J Vet Intern Med. 2008;22: 472–475.

10. Kuwamura M, Hattori R, Yamate J, Kotani T, Sasai K. Neuronal ceroid-lipofuscinosis and hydrocephalus in a chihuahua. J Small Anim Pract. 2003;44:227–230.

11. Franks JN, Dewey CW, Walker MA, Storts RW. Computed tomographic findings of ceroid lipofuscinosis in a dog. J Am Anim Hosp Assoc. 1999;35:430–435.

12. Asakawa MG, MacKillop E, Olby NJ, Robertson ID, Cullen JM. Imaging diagnosis – neuronal ceroid lipofuscinosis with a chronic subdural hematoma. Vet Radiol Ultrasound. 2010;51:155–158.

13. Suzuki K, Suzuki K. Lysosomal Diseases. In: Love S, Louis DN (eds): Greenfield's Neuropathology. London: Hodder Arnold, 2008;561.

14. Knowles K, Alroy J, Castagnaro M, Raghavan SS, Jakowski RM, Freden GO. Adult-onset lysosomal storage disease in a Schipperke dog: clinical, morphological and biochemical studies. Acta Neuropathol. 1993;86:306–312.

15. Markovich JE, Heinze CR, Freeman LM. Thiamine deficiency in dogs and cats. J Am Vet Med Assoc. 2013;243:649–656.

16. Malik R, Sibraa D. Thiamine deficiency due to sulphur dioxide preservative in 'pet meat' – a case of deja vu. Aust Vet J. 2005;83: 408–411.

17. Studdert VP, Labuc RH. Thiamin deficiency in cats and dogs associated with feeding meat preserved with sulphur dioxide. Aust Vet J. 1991;68:54–57.

18. Read DH, Harrington DD. Experimentally induced thiamine deficiency in beagle dogs: pathologic changes of the central nervous system. Am J Vet Res. 1986;47:2281–2289.

19. Read DH, Jolly RD, Alley MR. Polioencephalomalacia of dogs with thiamine deficiency. Vet Pathol. 1977;14:103–112.

20. Zachary JF. Nervous System. In: McGavin MD, Zachary JF (eds): Pathologic Basis of Veterinary Disease. St. Louis: Mosby Elsevier, 2007;912–913.

21. Garosi LS, Dennis R, Platt SR, Corletto F, de Lahunta A, Jakobs C. Thiamine deficiency in a dog: clinical, clinicopathologic, and magnetic resonance imaging findings. J Vet Intern Med. 2003; 17:719–723.

22. Penderis J, McConnell JF, Calvin J. Magnetic resonance imaging features of thiamine deficiency in a cat. Vet Rec. 2007;160: 270–272.

23. Torisu S, Washizu M, Hasegawa D, Orima H. Brain magnetic resonance imaging characteristics in dogs and cats with congenital portosystemic shunts. Vet Radiol Ultrasound. 2005;46:447–451.

24. Torisu S, Washizu M, Hasegawa D, Orima H. Measurement of brain trace elements in a dog with a portosystemic shunt: relation between hyperintensity on T1-weighted magnetic resonance images in lentiform nuclei and brain trace elements. J Vet Med Sci. 2008;70:1391–1393.

25. Bindu PS, Sinha S, Taly AB, Christopher R, Kovoor JM. Cranial MRI in acute hyperammonemic encephalopathy. Pediatr Neurol. 2009;41:139–142.

26. Choi JM, Kim YH, Roh SY. Acute hepatic encephalopathy presenting as cortical laminar necrosis: case report. Korean J Radiol. 2013;14:324–328.

27. Rosario M, McMahon K, Finelli PF. Diffusion-weighted imaging in acute hyperammonemic encephalopathy. Neurohospitalist. 2013;3:125–130.

28. Oborn AG. Diagnostic Imaging: Brain. Salt Lake City: Amirsis Inc., 2005.

29. Moon SJ, Kim JW, Kang BT, Lim CY, Park HM. Magnetic resonance imaging findings of hepatic encephalopathy in a dog with a portosystemic shunt. J Vet Med Sci. 2012;74:361–366.

30. Brown WD. Osmotic demyelination disorders: central pontine and extrapontine myelinolysis. Curr Opin Neurol. 2000;13:691–697.

31. Garcia-Monco JC, Cortina IE, Ferreira E, Martinez A, Ruiz L, Cabrera A, et al. Reversible splenial lesion syndrome (RESLES): what's in a name? J Neuroimaging. 2011;21:e1–14.

32. Go M, Amino A, Shindo K, Tsunoda S, Shiozawa Z. [A case of central pontine myelinolysis and extrapontine myelinolysis during rapid correction of hypernatremia]. Rinsho Shinkeigaku. 1994;34:1130–1135.

33. Ismail FY, Szollics A, Szolics M, Nagelkerke N, Ljubisavljevic M. Clinical semiology and neuroradiologic correlates of acute hypernatremic osmotic challenge in adults: a literature review. AJNR Am J Neuroradiol. 2013;34:225–2232.

34. King JD, Rosner MH. Osmotic demyelination syndrome. Am J Med Sci. 2010;339:561–567.

35. Kleinschmidt-Demasters BK, Rojiani AM, Filley CM. Central and extrapontine myelinolysis: then…and now. J Neuropathol Exp Neurol. 2006;65:1–11.

36. Lampl C, Yazdi K. Central pontine myelinolysis. Eur Neurol. 2002;47:3–10.

37. Lin SH, Hsu YJ, Chiu JS, Chu SJ, Davids MR, Halperin ML. Osmotic demyelination syndrome: a potentially avoidable disaster. QJM. 2003;96:935–947.

38. Martin RJ. Central pontine and extrapontine myelinolysis: the osmotic demyelination syndromes. J Neurol Neurosurg Psychiatry. 2004;75 Suppl 3:22–28.

39. Vaidya C, Ho W, Freda BJ. Management of hyponatremia: providing treatment and avoiding harm. Cleve Clin J Med. 2010;77: 715–726.

40. O'Brien DP, Kroll RA, Johnson GC, Covert SJ, Nelson MJ. Myelinolysis after correction of hyponatremia in two dogs. J Vet Intern Med. 1994;8:40–48.

41. Poncelet L, Salmon I, Jolly S, Summers BA. Primary bilateral pontine demyelination in a cat with similarity to central pontine myelinolysis. Vet Pathol. 2011;48:751–753.

42. Kim JA, Chung JI, Yoon PH, Kim DI, Chung TS, Kim EJ, et al. Transient MR signal changes in patients with generalized tonicoclonic seizure or status epilepticus: periictal diffusion-weighted imaging. AJNR Am J Neuroradiol. 2001;22: 1149–1160.

43. Mellema LM, Koblik PD, Kortz GD, LeCouteur RA, Chechowitz MA, Dickinson PJ. Reversible magnetic resonance imaging abnormalities in dogs following seizures. Vet Radiol Ultrasound. 1999;40:588–595.

44. Kim JH, Brown SL, Jenrow KA, Ryu S. Mechanisms of radiation-induced brain toxicity and implications for future clinical trials. J Neurooncol. 2008;87:279–286.

45. Siu A, Wind JJ, Iorgulescu JB, Chan TA, Yamada Y, Sherman JH. Radiation necrosis following treatment of high grade glioma – a review of the literature and current understanding. Acta Neurochir (Wien). 2012;154:191–201.

46. Tanino T, Kanasaki Y, Tahara T, Michimoto K, Kodani K, Kakite S, et al. Radiation-induced microbleeds after cranial irradiation: evaluation by phase-sensitive magnetic resonance imaging with 3.0 tesla. Yonago Acta Med. 2013;56:7–12.

47. Caylor KB, Cassimatis MK. Metronidazole neurotoxicosis in two cats. J Am Anim Hosp Assoc. 2001;37:258–262.

48. Dow SW, LeCouteur RA, Poss ML, Beadleston D. Central nervous system toxicosis associated with metronidazole treatment of dogs: five cases (1984–1987). J Am Vet Med Assoc. 1989;195:365–368.

49. Olson EJ, Morales SC, McVey AS, Hayden DW. Putative metronidazole neurotoxicosis in a cat. Vet Pathol. 2005;42:665–669.

50. Kuriyama A, Jackson JL, Doi A, Kamiya T. Metronidazole-induced central nervous system toxicity: a systematic review. Clin Neuropharmacol. 2011;34:241–247.

51. Patel K, Green-Hopkins I, Lu S, Tunkel AR. Cerebellar ataxia following prolonged use of metronidazole: case report and literature review. Int J Infect Dis. 2008;12:e111–114.

52. Dimakopoulos AC, Mayer RJ. Aspects of neurodegeneration in the canine brain. J Nutr. 2002;132:1579S–1582S.

53. Head E. Neurobiology of the aging dog. Age (Dordr). 2011;33:485–496.

54. Su MY, Tapp PD, Vu L, Chen YF, Chu Y, Muggenburg B, et al. A longitudinal study of brain morphometrics using serial magnetic resonance imaging analysis in a canine model of aging. Prog Neuropsychopharmacol Biol Psychiatry. 2005;29:389–397.

55. Tapp PD, Siwak CT, Gao FQ, Chiou JY, Black SE, Head E, et al. Frontal lobe volume, function, and beta-amyloid pathology in a canine model of aging. J Neurosci. 2004;24:8205–8213.

56. Pugliese M, Carrasco JL, Gomez-Anson B, Andrade C, Zamora A, Rodriguez MJ, et al. Magnetic resonance imaging of cerebral involutional changes in dogs as markers of aging: an innovative tool adapted from a human visual rating scale. Vet J. 2010;186:166–171.

57. Diaz JV, Duque C, Geisel R. Neuroaxonal dystrophy in dogs: case report in 2 litters of Papillon puppies. J Vet Intern Med. 2007;21:531–534.

58. Fyfe JC, Al-Tamimi RA, Castellani RJ, Rosenstein D, Goldowitz D, Henthorn PS. Inherited neuroaxonal dystrophy in dogs causing lethal, fetal-onset motor system dysfunction and cerebellar hypoplasia. J Comp Neurol. 2010;518:3771–3784.

59. Tamura S, Tamura Y, Uchida K. Magnetic resonance imaging findings of neuroaxonal dystrophy in a papillon puppy. J Small Anim Pract. 2007;48:458–461.

60. Eagleson JS, Kent M, Platt SR, Rech RR, Howerth EW. MRI findings in a rottweiler with leukoencephalomyelopathy. J Am Anim Hosp Assoc. 2013;49:255–261.

61. Gamble DA, Chrisman CL. A leukoencephalomyelopathy of rottweiler dogs. Vet Pathol. 1984;21:274–280.

62. Hirschvogel K, Matiasek K, Flatz K, Drogemuller M, Drogemuller C, Reiner B, et al. Magnetic resonance imaging and genetic investigation of a case of Rottweiler leukoencephalomyelopathy. BMC Vet Res. 2013;9:57.

63. Li FY, Cuddon PA, Song J, Wood SL, Patterson JS, Shelton GD, et al. Canine spongiform leukoencephalomyelopathy is associated with a missense mutation in cytochrome b. Neurobiol Dis. 2006;21:35–42.

64. Martin-Vaquero P, da Costa RC, Simmons JK, Beamer GL, Jaderlund KH, Oglesbee MJ. A novel spongiform leukoencephalomyelopathy in Border Terrier puppies. J Vet Intern Med. 2012;26:402–406.

65. Oevermann A, Bley T, Konar M, Lang J, Vandevelde M. A novel leukoencephalomyelopathy of Leonberger dogs. J Vet Intern Med. 2008;22:467–471.

66. Brenner O, Wakshlag JJ, Summers BA, de Lahunta A. Alaskan Husky encephalopathy–a canine neurodegenerative disorder resembling subacute necrotizing encephalomyelopathy (Leigh syndrome). Acta Neuropathol. 2000;100:50–62.

67. Vernau KM, Runstadler JA, Brown EA, Cameron JM, Huson HJ, Higgins RJ, et al. Genome-wide association analysis identifies a mutation in the thiamine transporter 2 (SLC19A3) gene associated with Alaskan Husky encephalopathy. PLoS One. 2013;8:e57195.

68. Wakshlag JJ, de Lahunta A, Robinson T, Cooper BJ, Brenner O, O'Toole TD, et al. Subacute necrotising encephalopathy in an Alaskan husky. J Small Anim Pract. 1999;40:585–589.

2.6

Noninfectious inflammatory disorders

Although a number of noninfectious inflammatory disorders of the brain of the dog and cat have been reported, two entities, granulomatous meningoencephalitis and necrotizing encephalitis, are the most common and best described.[1] Necrotizing encephalitis can be further subdivided into necrotizing meningoencephalitis and necrotizing leukoencephalitis, and it is possible that these represent different manifestations of the same disease. All three of these conditions are thought to be autoimmune disorders.

Granulomatous meningoencephalitis

Granulomatous meningoencephalitis (GME) is an idiopathic inflammatory disorder of the central nervous system, characterized by perivascular mononuclear cell infiltrates.[2] Young to middle-aged (4–5 years), female, small- and toy-breed dogs are predisposed, while the disorder is less common in large-breed dogs and rare in cats. Lesion distribution may be focal, disseminated (multifocal), or ocular, with the focal and disseminated forms predominating. Lesions primarily involve white matter, but gray matter and meninges may also be affected. This disorder most often affects the forebrain, brainstem, or spinal cord, with the cerebellum and optic nerves less frequently involved.[1–7]

Depending on the extent of associated edema, lesions may have ill-defined hypoattenuation on unenhanced CT images and will variably contrast enhance. Enhancement can be absent, heterogeneous and ill-defined, or may sometimes reveal a well-delineated mass. Lesions are typically T1 iso- to hypointense and T2 hyperintense and have similar contrast enhancement characteristics as described for CT (Figures 2.6.1, 2.6.2).[1,3,5]

Meningeal involvement is documented in many patients with GME, and abnormal imaging findings are sometimes limited to prominent meningeal enhancement (Figure 2.6.1). In a minority of patients, imaging may be normal or lesions may not contrast enhance.[1,5]

Necrotizing encephalitis

Necrotizing meningoencephalitis

Necrotizing meningoencephalitis, sometimes referred to as Pug dog encephalitis, is a nonsuppurative, necrotizing, inflammatory brain disorder.[8] Small- and toy-breed dogs are predisposed, and Pug, Maltese, and Chihuahua breeds are highly overrepresented. Median age of onset is 1.5–3 years, and females are affected more commonly than males. Lesions may be focal or asymmetrically multifocal and involve both gray and white matter of the cerebral hemispheres and overlying meninges.[1,8–10] Cerebellar and brainstem involvement, though uncommon, has been reported.[11] Grossly, lesions are frequently cavitary and associated with significant brain swelling from inflammation and edema.[8]

Lesions may be hypoattenuating on unenhanced CT images when cavitary or when associated with significant brain edema. Edema may also induce midline shift, brain herniation, and other features of mass effect. Contrast enhancement is variable on CT, ranging from absent to moderate, but when present, the enhancement pattern is heterogeneous and margins may be poorly delineated. On MR images, lesions are T1 iso- or hypointense and T2 hyperintense, involve the cerebral

Atlas of Small Animal CT and MRI, First Edition. Erik R. Wisner and Allison L. Zwingenberger.

gray and white matter, and typically have indistinct margins. About half to two thirds of lesions contrast enhance on MR, but enhancement is minimal to moderate and nonuniform, when present. Meningeal enhancement is evident in about 50% of patients (Figures 2.6.3, 2.6.4, 2.6.5).[11]

Necrotizing leukoencephalitis

Necrotizing leukoencephalitis is also a nonsuppurative, necrotizing, inflammatory brain disorder affecting both gray and white matter.[12–15] Grossly, there are subcortical regions of liquefaction and cavitation. Microscopically, lesions are characterized by mononuclear infiltrates, gitter

cells, and frank necrosis.[15] Descriptions of the anatomic distribution of this disorder are sparse, but lesions can be focal, asymmetrically multifocal, or regionally diffuse with a predilection for the cerebral hemispheres, although brainstem lesions have also been reported.[15,16]

Lesions are iso- to hypoattenuating on unenhanced CT images and may appear contiguous with the ventricles. Contrast enhancement is absent to moderate and nonuniform and ill defined, if present.[16] On MR images, brain lesions are T1 hypointense and T2 hyperintense and minimally to moderately contrast enhance. When enhancement is present, it is typically nonuniform and sometimes peripheral (Figures 2.6.6, 2.6.7).[15]

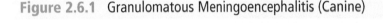

Figure 2.6.1   Granulomatous Meningoencephalitis (Canine)   MR

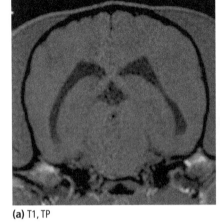
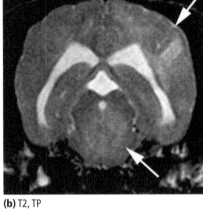

(a) T1, TP   **(b)** T2, TP   **(c)** FL, TP

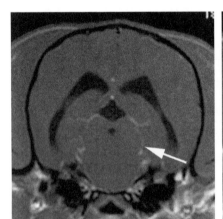
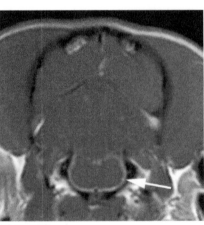
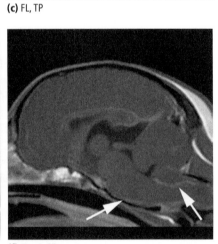

(d) T1+C, TP   **(e)** T1+C, TP   **(f)** T1+C, SP

4y MC Maltese with ataxia and lethargy of 2-week duration. Transverse images at the level of the midbrain (**a–c**) reveal predominantly left-sided T2 and FLAIR hyperintensity of the cerebral white matter and similar intensity changes in the midbrain (**b,c**: arrows). Following contrast administration, there is marked meningeal enhancement involving the left cerebrum and midbrain (**d**: arrow) and further caudally involving the cerebellum and brainstem (**e,f**: arrows). Postmortem examination confirmed a diagnosis of granulomatous meningoencephalitis.

Figure 2.6.2   Granulomatous Meningoencephalitis (Canine)   MR

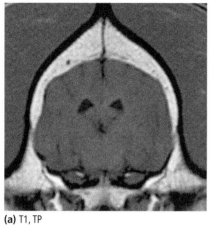

(a) T1, TP

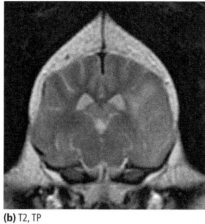

(b) T2, TP

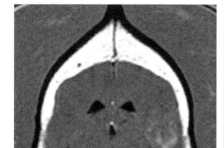

(c) T1+C, TP

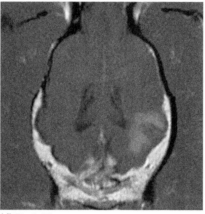

(d) T1+C, DP

5y MC Rottweiler cross with recent onset of seizures and disorientation. There is an ill-defined mass effect within the left temporo-occipital region, causing mild rightward midline shift. This region is T1 hypointense (**a**) and T2 hyperintense (**b**) with prominent surrounding edema. There is moderate non-uniform and amorphous contrast enhancement that appears to be distributed predominantly in white matter on contrast-enhanced T1 images (**c,d**). Postmortem examination revealed perivascular histiocytic and lymphoplasmacytic cuffing, consistent with granulomatous meningoencephalitis.

Figure 2.6.3 Necrotizing Meningoencephalitis (Canine)   MR

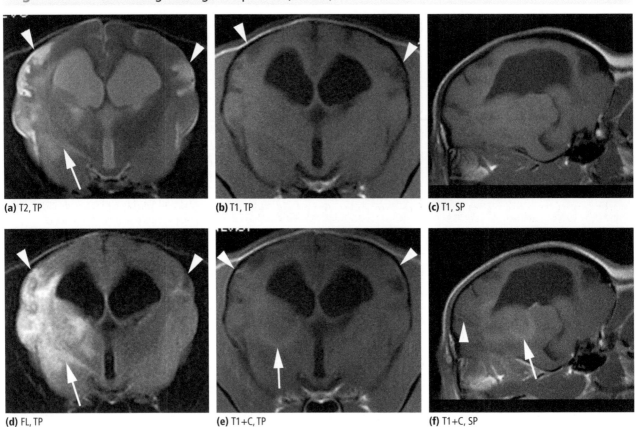

(a) T2, TP   (b) T1, TP   (c) T1, SP

(d) FL, TP   (e) T1+C, TP   (f) T1+C, SP

3y M Pomeranian with a recent history of seizures and circling to the left. There are multiple foci of marked T2 and FLAIR hyperintensity (**a**,**d**: arrowheads) and T1 hypointensity (**b**: arrowheads) involving the cerebral cortex and regional T2 hyperintensity of the white matter and caudate nucleus on the right (**a**,**d**: arrow). There is mild amorphous contrast enhancement of the right caudate nucleus (**e**,**f**: arrow) and of the meninges overlying the cerebral cortical lesions (**e**,**f**: arrowheads). Postmortem examination revealed extensive areas of cortical necrosis and encephalomalacia, consistent with necrotizing meningoencephalitis.

Figure 2.6.4 Necrotizing Meningoencephalitis (Canine)   MR

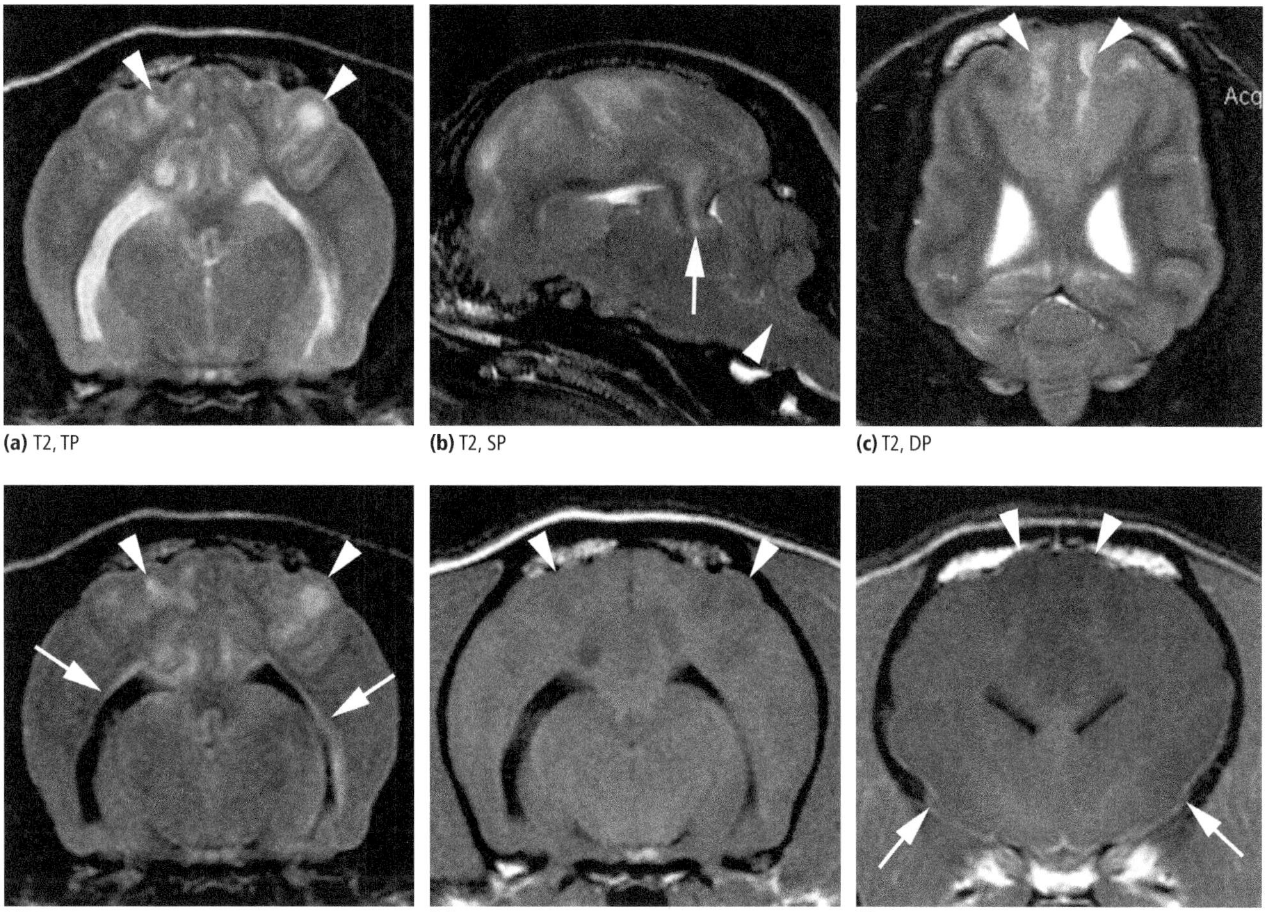

(a) T2, TP

(b) T2, SP

(c) T2, DP

(d) FL, TP

(e) T1, TP

(f) T1+C, TP

2y FS Pug with recent onset of lethargy. There is regional marked T2 and FLAIR hyperintensity (**a,c,d**: arrowheads) and T1 hypointensity (**e,f**: arrowheads) involving the frontoparietal cerebral cortex. Uncal (transtentorial) herniation (**b**: arrow), cerebellar herniation (**b**: arrowhead), and interstitial edema (**d**: arrows) are also present. Widespread meningeal enhancement is seen following contrast administration (**f**: arrows). Postmortem examination revealed meningitis and necrotizing encephalitis of gray and white matter predominately in the cerebral hemispheres, consistent with necrotizing meningoencephalitis.

Figure 2.6.5 Necrotizing Meningoencephalitis (Canine)   MR

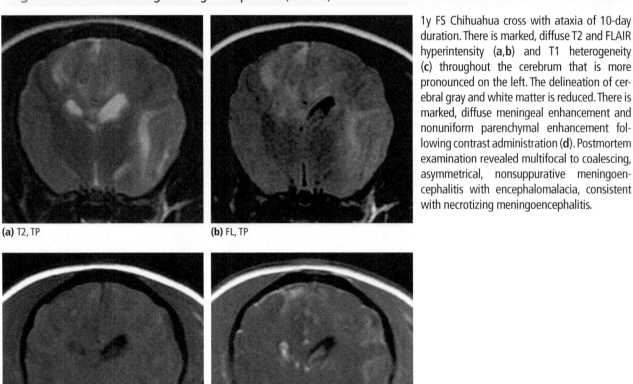

(a) T2, TP

(b) FL, TP

(c) T1, TP

(d) T1+C, TP

1y FS Chihuahua cross with ataxia of 10-day duration. There is marked, diffuse T2 and FLAIR hyperintensity (a,b) and T1 heterogeneity (c) throughout the cerebrum that is more pronounced on the left. The delineation of cerebral gray and white matter is reduced. There is marked, diffuse meningeal enhancement and nonuniform parenchymal enhancement following contrast administration (d). Postmortem examination revealed multifocal to coalescing, asymmetrical, nonsuppurative meningoencephalitis with encephalomalacia, consistent with necrotizing meningoencephalitis.

Figure 2.6.6 Necrotizing Leukoencephalitis (Canine)   MR

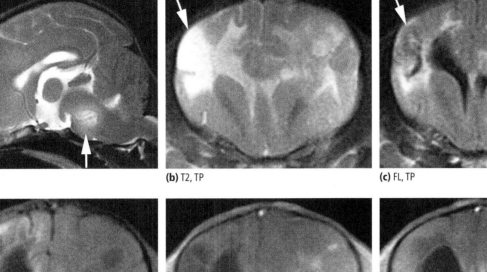

(a) T2, SP

(b) T2, TP

(c) FL, TP

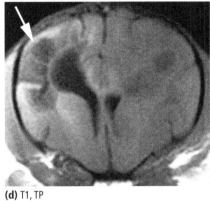
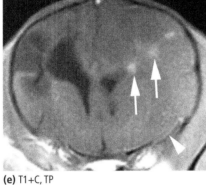
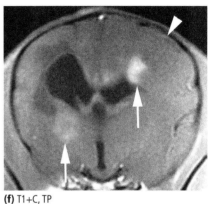

(d) T1, TP

(e) T1+C, TP

(f) T1+C, TP

2y MC Yorkshire Terrier with acute onset of ataxia, hypermetria, and obtundation. There is diffuse T2 and FLAIR white matter hyperintensity in both cerebral hemispheres, consistent with vasogenic edema (**b,c**). There is focal right hemispheric subcortical T2 hyperintensity, FLAIR mixed intensity, and T1 hypointensity, consistent with a focal fluid collection (**b–d**: arrow). An additional T2 hyperintense mass is present within the pons (**a**: arrow). Following contrast administration, multiple contrast-enhancing foci are seen in the parenchyma of the cerebrum and thalamus (**e,f**: arrows). Diffuse meningeal enhancement is also evident (**e,f**: arrowhead). Postmortem examination revealed widespread multifocal lymphohistiocytic leukoencephalitis with cystic malacia and necrosis, consistent with necrotizing leukoencephalitis.

Figure 2.6.7 Necrotizing Leukoencephalitis (Canine)   MR

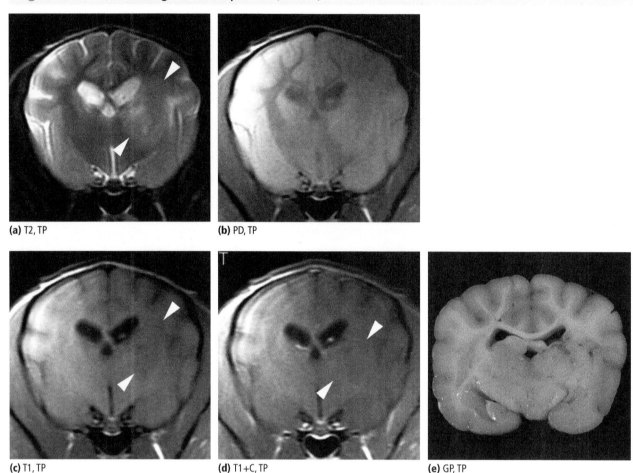

(a) T2, TP

(b) PD, TP

(c) T1, TP

(d) T1+C, TP

(e) GP, TP

2y FS Yorkshire Terrier with reduced mentation. The horizontal intensity gradient on all MR images is an artifact associated with the use of surface coils for image acquisition. There is an ill-defined region of T2 hyperintensity (**a**: arrowheads) and mild T1 hypointensity (**c**: arrowheads) involving the left cerebral white matter and thalamus, resulting in a loss of definition between gray and white matter (**b**). There is minimal peripheral enhancement of the lesion following contrast administration (**d**: arrowheads). Similar lesions were evident on other images (not shown). Postmortem examination confirmed inflammatory and malacic changes, consistent with necrotizing leukoencephalitis.

References

1. Granger N, Smith PM, Jeffery ND. Clinical findings and treatment of non-infectious meningoencephalomyelitis in dogs: a systematic review of 457 published cases from 1962 to 2008. Vet J. 2010;184:290–297.

2. Cordy DR. Canine granulomatous meningoencephalomyelitis. Vet Pathol. 1979;16:325–333.

3. Adamo PF, Adams WM, Steinberg H. Granulomatous meningoencephalomyelitis in dogs. Compend Contin Educ Vet. 2007;29:678–690.

4. Braund KG. Granulomatous meningoencephalomyelitis. J Am Vet Med Assoc. 1985;186:138–141.

5. Cherubini GB, Platt SR, Anderson TJ, Rusbridge C, Lorenzo V, Mantis P, et al. Characteristics of magnetic resonance images of granulomatous meningoencephalomyelitis in 11 dogs. Vet Rec. 2006;159:110–115.

6. Kitagawa M, Kanayama K, Satoh T, Sakai T. Cerebellar focal granulomatous meningoencephalitis in a dog: clinical findings and MR imaging. J Vet Med A Physiol Pathol Clin Med. 2004;51:277–279.

7. Kitagawa M, Okada M, Watari T, Sato T, Kanayama K, Sakai T. Ocular granulomatous meningoencephalomyelitis in a dog: magnetic resonance images and clinical findings. J Vet Med Sci. 2009;71:233–237.

8. Cordy DR, Holliday TA. A necrotizing meningoencephalitis of pug dogs. Vet Pathol. 1989;26:191–194.

9. Higgins RJ, Dickinson PJ, Kube SA, Moore PF, Couto SS, Vernau KM, et al. Necrotizing meningoencephalitis in five Chihuahua dogs. Vet Pathol. 2008;45:336–346.

10. Levine JM, Fosgate GT, Porter B, Schatzberg SJ, Greer K. Epidemiology of necrotizing meningoencephalitis in Pug dogs. J Vet Intern Med. 2008;22:961–968.

11. Young BD, Levine JM, Fosgate GT, de Lahunta A, Flegel T, Matiasek K, et al. Magnetic resonance imaging characteristics of necrotizing meningoencephalitis in Pug dogs. J Vet Intern Med. 2009;23:527–535.

12. Berrocal A, Montgomery DL, Pumarola M. Leukoencephalitis and vasculitis with perivascular demyelination in a Weimaraner dog. Vet Pathol. 2000;37:470–472.

13. Schatzberg SJ. Idiopathic granulomatous and necrotizing inflammatory disorders of the canine central nervous system. Vet Clin North Am Small Anim Pract. 2010;40:101–120.

14. Spitzbarth I, Schenk HC, Tipold A, Beineke A. Immunohistochemical characterization of inflammatory and glial responses in a case of necrotizing leucoencephalitis in a French bulldog. J Comp Pathol. 2010;142:235–241.

15. von Praun F, Matiasek K, Grevel V, Alef M, Flegel T. Magnetic resonance imaging and pathologic findings associated with necrotizing encephalitis in two Yorkshire terriers. Vet Radiol Ultrasound. 2006;47:260–264.

16. Ducote JM, Johnson KE, Dewey CW, Walker MA, Coates JR, Berridge BR. Computed tomography of necrotizing meningoencephalitis in 3 Yorkshire Terriers. Vet Radiol Ultrasound. 1999;40:617–621.

2.7

Infectious inflammatory disorders

Infectious causes of encephalitis and meningoencephalitis include viral, bacterial, mycotic, protozoal, and parasitic agents. Detailed imaging descriptions are sporadic, but features of the more common entities are included here.

Viral encephalitis

Canine distemper encephalitis

The canine distemper virus causes systemic illness in dogs and other species, with central nervous system involvement a common component in both the acute and chronic phases of the disease. Acute distemper encephalomyelitis is characterized by mild mononuclear inflammation and demyelination and is widely disseminated. Chronic encephalitis ("old dog encephalitis") may arise from long-term persistent viral infection and is characterized by nonsuppurative inflammation and demyelination involving primarily the brainstem and cerebral hemispheres.[1]

MR imaging features of acute distemper encephalitis include focal or regional T1 hypointense and T2 hyperintense lesions of the forebrain with little or no mass effect. The temporal lobes may be predisposed, and lesions are centered on cortical gray matter and the gray–white matter interface. Similar lesions have also been reported in the brainstem and cerebellum. Contrast enhancement is inconsistent and minimal when present (Figure 2.7.1).[2]

MR imaging features of chronic distemper encephalitis have been described in one case report and included T2 hyperintensity and loss of definition of the cerebral and cerebellar cortical gray–white matter interface as well as subtle T2 hyperintensity of the pons. Enhancement of the frontal and parietal lobe pachymeninges was evident on contrast-enhanced T1 images.[3] A loss of gray–white matter definition due to demyelination would likely be a prominent feature on proton density weighted images as well.

Feline infectious peritonitis meningoencephalitis

The feline infectious peritonitis (FIP) coronavirus causes systemic illness in domestic cats, with central nervous system involvement being a common component, particularly in cats with the dry or pyogranulomatous form of the disease. FIP infection causes an immune-complex pyogranulomatous vasculitis, and in the central nervous system (CNS), it targets the leptomeninges, choroid plexus, ependymal cells, brain parenchyma, and eyes.

Generalized or regional obstructive hydrocephalus may be present because of ependymal and choroid inflammation. Cerebrospinal fluid (CSF) may have variable T1 and FLAIR intensity depending on cellular and macromolecular content. The brain parenchyma may appear unremarkable on unenhanced T1 MR images, although cerebellar herniation may be evident in cats with obstructive hydrocephalus. Focal or multifocal regions of parenchymal hyperintensity may be evident on T2 images, and the meninges may appear thickened and T2 hyperintense. Choroidal, ependymal, and meningeal enhancement may be marked on contrast-enhanced T1 images (Figure 2.7.2).[4–7]

Atlas of Small Animal CT and MRI, First Edition. Erik R. Wisner and Allison L. Zwingenberger.

Bacterial meningoencephalopathy

Intracranial abscess

Intracranial abscesses are caused by penetrating injuries, such as migrating foreign bodies and bite wounds; extension of ear and nasal infections; or from bacteremia or septic emboli.[8-10] Their location within or adjacent to the brain is dependent on the initiating cause, with the brainstem most often affected by extension of otitis media/interna. Because of the inflammatory nature of the lesion and the often significant mass effect, surrounding vasogenic edema is usually pronounced. Epidural or subdural fluid collections may be present, particularly when the abscess is caused by penetrating injury. Obstructive hydrocephalus may occur, depending on abscess location.

Intracranial abscesses usually appear as solitary space-occupying masses of variable size and with a hypoattenuating center on unenhanced CT images. Depending on the thickness of the abscess capsule, this may appear as a distinct iso- or mildly hyperattenuating lesion rim surrounded by relatively hypoattenuating parenchymal edema. Abscesses are generally intensely peripherally enhancing, and regional meningeal enhancement may be present in some patients (Figure 2.7.3).

On MR images, abscesses are centrally T1 hypointense (but higher intensity than normal CSF) and T2 hyperintense because of the presence of abscess fluid and T1 hypointense and T2 hyperintense peripheral to the mass because of vasogenic edema. Abscess contents appear hyperintense on FLAIR sequences. A distinct T1 iso- to hyperintense abscess capsule may also be evident. Abscesses intensely peripherally contrast enhance and regional meningeal enhancement may be seen (Figures 2.7.4, 2.7.5).[8,9,11-14] Diffusion weighted imaging (DWI) typically reveals high signal intensity on the DWI map and low signal on the apparent diffusion coefficient (ADC) map, indicative of restricted water diffusion (Figure 2.7.5). This may be useful for differentiating abscesses from necrotic brain lesions and mucinous intra-axial tumors, such as oligodendroglioma.

Bacterial meningoencephalitis

Intracranial bacterial infections may also present as a diffuse or regional meningoencephalitis.[13,15]

Imaging features may be subtle or absent on unenhanced CT images. However, regional or diffuse parenchymal hypoattenuation from edema may be present, and pachymeninges may be visible if markedly thickened. Subdural or subarachnoid abscess may also be evident as a hypoattenuating crescent adjacent to the affected region of the brain. Meningeal contrast enhancement may be obscured because of the adjacent dense calvarial bone (Figure 2.7.6).

Affected parenchymas appear T1 hypointense and T2 hyperintense on MRI images because of the presence of vasogenic edema. Affected pachymeninges may be thickened and can appear T2 hyperintense. When present, subdural or subarachnoid abscess will appear as a T1 hypointense, T2 hyperintense crescent adjacent to the affected region of the brain. Affected meninges generally intensely contrast enhance, although affected brain parenchyma enhancement is variable and may be subtle (Figures 2.7.6, 2.7.7, 2.7.8).

Mycotic meningoencephalitis

A variety of mycotic species may cause central nervous system disease. Although reports are few, *Aspergillus*, *Cryptococcus*, *Cladophialophora*, and *Coccidioides* species are some of the organisms for which imaging features have been described.[6,16-20] *Prototheca* species, blue–green algae, have also been a reported cause of infectious meningoencephalitis.[21,22] In many patients, involvement of the brain, spinal cord, and meninges is part of a multiple organ system infection. Young, female German Shepherd Dogs are highly overrepresented, particularly for *Aspergillus* infections.[19] Most mycotic CNS infections occur through hematogenous spread, and they are therefore often diffuse or multifocal and asymmetrically distributed. Infections may involve both brain parenchyma and meninges, and parenchymal lesions may take the form of abscesses, solid granulomas, or diffuse infiltrative lesions.

Fungal meningoencephalitis may have CT and MR features similar to those described for bacterial abscess and meningoencephalitis, although more heterogeneous contrast enhancement will be evident in solid and complex granulomas. Contrast enhancement of infiltrative lesions may be diffuse and ill defined (Figures 2.7.9, 2.7.10, 2.7.11, 2.7.12, 2.7.13).[6,16-20]

Protozoal meningoencephalitis

Protozoal infection is a rare cause of encephalomyelitis, but imaging features of CNS lesions have been reported for *Toxoplasma* in cats and *Neospora*, *Leishmania*, and *Acanthamoeba* species in dogs.[23-27]

Because the veterinary imaging literature includes only single and small series case reports, characteristic features of protozoal CNS infection are not fully documented. However, imaging findings are generally consistent with those found with other inflammatory brain disorders and include focal, regional, multifocal, or diffuse asymmetrical distribution in white and gray matter; associated edema; variable meningeal involvement; and heterogeneous to homogeneous contrast enhancement. In addition to the general characteristics, cerebellitis with subsequent cerebellar atrophy has been linked to *Neospora caninum* infection (Figure 2.7.14), and a report of two canine patients with CNS leishmaniasis describes MR features consistent with multiple nonhemorrhagic infarcts.[24,25]

Helminth-induced meningoencephalopathy

Angiostrongylus vasorum

There are multiple reports of *Angiostrongylus vasorum*, the French heartworm, producing vasculitis and coagulopathy that lead to hemorrhagic inflammatory brain disease in dogs. Lesions include multifocal brain hemorrhages that may include large space-occupying hematomas. Lesion T1

and T2 signal intensity will vary depending on the age of the hemorrhage and is hypointense on T2* gradient echo sequences because of susceptibility effects.[28–31] MR imaging features consistent with meningitis have also been described with this disorder.[30]

Neurocysticercosis

Neurocysticercosis is a rare form of inflammatory brain disease caused by aberrant larval migration and development of *Taenia crassiceps*. One MR imaging report of neurocysticercosis in a dog describes cyst-like lesions in the subdural region of one occipital lobe and the brainstem. Cyst margins enhanced on contrast-enhanced T1 images.[32]

Figure 2.7.1 Canine Distemper Encephalitis (Canine)   MR

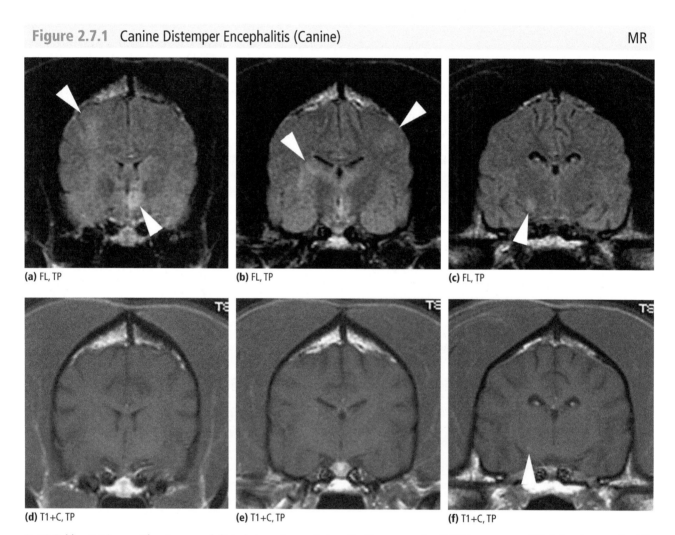

(a) FL, TP   **(b)** FL, TP   **(c)** FL, TP

(d) T1+C, TP   **(e)** T1+C, TP   **(f)** T1+C, TP

2y FS Golden Retriever with seizures and clinical signs of encephalopathy. Representative FLAIR images reveal ill-defined areas of mildly increased signal intensity, primarily in the cerebrum and thalamic regions (a–c: arrowheads). There is also mild asymmetrical hyperintensity of the parietal and temporal lobes. These areas do not contrast enhance with the exception of one focal lesion in the right thalamic region (f: arrowhead). Postmortem examination revealed severe generalized neuronal loss, axonal necrosis, and demyelination. Immunohistochemical staining documented abundant intralesional canine distemper virus antigen. The symmetrical parietal and temporal lobe changes were thought to be associated with recent seizures.

Figure 2.7.2   FIP-Associated Encephalitis and Ventriculitis (Feline)   MR

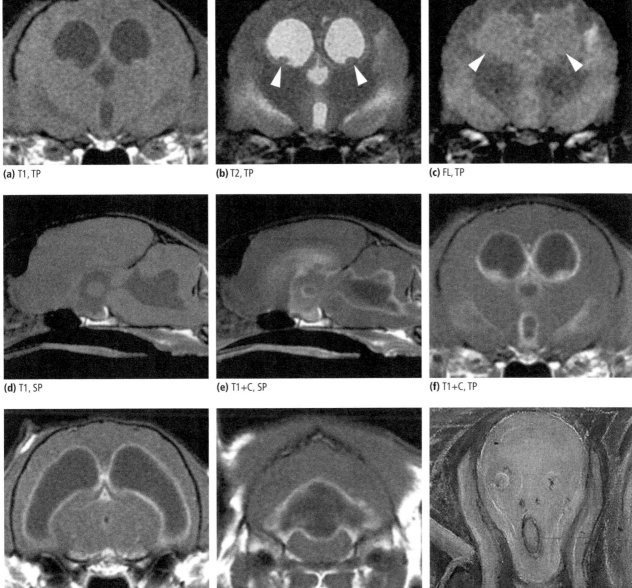

(a) T1, TP

(b) T2, TP

(c) FL, TP

(d) T1, SP

(e) T1+C, SP

(f) T1+C, TP

(g) T1+C, TP

(h) T1+C, TP

(i)

9mo MC Domestic Shorthair with 2-week history of lethargy, inappetence, and reduced motor function in the pelvic limbs. The ventricular system is markedly and uniformly enlarged, indicative of obstructive hydrocephalus (a–d). The choroid plexus of the floor of the lateral ventricles is enlarged (b: arrowheads). The cerebrospinal fluid (CSF) appears abnormally hyperintense on the FLAIR image, indicating a high cellularity or macromolecular content (c: arrowheads). There is nonuniform T2 and FLAIR hyperintensity of the white matter in both hemispheres consistent with the presence of vasogenic edema. Contrast-enhanced T1 images reveal uniform and intense enhancement of a thickened ependymal lining but no parenchymal enhancement (e–h). MR imaging findings characteristic of this disorder can be quite shocking (f,i). Based on the combination of clinical signs, MR findings, and CSF analysis, a clinical diagnosis of feline infectious peritonitis associated encephalitis and ventriculitis was made.

Figure 2.7.3   Intracranial Abscess (Feline)

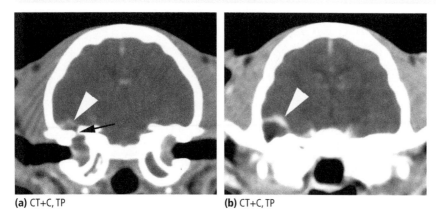

(a) CT+C, TP   **(b)** CT+C, TP

16y FS Abyssinian with bilateral ceruminous gland cystadenomas and otitis media. Recent onset of intracranial neurologic signs. Nonuniformly contrast-enhancing, soft-tissue attenuating material is present within both tympanic bullae (**a**). There is a peripherally contrast-enhancing intracranial mass, consistent with an abscess, adjacent to the internal margin of the petrous portion of the right temporal bone (**a,b**: arrowhead). The internal acoustic meatus can be seen (**a**: black arrow).

Figure 2.7.4   Intracranial Abscess (Feline)

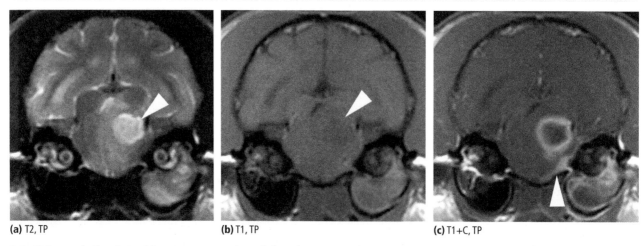

(a) T2, TP   **(b)** T1, TP   **(c)** T1+C, TP

2.5y FS Domestic Shorthair with acute onset ataxia and obtundation. T2 and T1 intensity within the left tympanic bulla is consistent with effusion (**a,b**). There is a T2 hyperintense, T1 hypointense mass adjacent to or within the left side of the brainstem (**a,b**: arrowhead), surrounded by a halo of T2 hyperintense edema (**a**). The mass intensely peripherally enhances following contrast administration, indicative of an abscess (**c**). Adjacent meninges also enhance and appear thickened, indicative of regional meningitis (**c**: arrowhead). The lining of the left tympanic cavity intensely enhances, consistent with otitis media (**c**). Biopsy and culture of the lining of the left middle ear confirmed suppurative otitis media. The intracranial abscess and meningitis was thought to have occurred by ascending infection through the internal acoustic meatus.

Figure 2.7.5 Intracranial Abscess (Canine)   MR

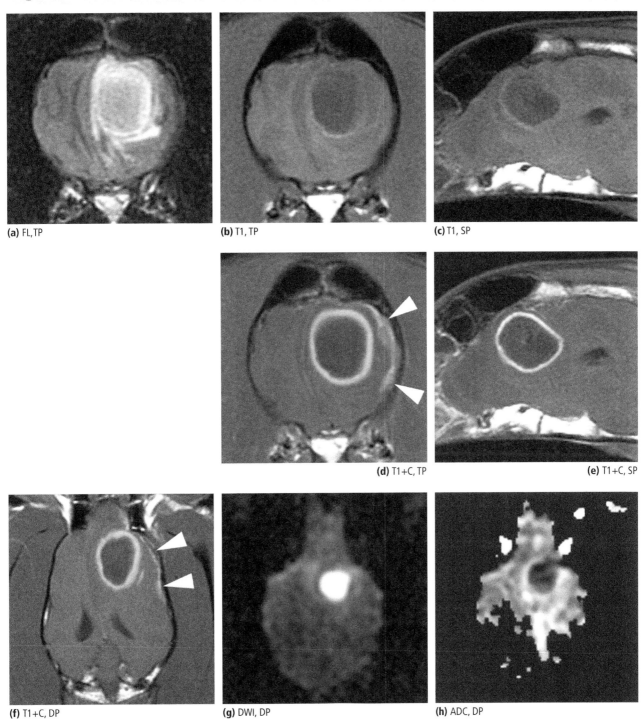

(a) FL,TP

(b) T1, TP

(c) T1, SP

(d) T1+C, TP

(e) T1+C, SP

(f) T1+C, DP

(g) DWI, DP

(h) ADC, DP

1y F Dalmatian with a 2-day history of progressive right-sided weakness and declining mentation. There is a large, well-delineated FLAIR hyperintense, T1 hypointense mass in the left frontal lobe causing a pronounced midline shift (**a–c**). The mass has a thin T1 hyperintense rim (**b,c**) and surrounding FLAIR hyperintensity consistent with vasogenic edema (**a**). Following contrast administration the mass intensely peripherally enhances (**d–f**). There is also marked enhancement of the adjacent meninges (**d,f**: arrowheads). The B_{1000} diffusion-weighted image (**g**) and ADC map (**h**) reveal focal hyperintensity and hypointensity, respectively, indicative of diffusion restriction and characteristic of a brain abscess. The diagnosis of brain abscess was confirmed by surgical exposure and drainage. A follow-up MR performed approximately 3 months after treatment revealed nearly complete resolution.

Figure 2.7.6   Bacterial Meningitis (Canine)   CT & MR

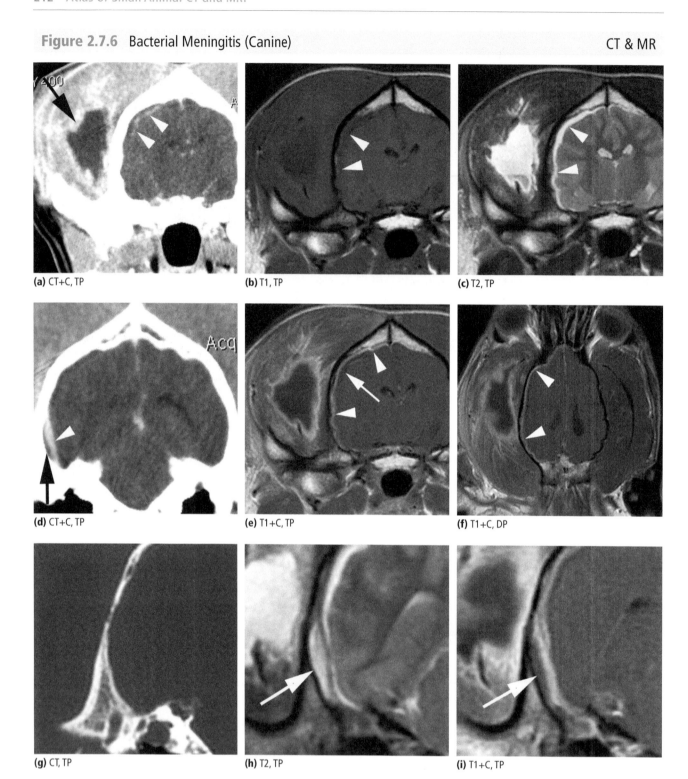

(a) CT+C, TP

(b) T1, TP

(c) T2, TP

(d) CT+C, TP

(e) T1+C, TP

(f) T1+C, DP

(g) CT, TP

(h) T2, TP

(i) T1+C, TP

3y F Labrador Retriever with recent onset of fever, altered behavior, and right cranial soft-tissue swelling. Contrast-enhanced CT images reveal a large abscess in the right temporalis muscle (**a**: arrow). There is also evidence of intracranial midline shift and enhancement as well as internal displacement of the right hemispheric meninges (**a,d**: arrowheads). Underlying temporal bone destruction is also seen (**g**). On MR images, the abscess is T1 hypointense (**b**) and T2 hyperintense (**c**). There is a curvilinear pattern of similar intensity adjacent and peripheral to the right cerebral hemisphere representing thickened meninges (**b,c**: arrowheads). There is marked irregular peripheral enhancement of the temporal abscess following contrast administration as well as more diffuse enhancement of the adjacent temporalis muscle (**e,f**). Right hemispheric meninges are prominent and enhance intensely (**e,f**: arrowheads). Epidural (**h,i**: arrow) and subdural (**e**: arrow) fluid collections appear T2 hyperintense and relatively T1 hypointense on enhanced MR images. The epidural fluid is also evident on the contrast-enhanced CT image (**d**: arrow). Cytologic evaluation of subdural fluid obtained during durotomy revealed septic suppurative inflammation with large numbers of intra- and extracellular cocci.

Figure 2.7.7   Bacterial Meningitis (Canine)   MR

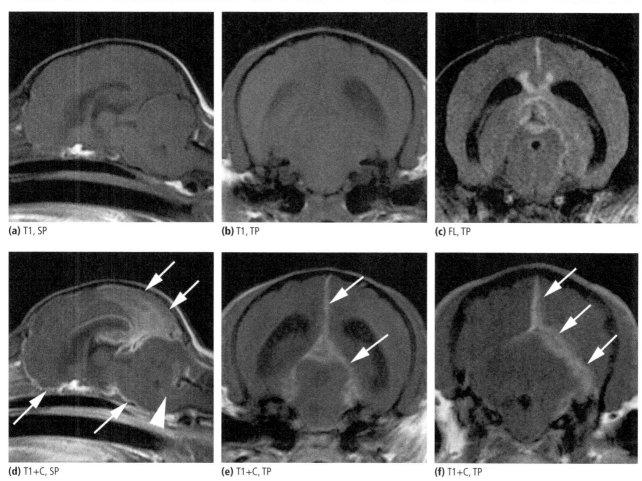

(a) T1, SP   **(b)** T1, TP   **(c)** FL, TP

(d) T1+C, SP   **(e)** T1+C, TP   **(f)** T1+C, TP

9mo F Dachshund with 2-week history of progressive weakness and lethargy. Cerebrospinal fluid analysis revealed marked suppurative inflammation and intracellular rod-shaped bacteria. Meningeal and periventricular hyperintensity is evident on the FLAIR image (**c**). The cerebellum appears enlarged with loss of cerebellar folia definition (**c**) and ventral foraminal herniation (**d**: arrowhead). There is marked thickening and regional enhancement of the meninges in the caudal aspect of the cranial vault (**d–f**: arrows). Cerebrospinal fluid analysis also revealed large numbers of neutrophils. A craniotomy was performed to reduce intracranial pressure. Meningeal biopsy confirmed severe suppurative meningitis.

Figure 2.7.8   Bacterial Meningoencephalitis (Feline)   MR

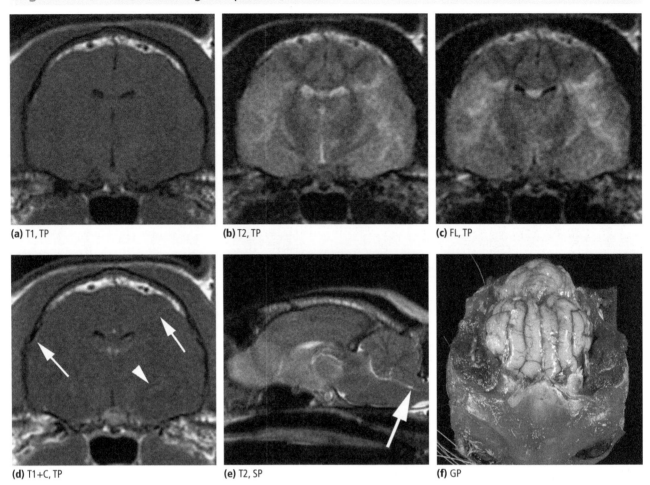

(a) T1, TP   **(b)** T2, TP   **(c)** FL, TP

(d) T1+C, TP   **(e)** T2, SP   **(f)** GP

14y FS Domestic Shorthair with a 5-day history of seizures and intracranial neurologic signs. T2 and FLAIR images show extensive cerebral edema affecting both white and gray matter (**b,c**). The caudal aspect of the cerebellum is herniated through the foramen magnum (**e**: arrow). There are multiple ill-defined focal areas of parenchymal enhancement (**d**: arrowhead), additional lesions present on other images (not shown), and meningeal enhancement following contrast administration (**d**: arrows). Postmortem examination confirmed hematogenous fibropurulent meningoencephalitis. *Klebsiella pneumoniae* was cultured from heart blood.

Figure 2.7.9   Mycotic Granulomatous Encephalitis (Canine)   MR

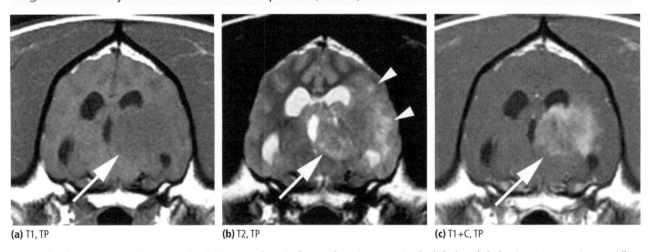

(a) T1, TP   **(b)** T2, TP   **(c)** T1+C, TP

6y FS Labrador Retriever with progressive lethargy and cervical pain. There is a mass in the left dorsal thalamic region causing a midline shift and compression of the third and left lateral ventricles. The mass is characterized by T1 hypointensity (**a**: arrow) with heterogeneous T2 intensity (**b**: arrow), and there is evidence of extensive perilesional edema (**b**: arrowheads). A similar-appearing lesion (not shown) was present in the left occipital lobe. The mass intensely and heterogeneously enhances following contrast administration, and mass margins are poorly defined and irregular (**c**: arrow). Postmortem examination confirmed granulomatous encephalitis from systemic aspergillosis. The disease was widely disseminated with multiple organ systems affected.

Figure 2.7.10   Mycotic Granulomatous Meningoencephalitis (Canine)   MR

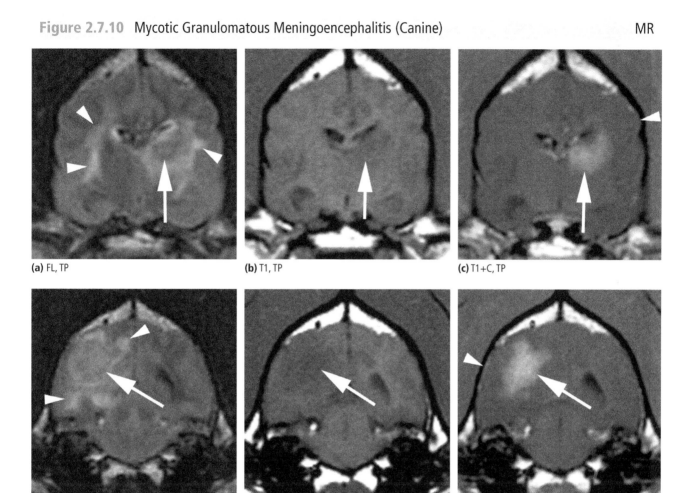

(a) FL, TP

(b) T1, TP

(c) T1+C, TP

(d) FL, TP

(e) T1, TP

(f) T1+C, TP

3y FS German Shepherd Dog with acute onset of seizures. There is an ill-defined, ovoid mass within the left thalamic region (**a–c**: arrow), which is heterogeneously T1 hypointense (**b**: arrow) and heterogeneously FLAIR hyperintense (**a**: arrow). A similar but larger mass is seen in the right occipital lobe (**d–f**: arrow). There is extensive bihemispheric white matter edema associated with both masses (**a**,**d**: arrowheads). The masses markedly contrast enhance, revealing ill-defined and irregular margins (**c**,**f**: arrow). There is also excessive meningeal enhancement evident adjacent to the masses (**c**,**f**: arrowhead). Postmortem examination confirmed granulomatous encephalitis from widely disseminated systemic aspergillosis.

Figure 2.7.11 Mycotic Granulomatous Meningoencephalitis (Canine)   MR

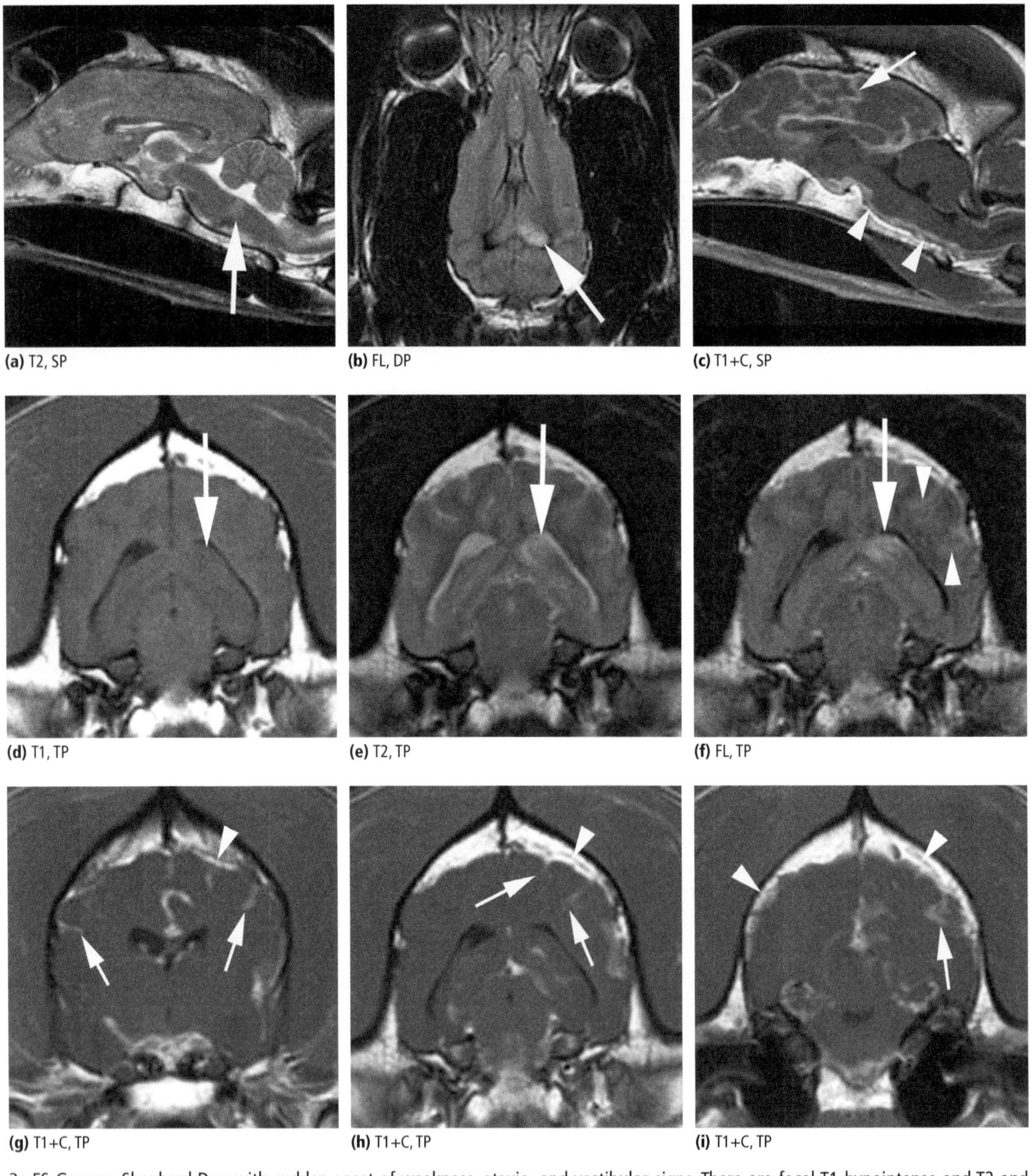

(a) T2, SP

(b) FL, DP

(c) T1+C, SP

(d) T1, TP

(e) T2, TP

(f) FL, TP

(g) T1+C, TP

(h) T1+C, TP

(i) T1+C, TP

3y FS German Shepherd Dog with sudden onset of weakness, ataxia, and vestibular signs. There are focal T1 hypointense and T2 and FLAIR hyperintense lesions seen in the brainstem (a: arrow) and left hippocampus (b,d–f: arrow). Unusual sulcal hyperintensity is also seen on the transverse FLAIR image (f: arrowheads). Marked meningeal enhancement is seen following contrast administration (c,g–i). Pachymeninges and leptomeninges are both affected, as evidenced by enhancement and thickening of the dura mater (c,g–i: arrowheads) as well as enhancement of the pia mater lining the sulci (c,g–i: arrows). Multiple focal parenchymal lesions also contrast enhanced (not shown). Postmortem examination confirmed granulomatous meningoencephalitis from widely disseminated systemic aspergillosis (*Aspergillus terreus*).

Figure 2.7.12 Mycotic Granulomatous Meningoencephalitis (Canine)   MR

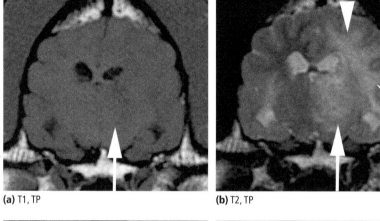
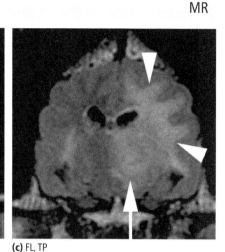

(a) T1, TP

(b) T2, TP

(c) FL, TP

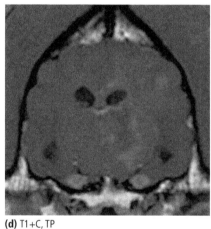
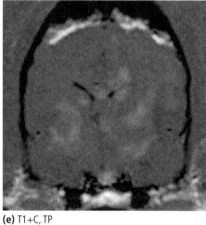
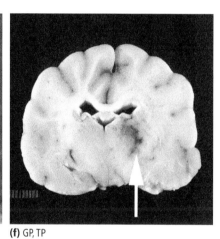

(d) T1+C, TP

(e) T1+C, TP

(f) GP, TP

2y FS German Shepherd Dog with abnormal ambulation and reduced mentation. There is a T1 hypointense and T2 and FLAIR hyperintense mass in the left thalamus that creates a moderate rightward midline shift (**a–c**: arrow). There is pronounced T2 and FLAIR hyperintensity involving the left hemispheric corona radiata, consistent with widespread edema (**b,c**: arrowheads). Additional, more subtle T2 hyperintense foci were identified, distributed randomly throughout the brain parenchyma (not shown). Following contrast administration, multiple ill-defined regions of contrast enhancement are present, distributed throughout the brain parenchyma, with the most prominent lesions seen in the thalamus bilaterally and surrounding the left lateral ventricle (**d,e**). Postmortem examination confirmed multisystemic granulomatous inflammatory disease caused by *Paecilomyces* sp. The thalamic mass detected on MR images corresponded to a cavitating granuloma seen on gross examination (**f**: arrow).

Figure 2.7.13   Mycotic Meningoencephalitis (Feline)   MR

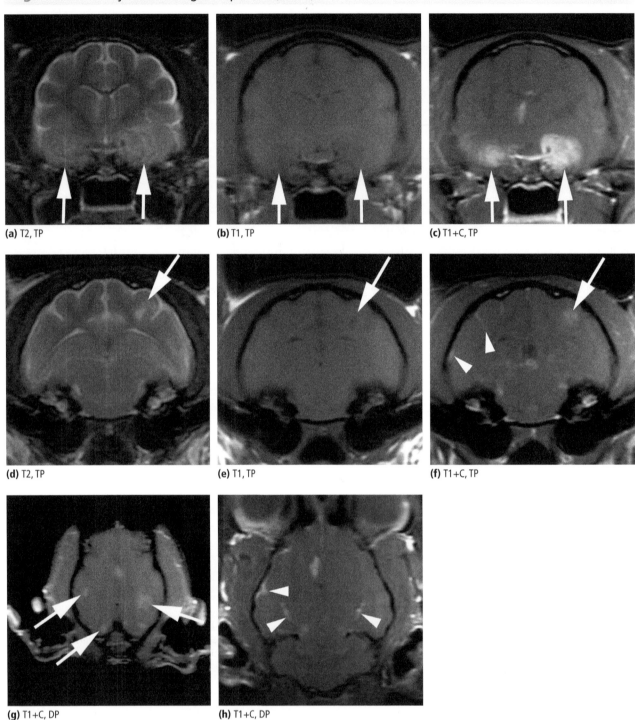

(a) T2, TP

(b) T1, TP

(c) T1+C, TP

(d) T2, TP

(e) T1, TP

(f) T1+C, TP

(g) T1+C, DP

(h) T1+C, DP

4y FS Bengal cross with pelvic limb weakness. Multiple ill-defined and variably sized T1 hypointense and T2 hyperintense foci are seen in the piriform lobes and parietal cortex (**a,b,d,e**: arrows; additional lesions not shown). These focal lesions heterogeneously enhance and have ill-defined margins following contrast administration (**c,f,g**: arrows). Prominent multifocal meningeal enhancement is also seen (**f,h**: arrowheads). Postmortem examination confirmed multisystemic inflammatory disease caused by *Cryptococcus gattii*. The chronic inflammatory response in the meninges and brain was histiocytic and lymphoplasmacytic with intralesional fungal elements.

Figure 2.7.14   Protozoal Granulomatous Cerebellitis (Canine)   MR

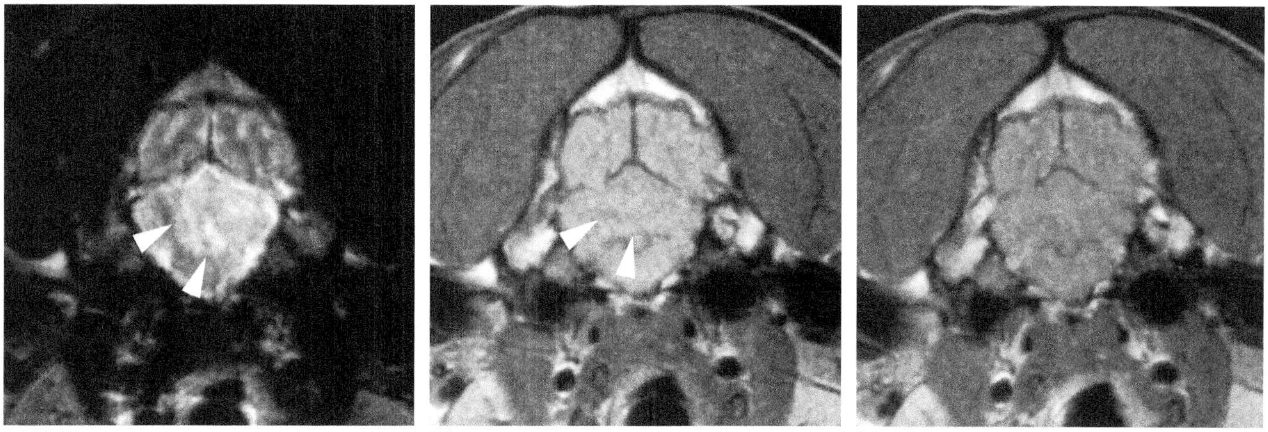

(a) T2, TP   **(b)** T1, TP   **(c)** T1+C, TP

6y M Rhodesian Ridgeback with a 4-day history of signs referable to cerebellar disease. There is a poorly margined, T1 isointense and T2 hyperintense region in the vermis and left hemisphere of the cerebellum (**a,b**: arrowheads), which is not associated with any significant mass effect. No enhancement of the lesion is seen following contrast administration. A fluorescent antibody test yielded a titer consistent with active *Neospora* infection. A postmortem examination performed approximately 3 months after initial diagnosis confirmed a diagnosis of necrotizing granulomatous cerebellitis with intralesional protozoa consistent with *Neospora*.

References

1. Sellon RK. Canine Viral Diseases. In: Ettinger SJ, Feldman EC (eds): Textbook of Veterinary Internal Medicine. Philadelphia: Elsevier Saunders, 2005;646–652.

2. Bathen-Noethen A, Stein VM, Puff C, Baumgaertner W, Tipold A. Magnetic resonance imaging findings in acute canine distemper virus infection. J Small Anim Pract. 2008;49:460–467.

3. Griffin JFt, Young BD, Levine JM. Imaging diagnosis – chronic canine distemper meningoencephalitis. Vet Radiol Ultrasound. 2009;50:182–184.

4. Foley JE, Lapointe JM, Koblik P, Poland A, Pedersen NC. Diagnostic features of clinical neurologic feline infectious peritonitis. J Vet Intern Med. 1998;12:415–423.

5. Kitagawa M, Okada M, Sato T, Kanayama K, Sakai T. A feline case of isolated fourth ventricle with syringomyelia suspected to be related with feline infectious peritonitis. J Vet Med Sci. 2007; 69:759–762.

6. Mellema LM, Samii VF, Vernau KM, LeCouteur RA. Meningeal enhancement on magnetic resonance imaging in 15 dogs and 3 cats. Vet Radiol Ultrasound. 2002;43:10–15.

7. Negrin A, Cherubini GB, Lamb C, Benigni L, Adams V, Platt S. Clinical signs, magnetic resonance imaging findings and outcome in 77 cats with vestibular disease: a retrospective study. J Feline Med Surg. 2010;12:291–299.

8. Costanzo C, Garosi LS, Glass EN, Rusbridge C, Stalin CE, Volk HA. Brain abscess in seven cats due to a bite wound: MRI findings, surgical management and outcome. J Feline Med Surg. 2011;13:672–680.

9. Mateo I, Lorenzo V, Munoz A, Pumarola M. Brainstem abscess due to plant foreign body in a dog. J Vet Intern Med. 2007;21: 535–538.

10. Sturges BK, Dickinson PJ, Kortz GD, Berry WL, Vernau KM, Wisner ER, et al. Clinical signs, magnetic resonance imaging features, and outcome after surgical and medical treatment of otogenic intracranial infection in 11 cats and 4 dogs. J Vet Intern Med. 2006;20:648–656.

11. Klopp LS, Hathcock JT, Sorjonen DC. Magnetic resonance imaging features of brain stem abscessation in two cats. Vet Radiol Ultrasound. 2000;41:300–307.

12. Negrin A, Lamb CR, Cappello R, Cherubini GB. Results of magnetic resonance imaging in 14 cats with meningoencephalitis. J Feline Med Surg. 2007;9:109–116.

13. Seiler G, Cizinauskas S, Scheidegger J, Lang J. Low-field magnetic resonance imaging of a pyocephalus and a suspected brain abscess in a German Shepherd dog. Vet Radiol Ultrasound. 2001;42: 417–422.

14. Wouters EG, Beukers M, Theyse LF. Surgical treatment of a cerebral brain abscess in a cat. Vet Comp Orthop Traumatol. 2011;24:72–75.

15. Radaelli ST, Platt SR. Bacterial meningoencephalomyelitis in dogs: a retrospective study of 23 cases (1990–1999). J Vet Intern Med. 2002;16:159–163.

16. Anor S, Sturges BK, Lafranco L, Jang SS, Higgins RJ, Koblik PD, et al. Systemic phaeohyphomycosis (*Cladophialophora bantiana*) in a dog – clinical diagnosis with stereotactic computed tomographic-guided brain biopsy. J Vet Intern Med. 2001;15: 257–261.

17. Bentley RT, Faissler D, Sutherland-Smith J. Successful management of an intracranial phaeohyphomycotic fungal granuloma in a dog. J Am Vet Med Assoc. 2011;239:480–485.

18. Foster SF, Charles JA, Parker G, Krockenberger M, Churcher RM, Malik R. Cerebral cryptococcal granuloma in a cat. J Feline Med Surg. 2001;3:39–44.

19. Schultz RM, Johnson EG, Wisner ER, Brown NA, Byrne BA, Sykes JE. Clinicopathologic and diagnostic imaging characteristics of systemic aspergillosis in 30 dogs. J Vet Intern Med. 2008;22:851–859.

20. Sykes JE, Sturges BK, Cannon MS, Gericota B, Higgins RJ, Trivedi SR, et al. Clinical signs, imaging features, neuropathology, and

outcome in cats and dogs with central nervous system cryptococcosis from California. J Vet Intern Med. 2010;24:1427–1438.

21. Marquez M, Rodenas S, Molin J, Rabanal RM, Fondevila D, Anor S, et al. Prototheal pyogranulomatous meningoencephalitis in a dog without evidence of disseminated infection. Vet Rec. 2012; 171:100.

22. Salvadori C, Gandini G, Ballarini A, Cantile C. Prototheal granulomatous meningoencephalitis in a dog. J Small Anim Pract. 2008;49:531–535.

23. Falzone C, Baroni M, De Lorenzi D, Mandara MT. Toxoplasma gondii brain granuloma in a cat: diagnosis using cytology from an intraoperative sample and sequential magnetic resonance imaging. J Small Anim Pract. 2008;49:95–99.

24. Garosi L, Dawson A, Couturier J, Matiasek L, de Stefani A, Davies E, et al. Necrotizing cerebellitis and cerebellar atrophy caused by Neospora caninum infection: magnetic resonance imaging and clinicopathologic findings in seven dogs. J Vet Intern Med. 2010; 24:571–578.

25. Jose-Lopez R, la Fuente CD, Anor S. Presumed brain infarctions in two dogs with systemic leishmaniasis. J Small Anim Pract. 2012;53:554–557.

26. Pfohl JC, Dewey CW. Intracranial *Toxoplasma gondii* granuloma in a cat. J Feline Med Surg. 2005;7:369–374.

27. Reed LT, Miller MA, Visvesvara GS, Gardiner CH, Logan MA, Packer RA. Diagnostic exercise. Cerebral mass in a puppy with respiratory distress and progressive neurologic signs. Vet Pathol. 2010;47:1116–1119.

28. Garosi LS, Platt SR, McConnell JF, Wrayt JD, Smith KC. Intracranial haemorrhage associated with *Angiostrongylus vasorum* infection in three dogs. J Small Anim Pract. 2005;46: 93–99.

29. Gredal H, Willesen JL, Jensen HE, Nielsen OL, Kristensen AT, Koch J, et al. Acute neurological signs as the predominant clinical manifestation in four dogs with *Angiostrongylus vasorum* infections in Denmark. Acta Vet Scand. 2011;53:43.

30. Negrin A, Cherubini GB, Steeves E. Angiostrongylus vasorum causing meningitis and detection of parasite larvae in the cerebrospinal fluid of a pug dog. J Small Anim Pract. 2008;49: 468–471.

31. Wessmann A, Lu D, Lamb CR, Smyth B, Mantis P, Chandler K, et al. Brain and spinal cord haemorrhages associated with *Angiostrongylus vasorum* infection in four dogs. Vet Rec. 2006;158:858–863.

32. Buback JL, Schulz KS, Walker MA, Snowden KF. Magnetic resonance imaging of the brain for diagnosis of neurocysticercosis in a dog. J Am Vet Med Assoc. 1996;208:1846–1848.

2.8

Neoplasia

Intracranial tumors can be characterized by anatomic location, distribution (intraaxial, intraventricular, extraaxial), CT density or MR signal characteristics, intensity and pattern of contrast enhancement, tumor margin definition, secondary mass effects, and the extent of associated brain edema. Although biopsy is necessary for definitive diagnosis, this constellation of imaging features can often lead to a specific or differential clinical diagnosis.[1] The tumor classification scheme used in this chapter is based on current WHO classification for central nervous system tumors in people.[2,3]

Neoplasms of the meninges

Meningioma

Meningiomas are the most common of the primary intracranial, extraaxial neoplasms in dogs and cats. German Shepherd Dogs, Collies, Golden Retrievers, and Boxers are overrepresented.[4,5] Meningiomas are derived from meningothelial cells and are divided into three grades: WHO grade I, benign; WHO grade II (atypical), which have intermediate histologic features; and WHO grade III, malignant. In a report of 112 canine meningiomas, 56% were grade I, 43% were grade II, and less than 1% were grade III.[6]

Meningiomas in dogs most frequently impinge on the olfactory bulbs and frontal lobes and are often of a macrocystic histological subtype. Other common sites include the cerebral or cerebellar convexity and cerebellopontine, basilar, tentorial, falcine, foraminal, or intraventricular locations.[6] Multiple meningiomas may be present simultaneously, particularly in older cats, and it is unclear whether these represent multicentric disease or metastasis from a single primary site.[7–9] Meningiomas may occasionally have a mineralized, cystic, or hemorrhagic component.

Meningiomas are typically iso- to mildly hyperattenuating to cortical gray matter on unenhanced CT images and can produce considerable mass effect. Cystic components appear hypoattenuating, as does surrounding peritumoral edema, which can be extensive (Figure 2.8.1). In some patients, hyperostosis of calvarial bone adjacent to a meningioma will appear thickened and hyperattenuating.

Solid meningiomas are usually uniformly T1 isointense on unenhanced MR images but are occasionally hypo- or hyperintense. Approximately 70% of meningiomas are T2 hyperintense, with the remainder being isointense. Despite the relatively benign biological behavior of the majority of meningiomas, about 95% are accompanied by edema, which may be peritumoral (40%) or diffuse (50%).[6] Edema in T2 or FLAIR images often clearly delineates the meningioma margin, confirming its extraaxial origin (Figures 2.8.2, 2.8.3, 2.8.4, 2.8.5, 2.8.6, 2.8.7). Signal void of adjacent calvarial bone due to reactive hyperostosis can sometimes be seen (Figure 2.8.4).[10]

On both CT and MR images, approximately 60–70% of meningiomas show marked, uniform contrast enhancement, with the remainder being heterogeneous and often associated with cystic, hemorrhagic, or mineralized components (Figure 2.8.5). Contrast enhancement usually reveals well-defined tumor margins; a globoid, plaque-like, or irregular shape; and a broad-based superficial margin conforming to the meningeal plane.[6,9,11–17] On contrast-enhanced MR images, thickening and intense

Atlas of Small Animal CT and MRI, First Edition. Erik R. Wisner and Allison L. Zwingenberger.
© 2015 John Wiley & Sons, Inc. Published 2015 by John Wiley & Sons, Inc.

enhancement of meninges adjacent to the tumor, often referred to as a dural tail sign, is a common imaging feature of meningiomas, although not pathognomonic for the disorder (Figure 2.8.2).[15,18] This feature may be difficult to recognize on contrast-enhanced CT images because of the hyperattenuation of adjacent bone.

Granular cell tumor

Granular cell tumors (GCT) are uncommon central nervous system neoplasms and are of uncertain origin. Astrocytic, pituicytic (modified astrocyte), meningeal cell, glial cell, and glial precursor cells have all been suggested as originating cell lines, and there is evidence that granular cell tumors represent a common phenotype of a variety of neoplasms. Granular cell tumors are included in this section because of the many imaging features they have in common with meningiomas. GCTs are usually well defined and extraaxial with a plaque-like, sessile distribution involving the meninges. They are preferentially located along the convexity of the cerebrum, the falx cerebri, or the floor of the cranial vault, and those involving the cerebrum can be quite extensive.[19]

Peritumoral edema and mass effect associated with these tumors can be seen on both CT and MR images. Granular cell tumors are mildly hyperattenuating on unenhanced CT images and mildly T1 hyperintense and T2 iso- to hyperintense on MR images. Granular cell tumors intensely and uniformly enhance on both CT and MR images following contrast administration, and tumor margins are usually well defined (Figure 2.8.8).[19,20]

Neoplasms of neuroepithelial origin

Astrocytoma

Astrocytomas are one of the most common of the intraaxial central nervous system (CNS) neoplasms.[21] Boxers and some other brachycephalic breeds are highly predisposed. Older dogs are most frequently affected, but astrocytomas also occur in young animals.[22] Although astrocytomas can originate from either white or gray matter, those that occur within the cerebrum appear to arise predominantly from white matter.[4,5] The frontal, piriform, and temporal lobes are the most common sites.

The current human WHO classification scheme grades astrocytomas based on cytological characteristics. Grade I and II astrocytomas (diffuse astrocytomas) are considered the least biologically aggressive forms and consist of a uniform, well-differentiated infiltrative cell population without mitotic activity. Grade III (anaplastic) astrocytomas have more nuclear atypia, a much higher cell density, and mitotic activity. Grade IV astrocytomas (glioblastoma multiforme) are the most malignant and infiltrative, frequently having regions of necrosis, microvascular proliferation, and sometimes intratumoral hemorrhage, which contribute heterogeneity to their MR imaging appearance in both humans and animals.[23] Astrocytomas may be globoid or irregularly shaped, and peritumoral edema is variable but usually minimal to moderate. Intratumoral hemorrhage may also occur in high-grade tumors. MR features of gliomas and presumed cerebrovascular accidents can be similar, although gliomas tend to be distributed primarily in the cerebrum, whereas vascular lesions are more likely to be located in the cerebellum, thalamus, midbrain, and brainstem. Diffusion-weighted imaging can be used to discriminate between these two disorders, with vascular lesions more likely to result in diffusion restriction.[24]

Astrocytomas are generally hypoattenuating on unenhanced CT images, and mass margins may be ill defined, particularly when surrounded by peritumoral edema or when biological grade is low (Figure 2.8.9).

Astrocytomas typically appear mildly to moderately T1 hypointense and moderately and heterogeneously T2 hyperintense. Surrounding edema may mask tumor margins on both T1 and T2 images.

With both CT and MR, the intensity of tumor enhancement following contrast administration reflects microvascular proliferation and blood–brain barrier disruption and tends to increase with astrocytoma grade. Low-grade astrocytomas typically do not enhance, or enhance minimally, whereas high-grade astrocytomas are more likely to show moderate or marked, nonuniform or peripheral contrast enhancement, although the degree of enhancement is not a reliable indicator of tumor grade (Figures 2.8.9, 2.8.10).[21,22,25–28]

Oligodendroglioma

Oligodendrogliomas occur with similar frequency to astrocytomas and affect older dogs, particularly Boxers and other brachycephalic breeds.[21] Oligodendrogliomas most frequently arise supratentorially in the frontal, piriform, and temporal lobes of the cerebrum and, less commonly, more caudally.

Oligodendrogliomas may be globoid or irregularly shaped, typically have a central mucinous core, and often encroach on or breach the ependymal lining of the ventricles.[28] Canine oligodendrogliomas are categorized as either low-grade (grades I or II) or high-grade (grade III), with grade III tumors predominating. Peripherally, low-grade oligodendrogliomas have a well-differentiated cell population and a well-defined interface with adjacent brain parenchyma, whereas the high-grade oligodendrogliomas are composed of more anaplastic cells with necrosis and microvascular proliferation. Intratumoral hemorrhage may also be present. As with astrocytomas, microvascular proliferation is associated with peripheral or nonuniform contrast enhancement.[23] Tumor-related production of vascular permeability factors, such as vascular endothelial growth factor, may also contribute to contrast enhancement in high-grade gliomas.[6]

The appearance of oligodendrogliomas on unenhanced CT images is similar to that of astrocytomas. They are typically hypoattenuating, and mass margins may be ill defined or lacking, particularly when peritumoral edema is present. Marked central hypoattenuation of some oligodendrogliomas, caused by the high water content of the mucinous core, may increase the index of suspicion for this tumor.

Oligodendrogliomas are moderately T1 hypointense and markedly T2 hyperintense, specifically when there is significant central mucinous content. Peritumoral edema ranges from minimal to moderate, although even large oligodendrogliomas may induce little edema formation.

Contrast enhancement of oligodendrogliomas on both CT and MR images is highly variable, ranging from none to marked, and when present it is often peripheral or nonuniform. Focal or regional contrast enhancement is often distributed centrally or eccentrically within the greater tumor volume and may have a serpentine shape.[21,27–29] Although high-grade oligodendrogliomas tend to contrast enhance to a greater degree than low-grade tumors, as with astrocytoma, this imaging feature is not a reliable indicator of biological grade (Figure 2.8.11, 2.8.12).

Mixed glial cell tumors

Canine mixed glial tumors are usually comprised of tumor cells with both astrocytic and oligodendrocytic features, or they may contain a combination of astrocytic and oligodendrocytic subpopulations. These tumors have MR imaging features similar to those of astrocytomas and oligodendrogliomas.

Ependymal tumors

Ependymomas are uncommon tumors that arise from the ependymal lining cells of the ventricular system and thus may occur within the ventricular system of the brain and spinal cord. Ependymomas usually affect older dogs and cats without breed predisposition. These tumors are predominantly intraventricular, although some invade the adjacent brain parenchyma, and they expand to fill the ventricular cavity in which they arise, causing distortion of the ventricle and obstructive hydrocephalus, depending on their size and location. Ependymomas may be well differentiated (WHO grade II) or anaplastic and aggressive (WHO grade III). Grossly, the tumors can be soft, lobular (papillary type), or solid (cellular subtype) and may contain cysts and/or hemorrhage.[4,5] Ependymomas may be accommodated by gradual ventricular dilation, hence edema is usually absent or minimal, unless the tumor invades the periventricular brain parenchyma or hydrocephalus causes periventricular interstitial edema.

Ependymomas are typically isoattenuating on unenhanced CT images, although they can have a heterogeneous appearance.

Ependymomas appear slightly T1 hypointense to slightly hyperintense on unenhanced images and moderately to markedly T2 hyperintense.

Contrast enhancement is usually marked and may be heterogeneous, which reflects the coarse texture of the tumor parenchyma, on both CT and MR images.[27,30,31] Heterogeneity may be even more pronounced when cysts or hemorrhage are present. Tumor margins are typically distinct, because the majority of the mass extends into a ventricular lumen (Figure 2.8.13).

Choroid plexus tumors

Choroid plexus tumors (CPT) are relatively common neoplasms that arise from the choroid plexus epithelium within the lateral, third, and fourth ventricles and the lateral recesses. About 50% originate in the fourth ventricle or lateral recesses. The average age of dogs at diagnosis is 6 years, which is earlier than most other intracranial tumors. Golden Retrievers appear to be highly overrepresented.[32] Classification of canine CPT distinguishes choroid plexus papillomas (CPP), comparable to WHO grade I and morphologically benign, from choroid plexus carcinomas (CPC), comparable to WHO grade III and histologically more abnormal and more likely to invade the brain or give rise to intraventricular or intrathecal metastases.[32] Mild to moderate edema is present in about 45% of CPP and about 70% of CPC.[32]

Choroid plexus tumors share many CT and MR imaging features with ependymomas. Initially, they may conform to the shape of the ventricle in which they grow, but enlargement may lead to hydrocephalus because of ventricular obstruction or, possibly, overproduction of CSF. Tumors have variable attenuation on unenhanced CT images and may be T1 hypo-, iso-, or hyperintense and T2 hyperintense on MR images. Choroid plexus tumors often appear heterogeneous, particularly when there is intratumoral hemorrhage.

Choroid plexus tumors usually show marked, uniform enhancement on both CT and MR images following contrast administration, which reflects the underlying papillary vascular architecture of these tumors (Figure 2.8.14). Intraventricular and intrathecal "drop metastases" may appear as intensely contrast-enhancing foci in the ventricles or subarachnoid space (Figure 2.8.15). Choroid plexus papillomas and carcinomas cannot be reliably distinguished by CT or MR imaging, although presence of drop metastases suggests CPC.[21,27,32–36]

Lymphoma and hematopoietic neoplasms

Lymphoma

Lymphoma is a relatively uncommon intracranial neoplasm that generally occurs in younger patients (3–7 years) than other intracranial tumors and without any apparent breed predisposition.[21] Intracranial lymphoma may be primary or metastatic within the CNS and of either B- or T-cell type. The majority of CNS lymphomas in dogs are due to metastasis of widely disseminated disease. In people, primary CNS lymphoma occurs most commonly in immunocompromised patients, is overwhelmingly B-cell phenotype, and presents as a solitary invasive periventricular mass. There are few published descriptions of MR features of intracranial lymphoma in dogs and cats, but the tumor can be either intraaxial or extraaxial and can be quite variable in appearance.[37] Canine primary intracranial lymphoma seems to frequently affect the thalamic/hypothalamic/sellar region, while metastatic lesions are disseminated in the meninges, choroid plexus, multiple cranial nerves, and pituitary gland.[37] Consistent with the variable manifestations of primary or metastatic lymphoma elsewhere, intracranial lymphoma may be mass-like, diffuse, or multicentric. Diagnosis of intracranial lymphoma is sometimes possible, based on cerebrospinal fluid cytology, which may eliminate the need for brain biopsy.

Most primary lesions have a mild to moderate mass effect. These tend to be iso- to hypoattenuating on unenhanced CT images, T1 iso- or hypointense, and variably T2 hyperintense with minimal to moderate peritumoral edema.[37]

Central nervous system lymphoma in dogs consistently enhances after contrast medium administration on both CT and MR images, but the degree of enhancement, tumor margin definition, and contrast distribution is variable (Figure 2.8.16).[38–43] Marked meningeal enhancement often occurs with the meningeal manifestation of the disorder (Figure 2.8.17). This is easily seen on enhanced MR images and can be recognized on CT images, particularly when there is significant pial enhancement.

Histiocytic tumors

Central nervous system histiocytic sarcoma is an uncommon neoplasm of the hematopoietic system with cellular features of malignancy and meningeal and brain parenchyma invasion, indicating biologically aggressive behavior.[44–46] On the basis of limited experience, it appears that histiocytic sarcoma tends to present as an extradural or intradural/extraaxial mass, although diffuse meningeal and intraaxial forms also occur.

Characteristic CT features of histiocytic sarcoma have not been documented, but these tumors are T1 iso- to hypointense and T2 iso- to hyperintense on unenhanced MR images and can cause a mass effect accompanied by regional or diffuse peritumoral edema.

Contrast enhancement on both CT and MR images is moderate to marked and can be either uniform or heterogeneous. As observed with meningiomas, the margins of extraaxial histiocytic sarcomas may appear well defined on T2 and enhanced T1 images, although the degree of contrast enhancement may sometimes be less than that of meningiomas and have a fine granular pattern (Figure 2.8.18). Dural tail signs have also been reported inconsistently with these tumors.[44]

Metastatic neoplasms

In a series of 177 secondary intracranial neoplasms in dogs, 29% were hemangiosarcomas and 12% were metastatic carcinomas.[40] Lymphoma and pituitary tumors were included in this study, but if these neoplasms are excluded, hemangiosarcoma and carcinomas account for 50% and 20% of secondary (metastatic) intracranial neoplasms, respectively.[40] Metastatic tumors appear to preferentially distribute to the gray–white matter interface, which may reflect the likelihood of tumor emboli lodging in the cortical arterioles where they narrow.[4,5] (Figures 2.8.19, 2.8.20, 2.8.21)

On MR images, metastatic hemangiosarcoma often appears as multiple mass lesions, although metastasis should still be considered when a solitary lesion is found. Hemangiosarcomas typically have a marked mass effect, mixed signal intensity on T1 and T2 sequences and heterogeneous intensity with susceptibility effects on T2* images because of intratumoral hemorrhage. Peritumoral edema may be marked. Contrast enhancement is variable and often peripheral (Figure 2.8.19). Metastatic carcinoma also appears as multiple variably contrast-enhancing ill-defined mass lesions with variable peritumoral edema, but typically without the intratumoral hemorrhage characteristic of hemangiosarcoma (Figure 2.8.20).

Figure 2.8.1   Meningioma (Canine)

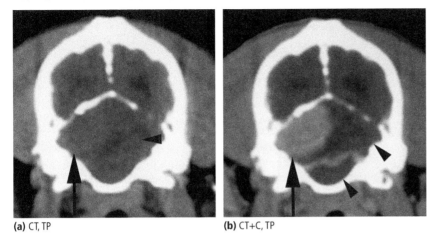

(a) CT, TP

(b) CT+C, TP

13y MC West Highland White Terrier with central vestibular signs. A soft-tissue mass, which is slightly hyperattenuating compared to occipital lobe cortex, is identified in the right caudal fossa adjacent to the ventral margin of the os tentorium (**a**: arrow). The left side of the cerebellum is hypoattenuating, suggesting the presence of perilesional edema (**a**: arrowhead). The mass intensely and uniformly enhances following contrast administration and is well margined and broad based, indicating an extraaxial origin (**b**: arrow). Adjacent cerebellum and brainstem are displaced and compressed (**b**: arrowheads). Postmortem examination confirmed a diagnosis of meningioma.

Figure 2.8.2   Meningioma (Canine)

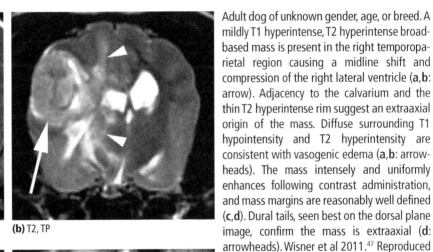

(a) T1, TP

(b) T2, TP

Adult dog of unknown gender, age, or breed. A mildly T1 hyperintense, T2 hyperintense broad-based mass is present in the right temporoparietal region causing a midline shift and compression of the right lateral ventricle (**a,b**: arrow). Adjacency to the calvarium and the thin T2 hyperintense rim suggest an extraaxial origin of the mass. Diffuse surrounding T1 hypointensity and T2 hyperintensity are consistent with vasogenic edema (**a,b**: arrowheads). The mass intensely and uniformly enhances following contrast administration, and mass margins are reasonably well defined (**c,d**). Dural tails, seen best on the dorsal plane image, confirm the mass is extraaxial (**d**: arrowheads). Wisner et al 2011.[47] Reproduced with permission from Wiley.

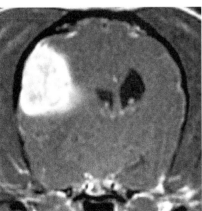

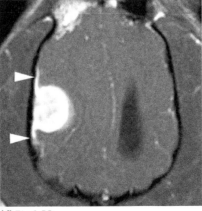

(c) T1+C, TP

(d) T1+C, DP

Figure 2.8.3 Macrocystic Meningioma (Canine)   MR

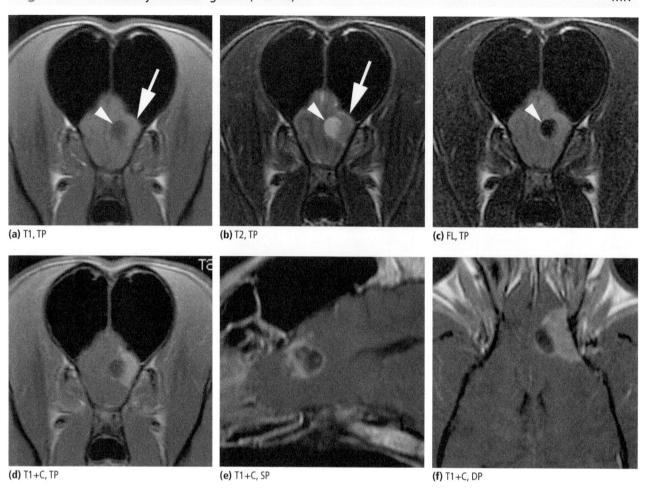

(a) T1, TP   **(b)** T2, TP   **(c)** FL, TP

(d) T1+C, TP   **(e)** T1+C, SP   **(f)** T1+C, DP

8y MC Golden Retriever with recent onset of seizures. There is a sessile T1 and T2 hyperintense mass involving the left olfactory bulb/frontal lobe region (**a**,**b**: arrow) with an adjacent T1 hypointense, T2 hyperintense, and FLAIR-nulling cystic component (**a–c**: arrowhead). The solid component of the mass intensely and uniformly enhances following contrast administration (**d–f**). There is a thin rim of enhancement in the cystic part, but it is otherwise unchanged.

Figure 2.8.4 Meningioma with Hyperostosis (Feline)   MR

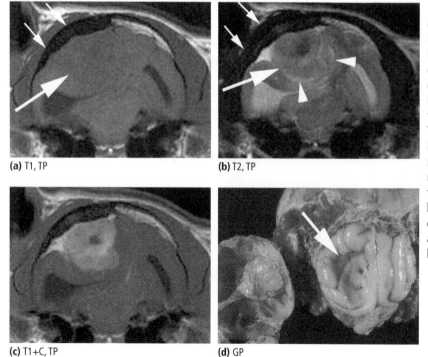

(a) T1, TP   **(b)** T2, TP

(c) T1+C, TP   **(d)** GP

15y FS Domestic Shorthair with acute onset of seizures. There is a broad-based, mildly T1 hypointense, T2 mixed-intensity mass involving the right frontoparietal region of the brain, causing marked displacement of the adjacent cerebrum (**a**,**b**: large arrow). The thin T2 hyperintense rim lends further evidence that this is an extraaxial mass (**b**: arrowheads). The overlying parietal bone is thickened and hypointense as a result of bone reactivity and resulting hyperostosis (**a**,**b**: small arrows). The mass intensely and heterogeneously enhances following contrast administration. Marked brain compression by the mass was evident on postmortem examination (**d**: arrow), and a diagnosis of meningioma was confirmed histologically.

Figure 2.8.5 Meningioma (Canine)

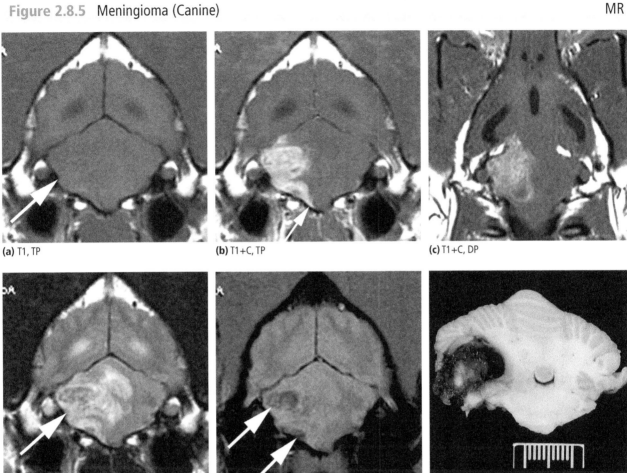

(a) T1, TP

(b) T1+C, TP

(c) T1+C, DP

(d) T2, TP

(e) T2*, TP

(f) GP, TP

13y FS Golden Retriever with recent onset central vestibular and brainstem signs. There is a T1 isointense, T2 mixed-intensity mass involving the right side of the cerebellum (**a,d**: arrow). The complex T2 intensity paired with the multifocal susceptibility effect present on the T2* image (**e**: arrows) is indicative of intralesional hemorrhage. The mass intensely, but nonuniformly, enhances following contrast administration (**b,c**), and a sessile base and dural tail (**b**: arrow) reflect an extraaxial origin. Gross postmortem examination revealed an extraaxial hemorrhagic caudal fossa mass that was histologically determined to be a meningioma.

Figure 2.8.6   Intraventricular Meningioma (Feline)   CT & MR

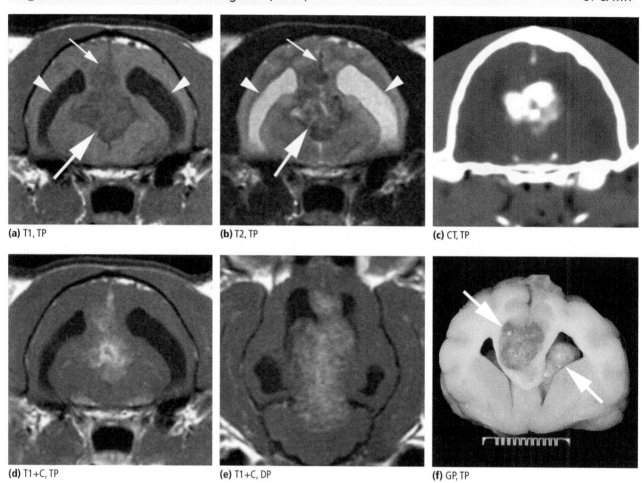

(a) T1, TP   **(b)** T2, TP   **(c)** CT, TP

(d) T1+C, TP   **(e)** T1+C, DP   **(f)** GP, TP

13y MC Domestic Shorthair with intracranial neurologic signs. There is a nonuniformly T1 hypointense, T2 mixed-intensity mass that distends the third ventricle (**a**,**b**: large arrow) and results in lateral ventriculomegaly (**a**,**b**: arrowheads). The mass also appears to have an extraventricular component involving the falx cerebri (**a**,**b**: small arrows). An unenhanced CT image (**c**) reveals the mass to be mineralized, which explains the heterogenous T1 and T2 hypointensity seen on MR images. There is moderate to marked nonuniform enhancement following contrast administration (**d**,**e**). Postmortem examination confirmed the presence of a predominantly intraventricular psammomatous meningioma (**f**: arrows).

Figure 2.8.7   Multiple Meningiomas (Canine)   MR

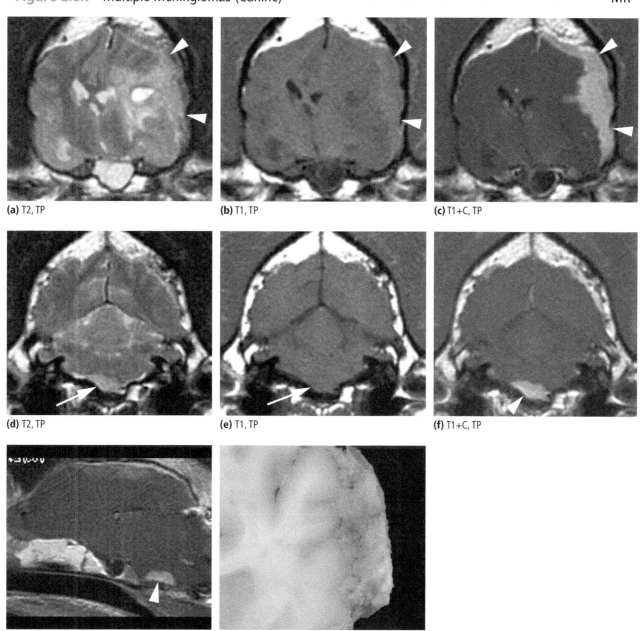

(a) T2, TP

(b) T1, TP

(c) T1+C, TP

(d) T2, TP

(e) T1, TP

(f) T1+C, TP

(g) T1+C, SP

(h) GP, TP

10y FS Labrador Retriever cross with recent onset of disorientation progressing to obtundation. There is a superficial plaque-like T1 and T2 hyperintense mass involving the entire left cerebrum, causing marked midline shift (**a,b**: arrowheads). Additional T2 hyperintensity in the corona radiata of the left hemisphere represents angiogenic edema (**a**). A similar, but smaller, sessile mass is present adjacent to the pons (**d,e**: arrow). Both masses intensely and uniformly enhance following contrast administration (**c,f,g**: arrowheads). Postmortem examination confirmed a diagnosis of multiple meningiomas. The gross specimen illustrates the extraaxial location of the larger meningioma (**h**). This is the same patient as in Figure 2.9.4 illustrating a pituitary cyst.

Figure 2.8.8 Granular Cell Tumor (Canine)   MR

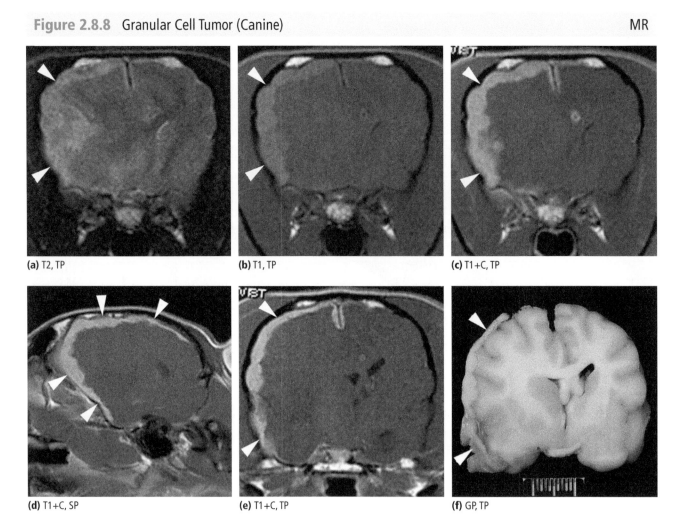

(a) T2, TP   (b) T1, TP   (c) T1+C, TP

(d) T1+C, SP   (e) T1+C, TP   (f) GP, TP

12y FS Miniature Poodle with vestibular signs. There is a thin, plaque-like, T1 and T2 hyperintense mass involving the entire right cerebral cortex, causing a pronounced midline shift (a,b: arrowheads). The mass intensely and uniformly enhances following contrast administration (c–e: arrowheads). A gross cross-sectional image, which correlates with MR image e, confirms the extraaxial origin of the tumor (e,f: arrowheads). The mass was histologically confirmed to be a granular cell tumor. Anwer et al 2013.[19] Reproduced with permission from Wiley.

Figure 2.8.9 Low-grade Astrocytoma (Canine) CT & MR

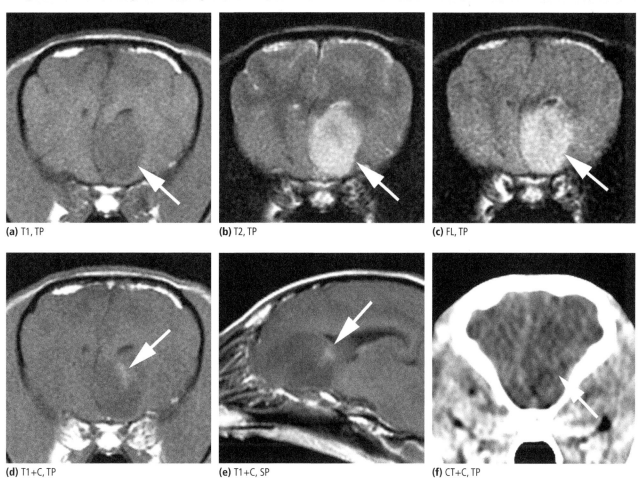

(a) T1, TP

(b) T2, TP

(c) FL, TP

(d) T1+C, TP

(e) T1+C, SP

(f) CT+C, TP

9y MC Toy Poodle with a 3-week history of seizures. A large, T1 hypointense, T2 and FLAIR hyperintense ovoid mass is seen in the ventral aspect of the left frontal lobe (**a–c**: arrow). There is mild enhancement in part of the mass following contrast administration (**d,e**: arrow). A more rostral contrast-enhanced CT image reveals a hypoattenuating mass effect in the left frontal lobe inducing midline shift (**f**: arrow). Biopsy revealed the mass to be a grade II astrocytoma.

Figure 2.8.10   Glioblastoma Multiforme (Canine)   MR

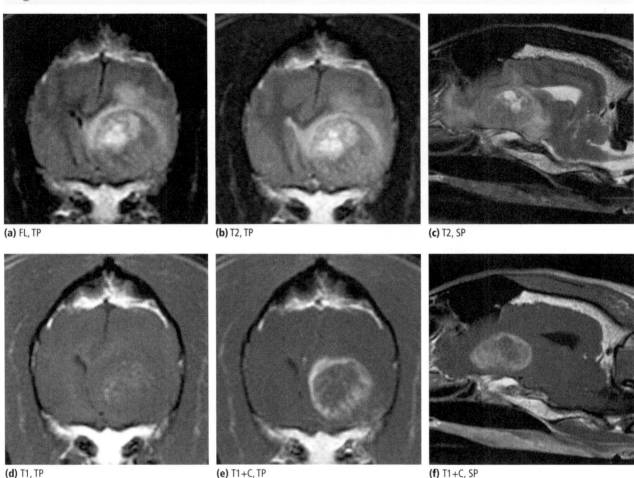

(a) FL, TP   **(b)** T2, TP   **(c)** T2, SP

(d) T1, TP   **(e)** T1+C, TP   **(f)** T1+C, SP

10y MC Australian Shepherd with recent onset of seizures. There is a large ovoid mass with mixed T1, T2, and FLAIR intensity in the left cerebrum. Mass margins are well defined on T2 and FLAIR images, and the halo of hyperintensity surrounding the mass on these sequences is indicative of vasogenic edema. The mass nonuniformly enhances following contrast administration, with more intense enhancement peripherally. Postmortem examination confirmed glioblastoma multiforme. There was extensive intratumoral hemorrhage consistent with the complex, mixed signal intensity seen on unenhanced images.

Figure 2.8.11   High-grade Oligodendroglioma (Canine)   CT

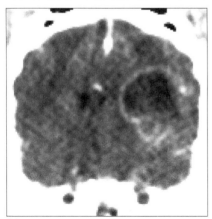

8y MC Labrador Retriever with recent onset of seizures and circling. There is a large, irregularly shaped, peripherally enhancing mass in the temporoparietal region of the left cerebrum. The center of the mass is hypoattenuating. Postmortem examination confirmed grade III oligodendroglioma.

(a) CT+C, TP

Figure 2.8.12   High-grade Oligodendroglioma (Canine)   MR

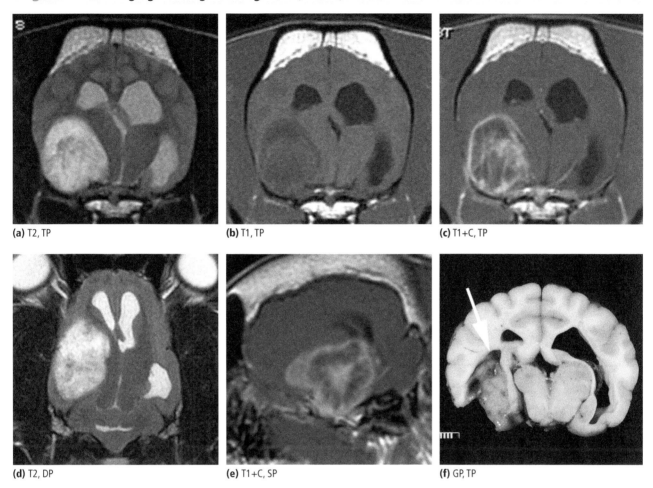

(a) T2, TP

(b) T1, TP

(c) T1+C, TP

(d) T2, DP

(e) T1+C, SP

(f) GP, TP

5y FS French Bulldog with inappetence, lethargy, and head tilt. There is a large, irregularly shaped T1 hypointense and T2 hyperintense mass in the right temporal–piriform region, resulting in midline shift and obscuration of the ventral aspect of the right lateral ventricle (**a,b,d**). Perilesional edema is conspicuously absent. The mass enhances nonuniformly following contrast administration, with a thin contrast rim defining the mass margins (**c,e**). Postmortem examination confirmed the mass to be a grade III oligodendroglioma with extension into the right lateral ventricle (**f**: arrow). The high water content of the mucinous center explains the T2 hyperintensity of the tumor.

Figure 2.8.13   Ependymoma (Canine)   MR

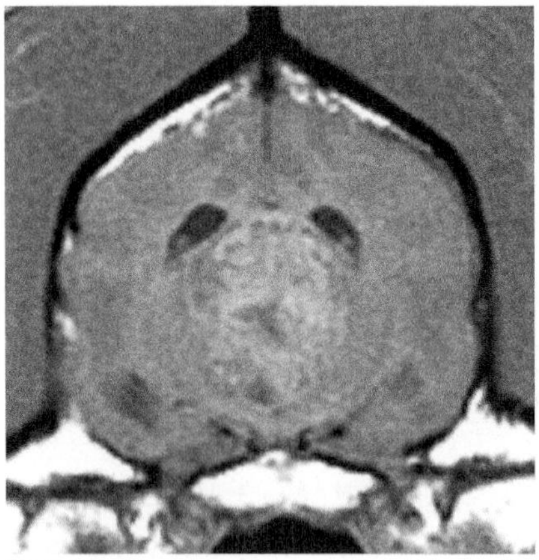

(a) T1, TP

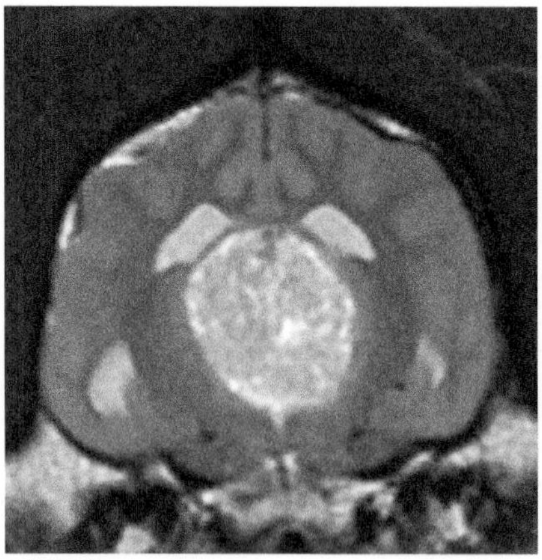

(b) T2, TP

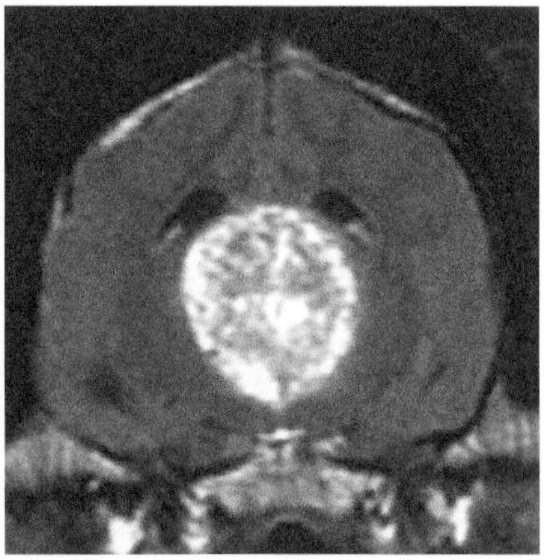

(c) FL, TP

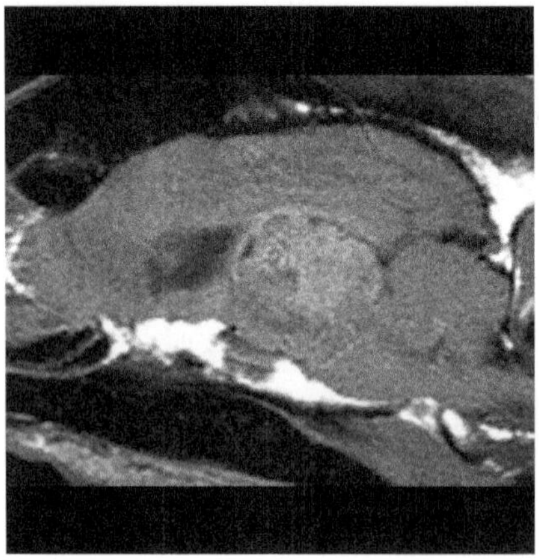

(d) T1, SP

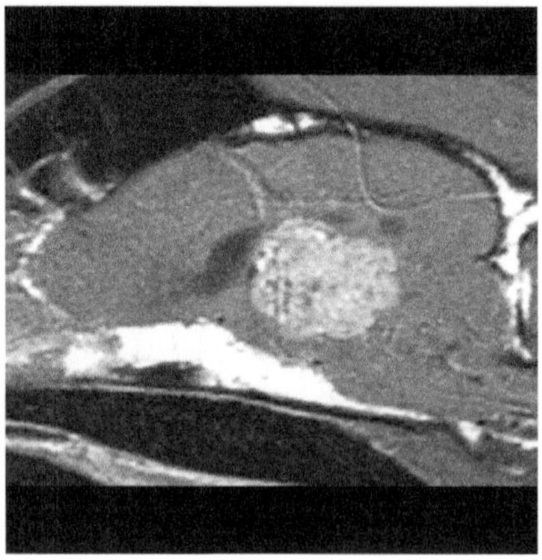

(e) T1+C, SP

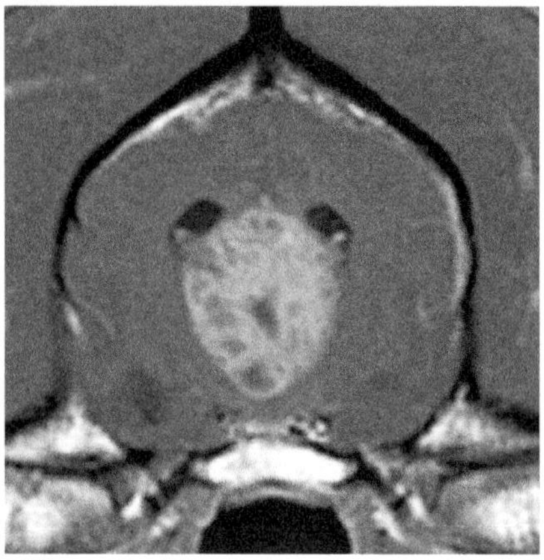

(f) T1+C, TP

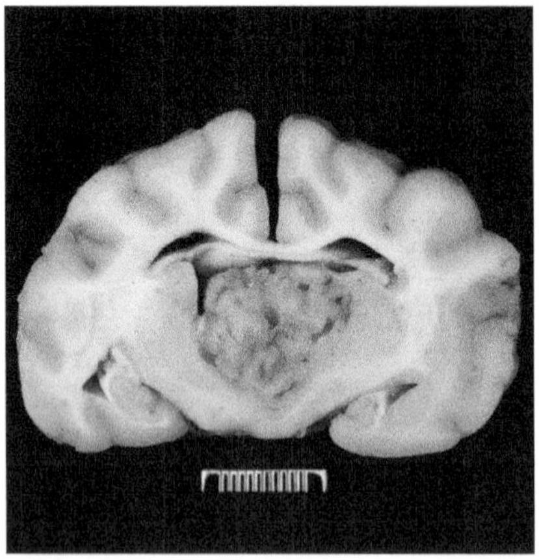

(g) GP, TP

7y MC German Shorthair Pointer with 2-week history of behavioral changes and neurologic deficits. There is a well-demarcated ovoid mass within the third ventricle, which is predominantly T1, T2, and FLAIR hyperintense (**a–d**). The mass deforms the lateral ventricles, but there is minimal hydrocephalus and no peritumoral edema. The mass intensely and nonuniformly enhances following contrast administration (**e,f**). Postmortem examination confirmed an ependymoma within the third ventricle (**g**). The granular appearance on cut surface correlates with the irregular cobblestone appearance of the tumor on MR images. An unrelated diagnosis of lymphoplasmacytic meningitis explains the meningeal contrast enhancement seen in image **f**.

Figure 2.8.14   Choroid Plexus Carcinoma (Canine)   MR

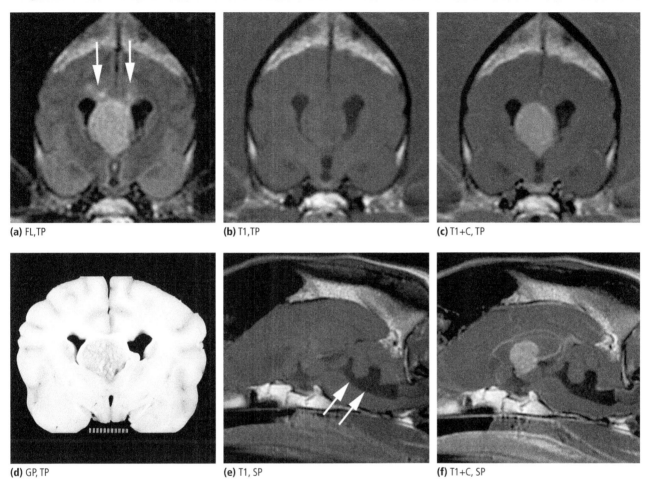

(a) FL,TP

(b) T1,TP

(c) T1+C, TP

(d) GP, TP

(e) T1, SP

(f) T1+C, SP

8y MC dog of unknown breed with a recent onset of depression progressing to obtundation. There is a mildly T1 hypointense, FLAIR hyperintense spherical mass in the third ventricle, causing displacement of the axial margins of the lateral ventricles (**a**,**b**). There is focal periventricular edema dorsal to the mass (**a**: arrows) and nonuniform ventriculomegaly, with the mesencephalic duct and fourth ventricle disproportionately enlarged (**e**: arrows). The mass intensely and uniformly enhances following contrast administration (**c**,**f**). Postmortem examination confirmed a choroid plexus carcinoma of the third ventricle (**d**). The irregular cut surface of the tumor correlates with the pattern of enhancement on MR images. The nonuniform hydrocephalus may be a result of either partial obstruction or overproduction of cerebrospinal fluid by the tumor. Westworth et al (2008).[32] Reproduced with permission from Wiley.

Figure 2.8.15   Choroid Plexus Carcinoma with Local Metastasis (Canine)   MR

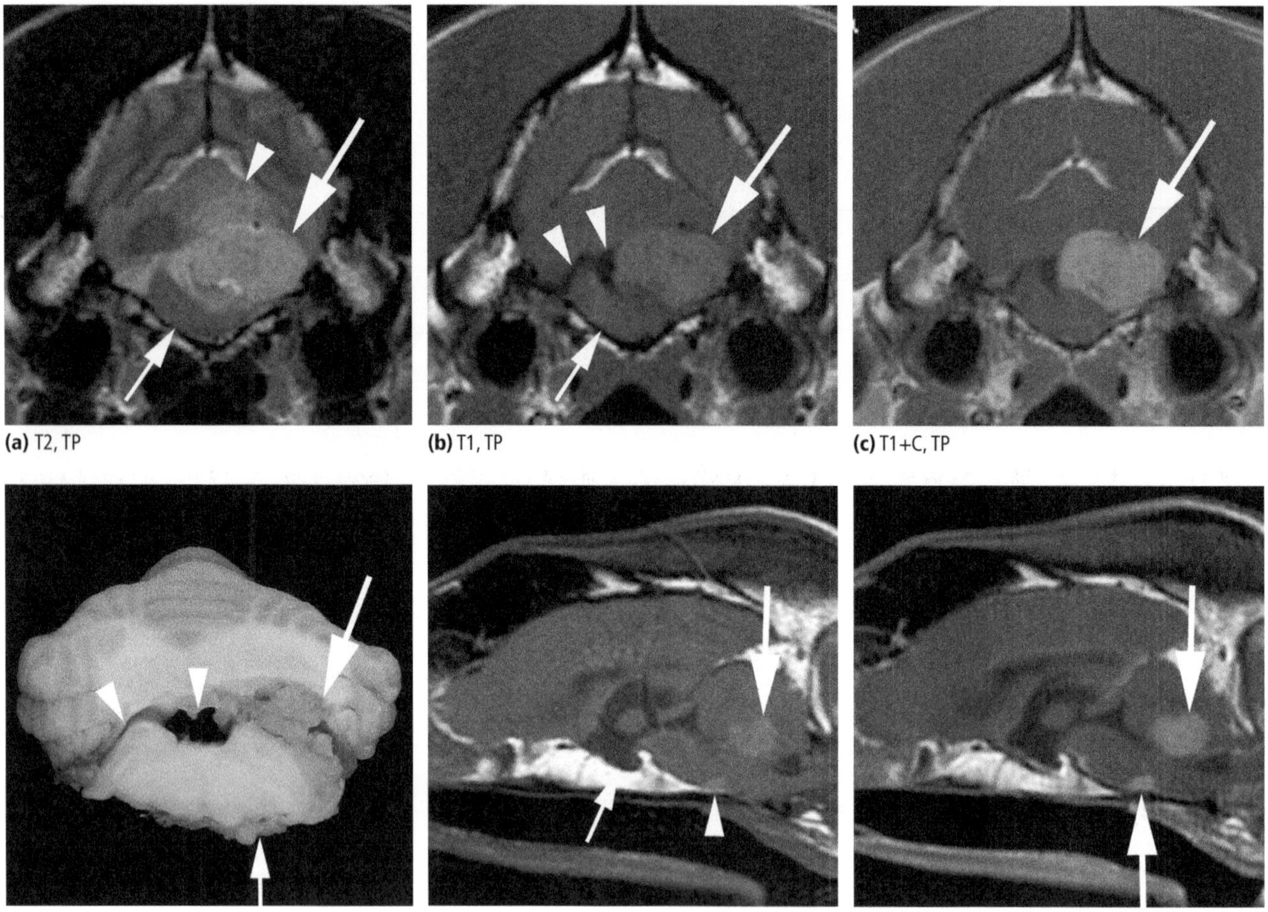

(a) T2, TP

(b) T1, TP

(c) T1+C, TP

(d) GP, TP

(e) T1, SP

(f) T1+C, SP

7y MC Chow with tetraparesis. There is a large, T1 and T2 hyperintense ovoid mass in the left lateral recess (**a,b,e**: large arrow) that encroaches on the fourth ventricle, distends the contralateral lateral recess (**b**: arrowheads), and displaces and compresses the brainstem (**a,b**: small arrow) and cerebellum (**a**: arrowhead). A smaller mass is seen ventral to the brainstem (**e**: arrowhead). Both masses intensely and uniformly enhance following contrast administration (**c,f**: arrows). Distension of the third ventricle and the infundibular recess (**e**: small arrow) is indicative of obstructive hydrocephalus. The large mass in the left lateral recess was confirmed to be a choroid plexus carcinoma (**d**: large arrow). The small mass was determined to be a local metastatic lesion (**d**: small arrow). The fourth ventricle and right lateral aperture were somewhat distended (**d**: arrowheads).

Figure 2.8.16   Lymphoma (Feline)   MR

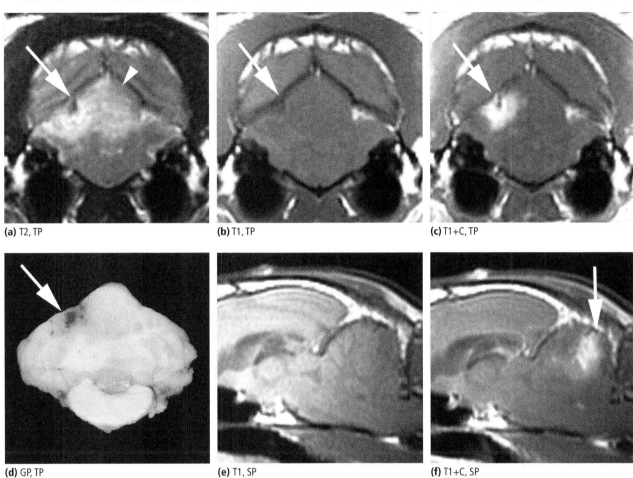

(a) T2, TP

(b) T1, TP

(c) T1+C, TP

(d) GP, TP

(e) T1, SP

(f) T1+C, SP

6y FS Domestic Shorthair with progressive obtundation and signs of intracranial disease. There is an ill-defined, mixed T1 and T2 signal intensity mass in the right cerebellar hemisphere (**a,b**: arrow) with T2 hyperintensity in the adjacent vermis, indicative of perilesional edema (**a**: arrowhead). The mass nonuniformly enhances following contrast administration, and mass margins are poorly defined (**c,f**: arrow). The cat had small intestinal T-cell lymphoma with metastasis to regional lymph nodes, liver, and cerebellum. Hemorrhage seen in the cut surface of the cerebellar mass (**d**: arrow) explains the mixed signal intensity seen on MR images.

Figure 2.8.17   Lymphoma (Canine)   MR

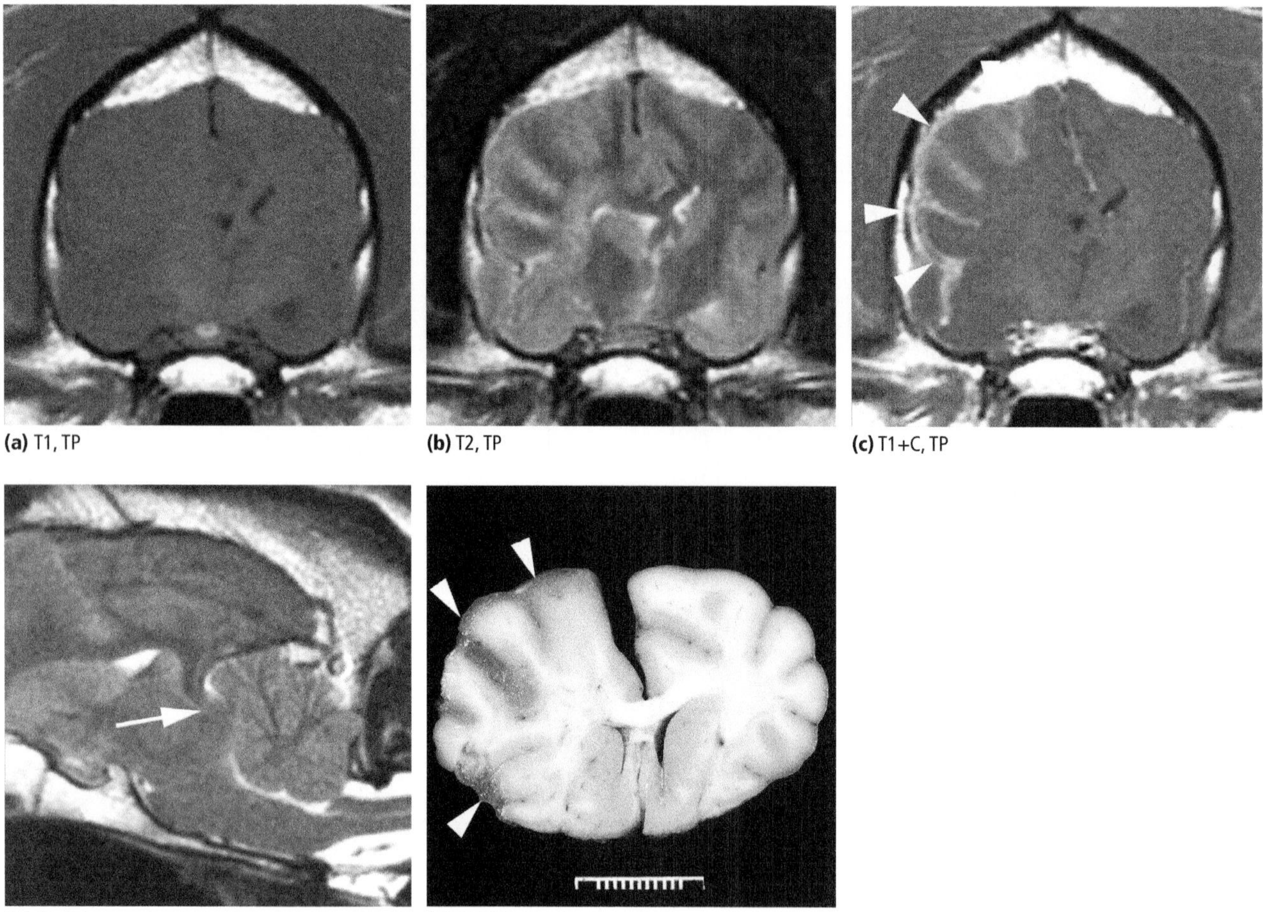

(a) T1, TP

(b) T2, TP

(c) T1+C, TP

(d) T2, SP

(e) GP, TP

10y FS Labrador Retriever with a 3-day history of progressive obtundation. There is a mass effect involving the right cerebral hemisphere, resulting in midline shift and compression and distortion of the ventricular system. The gray–white matter interface is indistinct on the right (**b**). White matter T2 hyperintensity on the right is indicative of vasogenic edema, and the sulci and gyri are effaced bilaterally. Subtentorial herniation is also evident (**d**: arrow). The meninges on the right moderately enhance and are markedly thickened following contrast administration (**c**: arrowheads). Pial involvement is recognized by the enhancement pattern that follows the contours of the brain surface. Multisystemic large-cell B-cell lymphoma was confirmed by postmortem examination. In addition to the meningeal involvement (**e**: arrowheads), there was widespread deep invasion of neoplastic cells from the leptomeninges and vessels to both cerebral hemispheres, the hippocampus, and the thalamus.

Figure 2.8.18   Histiocytic Sarcoma (Canine)   MR

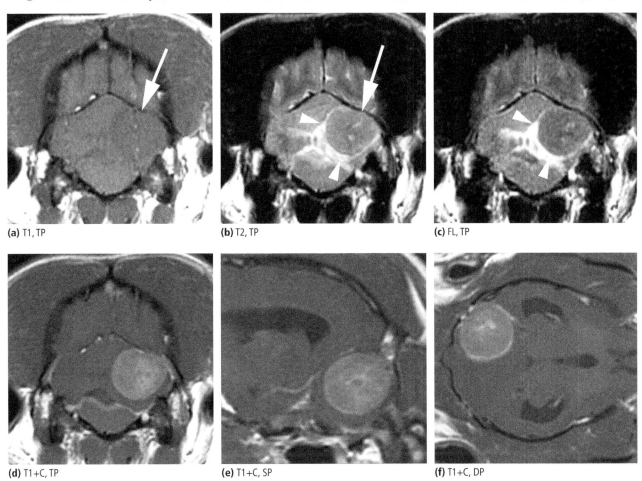

(a) T1, TP   (b) T2, TP   (c) FL, TP

(d) T1+C, TP   (e) T1+C, SP   (f) T1+C, DP

11y MC Shetland Sheepdog with recent onset of vestibular signs. There is a large T1 hypointense and T2 isointense spherical mass in the left side of the caudal fossa (**a**,**b**: arrow), causing displacement and compression of the cerebellum and brainstem. The T2 and FLAIR hyperintense rim surrounding the mass lends evidence that this is an extraaxial lesion (**b**,**c**: arrowheads). The mass enhances following contrast administration and has a subtle nonuniform "ground glass" enhancement pattern (**d–f**). The mass was confirmed to be a histiocytic sarcoma on postmortem examination. Microscopically, the mass was well demarcated, but unencapsulated, and invaded adjacent brain parenchyma from a broad meningeal base.

Figure 2.8.19   Metastatic Hemangiosarcoma (Canine)   MR

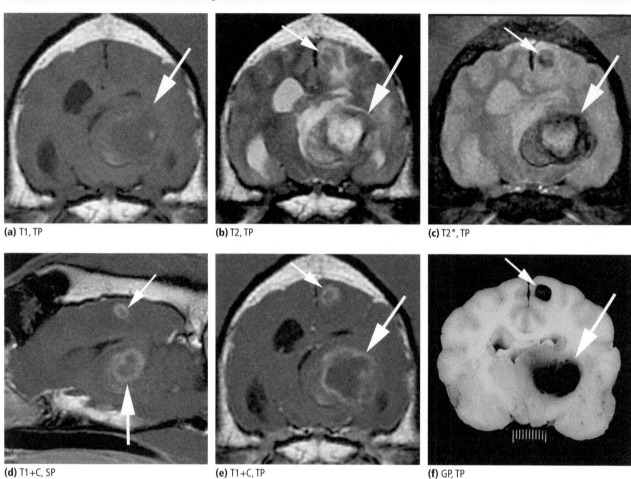

(a) T1, TP   **(b)** T2, TP   **(c)** T2*, TP

(d) T1+C, SP   **(e)** T1+C, TP   **(f)** GP, TP

11y MC Pit Bull Terrier with acute onset obtundation and tetraparesis. There is a large left thalamic mass of T1 and T2 mixed intensity, causing ventricular compression and distortion (**a,b**: large arrow). A second, smaller mass is seen in the left endomarginal gyrus, which also has mixed T2 intensity (**b**: small arrow). There is marked susceptibility effect within both masses on the gradient echo T2* image, indicative of hemorrhage (**c**: arrows). Both masses nonuniformly and peripherally enhance following contrast administration (**d,e**: arrows). Widespread hemangiosarcoma metastasis was confirmed by postmortem examination. Cut surfaces of the brain masses reveal extensive intratumoral hemorrhage, consistent with the complex intensity patterns seen on MR images (**f**: arrows). Anwer et al 2013.[19] Reproduced with permission from Wiley.

Figure 2.8.20   Metastatic Mammary Carcinoma (Canine)   MR

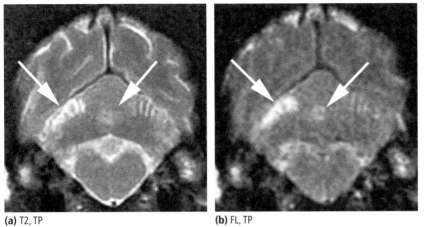

12y FS Dachshund with head tilt and seizures. There are multiple T2 and FLAIR hyperintense foci within the cerebellum (**a,b**: arrows). These lesions moderately and uniformly enhance following contrast administration (**c,d**: arrows), although margins are ill defined. Postmortem examination confirmed metastatic mammary carcinoma.

(a) T2, TP

(b) FL, TP

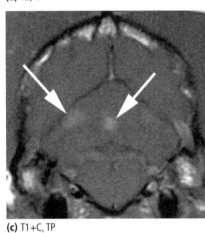

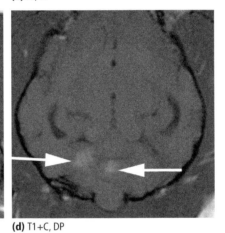

(c) T1+C, TP

(d) T1+C, DP

Figure 2.8.21   Metastatic Melanoma (Canine)   MR

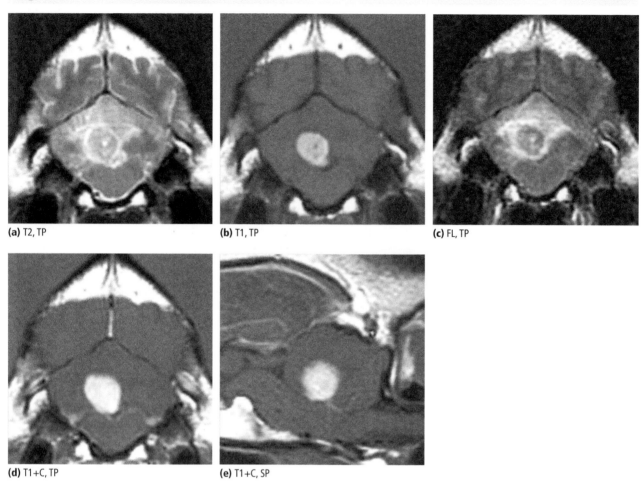

(a) T2, TP   **(b)** T1, TP   **(c)** FL, TP

(d) T1+C, TP   **(e)** T1+C, SP

7y MC Rottweiler with hypermetric gait, head tilt, and ataxia. The dog also has a lingual mass. There is a T1, T2, and FLAIR hyperintense mass involving the vermis of the cerebellum, associated with surrounding edema (**a–c**). The mass enhances following contrast administration, although the extent and uniformity of enhancement are indeterminate because of the underlying intensity present on unenhanced T1 images (**d,e**). The lingual mass proved to be a melanoma that had also metastasized to lung. The unusual hyperintensity of the mass on the unenhanced T1 image is a reported characteristic of melanotic melanomas.

References

1. Rodenas S, Pumarola M, Gaitero L, Zamora A, Anor S. Magnetic resonance imaging findings in 40 dogs with histologically confirmed intracranial tumours. Vet J. 2011;187:85–91.
2. Koestner A, Bilzer T, Fatzer R, Schulman FY, Summers BA, Van Winkle TJ. WHO International Histological Classification of Tumors of the Nervous System of Domestic Animals: Armed Forces Institute of Pathology and American Registry of Pathology, 1999.
3. Louis DN, Ohgaki H, Wiestler OD, Cavenee WK, Burger PC, Jouvet A, et al. The 2007 WHO classification of tumours of the central nervous system. Acta Neuropathol. 2007;114:97–109.
4. McGavin MD, Zachary, James F. (eds) Pathologic basis of veterinary disease. Elsevier Mosby, 2007.
5. Meuten DJ. (ed) Tumors in domestic animals. Iowa State Press, 2002.
6. Dickinson PJ, Sturges BK, Higgins RJ, Roberts BN, Leutenegger CM, Bollen AW, et al. Vascular endothelial growth factor mRNA expression and peritumoral edema in canine primary central nervous system tumors. Vet Pathol. 2008;45:131–139.
7. Forterre F, Tomek A, Konar M, Vandevelde M, Howard J, Jaggy A. Multiple meningiomas: clinical, radiological, surgical, and pathological findings with outcome in four cats. J Feline Med Surg. 2007;9:36–43.
8. McDonnell JJ, Kalbko K, Keating JH, Sato AF, Faissler D. Multiple meningiomas in three dogs. J Am Anim Hosp Assoc. 2007;43: 201–208.
9. Tomek A, Forterre E, Konar M, Vandevelde M, Jaggy A. Intracranial meningiomas associated with cervical syringohydromyelia in a cat. Schweiz Arch Tierheilkd. 2008;150:123–128.
10. Mercier M, Heller HL, Bischoff MG, Looper J, Bacmeister CX. Imaging diagnosis – hyperostosis associated with meningioma in a dog. Vet Radiol Ultrasound. 2007;48:421–423.

11. Hasegawa D, Kobayashi M, Fujita M, Uchida K, Orima H. A meningioma with hyperintensity on T1-weighted images in a dog. J Vet Med Sci. 2008;70:615–617.

12. Kitagawa M, Kanayama K, Sakai T. Cystic meningioma in a dog. J Small Anim Pract. 2002;43:272–274.

13. Kitagawa M, Kanayama K, Sakai T. Cerebellopontine angle meningioma expanding into the sella turcica in a dog. J Vet Med Sci. 2004;66:91–93.

14. Bagley RS, Silver GM, Gavin PR. Cerebellar cystic meningioma in a dog. J Am Anim Hosp Assoc. 2000;36:413–415.

15. Graham JP, Newell SM, Voges AK, Roberts GD, Harrison JM. The dural tail sign in the diagnosis of meningiomas. Vet Radiol Ultrasound. 1998;39:297–302.

16. Bagley RS, Kornegay JN, Lane SB, Thrall DL, Page RL. Cystic meningiomas in 2 dogs. J Vet Intern Med. 1996;10:72–75.

17. Zee CS, Chin T, Segall HD, Destian S, Ahmadi J. Magnetic resonance imaging of meningiomas. Semin Ultrasound CT MR. 1992;13:154–169.

18. Cherubini GB, Mantis P, Martinez TA, Lamb CR, Cappello R. Utility of magnetic resonance imaging for distinguishing neoplastic from non-neoplastic brain lesions in dogs and cats. Vet Radiol Ultrasound. 2005;46:384–387.

19. Anwer CC, Vernau KM, Higgins RJ, Dickinson PJ, Sturges BK, LeCouteur RA, et al. Magnetic resonance imaging features of intracranial granular cell tumors in six dogs. Vet Radiol Ultrasound. 2013;54:271–277.

20. Pizzoni C, Sarandria C, Pierangeli E. Clear-cell meningioma of the anterior cranial fossa. Case report and review of the literature. J Neurosurg Sci. 2009;53:113–117.

21. Snyder JM, Shofer FS, Van Winkle TJ, Massicotte C. Canine intracranial primary neoplasia: 173 cases (1986–2003). J Vet Intern Med. 2006;20:669–675.

22. Kube SA, Bruyette DS, Hanson SM. Astrocytomas in young dogs. J Am Anim Hosp Assoc. 2003;39:288–293.

23. Margain D, Peretti-Viton P, Arnaud O, Martini P, Salamon G. Astrocytic tumours. J Neuroradiol. 1991;18:141–152.

24. Cervera V, Mai W, Vite CH, Johnson V, Dayrell-Hart B, Seiler GS. Comparative magnetic resonance imaging findings between gliomas and presumed cerebrovascular accidents in dogs. Vet Radiol Ultrasound. 2011;52:33–40.

25. Lipsitz D, Higgins RJ, Kortz GD, Dickinson PJ, Bollen AW, Naydan DK, et al. Glioblastoma multiforme: clinical findings, magnetic resonance imaging, and pathology in five dogs. Vet Pathol. 2003;40:659–669.

26. Polizopoulou ZS, Koutinas AF, Souftas VD, Kaldrymidou E, Kazakos G, Papadopoulos G. Diagnostic correlation of CT-MRI and histopathology in 10 dogs with brain neoplasms. J Vet Med A Physiol Pathol Clin Med. 2004;51:226–231.

27. Kraft SL, Gavin PR, DeHaan C, Moore M, Wendling LR, Leathers CW. Retrospective review of 50 canine intracranial tumors evaluated by magnetic resonance imaging. J Vet Intern Med. 1997;11:218–225.

28. Young BD, Levine JM, Porter BF, Chen-Allen AV, Rossmeisl JH, Platt SR, et al. Magnetic resonance imaging features of intracranial astrocytomas and oligodendrogliomas in dogs. Vet Radiol Ultrasound. 2011;52:132–141.

29. Margain D, Peretti-Viton P, Perez-Castillo AM, Martini P, Salamon G. Oligodendrogliomas. J Neuroradiol. 1991;18:153–160.

30. Vural SA, Besalti O, Ilhan F, Ozak A, Haligur M. Ventricular ependymoma in a German Shepherd dog. Vet J. 2006;172: 185–187.

31. Yuh EL, Barkovich AJ, Gupta N. Imaging of ependymomas: MRI and CT. Childs Nerv Syst. 2009;25:1203–1213.

32. Westworth DR, Dickinson PJ, Vernau W, Johnson EG, Bollen AW, Kass PH, et al. Choroid plexus tumors in 56 dogs (1985–2007). J Vet Intern Med. 2008;22:1157–1165.

33. Lipsitz D, Levitski RE, Chauvet AE. Magnetic resonance imaging of a choroid plexus carcinoma and meningeal carcinomatosis in a dog. Vet Radiol Ultrasound. 1999;40:246–250.

34. Ohashi F, Kotani T, Onishi T, Katamoto H, Nakata E, Fritz-Zieroth B. Magnetic resonance imaging in a dog with choroid plexus carcinoma. J Vet Med Sci. 1993;55:875–876.

35. Wilson RB, Holscher MA, West WR. Choroid plexus carcinoma in a dog. J Comp Pathol. 1989;100:323–326.

36. Guermazi A, De Kerviler E, Zagdanski AM, Frija J. Diagnostic imaging of choroid plexus disease. Clin Radiol. 2000;55:503–516.

37. Palus V, Volk HA, Lamb CR, Targett MP, Cherubini GB. MRI features of CNS lymphoma in dogs and cats. Vet Radiol Ultrasound. 2012;53:44–49.

38. Kent M, Delahunta A, Tidwell AS. MR imaging findings in a dog with intravascular lymphoma in the brain. Vet Radiol Ultrasound. 2001;42:504–510.

39. Long SN, Johnston PE, Anderson TJ. Primary T-cell lymphoma of the central nervous system in a dog. J Am Vet Med Assoc. 2001;218:719–722.

40. Snyder JM, Lipitz L, Skorupski KA, Shofer FS, Van Winkle TJ. Secondary intracranial neoplasia in the dog: 177 cases (1986–2003). J Vet Intern Med. 2008;22:172–177.

41. Huang BY, Castillo M. Nonadenomatous tumors of the pituitary and sella turcica. Top Magn Reson Imaging. 2005;16:289–299.

42. Buhring U, Herrlinger U, Krings T, Thiex R, Weller M, Kuker W. MRI features of primary central nervous system lymphomas at presentation. Neurology. 2001;57:393–396.

43. Kuker W, Nagele T, Korfel A, Heckl S, Thiel E, Bamberg M, et al. Primary central nervous system lymphomas (PCNSL): MRI features at presentation in 100 patients. J Neurooncol. 2005;72: 169–177.

44. Tamura S, Tamura Y, Nakamoto Y, Ozawa T, Uchida K. MR imaging of histiocytic sarcoma of the canine brain. Vet Radiol Ultrasound. 2009;50:178–181.

45. Thio T, Hilbe M, Grest P, Pospischil A. Malignant histiocytosis of the brain in three dogs. J Comp Pathol. 2006;134:241–244.

46. Chandra AM, Ginn PE. Primary malignant histiocytosis of the brain in a dog. J Comp Pathol. 1999;121:77–82.

47. Wisner ER, Dickinson PJ, Higgins RJ. Magnetic resonance imaging features of canine intracranial neoplasia. Vet Radiol Ultrasound. 2011; 52(1Suppl 1):S52–61.

2.9

Sella and parasellar region

Normal pituitary gland

The sella turcica is the osseous boundary of the pituitary gland. It is comprised of the pituitary fossa ventrally and the rostral and caudal clinoid processes dorsally. The pituitary gland is located in the pituitary fossa of the basisphenoid bone. The pituitary gland is formed of two parts: the vascular, glandular adenohypophysis and the neurohypophysis. It is suspended from the hypothalamus by the infundibulum, which courses through an incomplete dural septum covering the dorsal aspect of the fossa. The ventral aspect of the third ventricle extends centrally through the infundibulum to the proximal neurohypophysis.[1]

The pituitary gland is perfused by branches of the internal carotid and communicating arteries of the circle of Willis, with venous drainage into the cavernous and intercavernous sinuses. The optic chiasm is located immediately rostral to the origin of the infundibulum, and the third cranial nerves arise caudal to, and course lateral to, the pituitary fossa.[1]

On unenhanced CT images, the pituitary gland is isoattenuating to deep gray matter and contiguous with the adjacent hypothalamus, with ventral margins well delineated by the basisphenoid bone. When the third ventricle is prominent, a relatively hypoattenuating infundibular recess may be visible extending to the proximal neurohypophysis. On contrast-enhanced CT and MR images, the pituitary gland markedly contrast enhances compared to brain tissue because of a rich vascular supply (Figure 2.9.1). Dynamic contrast imaging studies of the normal pituitary describe an initial central contrast blush, attributable to early enhancement of the neurohypophysis, followed by a slightly delayed peripheral enhancement of the adenohypophysis with diminished central enhancement.

On MR images, the normal pituitary gland usually has a focal T1 hyperintensity, which is thought to represent either vasopressin-containing neurosecretory granules or glial cell lipid droplets in the neurohypophysis.[2] T2 intensity is similar to cortical gray matter. The lipid-rich marrow of the basisphenoid bone is hyperintense on both T1 and T2 images (Figure 2.9.2).

Normal canine pituitary size on CT images is approximately 4.5 mm in height and 6 mm in width. On MR images, it is reported to be $5.1 \pm .9$ mm in height and 6.4 ± 1.0 mm in width, with little correlation to brain measurements or body weight.[3,4] Normal feline pituitary size has been estimated to be approximately 5 mm in height and 3.5 mm in width on both CT and MR imaging.[5,6] While these dimensions may be useful as general guidelines, they are not particularly useful for diagnosis of microadenomas. With both imaging modalities, the presence of a prominent convexity to the dorsal pituitary margin and elevation of the dorsal margin above the sella turcica on a sagittal plane image are additional qualitative imaging features that are suggestive of a pituitary disorder.

Dynamic CT and MR protocols

Dynamic contrast CT protocols have been used to detect small (micro) hypophyseal masses. However, the current trend in human and veterinary medicine has been toward the use of MR for diagnosis and characterization of pituitary disorders. Dynamic CT and MR procedures

Atlas of Small Animal CT and MRI, First Edition. Erik R. Wisner and Allison L. Zwingenberger.
© 2015 John Wiley & Sons, Inc. Published 2015 by John Wiley & Sons, Inc.

described in the veterinary literature involve dynamic thinly collimated image acquisition through the pituitary gland every few seconds for 2–5 minutes following intravenous bolus contrast administration to detect neurohypophysis displacement by adenohypophyseal tumors.[5,7–10]

Empty sella syndrome

Empty sella syndrome may occur when cerebrospinal fluid herniates through the fenestration in the dural septum that covers the dorsal part of the pituitary fossa and compresses the pituitary gland or as the result of pituitary volume reduction from a primary disease. Empty sella syndrome is an imaging finding rather than a specific pituitary disorder. If the pituitary gland shrinks for any reason or is compressed dorsally, this leads to an appearance of an empty sella turcica, which is usually best seen on sagittal plane MR sequences as focal T1 hypointensity and T2 hypointensity in the pituitary fossa (Figure 2.9.3) and as focal fluid attenuation on CT images. This entity is periodically seen as an incidental or clinically silent finding.[11]

Pituitary cysts

Pituitary cysts may be developmental or acquired and are often clinically silent. Degenerative cysts associated with pituitary adenomatous neoplasia are common and described below. Rathke's cleft cysts are fluid-filled, epithelial-lined cysts that arise from a remnant of the craniopharyngeal duct during development. Rathke's cleft cysts are rare, with few reports in the veterinary literature. Given the predominantly fluid content of these thin-walled cysts, they will appear hyperintense on T2 images and of variable intensity on T1 images, depending on the macromolecular and cellular content of the fluid.[12] Other cystic lesions of the sellar and parasellar region include craniopharyngioma, suprasellar arachnoid cyst, and suprasellar epidermoid cyst (Figure 2.9.4).

Pituitary hemorrhage/pituitary apoplexy

Although rare, acute pituitary hemorrhage may occur either spontaneously or secondary to infarction of a pituitary tumor or other underlying pathology. When the hemorrhage is associated with acute clinical signs of obtundation, nausea, vomiting, or visual and other cranial nerve deficits resulting from increased parasellar and intracranial pressure, the disorder is referred to as pituitary apoplexy. CT and MR features include a suprasellar mass or mass effect, particularly when an underlying pituitary tumor or a substantial hematoma is present, and evidence of acute hemorrhage within the pituitary gland and/or suprasellar mass. On CT images, this may appear as amorphous hyperattenuation on

unenhanced images and variable T1 and T2 intensity on MR images, depending on the specific age of the hemorrhage (Figure 2.9.5). With both modalities, contrast enhancement may occur if residual viable pituitary parenchyma remains, an underlying pituitary tumor is present, or if hemorrhage is active.[13]

Hypophysitis

Immune-mediated hypophysitis

Lymphocytic hypophysitis is an uncommon disorder in people associated with a variety of endocrinopathies and has been sporadically reported in dogs.[14,15] Although imaging features have not been described in the veterinary literature, MR findings in people include symmetrical pituitary enlargement, loss of neurohypophyseal T1 hyperintensity, homogeneous contrast enhancement, and empty sella as a late event.[16]

Infectious hypophysitis

Hypophysitis can occur through extension of bacterial, fungal, and other infectious meningoencephalitides. Imaging features will be dependent on the characteristics and distribution of the underlying infection. In those patients with a significant meningeal component, MR findings may include prominence of the dural layer within the pituitary fossa and intense meningeal contrast enhancement (Figure 2.9.6).

Neoplasia

Neoplasms of the adenohypophysis

Primary tumors arising from the adenohypophysis are common and frequently associated with endocrinopathies, such as feline acromegaly (see Chapter 1.4), whereas those arising from the neurohypophysis are rare. Adenohypophyseal neoplasms are histologically classified as adenomas or adenocarcinomas. Small tumors that do not appreciably alter total pituitary volume, generally those that are less than 10 mm in total pituitary height, are categorized as microtumors, whereas those greater than or equal to 10 mm in height are classified as macrotumors. Macroadenomas can be further differentiated as either noninvasive or biologically more aggressive and invasive into adjacent bone.[17,18]

Pituitary microtumors are challenging to diagnose based on imaging features alone (Figures 2.9.7). On MR images, the focal T1 hyperintensity within the neurohypophysis may be displaced caudally, dorsally, and laterally because of expansion of the adenohypophysis (Figures 2.9.8, 2.9.9). Marked convexity of the dorsal pituitary margin and elevation of the dorsal pituitary margin above the dorsal rim of the sella turcica may lend additional support for diagnosis of microtumor. Dynamic contrast-assisted CT and MRI may be used to more clearly identify pituitary microtumors by temporal differences in enhancement of the neurohypophysis and adenohypophyseal mass.[9,19,20]

Imaging features of adenomas, invasive adenomas, and adenocarcinomas are not sufficiently different to reliably differentiate these entities (Figures 2.9.10, 2.9.11, 2.9.12, 2.9.13, 2.9.14, 2.9.15, 2.9.16, 2.9.17).[17,21,22] Pituitary macroadenomas and adenocarcinomas are greater than 10 mm in height and arise from the sellar region. Although invasive adenomas are on average larger than noninvasive adenomas (1.9 cm vs. 1.2 cm mean height in one study), this is not a reliable criterion for differentiating the two. Both macroadenomas and adenocarcinomas can have smooth or irregular margins, can contain cysts or hemorrhage, and can occasionally be mineralized.

On CT images, macrotumors can be isoattenuating or slightly hypo- or hyperattenuating to adjacent brain parenchyma. Intratumoral cysts may be present as hypoattenuating foci, and mineralization is hyperattenuating. When present, paratumoral edema can appear hypoattenuating to normal brain parenchyma. On MR images, pituitary macrotumors are typically T1 isointense, variably T2 hyperintense, and may be accompanied by surrounding T2 hyperintense hypothalamic and thalamic edema. Macrotumors are generally intensely and uniformly contrast enhancing on both CT and MR images because of the rich vascular supply of the gland.[10,22]

Other sellar region tumors

Other sellar and parasellar neoplasms that must be considered as part of an imaging assessment include meningioma, primary or secondary lymphoma, ependymoma, granular cell tumors, and germ cell tumors, among others (Figures 2.9.18, 2.9.19). Tumors that arise from the neurohypophysis and other sellar tumors, such as craniopharyngiomas, are rare.

Figure 2.9.1   Normal Pituitary Gland (Canine)   CT

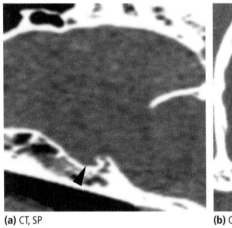

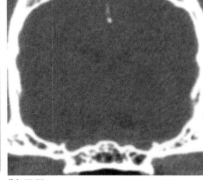

7y MC Rottweiler. Images **a–b** are representative sagittal and transverse images of the brain that include the sella and parasellar regions. The pituitary fossa is well delineated on the sagittal image (**a**: arrowhead), and the pituitary gland attenuation is similar to that of adjacent hypothalamus. Images **c–d** are comparable images acquired following intravenous iodinated contrast administration. The pituitary gland intensely and uniformly contrast enhances (**c,d**: arrow). The pituitary gland is contained within the pituitary fossa and does not extend above the dorsal rim of the sella turcica.

(a) CT, SP

(b) CT, TP

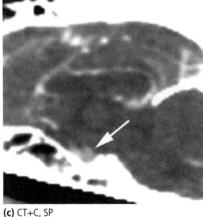

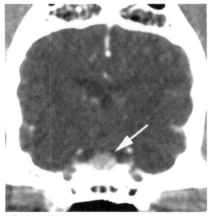

(c) CT+C, SP

(d) CT+C, TP

Figure 2.9.2   Normal Pituitary Gland (Canine)   MR

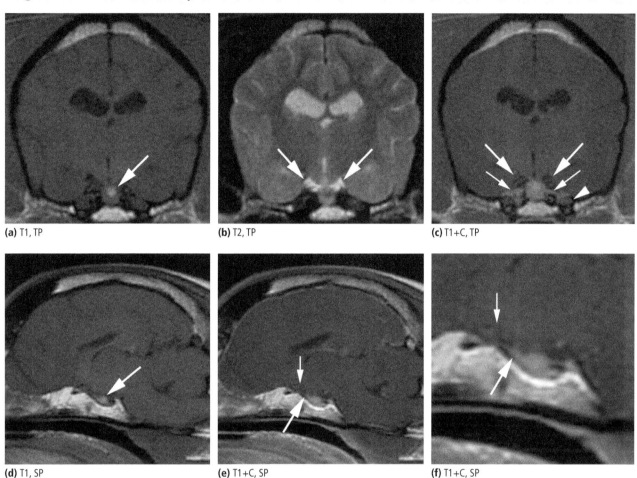

(a) T1, TP   **(b)** T2, TP   **(c)** T1+C, TP

(d) T1, SP   **(e)** T1+C, SP   **(f)** T1+C, SP

10y FS Beagle. Images **a–c** are representative transverse images at the level of the pituitary fossa. Images **d–e** are comparable sagittal images, and image **f** is a magnified view of image **e**. The pituitary gland is positioned within the pituitary fossa (height = 4 mm, width = 6 mm) and has a relatively flat dorsal margin that does not extend above the dorsal limits of the sella turcica (**d–f**). The pituitary gland is partly T1 hyperintense because of the presence of secretory granules in the neurohyphysis that result in T1 shortening (**a,d**: arrow). The normal pituitary gland is markedly contrast enhancing as a result of the high vascular density of the gland (**e,f**), and the pituitary stalk is also evident (**e,f**: large arrow). Cerebrospinal fluid in the chiasmatic cistern is evident dorsolateral to the pituitary gland and is T1 hypointense and T2 hyperintense (**b,c**: large arrows). The cavernous sinus enhances on the contrast-enhanced T1 image (**c**: small arrows), and circular hypointense signal voids can be seen within the sinus, representing flow voids in the internal carotid and/or communicating arteries. The optic chiasm is located rostral to the pituitary gland (**e,f**: small arrow) and can be encroached upon by expansile pituitary masses. Part of the mandibular branch of the left trigeminal nerve can also be seen (**c**: arrowhead).

Figure 2.9.3   Empty Sella Syndrome (Canine)

MR

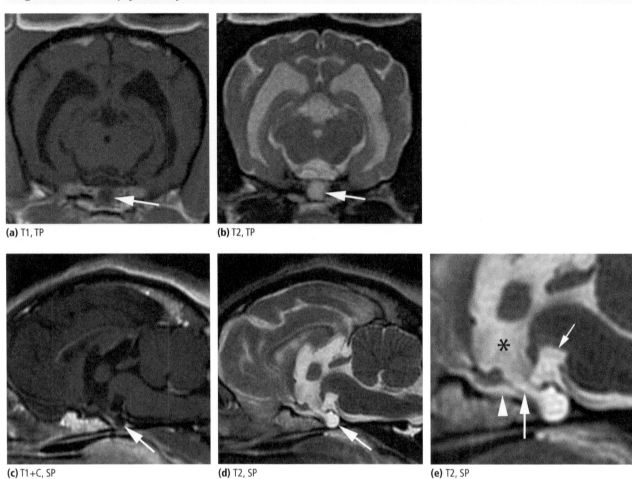

(a) T1, TP

(b) T2, TP

(c) T1+C, SP

(d) T2, SP

(e) T2, SP

10y FS Pekinese acutely nonambulatory with neurologic deficits referable to a cerebrothalamic lesion. The dog had no clinical or clinical chemistry evidence of central endocrinopathy. Images **a** and **b** are representative transverse images at the level of the pituitary fossa. Images **c–e** are comparable images oriented in the sagittal plane, and image **e** is a magnified view of image **d**. There is diffuse brain atrophy resulting in enlargement of the ventricular system and subarachnoid space (**a–e**). The pituitary fossa is fluid filled and appears T1 hypointense and T2 hyperintense (**a–d**: arrow). This fluid collection appears to communicate with the third ventricle (**e**: asterisk) by way of the infundibular recess (**e**: large arrow). The interpeduncular (**e**: small arrow) and chiasmatic (**e**: arrowhead) cisterns are also prominent.

Figure 2.9.4   Pituitary Cyst (Canine)

MR

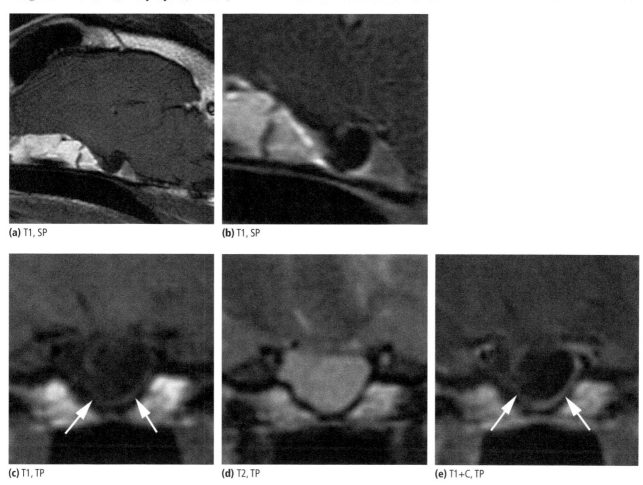

(a) T1, SP

(b) T1, SP

(c) T1, TP

(d) T2, TP

(e) T1+C, TP

10y FS Labrador Retriever with acute obtundation and disorientation. The dog had multiple meningiomas involving the right cerebrum and pons, causing the clinical signs, and the cystic pituitary gland was an incidental finding. Image **b** represents a magnified view of image **a**. Images **c–e** are representative close-up views of the pituitary fossa in the transverse plane. The pituitary fossa contains a predominantly T1 hypointense and T2 hyperintense cyst (**a–d**) with a thin rim that is isointense to adjacent deep gray matter (**c**: arrows). The cyst enhances peripherally (**e**: arrows). Ill-defined T2 hyperintense edema is present in the hypothalamus (**d**) because of the meningiomas.

Figure 2.9.5 Pituitary Hemorrhage (Apoplexy) (Canine)   MR

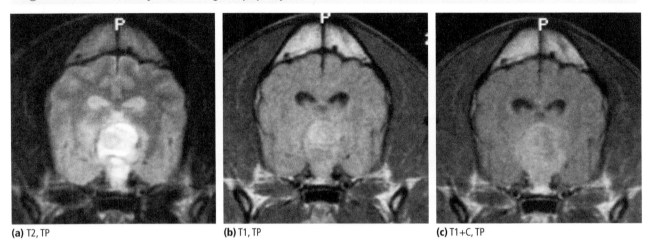

(a) T2, TP   **(b)** T1, TP   **(c)** T1+C, TP

10y MC Chow cross with neurologic signs consistent with increased intracranial pressure. The dog also had concurrent thrombocytopenia. A large, T1 and T2 hyperintense, heterogeneous mass is present involving the pituitary, hypothalamic, and thalamic regions (a,b). The mixed-signal pattern is consistent with intraparenchymal hemorrhage. The mass moderately and heterogeneously contrast enhances (c). Postmortem examination found that the pituitary was expanded, and in some regions obliterated, by lakes of free red blood cells and a mass composed of red blood cells, fibrin, and degenerate cells (hematoma).

Figure 2.9.6 Hypophysitis (Canine)   MR

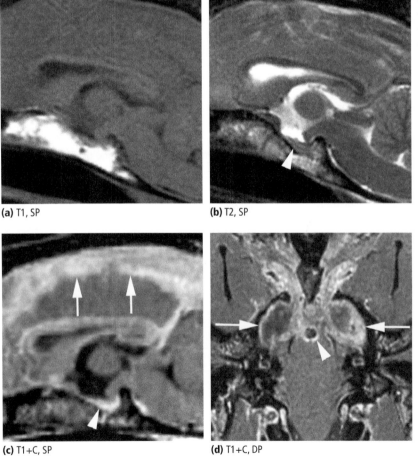

(a) T1, SP   **(b)** T2, SP

(c) T1+C, SP   **(d)** T1+C, DP

6y FS Greyhound with progressive obtundation. The meningeal lining of the pituitary fossa is T2 hyperintense (b: arrowhead), and the meninges of the fossa and dural septum intensely contrast enhance (c,d: arrowhead). More diffuse meningeal enhancement is evident, involving the meninges of the falx cerebri and the basilar regions of the piriform lobes (c,d: arrows). Postmortem examination revealed diffuse meningoencephalitis with marked chronic granulomatous and lymphoplasmacytic hypophysitis.

Figure 2.9.7   Pituitary Microadenoma (Canine)   CT

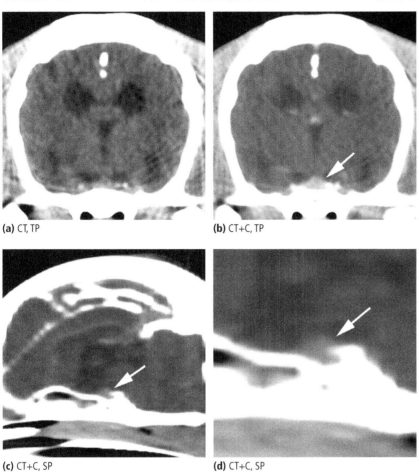

(a) CT, TP

(b) CT+C, TP

(c) CT+C, SP

(d) CT+C, SP

12y FS Border Terrier with confirmed pituitary-dependent hyperadrenocorticism. Images **a** and **b** are representative transverse images at the level of the pituitary fossa. Image **d** is a magnified view of image **c**. A uniformly contrast-enhancing and symmetrical pituitary gland is evident (**b–d**: arrow). The gland is considered within normal limits for size (height = 4 mm, width = 6 mm), but the dorsal margin is convex and extends beyond the dorsal extent of the sella turcica.

Figure 2.9.8 Pituitary Microadenoma (Canine)   MR

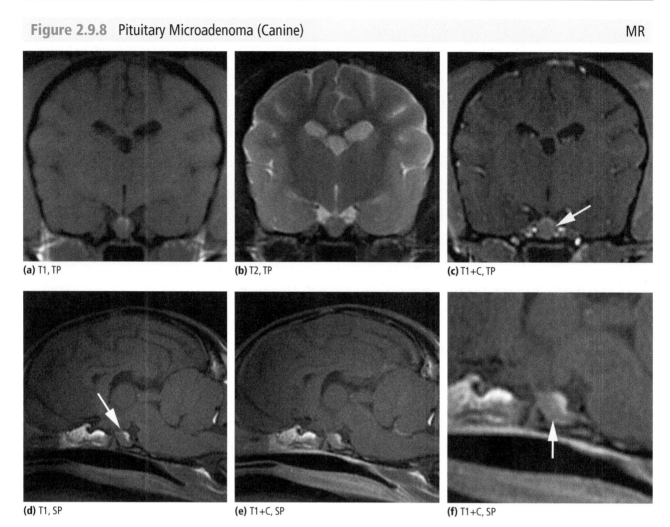

(a) T1, TP   **(b)** T2, TP   **(c)** T1+C, TP

(d) T1, SP   **(e)** T1+C, SP   **(f)** T1+C, SP

3y MC Corgi with confirmed pituitary-dependent hyperadrenocorticism. Images **a–c** are representative transverse images at the level of the pituitary fossa. Image **f** is a magnified view of image **e**. The pituitary gland has nonuniform mixed T1 intensity and T2 signal that is isointense with that of deep gray matter. Although the gland measures within normal limits for size (height = 5 mm, width = 5 mm), the adenohypophysis appears prominent, displaces the more hyperintense neurohypophysis dorsally, and extends beyond the dorsal extent of the sella turcica (**d**: arrow). The adenohypophysis enhances uniformly following contrast administration (**c,f**: arrow). History, clinical signs, and results of a low-dose dexamethasone suppression test were indicative of pituitary-dependent hyperadrenocorticism.

Figure 2.9.9   Pituitary Microadenoma (Canine)   MR

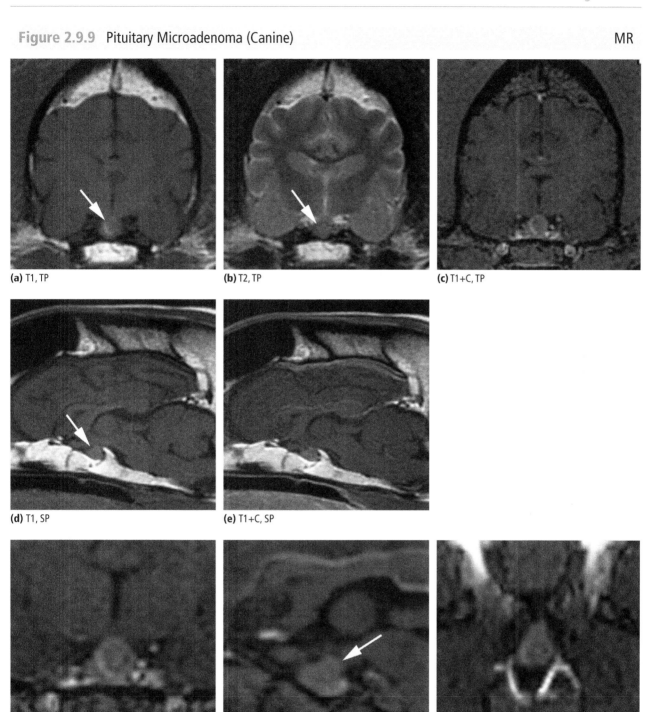

(a) T1, TP

(b) T2, TP

(c) T1+C, TP

(d) T1, SP

(e) T1+C, SP

(f) T1+C, SPGR, TP

(g) T1+C, SPGR, SP

(h) T1+C, SPGR, DP

8y MC Australian Shepherd with confirmed pituitary-dependent hyperadrenocorticism. Images **a–c** are representative transverse images at the level of the pituitary fossa, and images **f–h** represent thin contrast-enhanced T1 images of the pituitary gland in the three major planes. The pituitary gland has nonuniform, mixed T1 intensity (**a,d**: arrow) and T2 signal that is isointense (**b**: arrow) with that of deep gray matter. Hyperintense secretory granules within the neurohypophysis are displaced to the right in image **a**. The pituitary enhances nonuniformly following contrast administration (**c,e,f–h**). Although the gland measures within normal limits for size (height = 7 mm, depth = 8 mm), the dorsal pituitary margin is irregular, convex, and extends beyond the dorsal extent of the sella turcica (**g**: arrow). History, clinical signs, and results of a low-dose dexamethasone suppression test were indicative of pituitary-dependent hyperadrenocorticism.

Figure 2.9.10   Pituitary Mass with Acromegaly (Feline)   CT

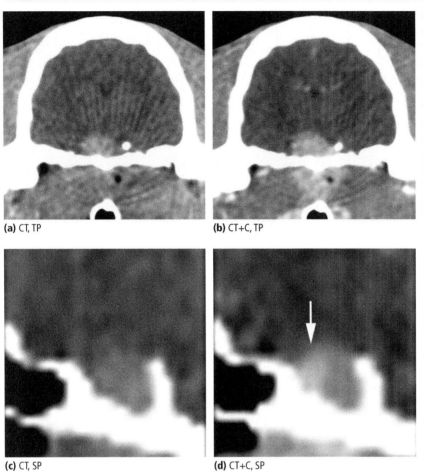

(a) CT, TP

(b) CT+C, TP

(c) CT, SP

(d) CT+C, SP

8y FS Siamese with confirmed acromegaly and diabetes mellitus. Images **a** and **b** represent transverse images at the level of the pituitary. Images **c** and **d** are magnified images of the pituitary fossa. A hyperattenuating and mildly asymmetrical pituitary mass is evident on the unenhanced images (**a**,**c**). The mass moderately and nonuniformly enhances, with enhancement more pronounced rostrally (**d**: arrow). The mass is 6 mm in height and 6 mm in depth and has a convex dorsal margin that extends beyond the dorsal aspect of the sella turcica. Postmortem examination confirmed the presence of a pars intermedia adenoma.

Figure 2.9.11   Mineralized Functional Pituitary Macrotumor (Canine)   CT

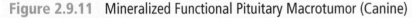

(a) CT, TP

(b) CT+C, TP

(c) CT+C, SP

8y FS Dachshund with confirmed pituitary-dependent hyperadrenocorticism. Images **a** and **b** represent transverse images at the level of the pituitary. Image **c** is a magnified image of the pituitary fossa. An ill-defined, partially mineralized pituitary/hypothalamic mass is evident on the unenhanced image (**a**). The mass is uniformly contrast enhancing and measures 11 mm in height and 10 mm in width. History, clinical signs, and results of a low-dose dexamethasone suppression test were indicative of pituitary-dependent hyperadrenocorticism.

Figure 2.9.12 Pituitary Adenoma (Canine)   MR

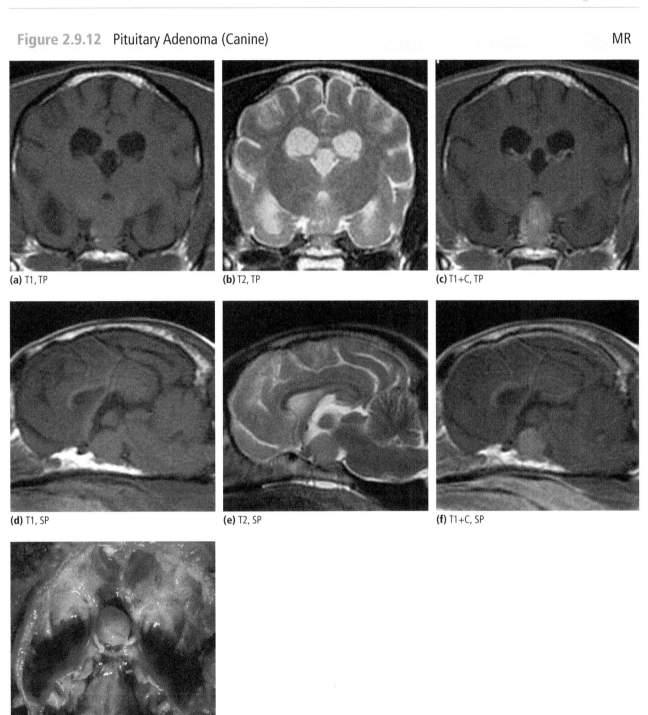

(a) T1, TP

(b) T2, TP

(c) T1+C, TP

(d) T1, SP

(e) T2, SP

(f) T1+C, SP

(g) GP, VENT

14y FS Spitz with head tilt and recent onset of circling to the right. Images **a–c** are representative transverse images at the level of the pituitary fossa. Images **d–f** are comparable images oriented in the sagittal plane. The pituitary gland is markedly enlarged (height = 10 mm, width = 10 mm) and is T1 isointense (**a,d**) and mildly T2 hyperintense (**b,e**) compared to deep gray matter. Ventriculomegaly is also evident and may be due to partial obstruction. The pituitary gland is uniformly contrast enhancing (**c,f**) and appears as a well-defined spherical mass on postmortem examination (**g**). The mass was confirmed to be a pituitary macroadenoma.

Figure 2.9.13   Pituitary Adenoma (Canine)   MR

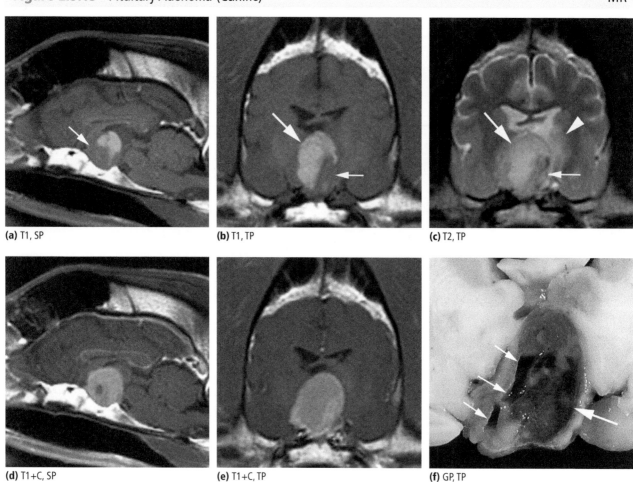

(a) T1, SP   **(b)** T1, TP   **(c)** T2, TP

(d) T1+C, SP   **(e)** T1+C, TP   **(f)** GP, TP

10y MC Golden Retriever with a 6-day history of progressive obtundation. Images **b**, **c**, and **e** are representative transverse images at the level of the pituitary fossa. Images **a** and **d** are comparable images oriented in the sagittal plane. The pituitary gland is markedly enlarged (height = 20 mm, width = 19 mm) and has a cystic component that is both T1 and T2 hyperintense (**b**,**c**: large arrow). The peripheral parenchymal component of the mass is T1 isointense compared to deep gray matter (**a**,**b**: small arrow) and is of mixed, but low, T2 intensity (**c**: small arrow). Mild peripheral edema is also evident (**c**: arrowhead). A deflated cystic cavity (**f**: small arrows) and hemorrhage within the remaining pituitary parenchyma (**f**: large arrow) are seen on the transected gross specimen. Imaging features are consistent with a large cystic pituitary mass with hemorrhage in the parenchymal component. The cyst fluid is hyperintense on both T1 and T2, likely due to high lipid content or T1 shortening solutes. The mass was determined to be a nonfunctional macroadenoma arising from the pars intermedia.

Figure 2.9.14   Pituitary Adenoma (Canine)

MR

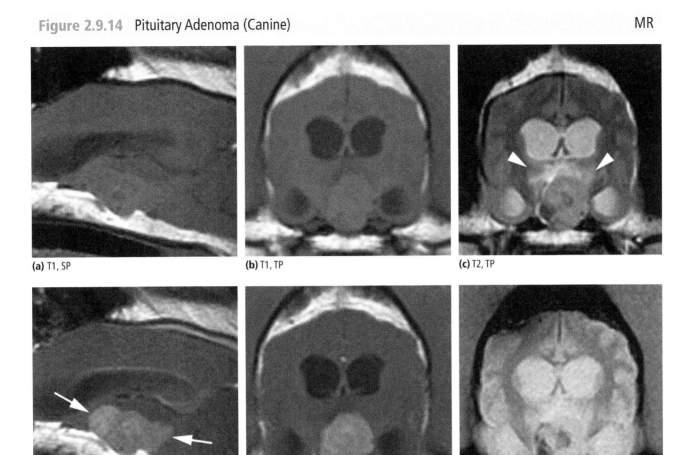

(a) T1, SP   (b) T1, TP   (c) T2, TP

(d) T1+C, SP   (e) T1+C, TP   (f) T2*, TP

11y FS Great Dane with recent-onset abnormal behavior and difficulty walking. Images **b**, **c**, **e**, and **f** are representative transverse images at the level of the pituitary fossa. Images **a** and **d** are comparable images oriented in the sagittal plane. The pituitary gland is markedly enlarged (height = 17 mm, width = 30 mm), extends dorsally into the hypothalamic and thalamic regions, and is mildly T1 and T2 hyperintense compared to deep gray matter (**a–c**). The mass is uniformly contrast enhancing, and margins are irregular and extend well beyond the rostral and caudal extent of the pituitary fossa (**d**: arrows). Central mixed T2 intensity (**c**) and multifocal signal voids on the gradient echo sequence (**f**) are indicative of parenchymal hemorrhage. Moderate peripheral edema is also evident on the T2 sequence (**c**: arrowheads). The mass was confirmed to be a pituitary adenoma on postmortem examination.

Figure 2.9.15   Pituitary Carcinoma (Canine)   MR

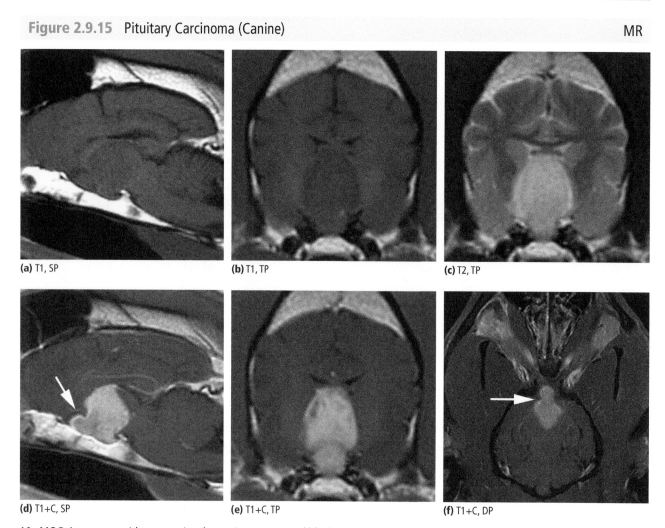

(a) T1, SP

(b) T1, TP

(c) T2, TP

(d) T1+C, SP

(e) T1+C, TP

(f) T1+C, DP

10y MC Pointer cross with progressive depression, ataxia, and blindness. Images **b**, **c**, and **e** are representative transverse images at the level of the pituitary fossa. Images **a** and **d** are comparable images oriented in the sagittal plane. Image **f** is a representative dorsal plane image that includes the optic chiasm. The pituitary gland is markedly enlarged (height = 22 mm, depth = 22 mm), extends dorsally into the hypothalamic and thalamic regions, and is mildly T1 hypointense and T2 hyperintense compared to deep gray matter (**a–c**). The mass is uniformly contrast enhancing, and margins are irregular and extend well beyond the rostral extent of the pituitary fossa (**d**: arrow), encroaching on the optic chiasm (**d,f**: arrow). The mass was confirmed to be a pituitary adenocarcinoma on postmortem examination.

Figure 2.9.16   Pituitary Carcinoma (Feline)

MR

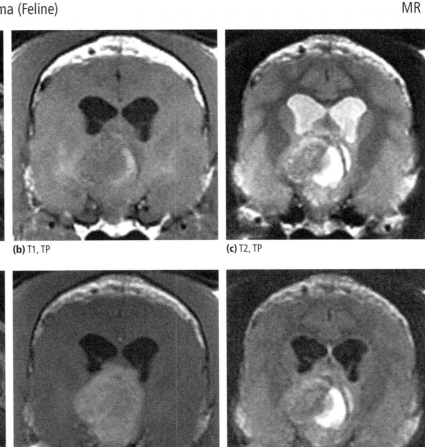

(a) T1, SP

(b) T1, TP

(c) T2, TP

(d) T1+C, SP

(e) T1+C, TP

(f) FL, TP

14y MC Domestic Longhair with neurologic signs referable to a right-sided cerebrothalamic lesion. Images **b**, **c**, **e**, and **f** are representative transverse images at the level of the pituitary fossa. Images **a** and **d** are comparable images oriented in the sagittal plane. The pituitary gland is markedly enlarged (height = 17 mm, depth = 18 mm) and extends dorsally into the hypothalamic and thalamic regions. The mass has mixed T1 and T2 intensity compared to deep gray matter (**a**–**c**,**f**), suggesting intralesional hemorrhage; is nonuniformly contrast enhancing; and has irregular margins that extend well beyond the rostral and caudal extent of the pituitary fossa. The mass was confirmed to be a pituitary carcinoma on postmortem examination.

Figure 2.9.17   Pituitary Carcinoma (Canine)   MR

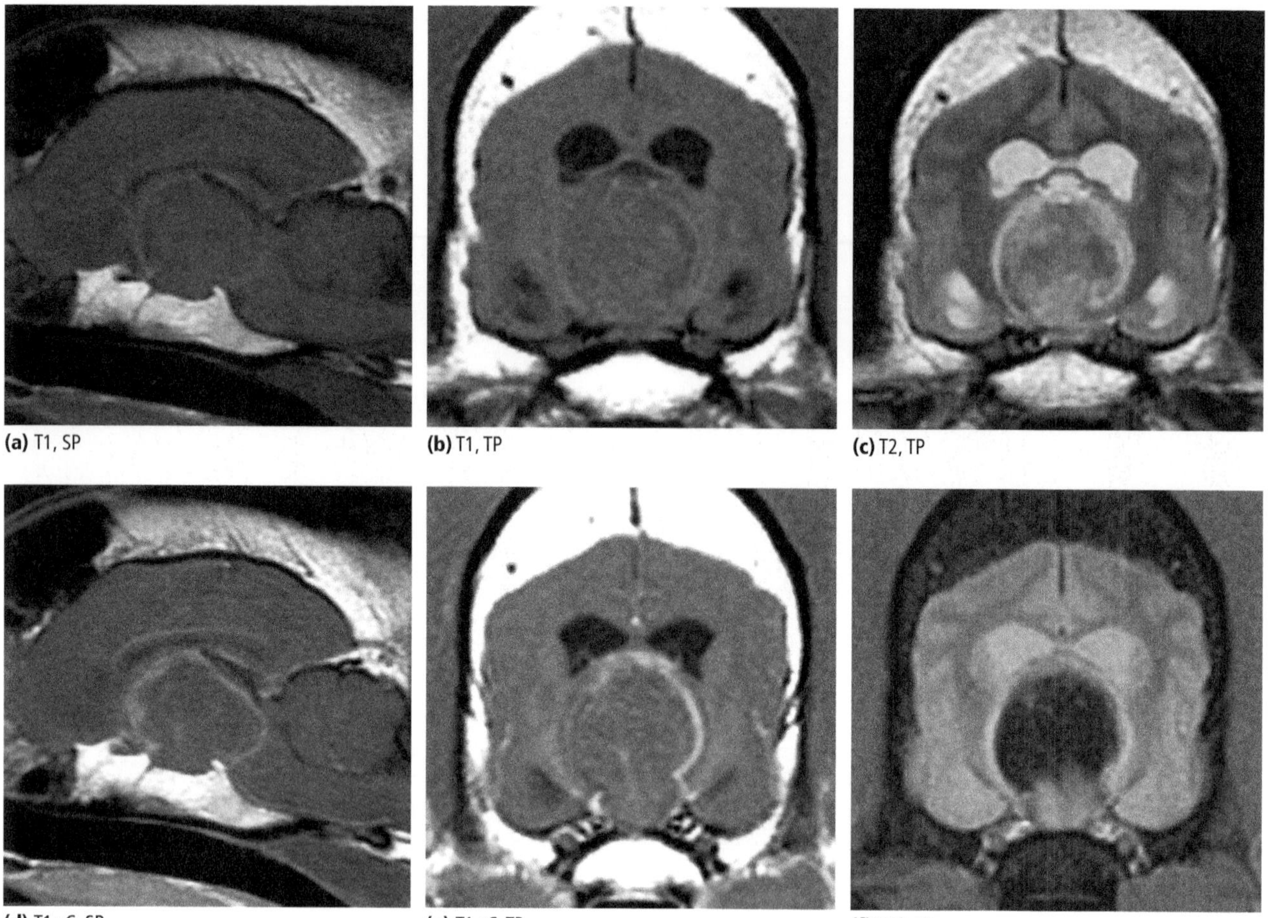

(a) T1, SP

(b) T1, TP

(c) T2, TP

(d) T1+C, SP

(e) T1+C, TP

(f) T2*, TP

6y MC Pit Bull Terrier with progressive disorientation. Images **b**, **c**, **e**, and **f** are representative transverse images at the level of the pituitary fossa. Images **a** and **d** are comparable images oriented in the sagittal plane. The pituitary gland is markedly enlarged (height = 23 mm, depth = 29 mm) and extends dorsally into the hypothalamic and thalamic regions. The mass has mixed T1 and T2 intensity compared to deep gray matter (**a–c**) and signal void on the gradient echo sequence (**f**), indicative of diffuse intralesional hemorrhage. The mass is peripherally contrast enhancing, suggesting poor perfusion centrally. This was confirmed to be a pituitary adeno-carcinoma with central hemorrhage and necrosis on postmortem examination.

Figure 2.9.18   Meningioma (Canine)   MR

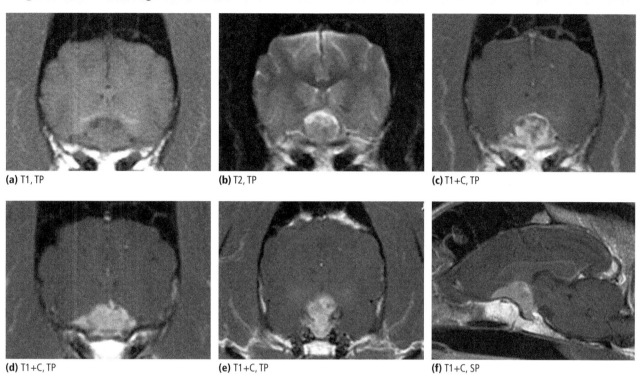

(a) T1, TP   **(b)** T2, TP   **(c)** T1+C, TP

(d) T1+C, TP   **(e)** T1+C, TP   **(f)** T1+C, SP

7y MC Golden Retriever with recent onset of blindness. Images **a–c** are representative transverse images just rostral to the pituitary fossa. Images **d** and **e** are additional representative contrast-enhanced images rostral and caudal to image **c**, respectively. Image **f** is a comparable image oriented in the sagittal plane. A large sessile mass is evident, centered on the region of the optic chiasm. The mass has mixed T1 and T2 signal intensity (**a,b**) and is nonuniformly but intensely contrast enhancing (**c–f**). The mass appears to fill the pituitary fossa (**e,f**), and the pituitary gland is not delineated from the mass. Although this lesion has some imaging features similar to those of a primary pituitary neoplasm, the sessile appearance, with extension well beyond the pituitary fossa and hypothalamus, and the intense contrast enhancement suggest an extraaxial neoplasm, such as meningioma. CT-guided biopsy was interpreted as probable meningioma.

Figure 2.9.19   Granular Cell Tumor (Canine)   MR

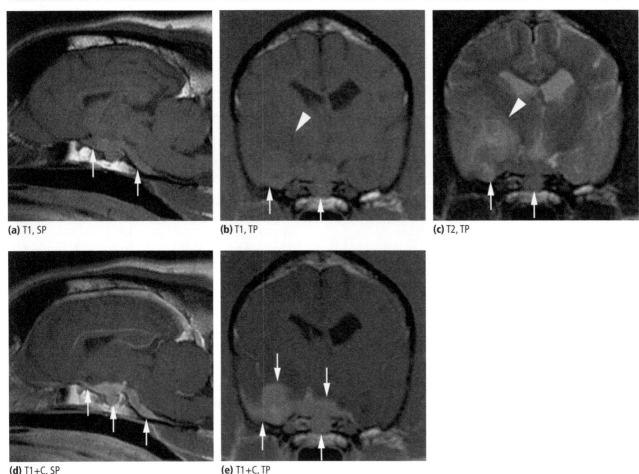

(a) T1, SP   **(b)** T1, TP   **(c)** T2, TP

(d) T1+C, SP   **(e)** T1+C, TP

11y M Fox Terrier a 2-week history of seizures. Images **b**, **c**, and **e** are representative transverse images at the level of the pituitary fossa. Images **a** and **d** are comparable images oriented in the sagittal plane. A large, plaque-like, sessile mass is distributed along the floor of the calvarium and extends into the pituitary fossa, the hypothalamus, and the right piriform lobe (**d,e**: arrows). The mass is mildly T1 hyperintense and T2 isointense to deep gray matter (**a–c**: arrows) and is uniformly and intensely contrast enhancing (**d,e**). Perilesional edema is also evident (**b,c**: arrowhead). Although the mass involves the pituitary fossa and the pituitary gland is not evident, the constellation of imaging features of this lesion is more consistent with a nonpituitary extraaxial neoplasm. The lesion was confirmed to be a granular cell tumor on postmortem examination.

References

1. Hullinger RL. The Endocrine System. In: Evans HE (ed): Miller's Anatomy of the Dog. Philadelphia: W. B. Saunders Company, 1993.
2. Kucharczyk J, Kucharczyk W, Berry I, de Groot J, Kelly W, Norman D, et al. Histochemical characterization and functional significance of the hyperintense signal on MR images of the posterior pituitary. AJR Am J Roentgenol. 1989;152:153–157.
3. van der Vlugt-Meijer RH, Meij BP, Voorhout G. Intraobserver and interobserver agreement, reproducibility, and accuracy of computed tomographic measurements of pituitary gland dimensions in healthy dogs. Am J Vet Res. 2006;67:1750–1755.
4. Kippenes H, Gavin PR, Kraft SL, Sande RD, Tucker RL. Mensuration of the normal pituitary gland from magnetic resonance images in 96 dogs. Vet Radiol Ultrasound. 2001;42:130–133.
5. Tyson R, Graham JP, Bermingham E, Randall S, Berry CR. Dynamic computed tomography of the normal feline hypophysis cerebri (Glandula pituitaria). Vet Radiol Ultrasound. 2005;46: 33–38.
6. Wallack ST, Wisner ER, Feldman EC. Mensuration of the pituitary gland from magnetic resonance images in 17 cats. Vet Radiol Ultrasound. 2003;44:278–282.
7. Graham JP, Roberts GD, Newell SM. Dynamic magnetic resonance imaging of the normal canine pituitary gland. Vet Radiol Ultrasound. 2000;41:35–40.
8. Love NE, Fisher P, Hudson L. The computed tomographic enhancement pattern of the normal canine pituitary gland. Vet Radiol Ultrasound. 2000;41:507–510.
9. Van der Vlugt-Meijer RH, Meij BP, Voorhout G. Dynamic helical computed tomography of the pituitary gland in healthy dogs. Vet Radiol Ultrasound. 2007;48:118–124.

10. van der Vlugt-Meijer RH, Voorhout G, Meij BP. Imaging of the pituitary gland in dogs with pituitary-dependent hyperadrenocorticism. Mol Cell Endocrinol. 2002;197:81–87.

11. Konar M, Burgener IA, Lang J. Magnetic resonance imaging features of empty sella in dogs. Vet Radiol Ultrasound. 2008;49: 339–342.

12. Hasegawa D, Uchida K, Kobayashi M, Kuwabara T, Ide T, Ogawa F, et al. Imaging diagnosis – Rathke's cleft cyst. Vet Radiol Ultrasound. 2009;50:298–300.

13. Bertolini G, Rossetti E, Caldin M. Pituitary apoplexy-like disease in 4 dogs. J Vet Intern Med. 2007;21:1251–1257.

14. Meij BP, Voorhout G, Gerritsen RJ, Grinwis GC, Ijzer J. Lymphocytic hypophysitis in a dog with diabetes insipidus. J Comp Pathol. 2012;147(4):503–507.

15. Wolfesberger B, Fuchs-Baumgartinger A, Schwendenwein I, Zeugswetter F, Shibly S. Sudden death in a dog with lymphoplasmacytic hypophysitis. J Comp Pathol. 2011;145:231–234.

16. Glezer A, Bronstein MD. Pituitary autoimmune disease: nuances in clinical presentation. Endocrine. 2012;42:74–79.

17. Pollard RE, Reilly CM, Uerling MR, Wood FD, Feldman EC. Cross-sectional imaging characteristics of pituitary adenomas, invasive adenomas and adenocarcinomas in dogs: 33 cases (1988–2006). J Vet Intern Med. 2010;24:160–165.

18. Posch B, Dobson J, Herrtage M. Magnetic resonance imaging findings in 15 acromegalic cats. Vet Radiol Ultrasound. 2011;52: 422–427.

19. Taoda T, Hara Y, Masuda H, Teshima T, Nezu Y, Teramoto A, et al. Magnetic resonance imaging assessment of pituitary posterior lobe displacement in dogs with pituitary-dependent hyperadrenocorticism. J Vet Med Sci. 2011;73:725–731.

20. van der Vlugt-Meijer RH, Meij BP, van den Ingh TS, Rijnberk A, Voorhout G. Dynamic computed tomography of the pituitary gland in dogs with pituitary-dependent hyperadrenocorticism. J Vet Intern Med. 2003;17:773–780.

21. Auriemma E, Barthez PY, van der Vlugt-Meijer RH, Voorhout G, Meij BP. Computed tomography and low-field magnetic resonance imaging of the pituitary gland in dogs with pituitary-dependent hyperadrenocorticism: 11 cases (2001–2003). J Am Vet Med Assoc. 2009;235:409–414.

22. Duesberg CA, Feldman EC, Nelson RW, Bertoy EH, Dublin AB, Reid MH. Magnetic resonance imaging for diagnosis of pituitary macrotumors in dogs. J Am Vet Med Assoc. 1995;206:657–662.

2.10

Cranial nerves

For an in-depth description of the imaging anatomy of the skull and cranial nerves, the reader is referred to a number of studies detailing the CT and MR appearance of the normal cranial nerves and the skull foramina from which they emerge.[1-4] This chapter is limited to a discussion of the most common clinical disorders involving the cranial nerves.

Cranial nerves

Cranial nerve II

The optic nerve, or cranial nerve II, is a tract of the brain and is unique among the cranial nerves in that it has a meningeal covering and a subarachnoid space. Axons arising from retinal ganglion cells form the optic nerve after collecting and exiting at the optic disc of the eye. The nerve extends caudally in the retrobulbar space and enters the cranium through the optic canal. The paired nerves partially decussate at the optic chiasm, with the resulting optic tracts terminating in the lateral geniculate nucleus and other nuclei with vision functions. The normal canine optic nerve has been reported to be between 1.2 and 2.4 mm in diameter.[5]

The normal optic nerve is isoattenuating to brain parenchyma on unenhanced CT images and is T1 and T2 isointense to normal white matter on MR images. The margins of the nerve are usually well delineated because of orbital fat within the retrobulbar space on both modalities and as a result of surrounding CSF on MR images. The normal optic nerve can be followed from the optic chiasm, through the optic canal, and into the retrobulbar space. Thin-collimation CT imaging and volume-acquisition MR techniques can be used to define reformatted imaging planes that parallel the path of a nerve (Figure 2.10.1).

The normal optic nerve may have a striated "tram-track" appearance following contrast medium administration on both imaging modalities as a result of the relatively greater enhancement of the surrounding dural sheath compared to the nerve. Fat-suppression techniques are particularly useful for increasing the conspicuity of the optic nerve on contrast-enhanced MR sequences.

Cranial nerve V

The trigeminal nerves arise from either side of the pons and exit the cranium through the trigeminal canal of the temporal bone. Within the temporal bone, sensory components of the nerve form the large trigeminal ganglion. The nerve divides to form three major peripheral branches, the ophthalmic, maxillary, and mandibular nerves, that exit through the orbital fissure, round foramen, and oval foramen, respectively.

In a review of MR contrast enhancement patterns of cranial nerve V in 42 dogs without clinical signs referable to trigeminal nerve dysfunction, the entire nerve enhanced in over 90% of dogs, and enhancement was limited to the region of the trigeminal ganglion in the remaining dogs. Intensity of enhancement was subjectively determined to be less than that of the pituitary gland.[6]

Cranial nerves VII and VIII

Cranial nerve VII, the facial nerve, arises in the medulla oblongata and emerges from the trapezoid body. The nerve exits the cranial cavity through the

Atlas of Small Animal CT and MRI, First Edition. Erik R. Wisner and Allison L. Zwingenberger.
© 2015 John Wiley & Sons, Inc. Published 2015 by John Wiley & Sons, Inc.

internal acoustic meatus, courses through the facial canal in the temporal bone, and exits through the stylomastoid foramen.

The origin and intracranial path of cranial nerve VIII, the vestibulocochlear nerve, is similar to that of the facial nerve, emerging from the trapezoid body adjacent and dorsal to the emergence of the facial nerve. The nerve also exits the cranial cavity through the internal acoustic meatus. Because of the close proximity of intracranial parts of these nerves, disorders affecting one can often also affect the other.

Inflammatory and idiopathic disorders

Noninfectious disorders

Idiopathic cranial neuropathy

Idiopathic trigeminal neuropathy is peripheral, often bilateral, and is the most common cause of masticatory muscle paralysis in the dog. This disorder causes dropped jaw from dysfunction of the mandibular branch motor innervation of the masticatory muscles. Variable facial sensory deficits may also be present.[7]

Idiopathic facial paralysis is the most common cause of acute facial nerve neuropathy in the dog and is also seen in cats. This disorder is peripheral in origin and is most often unilateral but can be bilateral. Clinical signs include: palsy of the external ear, lips, and cheek; a lack of palpebral closure; and ptyalism.[8]

Idiopathic trigeminal neuropathy imaging characteristics include diffuse nerve enlargement that is T1 isointense and T2 iso- to hyperintense on MR images. Affected nerves consistently enhance following contrast administration (Figure 2.10.2).[9]

Imaging diagnosis of idiopathic facial neuropathy may be more challenging. The nerve is visible on unenhanced images, but features may be unremarkable. Affected nerves variably enhance following contrast administration.[8] Contrast-enhanced ultrafast gradient echo sequences have been reported to increase sensitivity of detection of nerve enhancement in dogs with facial nerve neuropathy.[10]

Ocular granulomatous meningoencephalitis

The ocular form of granulomatous meningoencephalitis (GME) is uncommon compared to disseminated and focal forms. Features of GME are more fully described in Chapter 2.6, but the ocular manifestation is characterized clinically by blindness and optic neuritis and may occur as a component of more widespread disease. Ocular and optic nerve involvement is most often bilateral. Magnetic resonance imaging features have been reported to include T1 and T2 isointensity with enhancement following contrast administration (Figure 2.10.3).[11]

In our experience, ocular granulomatous meningoencephalitis can often have subtle MR imaging features.

Infectious inflammatory disorders

Infectious cranial neuritis can be viral, bacterial, mycotic, or protozoal. Imaging descriptions of infectious inflammatory cranial neuropathies are sparse, but expected features would include nerve enlargement, variable T1 and T2 intensity on unenhanced MR images, and some degree of enhancement following contrast administration. Mass lesions may also be seen when a suppurative or granulomatous inflammatory response is present (Figure 2.10.4).

Seventh and eighth cranial neuropathy often occurs from intracranial extension of bacterial otitis media/interna, and neuritis may be accompanied by regional meningitis and abscess formation (see Chapter 1.2, Figure 1.2.10).[12]

Neoplasia

Optic nerve meningioma

Because the meninges cover the optic nerves, retrobulbar meningiomas can occur either *in situ* or by expansion of an intracranial meningioma through the optic canal. Imaging features of meningiomas are described in Chapter 2.8. Optic nerve meningiomas can have both extracranial and intracranial components and cause exophthalmos. Owing to location, dural tails are not a feature of extracranial meningiomas (Figures 2.10.5, 2.10.6).

Peripheral nerve sheath tumor

Peripheral nerve sheath tumors most commonly affect the origin and branches of the trigeminal nerve. These tumors may be benign or malignant. Clinical signs associated with cranial nerve V nerve sheath tumor are unilateral and include atrophy of the temporalis and masseter muscles.

Trigeminal nerve sheath tumors appear as an isoattenuating extraaxial mass, usually in the region of the origin of the nerve lateral to the pons. The ophthalmic, maxillary, and mandibular branches of the nerve can all be involved. Trigeminal nerve sheath tumors appear T1 isointense and T2 iso- or hyperintense on MR images. These tumors generally intensely, and uniformly contrast enhance on both CT and MR images (Figures 2.10.7, 2.10.8). Affected cranial nerve V branches are enlarged and have a similar enhancement pattern as the central tumor mass. The trigeminal canal, the orbital fissure, and the round and oval foramina are often enlarged as a result of bone resorption resulting from expansion of the nerve branches (Figure 2.10.9). Marked unilateral temporalis and masseter muscle atrophy is most often also present. On MR images, the affected muscle is T1 and T2 hyperintense, because of fatty infiltration from denervation, and mildly to moderately contrast enhances.

Lymphoma

Lymphoma can occasionally involve the cranial nerves, either locally or as part of a more widespread central nervous system or systemic distribution. One or more cranial nerves can be affected, and nerve involvement is often bilateral. Affected nerves are generally enlarged and T1 iso- to hypointense and T2 iso- to hyperintense. Uniform moderate to marked enhancement is seen following contrast administration (Figures 2.10.10, 2.10.11).

Cavernous sinus syndrome

The cavernous sinuses are located on either side of the sella turcica and contain the internal carotid arteries and their associated sympathetic plexuses; the third, fourth, and sixth cranial nerves; and branches of the fifth cranial nerve. Mass lesions that encroach on or invade the cavernous sinuses will therefore often cause a cranial poly-neuropathy with clinical signs referable to the functions of these cranial nerves. Both neoplastic and inflammatory causes have been reported. Imaging features will depend on the inciting lesion but often include the presence of a space-occupying mass within or near the pituitary fossa with evidence of invasion or compression of the sinuses (Figure 2.10.12).[13–15]

Figure 2.10.1   Normal Cranial Nerve II (Canine)   CT & MR

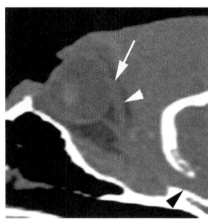 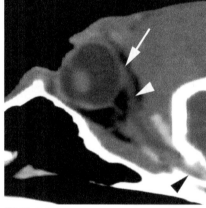 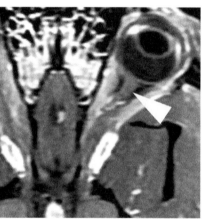

(a) CT, OP   **(b)** CT+C, OP   **(c)** T1+C FS, DP

The normal optic nerve (**a,b**: white arrowhead) can usually be identified on CT images from the optic canal (**a,b**: black arrowhead) to the optic disc (**a,b**: arrow). The normal optic nerve can also be seen on MR images (**c**: arrowhead). Because the nerve takes a tortuous path through the retrobulbar space, it is usually not possible to see the entire length of the extracranial part of the nerve on a single image.

Figure 2.10.2   Idiopathic Trigeminal Neuropathy (Canine)   MR

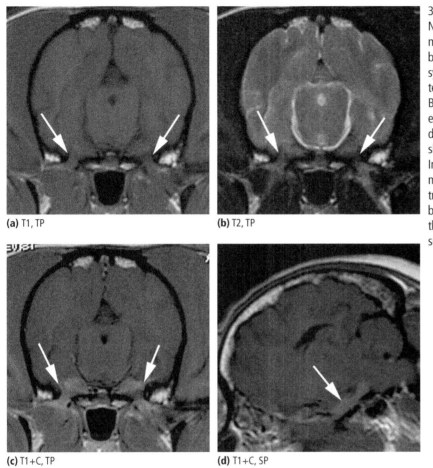

(a) T1, TP

(b) T2, TP

(c) T1+C, TP

(d) T1+C, SP

3y F Pug with a 6-day history of dropped jaw. Neurologic deficits were limited to cranial nerve V motor function bilaterally. The mandibular branches of the fifth cranial nerves are symmetrically enlarged and are T1 and T2 isointense on unenhanced images (**a**,**b**: arrows). Both nerves uniformly and intensely contrast enhance, defining enlarged intracranial and distal components that exit the base of the skull through the oval foramina (**c**,**d**: arrows). Image **d** is a parasagittal view of one of the mandibular nerves. A diagnosis of idiopathic trigeminal neuropathy was made in this patient based on the lack of any identifiable cause for the neuropathy and gradual improvement with supportive care.

Figure 2.10.3   Cranial Nerve II Granulomatous Meningoencephalitis (Canine)   MR

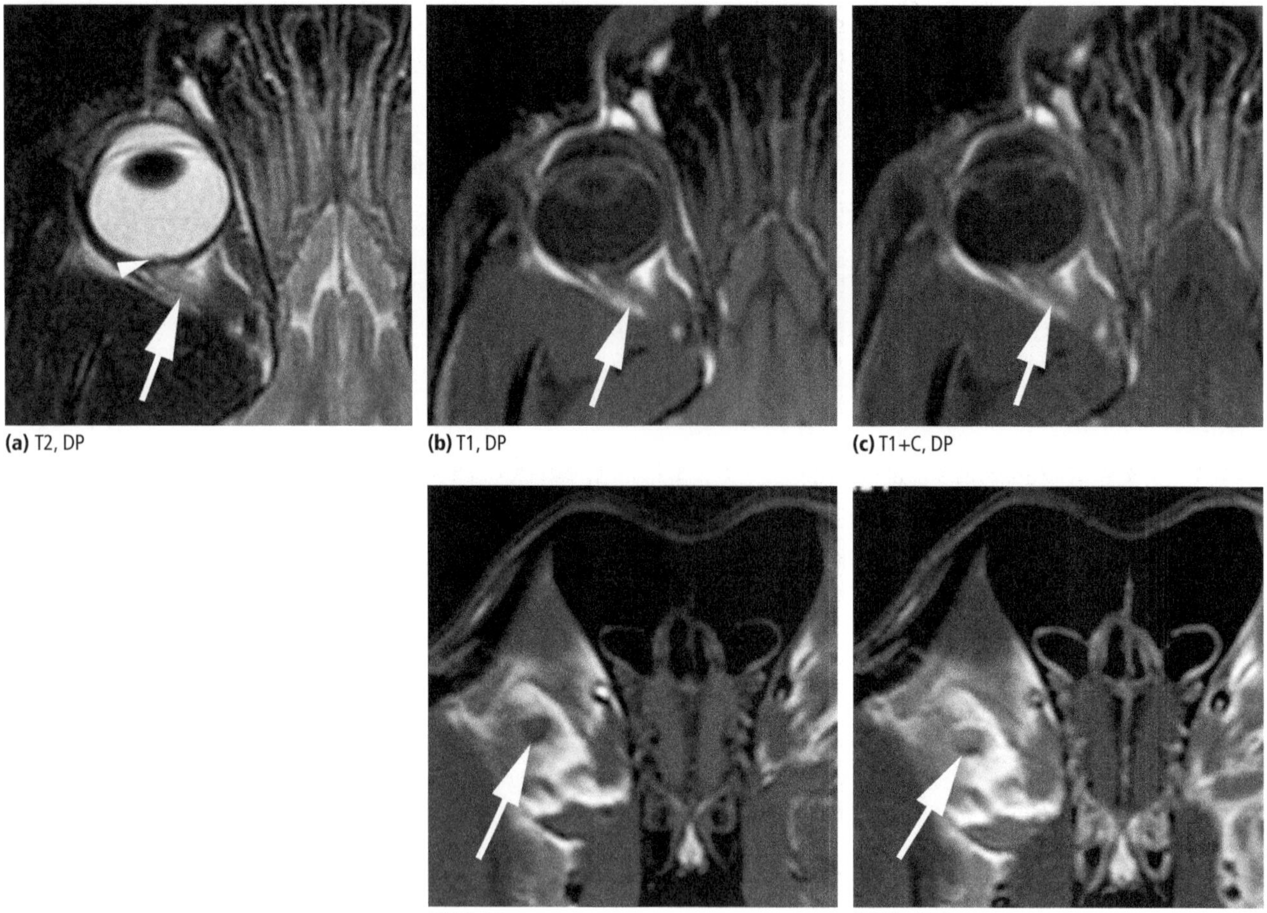

(a) T2, DP

(b) T1, DP

(c) T1+C, DP

(d) T1, TP

(e) T1+C, TP

4y MC Golden Retriever with ataxia and weakness. The right optic nerve is mildly enlarged and is T1 isointense and T2 hyperintense (a,b,d: arrow). There is also a slight bulge of the optic disc, best seen on the dorsal plane T2 image (a: arrowhead). The nerve moderately enhances following contrast administration (c,e: arrow). Postmortem examination confirmed granulomatous meningoencephalitis involving the brain and the right optic nerve. The MR features of the optic nerve lesion are subtle in this patient.

Figure 2.10.4   Cranial Nerve II Chronic Suppurative Neuritis (Feline)   MR

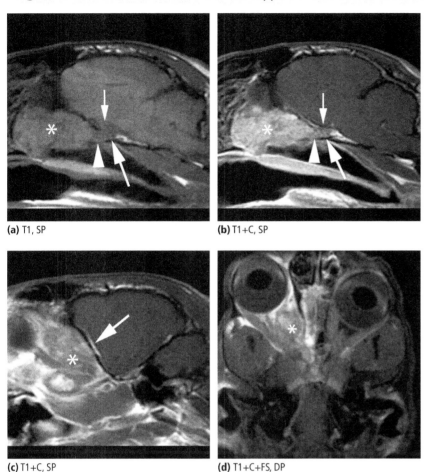

(a) T1, SP

(b) T1+C, SP

(c) T1+C, SP

(d) T1+C+FS, DP

12y MC Domestic Shorthair with progressive left-sided exophthalmos. Images **a** and **b** are to the left of midline in the parasagittal plane at the level of the optic canal. Image **c** is somewhat more lateral in the same plane. A large left retrobulbar mass (**a–d**: asterisk) results in rostral displacement of the ipsilateral globe. The mass extends caudally through the left optic canal (**a,b**: large arrow) and incorporates the optic chiasm (**a,b**: small arrow). Regional meningeal enhancement is also evident (**c**: arrow). The left optic nerve is not well delineated, but neural enlargement is assumed from the parasagittal images (**a,b**: arrowhead). Postmortem examination revealed severe chronic suppurative optic neuritis and meningitis.

Figure 2.10.5 Cranial Nerve II Meningioma (Canine)   CT & MR

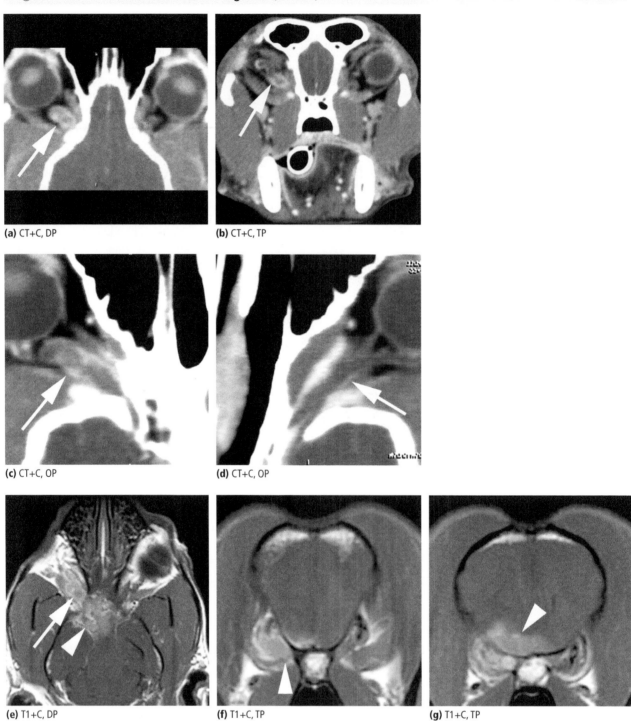

(a) CT+C, DP

(b) CT+C, TP

(c) CT+C, OP

(d) CT+C, OP

(e) T1+C, DP

(f) T1+C, TP

(g) T1+C, TP

10y FS Kelpie with right exophthalmia and absent menace response of 3-week duration. The right optic nerve is enlarged and has a nonuniform diameter (a–c: arrow). The meningeal sheath intensely enhances. Oblique plane images were generated to approximate the path of the right (c) and left (d) optic nerves through their respective optic canals (c, d: arrow). A right orbital exenteration was performed, and a right optic nerve meningioma was confirmed histologically.

The dog returned 2 years later with clinical signs referable to intracranial neurologic disease. The proximal remnant of the right optic nerve is enlarged, irregularly margined, and nonuniformly contrast enhances (e: arrow). The mass now includes both retrobulbar and intracranial components (e–g: arrowhead).

Figure 2.10.6   Cranial Nerve II Meningioma (Feline)

MR

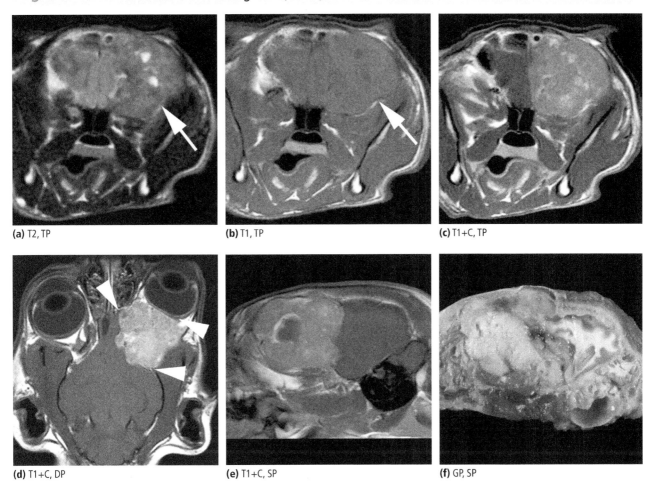

(a) T2, TP

(b) T1, TP

(c) T1+C, TP

(d) T1+C, DP

(e) T1+C, SP

(f) GP, SP

8y FS Domestic Shorthair with left-sided exophthalmos. There is a large T1 isointense, T2 mixed-intensity mass in the left retrobulbar space (**a**,**b**: arrow). The mass displaces the left eye rostrally and has eroded through the frontal, ethmoid, and lacrimal bones, compressing the left frontal lobe axially (**d**: arrowheads). The mass intensely contrast enhances (**c–e**) and has a large central cavitary component (**e**). Postmortem examination confirmed meningioma arising from the left optic nerve.

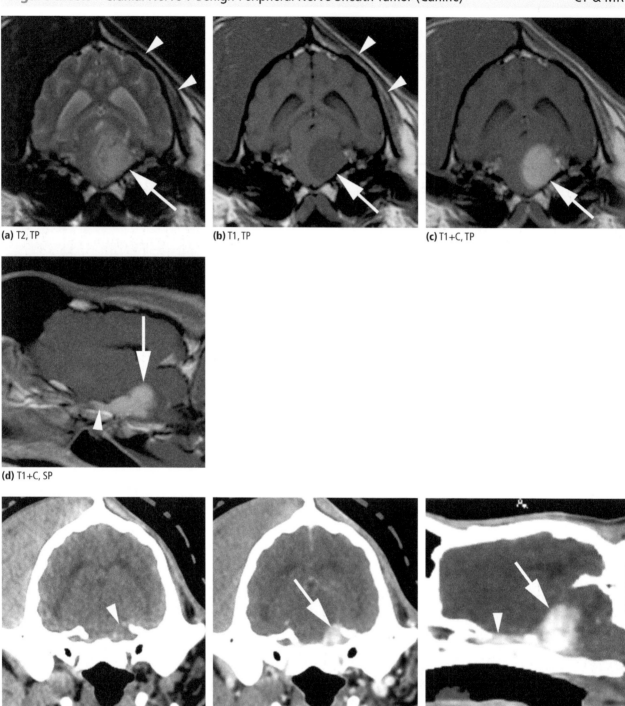

(a) T2, TP

(b) T1, TP

(c) T1+C, TP

(d) T1+C, SP

(e) CT, TP

(f) CT+C, TP

(g) CT+C, SP

7y MC Shetland Sheepdog with left-sided masticatory muscle atrophy and other signs of left trigeminal nerve dysfunction. MR images reveal a large, well-delineated, T1 hypointense, T2 hyperintense left-sided extraaxial mass causing compression of the brainstem and cerebellum (a–d: arrow). The mass intensely and uniformly contrast enhances and extends rostrally through the trigeminal canal (d: arrowhead). There is also marked atrophy and T1 and T2 hyperintensity of the left masseter muscle, consistent with fatty infiltration from chronic denervation (a,b: arrowheads). A CT examination was performed for radiation treatment planning. Images e and f are unenhanced and enhanced images acquired at the level of the trigeminal canal. Images h and i (next page) are more caudal, centered at the level of the mass. There is destruction of the temporal bone pyramid that forms the trigeminal canal (e: arrowhead). Note that the mass is not seen on the unenhanced CT images (h). The previously identified mass intensely but nonuniformly enhances (f,g,i: arrow). The globoid part of the mass is located in the caudal fossa (g,i: arrow) but extends rostrally through the trigeminal canal (g: arrowhead). Postmortem examination confirmed the presence and location of the extraaxial mass (j: arrowheads). Microscopic diagnosis was left trigeminal nerve neurofibroma.

Figure 2.10.7   (*Continued*)   CT & MR

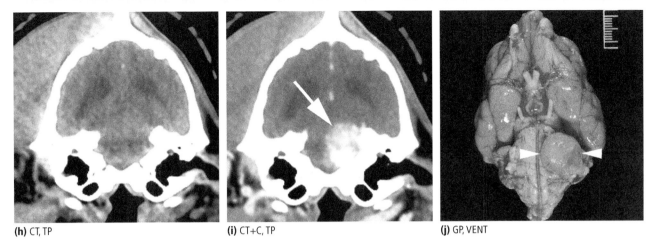

(h) CT, TP   **(i)** CT+C, TP   **(j)** GP, VENT

Figure 2.10.8   Cranial Nerve V Malignant Peripheral Nerve Sheath Tumor (Canine)   MR

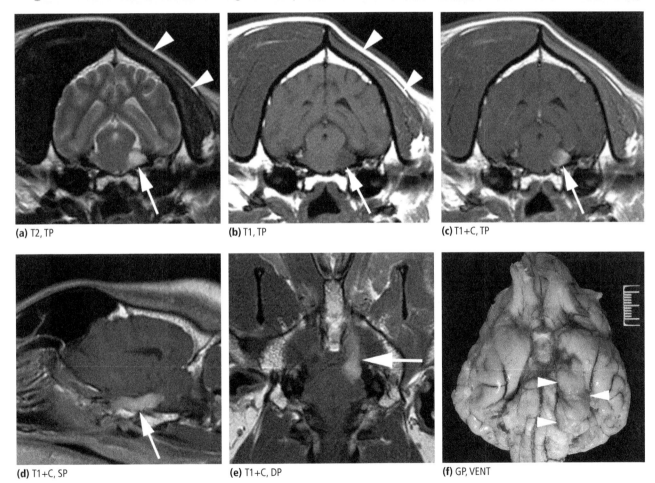

(a) T2, TP   **(b)** T1, TP   **(c)** T1+C, TP

(d) T1+C, SP   **(e)** T1+C, DP   **(f)** GP, VENT

7y FS Labrador Retriever with neurologic deficits localized to the mandibular branch of the left trigeminal nerve. There is a large, T1 hypointense, T2 hyperintense tubular mass that arises at the origin of the left trigeminal nerve and extends rostrally through the trigeminal canal of the temporal bone (a–e: arrow). There is marked left temporal muscle atrophy consistent with mandibular nerve motor dysfunction, and the muscle is mildly T1 and T2 hyperintense compared to the contralateral temporal muscle as a result of fatty infiltration from chronic denervation (a,b: arrowheads). The mass intensely and uniformly enhances following contrast administration (c–e: arrow). Postmortem examination confirmed a peripheral nerve sheath tumor of the origin and mandibular branch of the left trigeminal nerve (f: arrowheads).

Figure 2.10.9   Presumptive Nerve Sheath Tumor (V) with Oval Foramen Enlargement (Canine)   CT & MR

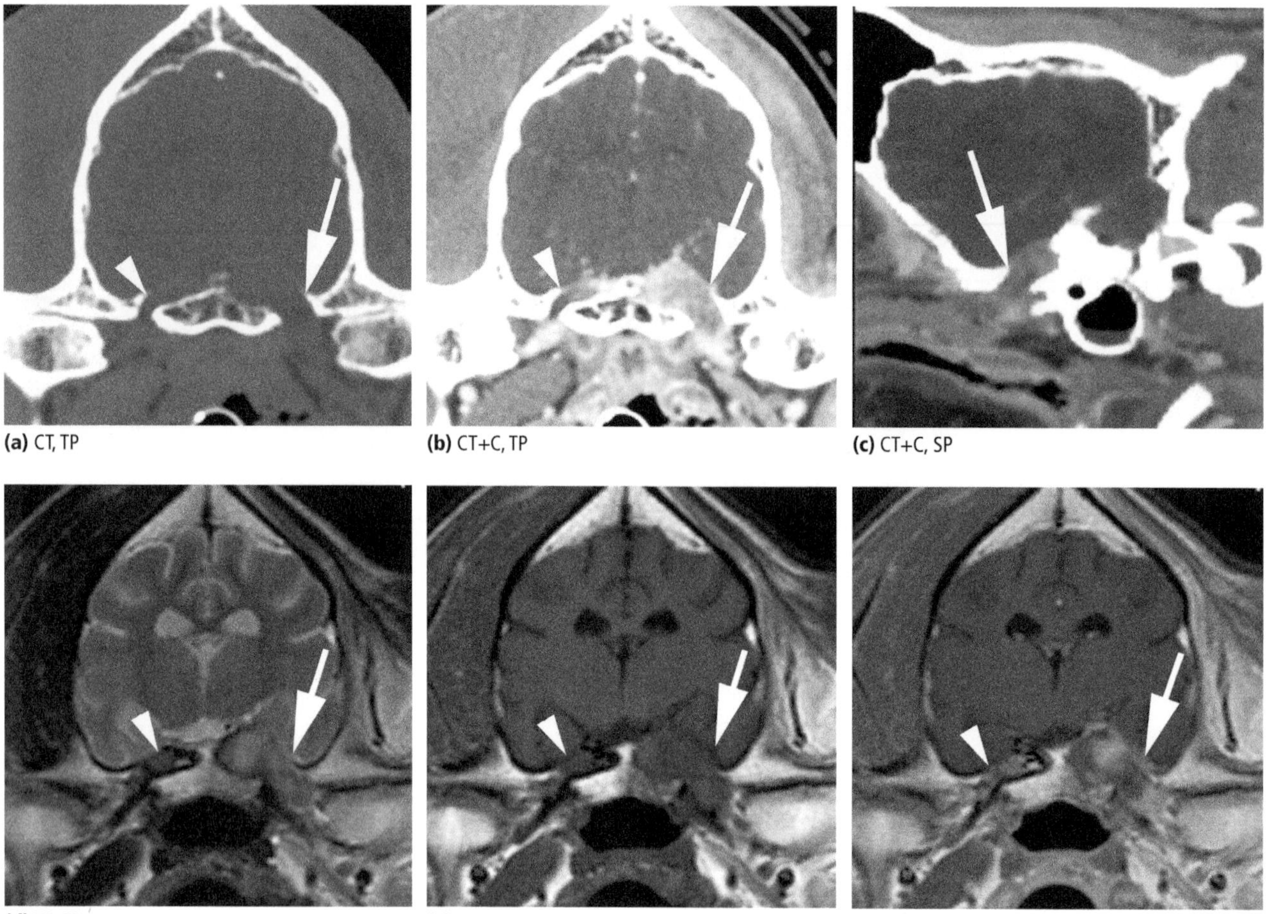

(a) CT, TP

(b) CT+C, TP

(c) CT+C, SP

(d) T2, TP

(e) T1, TP

(f) T1+C, TP

7y FS Golden Retriever with left-sided temporal muscle atrophy and enophthalmos. The left oval foramen is enlarged because of the presence of a peripheral nerve sheath tumor involving the mandibular branch of the left trigeminal nerve. (a–f: arrow) The normal right oval foramen is highlighted for comparison (a,b,d–f: arrowhead). The mass uniformly and intensely enhances on both CT and MR images following contrast administration. There is also marked left temporal muscle atrophy and tympanic bulla effusion. Affected muscle is T1 and T2 hyperintense and contrast enhances.

Figure 2.10.10 Cranial Nerve V Lymphoma (Canine)   MR

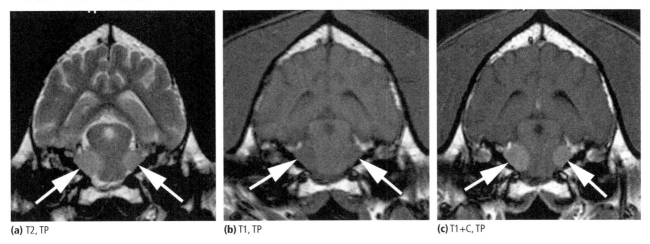

(a) T2, TP   **(b)** T1, TP   **(c)** T1+C, TP

7y MC German Shepherd Dog with multiple cranial nerve neuropathy, including pronounced bilateral trigeminal nerve involvement. Prominent, well-delineated, T1 hypointense, T2 hyperintense extraaxial masses are present on either side of the brainstem, causing axial compression bilaterally (**a,b**: arrows). The masses moderately and uniformly contrast enhance (**c**: arrows). Cerebrospinal fluid analysis revealed the presence of abnormal lymphocytes. The diagnosis of lymphoma was confirmed on postmortem examination performed 6 months following the MRI examination.

Figure 2.10.11 Multiple Cranial Nerve Lymphoma (Canine)   MR

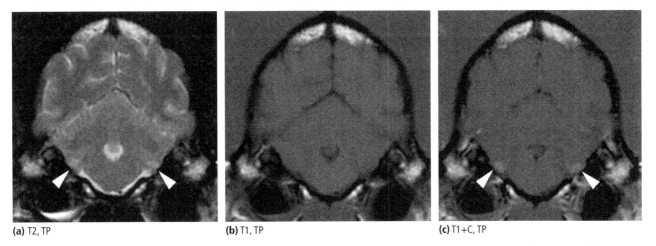

(a) T2, TP   **(b)** T1, TP   **(c)** T1+C, TP

5y FS Border Collie with progressive ataxia, head tilt, and dropped jaw. There is ill-defined T2 hyperintensity in the region of the origins of the seventh and eighth cranial nerves bilaterally (**a**: arrowheads). Moderate focal enhancement is evident in the same locations following contrast administration (**c**: arrowheads). There is also right-sided tympanic bulla effusion. Cerebrospinal fluid analysis confirmed a diagnosis of lymphoma.

Figure 2.10.12 Cavernous Sinus Syndrome (Canine)   MR

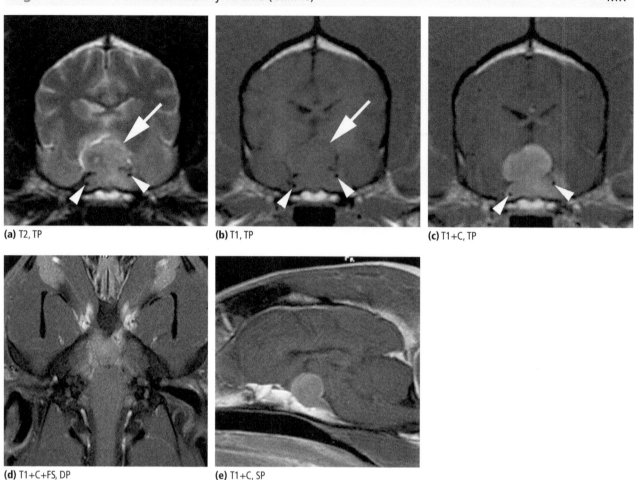

(a) T2, TP

(b) T1, TP

(c) T1+C, TP

(d) T1+C+FS, DP

(e) T1+C, SP

8y FS Shepherd cross with cranial nerve III, IV, V, VI, and ocular sympathetic innervation deficits consistent with cavernous sinus syndrome. There is a large, well-defined, T1 isointense, T2 hyperintense ovoid mass arising from the pituitary fossa (**a,b**: arrow). The carotid arteries are identified in cross-section and appear to be surrounded by the mass (**a,b**: arrowheads). Following contrast administration, the mass uniformly and intensely enhances, and the basilar part of the mass can be seen to invade the cavernous sinus bilaterally. Carotid arteries are confirmed to be incorporated into the mass (**c**: arrowheads). The cavernous sinus contains the carotid arteries, its sympathetic plexus, and the third, fourth, sixth, and some branches of the fifth cranial nerves. The invasion of the mass within the sinus explains the clinical signs.

References

1. Probst A, Kneissl S. Computed tomographic anatomy of the canine temporal bone. Anat Histol Embryol. 2006;35:19–22.
2. Parry AT, Volk HA. Imaging the cranial nerves. Vet Radiol Ultrasound. 2011;52:S32–41.
3. Gomes E, Degueurce C, Ruel Y, Dennis R, Begon D. Anatomic study of cranial nerve emergence and associated skull foramina in cats using CT and MRI. Vet Radiol Ultrasound. 2009;50:398–403.
4. Couturier L, Degueurce C, Ruel Y, Dennis R, Begon D. Anatomical study of cranial nerve emergence and skull foramina in the dog using magnetic resonance imaging and computed tomography. Vet Radiol Ultrasound. 2005;46:375–383.
5. Boroffka SA, Gorig C, Auriemma E, Passon-Vastenburg MH, Voorhout G, Barthez PY. Magnetic resonance imaging of the canine optic nerve. Vet Radiol Ultrasound. 2008;49:540–544.
6. Pettigrew R, Rylander H, Schwarz T. Magnetic resonance imaging contrast enhancement of the trigeminal nerve in dogs without evidence of trigeminal neuropathy. Vet Radiol Ultrasound. 2009; 50:276–278.
7. Mayhew PD, Bush WW, Glass EN. Trigeminal neuropathy in dogs: a retrospective study of 29 cases (1991–2000). J Am Anim Hosp Assoc. 2002;38:262–270.
8. Varejao AS, Munoz A, Lorenzo V. Magnetic resonance imaging of the intratemporal facial nerve in idiopathic facial paralysis in the dog. Vet Radiol Ultrasound. 2006;47:328–333.
9. Schultz RM, Tucker RL, Gavin PR, Bagley R, Saveraid TC, Berry CR. Magnetic resonance imaging of acquired trigeminal nerve disorders in six dogs. Vet Radiol Ultrasound. 2007;48:101–104.
10. Smith PM, Goncalves R, McConnell JF. Sensitivity and specificity of MRI for detecting facial nerve abnormalities in dogs with facial neuropathy. Vet Rec. 2012;171:349.

11. Kitagawa M, Okada M, Watari T, Sato T, Kanayama K, Sakai T. Ocular granulomatous meningoencephalomyelitis in a dog: magnetic resonance images and clinical findings. J Vet Med Sci. 2009;71:233–237.

12. Sturges BK, Dickinson PJ, Kortz GD, Berry WL, Vernau KM, Wisner ER, et al. Clinical signs, magnetic resonance imaging features, and outcome after surgical and medical treatment of otogenic intracranial infection in 11 cats and 4 dogs. J Vet Intern Med. 2006;20:648–656.

13. Theisen SK, Podell M, Schneider T, Wilkie DA, Fenner WR. A retrospective study of cavernous sinus syndrome in 4 dogs and 8 cats. J Vet Intern Med. 1996;10:65–71.

14. Hernandez-Guerra AM, Del Mar Lopez-Murcia M, Planells A, Corpa JM, Liste F. Computed tomographic diagnosis of unilateral cavernous sinus syndrome caused by a chondrosarcoma in a dog: a case report. Vet J. 2007;174:206–208.

15. Fransson B, Kippenes H, Silver GE, Gavin PR. Magnetic resonance diagnosis: cavernous sinus syndrome in a dog. Vet Radiol Ultrasound. 2000;41:536–538.

Section 3
Vertebral Column & Spinal Cord

3.1

Developmental disorders

Anomalies of the vertebral column

Vertebral malformation

Malformations of the vertebrae are common, and although some are clinically significant, many are seen as incidental findings on imaging studies. Malformations can be categorized as simple or complex, and a recent review of spinal anomalies proposed specific classification of anomalous vertebrae based on a similar scheme used in people.[1,2] Those anomalies that occur during the early embryonic period include centrum median cleft (butterfly vertebrae), true hemivertebrae, mediolateral wedged vertebrae, and transitional vertebrae. Anomalies that develop during the later fetal period include block vertebrae, articular process hypoplasia, and centrum hypoplasia or aplasia (dorsoventral wedged vertebrae).[1-3] Vertebral anomalies can be further classified as arising from defects in formation (e.g. wedged, hemi-, and butterfly vertebrae) versus incomplete or absent segmentation (e.g. block vertebrae).

German Shepherd Dogs are overrepresented for developing transitional vertebrae at the lumbosacral junction.[4] Certain screw-tailed breeds, such as Bulldogs, French Bulldogs, Pugs, and Boston Terriers, are highly predisposed to complex vertebral anomalies, particularly in the midthoracic region.[5] Vertebral anomalies can result in a combination of scoliosis, kyphosis, lordosis, or rotational spinal abnormalities; can cause spinal canal stenosis; and may predispose to spinal injury from what might otherwise be clinically insignificant trauma. In animals with vertebral canal stenosis, spinal cord diameter is often focally decreased as a result of chronic compression atrophy, even in patients without overt neurologic deficits. An uncommon vertebral anomaly, caudal articular facet hypoplasia or aplasia in the thoracolumbar vertebral column, has been reported with spinal cord compression due to contralateral facet and ligamentum flavum hypertrophy.[6]

The CT appearance of vertebral anomalies will vary depending on the specific malformation, but common findings include alteration in vertebral shape, reduced attenuation when mineralization is incomplete, and vertebral column curvature abnormalities. Vertebral canal stenosis suggests spinal cord impingement or compression, which can be documented using CT myelography (Figures 3.1.1, 3.1.2). Lumbosacral transitional vertebrae can predispose to cauda equina syndrome (Chapter 3.5), and asymmetrical transitional vertebra at this level can result in pelvic rotation leading to coxofemoral malarticulation (Figure 3.1.3).

MR features are similar to those seen with CT, and spinal cord pathology is often more clearly detected (Figure 3.1.2).

Craniocervical junction malformation

The term craniocervical junction malformation includes anomalies of the occipital bone and the first two cervical vertebrae.[7] The most common of these disorders, Chiari-like malformation, is discussed in Chapter 2.3. Other malformations involving the occipital bone and atlanto-occipital overlap are described in Chapter 1.4. Chiari-like malformation aside, craniocervical junction malformations primarily affect

---

Atlas of Small Animal CT and MRI, First Edition. Erik R. Wisner and Allison L. Zwingenberger.
© 2015 John Wiley & Sons, Inc. Published 2015 by John Wiley & Sons, Inc.

small and toy breed dogs, with clinical signs often occurring at an early age.[7,8]

Atlantoaxial instability

Atlantoaxial instability can be caused by malformation of either or both of the first two cervical vertebrae, with dorsal subluxation of the axis in relation to the atlas causing spinal cord compression.[8] Malformations can include fusion of adjacent vertebrae, grossly abnormal vertebral shape, and hypoplastic, aplastic, or misshaped dens. The latter feature is associated with abnormalities of ligaments of the dens, which in turn exacerbate instability.[8-12] Caution should be used when imaging patients with suspected craniocervical junction malformations since abnormalities are often unstable.

CT imaging features of atlantoaxial malformations include the abnormalities described above as well as separation of the cranial part of the spinous process of the atlas from the dorsal arch of the atlas with mild cervical flexion. Abnormalities of the dens can sometimes be more clearly seen on sagittal or dorsal plane reformatted images. Dorsal subluxation of the axis in relation to the atlas also results in decreased vertebral canal diameter (Figure 3.1.4).

MR features of atlantoaxial malformations include those described for CT imaging. Spinal cord compression can also be seen as a narrowing of the hyperintense subarachnoid column on T2 images and narrowed spinal cord diameter due to dorsal–ventral cord compression (Figure 3.1.5). The MR appearance of the ligamentous structures of the normal canine occipitoatlantoaxial region has been described in a cadaveric study, but they can be challenging to accurately identify in small patients.[10]

Chiari-like malformation

Although imaging features of Chiari-like malformation are detailed in Chapter 2.3, a striking imaging feature of the disorder worth mentioning here is the often pronounced saccular syringohydromyelia that can result from altered cerebrospinal fluid dynamics and is best seen on T2 images as a hyperintense dilatation of the central canal (Figure 3.1.6).[13]

Cervical spondylomyelopathy

Canine cervical spondylomyelopathy (CSM) is challenging to concisely summarize because the etiology is unclear, the underlying pathology is variable, and the clinical presentation varies with breed and age of the patient. Genetic, congenital, body conformational, and nutritional etiologies have all been postulated, and the disorder may stem from a combination of these factors. CSM usually occurs in large- to giant-breed dogs

between 2 and 8 years of age, and Doberman Pinschers are overrepresented. Although the disorder appears to occur more often in males, there is no confirmed sex predilection. Clinical signs include cervical pain and spinal cord compressive myelopathy that is neuroanatomically localized to the cervical region. Cord compression is due to some combination of three distinct mechanisms. Compression can occur from intervertebral disk protrusion, which tends to occur most frequently between C5 and C7. This manifestation of the disorder occurs in older large-breed dogs and is common in Doberman Pinschers. Osseous stenotic compression is due to inherent vertebral canal stenosis and from proliferative new bone formation occurring on the lamina, pedicles, and articular facet margins of affected vertebrae. This manifestation occurs in younger large- and giant-breed dogs and often involves many of the cervical vertebrae. Intermittent or dynamic compression can also occur with change in cervical spine position, usually in extension.[14,15]

CT imaging features can include angulation of the endplate subchondral bone margin, associated with vertebral bodies having a rhomboidal rather than rectangular shape as viewed on sagittal images. Dogs with a component of intervertebral disk disease will have imaging signs referable to intervertebral disk protrusion (see Chapter 3.5). In dogs with osseous stenotic manifestations, bone-attenuating proliferative changes are seen involving the lamina, pedicles, and articular facets, resulting in decreased vertebral canal diameter, which is most pronounced in the lateromedial direction. This results in a change of canal cross-sectional shape from round to rectangular or triangular and causes predominantly lateral or dorsolateral spinal cord compression and atrophy, which can be documented using CT myelography (Figure 3.1.7, 3.1.8, 3.1.9). In those dogs with a dynamic component to spinal cord compression, traction studies can be used to document reduction.[14,16,17]

Anatomical features of CSM on MR images are similar to those in CT. Dense new bone will appear T1 and T2 hypointense. Spinal cord compression is usually clearly defined by attenuation of the subarachnoid column and cord flattening, seen best on T2 images. The affected region of the spinal cord may be reduced in diameter from atrophy, and change in signal intensity sometimes occurs as a result of central canal dilation, edema, or gliosis (Figure 3.1.9, 3.1.10).[14,18-22]

Osteochondrosis

Osteochondrosis involving the lumbosacral junction has been reported in dogs, and articular facet subchondral bone fragmentation is occasionally seen either in isolation or as a sequela to other disorders, such as cervical spondylomyelopathy.[23-25] For lumbosacral osteochondrosis, male dogs and Boxer, Rottweiler, and German Shepherd Dog breeds are overrepresented. Clinical signs are those of cauda equina neuropathy, and mean age at presentation is 6.3 years. Approximately 90% of lesions involve the craniodorsal margin of the body of the sacrum, while the remainder involve the caudodorsal margin of the body of the last lumbar vertebra.[23]

On CT images, lumbosacral osteochondrosis lesions appear as one or more separate, bone-attenuating bodies associated with an underlying defect within the subchondral bone of the parent vertebra. Osteochondrosis lesions may be isolated or associated with other developmental or degenerative processes of the lumbosacral junction (Figure 3.1.11).[24]

In a report of MR features of lumbosacral osteochondrosis in seven dogs, affected endplates were predominantly T1 spin-echo hypointense, T1 gradient-echo hyperintense, variably T2 hyperintense, and contrast enhanced. Concurrent intervertebral disk disease was present in five of seven dogs.[26]

Intradural arachnoid diverticula

Intradural arachnoid diverticula, sometimes termed arachnoid or subarachnoid cysts, are focal, subdural, and usually dorsally located dilatations containing cerebrospinal fluid and most often confluent with the subarachnoid space. The etiology of intradural arachnoid diverticula is not known, but when seen in young animals they are thought to be developmental.[27] A broader discussion of the various forms of arachnoid diverticula, both developmental and acquired, is included in Chapter 3.5. In young dogs, presumed developmental arachnoid diverticula commonly occur in the C2–C4 region in large breeds and in the thoracolumbar region in all breeds.[28–31] Male dogs and Pug, French Bulldog, and Rottweiler breeds are overrepresented.[27] Imaging features of intradural arachnoid diverticula are described in Chapter 3.5 (Figure 3.1.12).

Spinal neural tube defects (spinal dysraphism)

Neural tube defects result from abnormal closure or failure of closure of the developing neural tube. Closure errors in the rostral part of the tube lead to cranial defects, while those that occur caudally lead to vertebral column and spinal cord anomalies. Folate deficiency is one well-established cause of the disorder in people, and a hereditary link has been identified in neural tube defects described in Weimaraner dogs.[32–35]

Terminology and classification of the various spinal neural tube defects are both inconsistent and confusing, and we choose to use a simplified scheme for this discussion. Errors of ectoderm, mesoderm, and neuroectoderm development and differentiation, primarily associated with incomplete dorsal migration and closure, result in a grouping of related disorders under the overarching term spina bifida, which often involves the caudal lumbar and sacral region.

Spina bifida can be further subclassified as spina bifida occulta or spina bifida cystica. Spina bifida occulta is limited to incomplete dorsal closure of affected vertebra and is periodically seen on imaging studies as an incidental finding. Spina bifida cystica includes dorsal meningeal defects leading to meningocele alone or the most clinically significant form that includes defective meningeal and cord development resulting in myelomeningocele. Spina bifida can further be characterized as closed or open to the external environment.

Sacrocaudal dysgenesis of the Manx cat is a complex spinal neural tube defect that includes developmental abnormalities of the sacral and caudal vertebrae and associated spinal cord segments, which can include meningomyelocele and can be closed or open.[36] Other manifestations of abnormal neural tube development, such as spinal duplication, are rare.[37]

Spina bifida occulta

The specific CT or MR imaging feature of spina bifida occulta is incomplete closure of the dorsal arch and spinous process of one or more vertebrae (Figure 3.1.13). The meninges and spinal cord should appear unaffected.

Spina bifida cystica

MR imaging features of meningocele include T1 hypointense, STIR and T2 hyperintense dorsal dilation of the subarachnoid space in the region of the lumbosacral junction. The terminal spinal cord and associated spinal nerves remain within the vertebral canal. Meningocele is also present in patients with myelomeningocele, but the terminal spinal cord or the associated spinal nerves are displaced dorsally into the meningocele. If the lesion is open, sagittal or transverse STIR or T2 images can be used to document a communicating tract as a linear hyperintensity (Figures 3.1.14, 3.1.15).

Spinal dermoid sinus

Dermoid sinus is an uncommon disorder that also results from neural tube closure errors. Failure of normal cell separation and differentiation into developing spine and skin leads to a dorsal sinus that histologically contains skin elements, such as hair follicles and sebaceous glands. The sinus can have a closed end at its most internal extent or connect to the meninges or spinal cord via a closed or patent tract. A grading scheme has been proposed, ranging from I to IV depending on the internal extent and character of the sinus, with increasing grade reflecting a more invasive lesion.[38] Of the few reported cases, most are at the level of the cervical or cranial thoracic vertebral column. Dermoid sinuses have been reported in dogs and cats, and Rhodesian Ridgebacks are predisposed.[39–43]

CT imaging features may be unremarkable other than a possible skin surface defect. Conventional radiographic sinusography has been used to determine the internal margin of the sinus and assess its association to the underlying vertebral column, meninges, and spinal cord, and CT would likely be of similar value. Reported MR imaging features include superficial mass with mixed T1 intensity, mild T2 hyperintensity, and STIR hyperintensity. In some instances, a sinus tract was not seen, and the depth of the lesion was underestimated. In one other patient, a T2 hyperintense tract was clearly identified coursing from the superficial mass to the dura matter.[2,44,45]

Vascular anomalies

Although vascular anomalies involving the spinal cord are rare in dogs and cats, various disorders have been sporadically reported as single case reports or small case studies. Abnormalities have included arterial malformation, arteriovenous malformation, hemangioma, intramedullary cavernous malformation, and hamartoma. Intrinsic vascular anomalies can displace spinal cord parenchyma, and both intrinsic and extrinsic anomalies can cause cord compression.[46–51]

CT and MR imaging features are dependent on the type and location of the anomaly. Large vessel anomalies can clearly be seen on contrast-enhanced imaging studies (Figure 3.1.16). Imaging signs of intrinsic spinal cord disease can be seen with intramedullary lesions, and T2* sequences may be helpful in characterizing thrombotic disease.

Figure 3.1.1 Complex Vertebral Anomalies (Canine)   CT

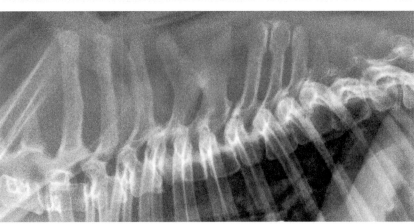

(a) DX, LAT

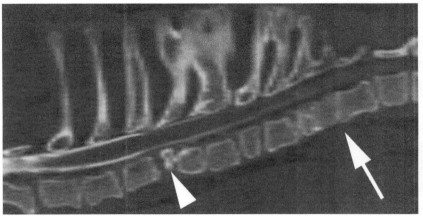

(b) CT+C, SP

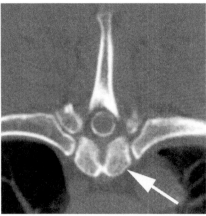

(c) CT+C, TP

6y MC French Bulldog with T3–L3 myelopathy. Survey radiographs show multiple vertebral anomalies affecting most of the thoracic vertebral column (**a**). CT myelographic images more clearly define multiple incomplete and misshapen vertebra and fusion of multiple adjacent spinous processes. Wedged (**b**: arrowhead), block (**b**: arrow), and butterfly (**c**: arrow) vertebrae are clearly identified.

Figure 3.1.2   Complex Vertebral Anomalies (Canine)   CT & MR

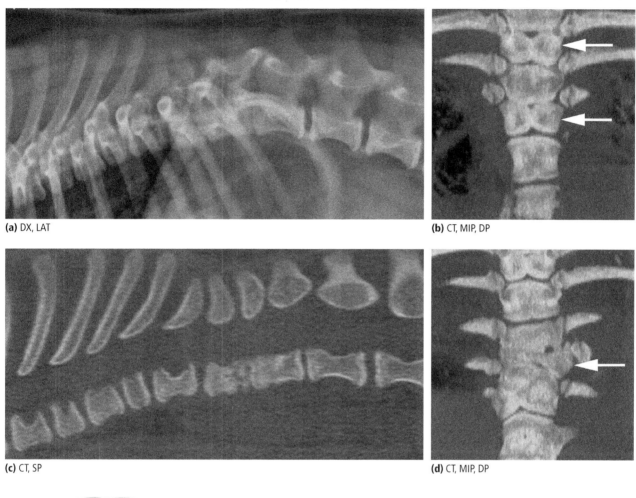

(a) DX, LAT

(b) CT, MIP, DP

(c) CT, SP

(d) CT, MIP, DP

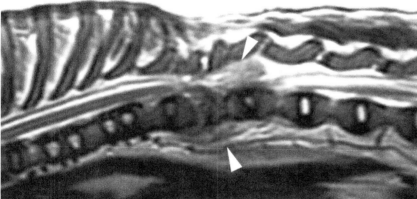

(e) T2, SP

1y M English Bulldog with epidural space empyema. Survey radiographs and CT images show multiple vertebral anomalies of the mid and caudal thoracic vertebral column (**a–d**). Anomalous butterfly vertebrae (**b**: arrows) and hemivertebrae (**d**: arrow) are clearly defined. Similar features are seen on a T2 MR image (**e**). The complex intensity pattern (**e**: arrowheads) in the soft tissues are likely related to the empyema.

Figure 3.1.3   Asymmetrical Transitional Vertebra (Canine) CT

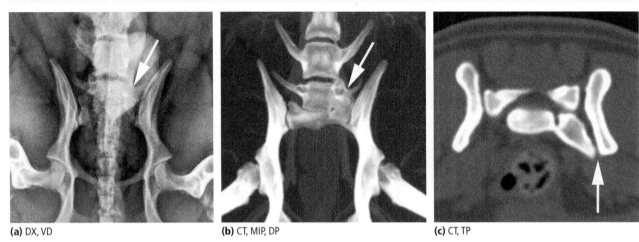

(a) DX, VD   **(b)** CT, MIP, DP   **(c)** CT, TP

1y M Pekingese. The CT examination was acquired for anatomic characterization of a previously diagnosed portosystemic shunt. Survey radiographs reveal an asymmetrical transitional vertebra with left-sided sacralization at the lumbosacral junction (**a**: arrow). The degree of asymmetry and the left-sided sacral articulation is clearly defined on CT images (**b**,**c**: arrow).

Figure 3.1.4   Atlantoaxial Instability (Canine) CT

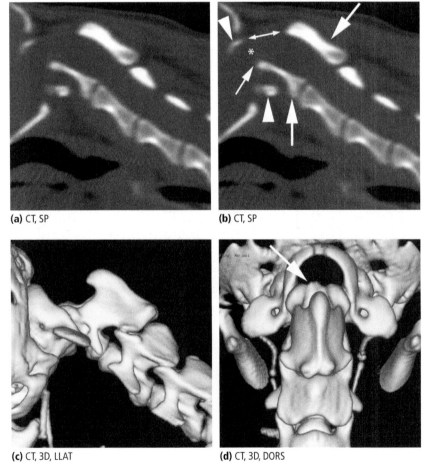

(a) CT, SP   **(b)** CT, SP

(c) CT, 3D, LLAT   **(d)** CT, 3D, DORS

5mo MC Yorkshire Terrier with acute onset cervical pain of 1-week duration. Image **a** is the same as image **b** without annotations. Dorsal subluxation of the axis (**b**: large arrows) is present in relation to the atlas (**b**: arrowheads), causing marked narrowing of the vertebral canal in the dorsal–ventral axis (**b**: asterisk). The angulation of the vertebral column at the atlantoaxial joint, the gap between the caudal margin of the dorsal arch of the atlas, and the cranial margin of the spinous process of the axis (**b**: two-headed arrow) are further evidence of atlantoaxial instability. The dens is also absent (**b**: small arrow). The abnormal relationship of the atlas and axis is also clearly seen on 3D renderings (**c**,**d**). Aplasia of the dens is best seen from the dorsal view (**d**: arrow).

Figure 3.1.5   Atlantoaxial Instability (Canine)   MR

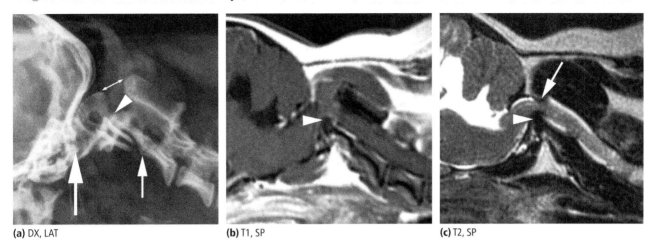

(a) DX, LAT   **(b)** T1, SP   **(c)** T2, SP

7y FS Maltese with a 4-day history of lethargy and tetraparesis. The survey radiographic image shows a complex craniocervical junction malformation with occipital malformation and abnormal atlantooccipital articulation (**a**: large arrow), hypoplastic dens (**a**: arrowhead), misshapen axis with caudal fusion to the third cervical vertebra (**a**: small arrow), and dorsal subluxation of the atlantoaxial joint. There is widening of the space between the caudal margin of the dorsal arch of the atlas and the cranial margin of the spinous process of the axis (**a**: two-headed arrow). Atlantoaxial subluxation and dens hypoplasia (**b,c**: arrowhead) are also seen on the MR images, and spinal cord compression can be seen at the site of atlantoaxial subluxation (**c**: arrow).

Figure 3.1.6   Chiari-like Malformation with Syringohydromyelia (Canine)   MR

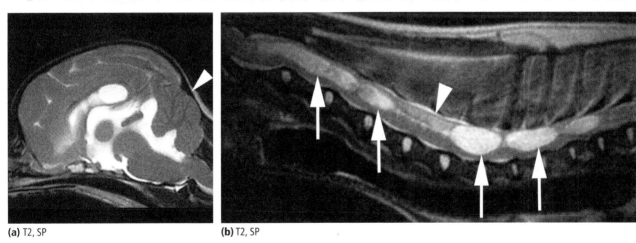

(a) T2, SP   **(b)** T2, SP

1.5y F Chihuahua with recent-onset paroxysmal episodes. The caudal cranial vault is small as a result of occipital hypoplasia (**a**: arrowhead), and moderate generalized hydrocephalus is evident (**a**). Marked saccular syringohydromyelia is present throughout the cervical and cranial thoracic spinal cord (**b**: arrows). There is also T2 hyperintensity within cord parenchyma, which is likely due to edema (**b**: arrowhead). A diagnosis of Chiari-like malformation with syringohydromyelia was made based on clinical and imaging findings.

Figure 3.1.7 Cervical Spondylomyelopathy (Canine)   CT

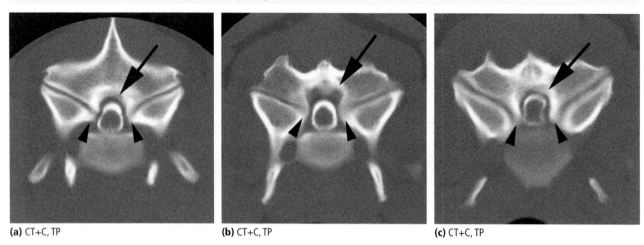

(a) CT+C, TP   **(b)** CT+C, TP   **(c)** CT+C, TP

3y MC Mastiff with hypermetria in all limbs. CT myelographic images **a**, **b**, and **c** are at the approximate level of the C2–3, C3–4, and C4–5 intervertebral disk spaces, respectively. Hyperattenuating new bone of the lamina (**a–c**: arrow) and articular facets (**a–c**: arrowheads) at all three levels results in reduction of vertebral canal cross-sectional area and change in shape, with greatest narrowing occurring in the horizontal axis. Remodeled articular facet margins impinge on the spinal cord to the greatest extent at C4–5, although a thin subarachnoid contrast column is retained (**c**). Additional sites with similar abnormalities were present more caudally (not shown).

Figure 3.1.8 Cervical Spondylomyelopathy (Canine)   CT

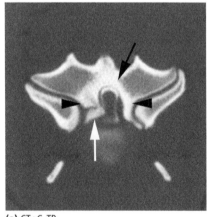

3y MC Labrador Retriever with myelopathy neuroanatomically localized to C1–5. The CT myelographic image is at the level of C4–5. Hyperattenuating new bone of the lamina (black arrow) and articular facets (arrowheads) results in reduction of vertebral canal cross-sectional area and change in shape, with greatest narrowing occurring in the horizontal axis. The spinal cord is grossly distorted by bilateral compression from hypertrophied articular facets. There is also a separate osseous fragment associated with the distal margin of the right caudal aspect of the fourth cervical articular facet (white arrow), consistent with osteochondrosis.

(a) CT+C, TP

Figure 3.1.9 Cervical Spondylomyelopathy (Canine)   CT & MR

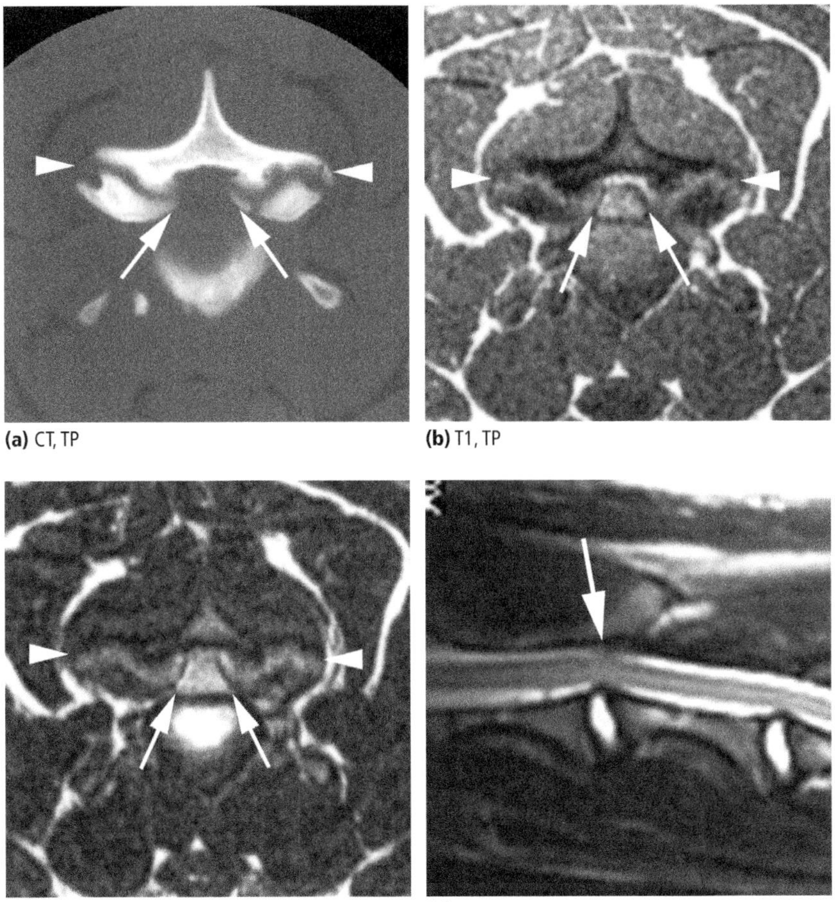

(a) CT, TP

(b) T1, TP

(c) T2, TP

(d) T2, SP

10mo MC Rhodesian Ridgeback with myelopathy neuroanatomically localized to C1–5. Transverse images are at the level of C2–3. Marked hypertrophy and remodeling of the C2 and C3 articular facets is seen on the CT image, associated with subchondral bone defects (**a**: arrowheads) and encroachment of new bone into the vertebral canal (**a**: arrows). Comparable MR images similarly document facet hypertrophy (**b**,**c**: arrowheads) and encroachment into the vertebral canal causing primarily lateral spinal cord compression (**b**,**c**: arrows). The sagittal plane image shows attenuation of the dorsal and ventral subarachnoid columns but no significant change in cord diameter in this plane (**d**: arrow). A hemilaminectomy was performed to relieve compression.

Figure 3.1.10 Cervical Spondylomyelopathy (Canine)

MR

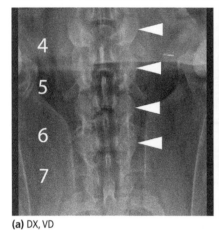

(a) DX, VD

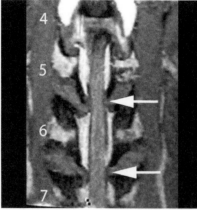

(b) T1, SPGR, DP

2y MC Saint Bernard with recent onset of ataxia. Images **c** and **d** are at the midbody of C5 and the C5–6 intervertebral disk space, respectively. Marked enlargement of all cervical articular facets is seen on a survey radiographic image (**a**: arrowheads). The spinal cord appears normal and is surrounded by a hyperintense halo of epidural fat in the midbody of the fifth cervical vertebra (**c**). Articular facet remodeling (**d**: arrowheads) results in encroachment of bone on the lateral aspects of the vertebral canal, causing narrowing of the canal diameter and spinal cord compression in the horizontal axis at multiple sites (**b,d**: arrows).

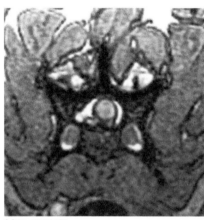

(c) T1, SPGR, TP

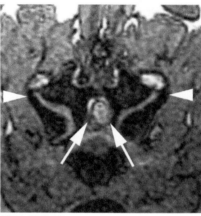

(d) T1, SPGR, TP

Figure 3.1.11 Sacral Osteochondrosis (Canine)

CT

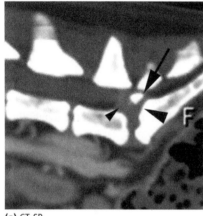

(a) CT, SP

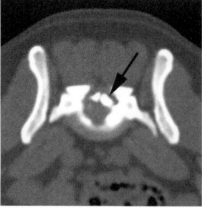

(b) CT, TP

4y FS Miniature Schnauzer with a diagnosis of portosystemic shunt and no neurologic abnormalities. A CT examination was performed for surgical planning. Multiple small but highly attenuating osseous fragments are seen within the vertebral canal at the level of the lumbosacral junction (**a,b**: arrow). There is an underlying defect of the craniodorsal margin of the first sacral body, manifest as an angular flattening of the bone (**a**: large arrowhead). The lumbosacral intervertebral disk space is widened, and a soft-tissue mass containing the fragmented bone protrudes into the vertebral canal, indicative of intervertebral disk herniation (**a**: small arrowhead) and possible dorsal longitudinal ligament hypertrophy.

Figure 3.1.12 Intradural Arachnoid Diverticulum (Canine)   CT

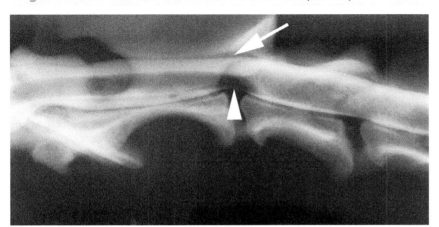

(a) DX+C, LAT

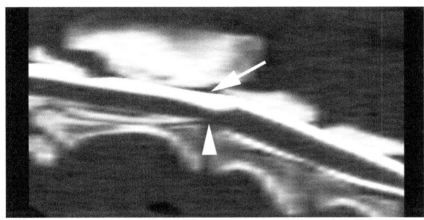

(b) CT+C, SP

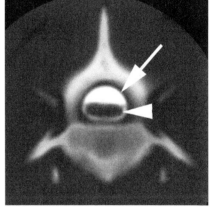

(c) CT+C, TP

10mo FS Boxer cross with myelopathy neuroanatomically localized to C1–5. Conventional and CT myelographic images show an elongated teardrop-shaped dilation of the dorsal subarachnoid space at the level of the second cervical vertebra (**a–c**: arrow), resulting in pronounced spinal cord compression (**a–c**: arrowhead). Contrast enhancement within this focal dilation is evidence that it communicates with the rest of the subarachnoid space. A large cyst-like structure was surgically removed following durotomy and was histologically confirmed to be an arachnoid diverticulum.

Figure 3.1.13 Spina Bifida Occulta (Canine)   CT

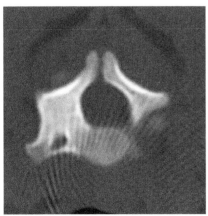

4mo M English Bulldog with cervical pain. The dorsum of the fourth cervical vertebra has not fused. The spiral pattern is an artifact due to a metallic marker within the endotracheal catheter (outside the field of view). Cerebrospinal fluid cytology revealed an inflammatory response, and *Bordetella* sp. was cultured from the sample. The dog responded to antibiotic therapy, and the spina bifida occulta was deemed an incidental finding.

(a) CT, TP

Figure 3.1.14 Myelomeningocele (Canine)

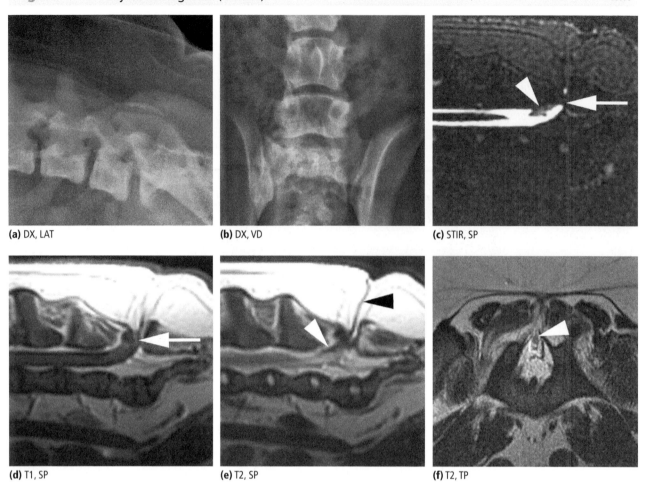

(a) DX, LAT

(b) DX, VD

(c) STIR, SP

(d) T1, SP

(e) T2, SP

(f) T2, TP

6mo M English Bulldog with urinary and fecal incontinence since birth. The spinous process and pedicle margins of the caudal-most lumbar vertebra are missing, consistent with spina bifida (a,b). There is dorsal deviation of the dural sac (c,d: arrow), which contains neural elements (c,e,f: white arrowhead), defining this as a myelomeningocele. A thin stalk (e: black arrowhead) extends from the dorsum of the myelomeningocele to the skin surface, which is dimpled. The hyperintensity in image c defining the volume of the meningocele does not extend dorsally within the stalk, and clinically this was determined to be a closed meningomyelocele.

Figure 3.1.15 Myelomeningocele (Canine)

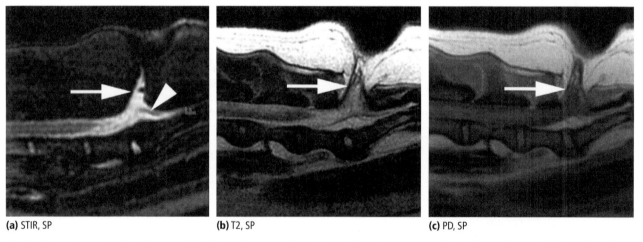

(a) STIR, SP

(b) T2, SP

(c) PD, SP

Adult mixed-breed dog with urinary and fecal incontinence and no tail tone. There is pronounced dorsal deviation and dilation of the dural sac at the level of the lumbosacral junction that extends nearly, but not to, the skin surface (a–c: arrow). Neural elements elevate dorsally into the basilar part of the meningocele (a: arrowhead), defining this as a closed myelomeningocele. Russell H Morgan Department of Radiology and Radiological Science, Johns Hopkins University, Baltimore, MD, 2014. Reproduced with permission from Johns Hopkins Uinversity.

Figure 3.1.16 Vascular Anomaly (Canine)   CT

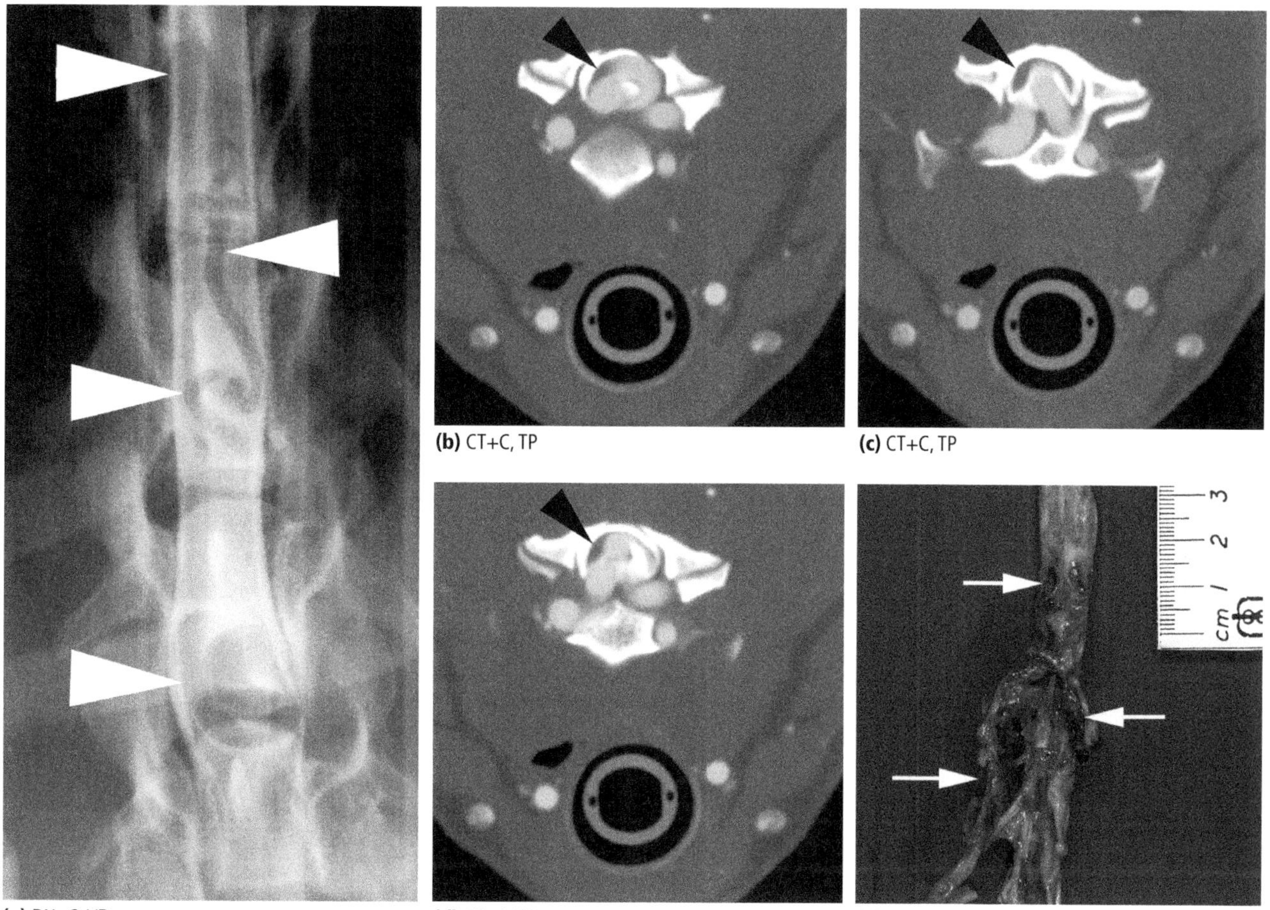

(a) DX+C, VD

(b) CT+C, TP

(c) CT+C, TP

(d) CT+C, TP

(e) GP, VENT

3y FS German Shorthair Pointer with a 1-month history of ataxia and collapsing. A complex tubular contrast-filling defect is seen within the cervical subarachnoid space on a conventional myelographic examination (a: arrowheads). A complex of dilated, coiled blood vessels is seen in the cervical region on a CT myelogram following intravenous contrast administration. Vessels within and external to the vertebral canal cause spinal cord displacement and compression (b–d: arrowhead). Selective angiography (not shown) revealed absence of the right subclavian artery, causing redirected arterial flow from the left vertebral artery through the vertebral canal to the right side. Postmortem examination documented the extent of vascular dilation and impingement on the cervical spinal cord (e: arrows). Westworth et al 2006.[51] Reproduced with permission from Wiley.

References

1. Tsou PM, Yau A, Hodgson AR. Embryogenesis and prenatal development of congenital vertebral anomalies and their classification. Clin Orthop Relat Res. 1980:211–231.

2. Westworth DR, Sturges BK. Congenital spinal malformations in small animals. Vet Clin North Am Small Anim Pract. 2010;40:951–981.

3. Grimme JD, Castillo M. Congenital anomalies of the spine. Neuroimaging Clin N Am. 2007;17:1–16.

4. Lappalainen AK, Salomaa R, Junnila J, Snellman M, Laitinen-Vapaavuori O. Alternative classification and screening protocol for transitional lumbosacral vertebra in German shepherd dogs. Acta Vet Scand. 2012;54:27.

5. Done SH, Drew RA, Robins GM, Lane JG. Hemivertebra in the dog: clinical and pathological observations. Vet Rec. 1975;96: 313–317.

6. Penderis J, Schwarz T, McConnell JF, Garosi LS, Thomson CE, Dennis R. Dysplasia of the caudal vertebral articular facets in four dogs: results of radiographic, myelographic and magnetic resonance imaging investigations. Vet Rec. 2005;156:601–605.

7. Dewey CW, Marino DJ, Loughin CA. Craniocervical junction abnormalities in dogs. N Z Vet J. 2013;61:202–211.

8. Cerda-Gonzalez S, Dewey CW. Congenital diseases of the craniocervical junction in the dog. Vet Clin North Am Small Anim Pract. 2010;40:121–141.

9. Cerda-Gonzalez S, Dewey CW, Scrivani PV, Kline KL. Imaging features of atlanto-occipital overlapping in dogs. Vet Radiol Ultrasound. 2009;50:264–268.

10. Middleton G, Hillmann DJ, Trichel J, Bragulla HH, Gaschen L. Magnetic resonance imaging of the ligamentous structures of the occipitoatlantoaxial region in the dog. Vet Radiol Ultrasound. 2012;53:545–551.

11. Parry AT, Upjohn MM, Schlegl K, Kneissl S, Lamb CR. Computed tomography variations in morphology of the canine atlas in dogs with and without atlantoaxial subluxation. Vet Radiol Ultrasound. 2010;51:596–600.

12. Thomas WB, Sorjonen DC, Simpson ST. Surgical management of atlantoaxial subluxation in 23 dogs. Vet Surg. 1991;20:409–412.

13. Driver CJ, Volk HA, Rusbridge C, Van Ham LM. An update on the pathogenesis of syringomyelia secondary to Chiari-like malformations in dogs. Vet J. 2013;198:551–559.

14. da Costa RC. Cervical spondylomyelopathy (wobbler syndrome) in dogs. Vet Clin North Am Small Anim Pract. 2010;40:881–913.

15. De Decker S, da Costa RC, Volk HA, Van Ham LM. Current insights and controversies in the pathogenesis and diagnosis of disc-associated cervical spondylomyelopathy in dogs. Vet Rec. 2012;171:531–537.

16. da Costa RC, Echandi RL, Beauchamp D. Computed tomography myelographic findings in dogs with cervical spondylomyelopathy. Vet Radiol Ultrasound. 2012;53:64–70.

17. De Decker S, Gielen IM, Duchateau L, Corzo-Menendez N, van Bree HJ, Kromhout K, et al. Intraobserver, interobserver, and intermethod agreement for results of myelography, computed tomography-myelography, and low-field magnetic resonance imaging in dogs with disk-associated wobbler syndrome. J Am Vet Med Assoc. 2011;238:1601–1608.

18. da Costa RC, Parent JM, Partlow G, Dobson H, Holmberg DL, Lamarre J. Morphologic and morphometric magnetic resonance imaging features of Doberman Pinschers with and without clinical signs of cervical spondylomyelopathy. Am J Vet Res. 2006;67:1601–1612.

19. De Decker S, Gielen IM, Duchateau L, Saunders JH, van Bree HJ, Polis I, et al. Magnetic resonance imaging vertebral canal and body ratios in Doberman Pinschers with and without disk-associated cervical spondylomyelopathy and clinically normal English Foxhounds. Am J Vet Res. 2011;72:1496–1504.

20. Eagleson JS, Diaz J, Platt SR, Kent M, Levine JM, Sharp NJ, et al. Cervical vertebral malformation–malarticulation syndrome in the Bernese mountain dog: clinical and magnetic resonance imaging features. J Small Anim Pract. 2009;50:186–193.

21. Gutierrez-Quintana R, Penderis J. MRI features of cervical articular process degenerative joint disease in Great Dane dogs with cervical spondylomyelopathy. Vet Radiol Ultrasound. 2012;53:304–311.

22. Penderis J, Dennis R. Use of traction during magnetic resonance imaging of caudal cervical spondylomyelopathy ("wobbler syndrome") in the dog. Vet Radiol Ultrasound. 2004;45:216–219.

23. Hanna FY. Lumbosacral osteochondrosis: radiological features and surgical management in 34 dogs. J Small Anim Pract. 2001;42:272–278.

24. Mathis KR, Havlicek M, Beck JB, Eaton-Wells RD, Park FM. Sacral osteochondrosis in two German Shepherd Dogs. Aust Vet J. 2009;87:249–252.

25. Snaps FR, Heimann M, Saunders J, Beths T, Balligand M, Breton L. Osteochondrosis of the sacral bone in a mastiff dog. Vet Rec. 1998;143:476–477.

26. Gendron K, Doherr MG, Gavin P, Lang J. Magnetic resonance imaging characterization of vertebral endplate changes in the dog. Vet Radiol Ultrasound. 2012;53:50–56.

27. Mauler DA, De Decker S, De Risio L, Volk HA, Dennis R, Gielen I, et al. Signalment, clinical presentation, and diagnostic findings in 122 dogs with spinal arachnoid diverticula. J Vet Intern Med. 2014;28:175–181.

28. Gnirs K, Ruel Y, Blot S, Begon D, Rault D, Delisle F, et al. Spinal subarachnoid cysts in 13 dogs. Vet Radiol Ultrasound. 2003;44:402–408.

29. Jurina K, Grevel V. Spinal arachnoid pseudocysts in 10 rottweilers. J Small Anim Pract. 2004;45:9–15.

30. Rylander H, Lipsitz D, Berry WL, Sturges BK, Vernau KM, Dickinson PJ, et al. Retrospective analysis of spinal arachnoid cysts in 14 dogs. J Vet Intern Med. 2002;16:690–696.

31. Skeen TM, Olby NJ, Munana KR, Sharp NJ. Spinal arachnoid cysts in 17 dogs. J Am Anim Hosp Assoc. 2003;39:271–282.

32. Confer AW, Ward BC. Spinal dysraphism: a congenital myelodysplasia in the Weimaraner. J Am Vet Med Assoc. 1972;160:1423–1426.

33. Engel HN, Draper DD. Comparative prenatal development of the spinal cord in normal and dysraphic dogs: embryonic stage. Am J Vet Res. 1982;43:1729–1734.

34. Osterhues A, Ali NS, Michels KB. The role of folic acid fortification in neural tube defects: a review. Crit Rev Food Sci Nutr. 2013;53:1180–1190.

35. Safra N, Bassuk AG, Ferguson PJ, Aguilar M, Coulson RL, Thomas N, et al. Genome-wide association mapping in dogs enables identification of the homeobox gene, NKX2-8, as a genetic component of neural tube defects in humans. PLoS Genet. 2013;9:e1003646.

36. Leipold HW, Huston K, Blauch B, Guffy MM. Congenital defects on the caudal vertebral column and spinal cord in Manx cats. J Am Vet Med Assoc. 1974;164:520–523.

37. Allett B, Broome MR, Hager D. MRI of a split cord malformation in a German shepherd dog. J Am Anim Hosp Assoc. 2012;48:344–351.

38. Mann GE, Stratton J. Dermoid sinus in the Rhodesian Ridgeback. J Small Anim Pract. 1966;7:631–642.

39. Colon JA, Maritato KC, Mauterer JV. Dermoid sinus and bone defects of the fifth thoracic vertebrae in a shih-tzu. J Small Anim Pract. 2007;48:180.

40. Cornegliani L, Jommi E, Vercelli A. Dermoid sinus in a golden retriever. J Small Anim Pract. 2001;42:514–516.

41. Kiviranta AM, Lappalainen AK, Hagner K, Jokinen T. Dermoid sinus and spina bifida in three dogs and a cat. J Small Anim Pract. 2011;52:319–324.

42. Lambrechts N. Dermoid sinus in a crossbred Rhodesian ridgeback dog involving the second cervical vertebra. J S Afr Vet Assoc. 1996;67:155–157.

43. Motta L, Skerritt G, Denk D, Leeming G, Saulnier F. Dermoid sinus type IV associated with spina bifida in a young Victorian bulldog. Vet Rec. 2012;170:127.

44. Davies ES, Fransson BA, Gavin PR. A confusing magnetic resonance imaging observation complicating surgery for a dermoid cyst in a Rhodesian Ridgeback. Vet Radiol Ultrasound. 2004;45:307–309.

45. Rahal S, Mortari AC, Yamashita S, Filho MM, Hatschbac E, Sequeira JL. Magnetic resonance imaging in the diagnosis of type 1 dermoid sinus in two Rhodesian ridgeback dogs. Can Vet J. 2008;49:871–876.

46. Alexander K, Huneault L, Foster R, d'Anjou MA. Magnetic resonance imaging and marsupialization of a hemorrhagic intramedullary vascular anomaly in the cervical portion of the spinal cord of a dog. J Am Vet Med Assoc. 2008;232:399–404.

47. Cordy DR. Vascular malformations and hemangiomas of the canine spinal cord. Vet Pathol. 1979;16:275–282.

48. Hayashida E, Ochiai K, Kadosawa T, Kimura T, Umemura T. Arteriovenous malformation of the cervical spinal cord in a dog. J Comp Pathol. 1999;121:71–76.

49. MacKillop E, Olby NJ, Linder KE, Brown TT. Intramedullary cavernous malformation of the spinal cord in two dogs. Vet Pathol. 2007;44:528–532.

50. Sanders SG, Bagley RS, Gavin PR, Konzik RL, Cantor GH. Surgical treatment of an intramedullary spinal cord hamartoma in a dog. J Am Vet Med Assoc. 2002;221:659–661, 643–654.

51. Westworth DR, Vernau KM, Cullen SP, Long CD, Van Halbach V, LeCouteur RA. Vascular anomaly causing subclavian steal and cervical myelopathy in a dog: diagnosis and endovascular management. Vet Radiol Ultrasound. 2006;47:265–269.

3.2

Traumatic and vascular disorders

Vertebral column trauma

Fracture/luxation

Fractures and luxations vary widely in location and appearance but generally occur as a result of compressive, rotational, translational, hyperflexion, or hyperextension forces caused by blunt or penetrating trauma.[1] Because vertebral column injuries are often unstable, care should be taken to minimize patient movement even when image quality is compromised. Patients are often placed on a backboard and maintained in lateral recumbency for imaging studies. The most significant clinical questions to address in patients with vertebral column trauma are whether spinal cord compression is present and whether the injury is stable or unstable.[2,3] Although survey radiography is an excellent screening tool, sensitivity is only 72% for fracture detection and 77.5% for subluxation detection as compared to CT.[4] Imaging studies should be viewed carefully and completely since a significant minority of patients with vertebral fracture/luxation disorders sustain multiple injuries.

Fractures and luxations are both clearly delineated on CT images, and multiplanar or 3D reformatting is often useful to better characterize complex injuries. CT myelography can be employed to define the presence and extent of spinal cord compression due to fracture displacement or hemorrhage. Although MRI is superior to CT for detecting spinal cord and other soft tissue injury, it is less sensitive and specific for detecting and characterizing vertebral fractures or subluxations. Gradient echo volume-acquisition sequences can be used to better delineate bone (signal void) from surrounding soft tissues, and thin-collimation and reformatted images can aid fracture diagnosis.[5]

It can be clinically useful to characterize thoracolumbar vertebral fractures using a variation of the three-column model used in people.[6] In this scheme, the dorsal column includes the lamina, pedicles, and articular facets; the middle column includes the dorsal half of the vertebral body; and the disk and the ventral column includes the ventral half of the vertebral body (Figure 3.2.1). In people, middle column trauma is more likely to be associated with instability and neurologic deficits.[6]

Cervical vertebral fracture/luxation

Fractures occur less frequently in the cervical region than in other parts of the vertebral column in dogs and cats. When present, they most often involve the atlas (25%) or axis (52%), and multiple cervical vertebrae are frequently affected.[7-10] Most cervical vertebral fractures are caused by either automobile collision or bite injury, and almost half of these patients have other clinically significant injuries.[9]

Occipital condylar fractures and luxations

Occipital condylar fracture or atlanto-occipital luxation can occasionally occur as the result of high-impact trauma and is associated with significant neurologic deficits (Figure 3.2.2).[11]

Atlantal (C1) fractures

Atlantal trauma caused by compression forces generally results in multiple fractures through the body and arch and these are sometimes referred to as burst fractures

Atlas of Small Animal CT and MRI, First Edition. Erik R. Wisner and Allison L. Zwingenberger.
© 2015 John Wiley & Sons, Inc. Published 2015 by John Wiley & Sons, Inc.

because of the peripheral displacement of fracture fragments (Figure 3.2.3). Atlantal wing fractures are often mildly displaced as the result of traction forces from muscle attachments (Figure 3.2.4).

Axial (C2) fractures

Odontoid process (dens) fractures are usually caused by cervical hyperflexion/hyperextension and atlantoaxial malformations with pre-existing instability predisposed to the injury. Fractures of the odontoid process are easily detected on both CT and MR images because the cranial fracture fragment is often displaced (Figures 3.2.5, 3.2.6). The MR appearance of the ligaments of the normal canine occipitoatlantoaxial region has been described, and ligaments were hypointense on all sequences.[12] Close inspection of the integrity of the ligaments may be useful in determining the stability of traumatic lesions in this region.

Fractures of the axial body, arch, and spinous process also occur, with the integrity of atlantoaxial stability dependent on the specific nature of the fracture (Figure 3.2.7). C2 fractures are referred to as burst fractures when comminuted and the result of compressive forces.

Caudal cervical (C3–C7) vertebral fractures and luxations

Fractures and luxations of the third through seventh cervical vertebrae are less common than C1 and C2 injuries and are caused more often by bite injury than motor vehicle trauma (Figures 3.2.8).[9]

Thoracolumbar fracture/luxation

Between 49% and 58% of vertebral fracture/luxations involve the T3–L3 region in dogs and cats, and 24–38% involve the L4–L7 region. Most fractures in this region are associated with clinically significant neurologic deficits.[8,13] Motor vehicle trauma has been reported as the most common cause for thoracolumbar fracture/luxation in dogs, whereas cats are just as likely to sustain injuries from a fall.[13] Although there are some differences between cats and dogs, vertebral luxation or fracture/luxation has been reported to be the most common injury for both, followed by wedge compression fractures, transverse fractures, and subluxation and hyperextension injuries. Multiple compartments are involved in the majority of injuries; endplate involvement is seen in approximately a third, and rotational displacement and intervertebral space involvement is present in more than half.[13] Fracture/luxation also occurs with greater frequency at junctions between mobile and less mobile regions of the vertebral column (Figures 3.2.9, 3.2.10, 3.2.11, 3.2.12, 3.2.13, 3.2.14).[14]

Sacral trauma

A sacral fracture classification system has been proposed, which classifies fractures as alar, foraminal, transverse, avulsion, and comminuted, with transverse fractures making up about half of all sacral fractures in both dogs and cats.[15] A simpler scheme distinguishes abaxial fractures, those that occur lateral to the sacral foramina, from axial fractures.[16] Fractures that involve the sacral foramina and canal are more likely to result in clinically significant neurologic deficits. A majority of patients with sacral fractures also have complex orthopedic injuries, including sacroiliac luxation and other pelvic fractures (Figures 3.2.15, 3.2.16).[15,16]

Traumatic intervertebral disk extrusion

Intervertebral disk extrusion can occur as the direct result of trauma and can be either compressive or noncompressive. Both normal disks and those with nuclear degeneration are at risk, but degenerate disks more often lead to spinal cord compression. Normal nucleus pulposis is composed predominantly of water, and when herniated through the annulus, fibrosis can dissipate into the epidural fat or through the dura mater and into the spinal cord. This can result in an intrinsic spinal cord lesion with no overt evidence of compression. Because degenerate nucleus pulposis contains more solid mass, traumatic extrusion is more likely to result in spinal cord compression.[17-19] CT features of traumatic intervertebral disk extrusion include disk space narrowing with or without extradural spinal cord compression. The latter feature is best seen using CT myelography. The MR features of traumatic intervertebral disk extrusion in dogs include reduced volume and T2 signal intensity of the affected disk and increased spinal cord T2 intensity at the level of disk extrusion. Extrusion of degenerate disk material is more likely to result in an extradural compressive mass (Figure 3.2.17).[17-19]

Spinal cord trauma

Contusion/hemorrhage

Spinal cord trauma is usually but not always accompanied by overt vertebral column trauma. Neurologic deficits range from clinically silent to complete spinal cord transection. In addition to the primary spinal cord injury that results directly from trauma, secondary injury occurs from vascular damage, local cytotoxic biochemical responses to injury, and inflammatory response, the combination of which can lead to progressive disease.[20] Postmortem examination of spinal cords of dogs and cats that sustained traumatic injury revealed thoracolumbar necrosis that correlated with the degree of static compression from vertebral column injury.[21] Cervical cord injury often included central hemorrhagic necrosis that was more consistent with transient impact trauma than static cord compression.

MR features of spinal cord contusion include focal to regional increased T2 intensity with mild to no enhancement following contrast administration (Figure 3.2.18). T2* sequences reveal parenchymal susceptibility effects when there is a hemorrhagic component. Syringohydromyelia is often a late sequela to spinal cord trauma and appears as a focal to regional and central to eccentric T2 hyperintensity.

Vascular disorders

Hematomyelia

Occasionally frank hematomyelia will be seen as a sequela to trauma, primary vascular disease, or an underlying bleeding diathesis. MR features are similar to those of spinal cord contusion; however, susceptibility effects may be a predominant sign (Figure 3.2.19).

Fibrocartilagenous embolism

Early reports indicated that fibrocartilaginous embolism (FCE) occurs primarily in middle-aged to older, large- and giant-breed dogs; however, a more recent review in which diagnosis was based on clinical signs and MR imaging findings suggests that small and medium-sized dogs are also commonly affected.[22–24] The disorder has also been reported in cats.[25] The clinical presentation is often a peracute onset of symmetrical or asymmetrical motor dysfunction immediately following exercise or minor trauma, with lower motor neuron

signs also present in some patients. Initial clinical signs can include transient pain and can be progressive for the first 2 hours but are often nonprogressive thereafter. The cervicothoracic (C5–T2) and lumbosacral (L3–S3) regions appear to be predisposed. Pathology in histologically confirmed patients includes spinal cord infarction and hemorrhage with cartilaginous emboli in meningeal or spinal vessels. In some patients, extensive myelomalacia may also be present, but pathology is likely to be more severe in those patients that were euthanized and confirmed as having FCE.[22–24] A poorer prognosis is seen in patients with involvement of the intumescences, symmetrical neurological signs, and decreased deep pain sensation.[23] A recent review of dogs with ischemic myelopathy found that a combination of lesion length greater than twice a vertebral length and cross-sectional involvement of greater than 67% had a positive correlation with an unsuccessful outcome.[26] Recovery rates for FCE are unclear since patients who do respond are not definitively diagnosed. However, a majority of patients with stable disease seem to partially or fully recover neurologic function.[22]

CT imaging features can be limited to a noncompressive focal increase in spinal cord diameter, indicative of an intrinsic lesion (Figure 3.2.20). MR features include focal T1 iso- to hypointensity and T2 hyperintensity within the affected spinal cord segments. Lesions preferentially affect gray matter and can be either symmetrical or asymmetrical. Spinal cord diameter can also appear locally enlarged but without compression. Intervertebral disk T2 signal intensity at the level of the spinal cord lesion is often less than that of adjacent disks (Figures 3.2.21, 3.2.22).[24]

Figure 3.2.1   Three Column Classification Model for Thoracolumbar Vertebral Trauma (Canine)

Cranial view of a thoracic vertebra. The dorsal column (D) includes lamina, pedicles, and articular facets. The middle column (M) includes the dorsal half of the vertebral body and the intervertebral disk. The ventral column (V) includes the ventral half of the vertebral body.

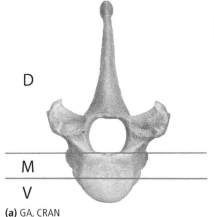

(a) GA, CRAN

Figure 3.2.2   Occipitoatlantal Luxation (Canine)

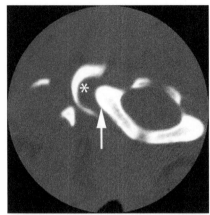

(a) CT, TP

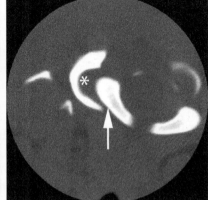

(b) CT, TP

1y FS Keeshond cross with acute cervical injury after being struck by an automobile earlier in the day. A CT examination was performed with the dog on a backboard in lateral recumbency. Images **a–c** were acquired at the level of the occipitoatlantal joint and are ordered from cranial to caudal. The right occipital condyle (**a–d**: arrow) is axially subluxated in relation to the cranial articular fovea of C1 (**a–c**: asterisk). The left occipital condyle is ventrally luxated (**c,d**: arrowhead). Closed reduction of the luxation was successfully performed using fluoroscopic guidance.

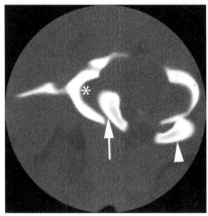

(c) CT, TP

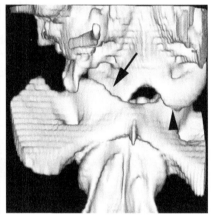

(d) CT, 3D, VENT

Figure 3.2.3 Chronic C1 Burst Fracture (Canine) CT & MR

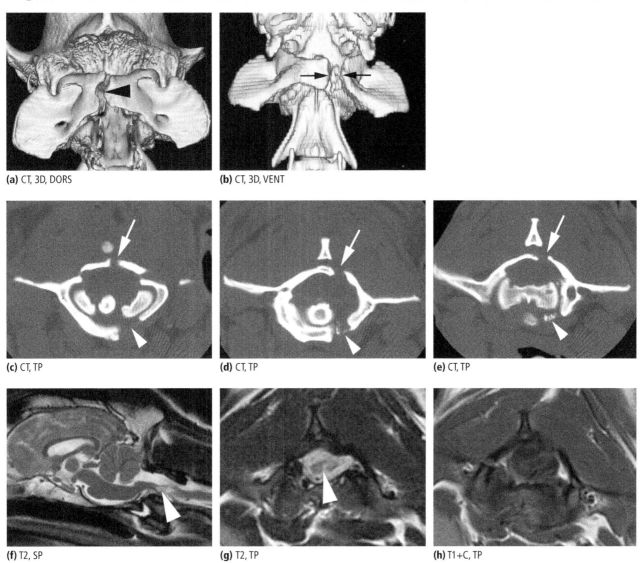

(a) CT, 3D, DORS

(b) CT, 3D, VENT

(c) CT, TP

(d) CT, TP

(e) CT, TP

(f) T2, SP

(g) T2, TP

(h) T1+C, TP

8y MC Chow cross with a 1-year history of progressive neurologic deficits and behavior change. The dog was struck by an automobile as a puppy and recovered but had unspecified spinal problems since that time. Dorsal (**a**) and ventral view 3D renderings of CT data reveal multiple smoothly margined displaced fractures of the dorsal arch (**a**: arrowhead) and body (**b**: arrows). Transverse CT images of C1 ordered from cranial to caudal also show the dorsal arch (**c–e**: arrowhead) and body (**c–e**: arrow) fractures. Sagittal (**f**) and transverse MR images (**g,h**) acquired at approximately the same level as (**d**) reveal marked abnormality of the shape of the vertebral canal and pronounced atrophy of the cervical spinal cord at the level of C1 (**f,g**: arrowhead), which are the sequelae of a C1 fracture that presumably occurred 7 years previously.

Figure 3.2.4   C1 Wing Fracture (Feline)   CT

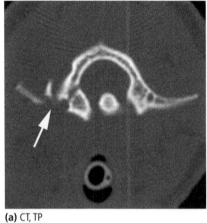

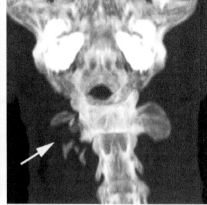

15y Norwegian Forest Cat attacked by a dog 5 days previously. The cat is now nonambulatory with signs of head trauma and a fractured mandible. There is a comminuted fracture of the right wing of the atlas with moderate displacement of fracture fragments (**a,b**: arrow). The atlas fracture was managed conservatively, and the cat had returned to normal neurologic status by 3 months after the initial trauma.

(a) CT, TP

(b) CT, MIP, DV

Figure 3.2.5   Odontoid Process Fracture (Canine)   CT

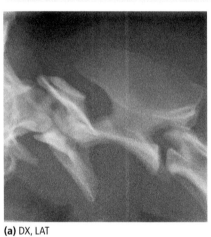

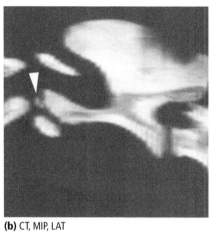

(a) DX, LAT

(b) CT, MIP, LAT

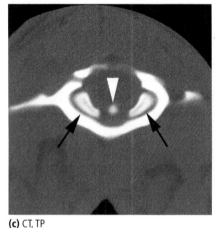

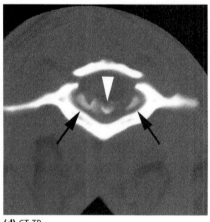

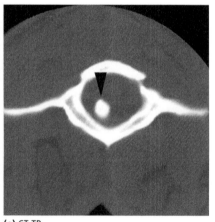

(c) CT, TP

(d) CT, TP

(e) CT, TP

Same dog as in Figure 3.2.2. A second CT study was acquired following reduction of the occipitoatlantal luxation. An apical fracture of the odontoid process is not seen on survey radiographs (**a**) but is easily detected on the CT examination (**b**: arrowhead). Transverse images through C1 ordered from cranial to caudal show the apical fracture fragment positioned on midline (**c,d**: white arrowhead) with the basilar part of the dens positioned to the left of midline (**e**: black arrowhead), indicative of fracture displacement and atlantoaxial instability. The occipitoatlantal luxation has been reduced (**c,d**: arrows). The odontoid process fracture was managed conservatively.

Figure 3.2.6   C2 Odontoid Process Fracture (Feline)   MR

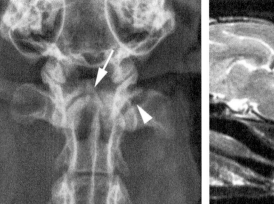

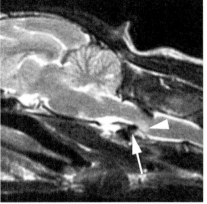

(a) DX, VD

(b) T2, SP

4y FS Bengal with generalized ataxia following trauma of unknown cause. A displaced odontoid process fracture (**a**: arrow) and a mildly displaced left C1 wing fracture (**a**: arrowhead) are seen on survey radiographs. The odontoid process fracture is also evident on MR images (**b–d**: arrow). Instability of the atlantoaxial joint results in spinal cord compression of the cranial cervical spinal cord, best seen on the sagittal images (**b,d**). There is an associated focal region of T2 hyperintensity within the ventral aspect of the spinal cord immediately dorsal to the fractured odontoid process and best seen on the T2 image (**b**: arrowhead).

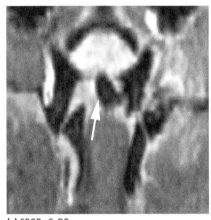

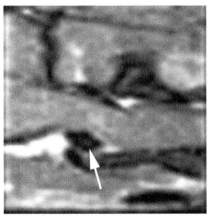

(c) SPGR+C, DP

(d) SPGR+C, SP

Figure 3.2.7 C2 Body Fracture (Canine)

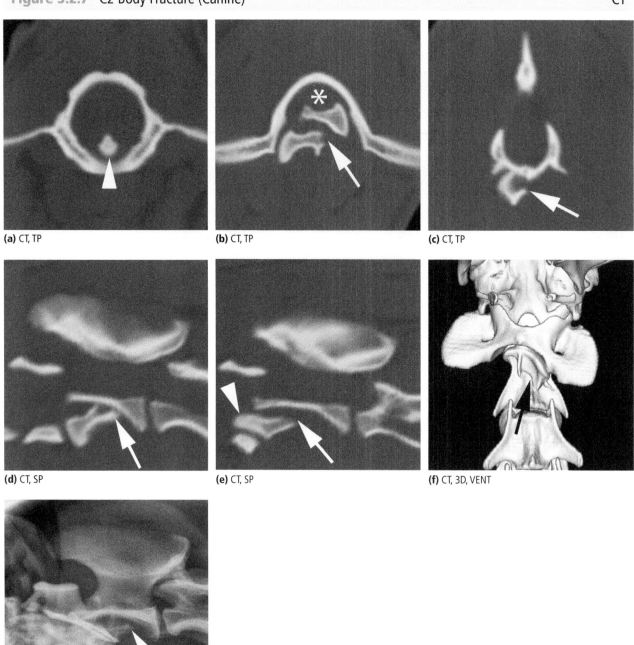

(a) CT, TP

(b) CT, TP

(c) CT, TP

(d) CT, SP

(e) CT, SP

(f) CT, 3D, VENT

(g) DX, LAT

2y FS Australian Shepherd with cervical pain but no neurologic deficits after running into a fence 9 days previously. Images **a–c** are ordered from cranial to caudal at the level of the odontoid process (**a**: arrowhead), cranial C2, and the midbody of C2. Image **d** is reformatted on sagittal midline, and image **e** is a parasagittal image that includes the odontoid process (**e**: arrowhead). A displaced, oblique fracture of the body of the axis is evident (**b–f**: arrow). Fracture fragment displacement relative to the atlas results in a marked decrease in vertebral canal diameter (**b**: asterisk). The fracture is detected on a radiographic image (**g**: arrowhead), but the level of vertebral canal compromise cannot be assessed as accurately as with CT. Given the time interval since the injury and the lack of neurologic signs, the patient was managed conservatively and was lost to follow-up.

Figure 3.2.8 Cervical Vertebral Subluxation with Articular Facet Fracture (Canine)   CT & MR

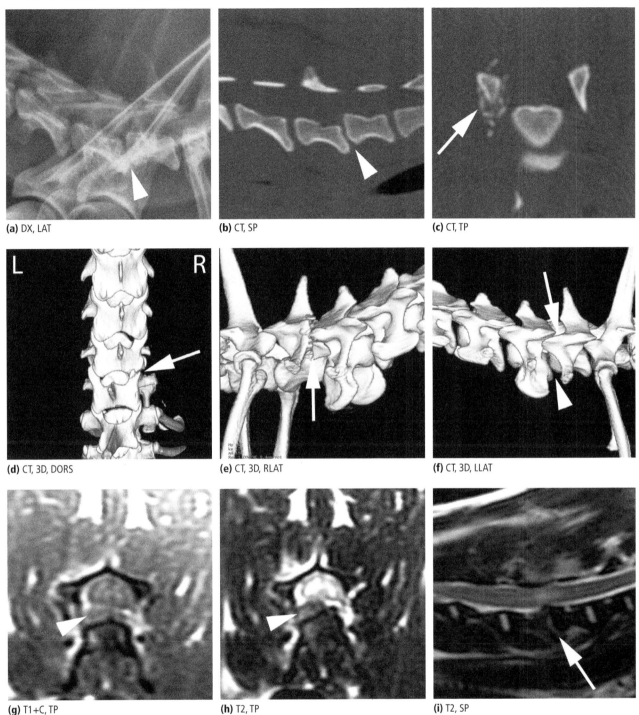

(a) DX, LAT

(b) CT, SP

(c) CT, TP

(d) CT, 3D, DORS

(e) CT, 3D, RLAT

(f) CT, 3D, LLAT

(g) T1+C, TP

(h) T2, TP

(i) T2, SP

5y F Terrier cross bitten in the cervical region by a larger dog earlier in the day. Currently has neurologic deficits neuroanatomically localized to C6–T2. Survey radiographs reveal dorsal subluxation of C7 relative to C6 and narrowing of the C6–7 intervertebral disk space (**a**: arrowhead). Similar findings are also seen on sagittal and 3D reformatted CT images (**b,f**: arrowhead). In addition, there is a highly comminuted and displaced fracture of the right cranial articular process of C7 (**c–e**: arrow). The left articular process is normal by comparison (**f**: arrow). On MR images, the C6–7 intervertebral disk space is reduced in width and T2 signal intensity (**i**: arrow), and extruded disk material is present in the right ventral vertebral canal (**g,h**: arrowhead). There is evidence of spinal cord compression (**g–i**) and spinal cord T2 hyperintensity at the level of C6–7 (**h,i**), indicative of an intrinsic component to the injury. Disk material was removed from the canal, and the subluxation was reduced and stabilized surgically.

Figure 3.2.9 T5 Salter-Harris Fracture (Canine)   CT

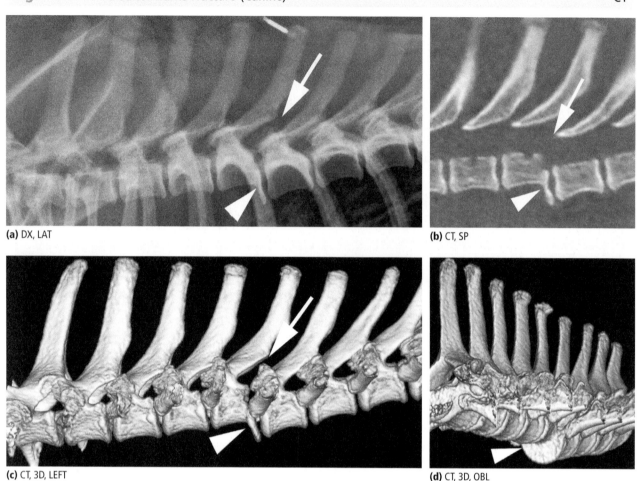

(a) DX, LAT

(b) CT, SP

(c) CT, 3D, LEFT

(d) CT, 3D, OBL

7mo FS Poodle cross with pain and T3–L3 neurologic deficits immediately after being hit with a pick-axe. A lateral thoracic spinal radiograph shows a Salter–Harris type 1 fracture of the caudal body physis of T5, with concurrent ventral displacement of T6 relative to T5 (**a**: arrowhead). These findings are seen on sagittal plane and 3D reformatted CT images (**b–d**: arrowheads). The T5–6 vertebral articulations are subluxated (**a,c**: arrow), and the vertebral canal diameter is reduced, indirectly indicative of spinal cord compression (**b**: arrow). The injury was reduced and stabilized surgically.

Figure 3.2.10 T12 Fracture and T10–T11 Subluxation (Canine)   CT

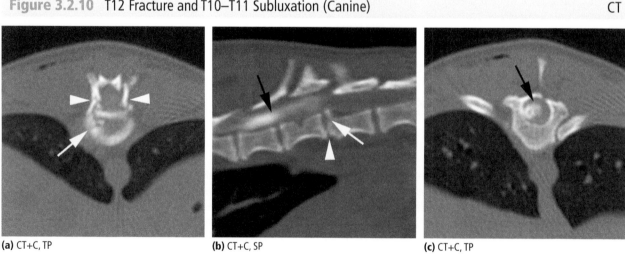

(a) CT+C, TP

(b) CT+C, SP

(c) CT+C, TP

1y M Chihuahua bitten by another dog 6 days previously. Now has neurologic deficits with neuroanatomical localization to T3–L3. A CT myelogram was performed. Comminuted fractures of the pedicles (**a**: arrowheads) and the cranial body (**a,b**: white arrow) of the 11th thoracic vertebra are present. T10–T11 intervertebral disk space narrowing and subluxation are also seen (**b**: arrowhead). Contrast medium administered intrathecally has absorbed into the spinal cord parenchyma, indicative of myelomalacia (**b,c**: black arrow). Spinal cord compression is also evident (**a,b**).

Figure 3.2.11   L3 Vertebral Compression Fracture (Canine)   CT

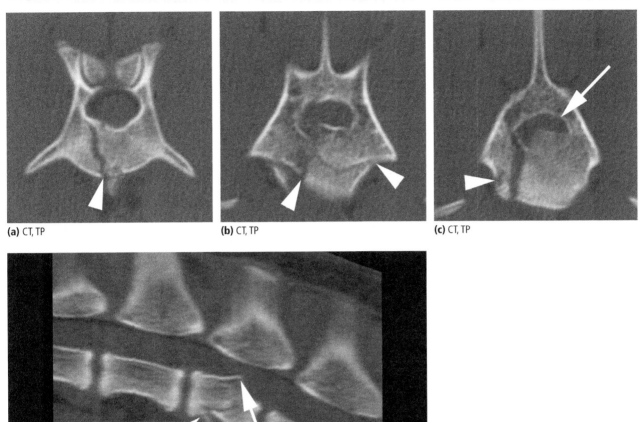

(a) CT, TP

(b) CT, TP

(c) CT, TP

(d) CT, SP

1y MC Labrador Retriever struck by an automobile earlier in the day. Currently has a nearly complete transverse myelopathy neuroanatomically localized to T3–L3. Images **a–c** are at the level of L3 and are ordered from cranial to caudal. There is a comminuted compression fracture of L3 (**a–d**: arrowheads) that results in marked reduction of the vertebral canal diameter (**c**: arrow). A sharp fracture margin from one of the larger fragments is displaced dorsally into the canal and impinges on the ventral margin of the spinal cord (**d**: arrow). This is likely contributing to the functional spinal cord transection. The injury was reduced and stabilized surgically, but there was minimal return of neurologic function over 6 months of rehabilitation.

Figure 3.2.12 L3 Lamina Depression Fracture (Feline)   CT & MR

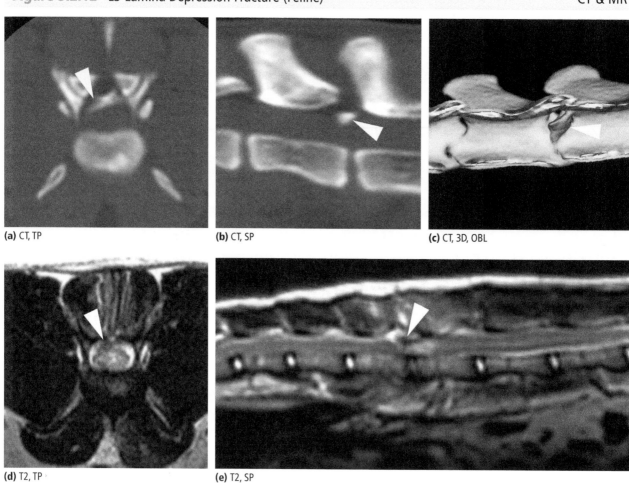

(a) CT, TP

(b) CT, SP

(c) CT, 3D, OBL

(d) T2, TP

(e) T2, SP

8y FS Domestic Shorthair bitten by a dog 2 days previously. Currently has a nonambulatory T3–L3 myelopathy. On CT images, a depression fracture arising from the cranial margin of the L3 lamina (**a,b**: arrowhead) impinges on the dorsal margin of the spinal cord. A ventral oblique 3D rendering with the vertebral bodies removed further illustrates the displacement of the fracture fragment into the canal (**c**: arrowhead). The fracture fragment is T2 hypointense on MR images (**d,e**: arrowhead) and impinges on the spinal cord, causing deformation and compression. There is also marked increase in spinal cord T2 signal intensity at this level due to intrinsic edema and hemorrhage. The T2 signal intensity of the L3–4 intervertebral disk is also reduced, suggesting possible traumatic intervertebral disk extrusion. Spinal cord compression was relieved with a hemilaminectomy, and the L3–4 vertebral column was stabilized, resulting in gradual return of neurologic function.

Figure 3.2.13   L6–L7 Luxation (Canine)   CT

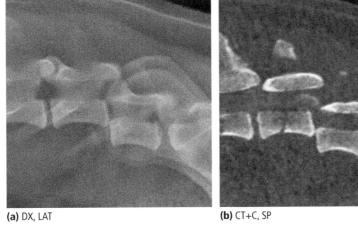
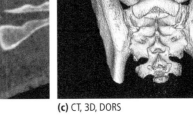

(a) DX, LAT

(b) CT+C, SP

(c) CT, 3D, DORS

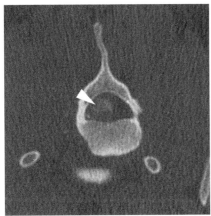
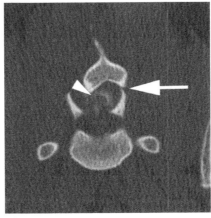
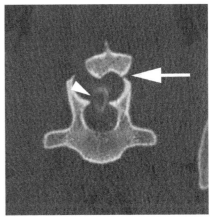

(d) CT+C, TP

(e) CT+C, TP

(f) CT+C, TP

4y FS Springer Spaniel with an L6–caudal neuropathy after being struck by an automobile earlier in the day. A lateral spinal radiograph shows an L6–L7 ventral luxation (**a**). A CT myelogram also shows the ventral subluxation and spinal cord compression (**b**). The vertical lucent line in the body of C6 in image **b** represents a normal vascular canal. A 3D rendering also reveals right lateral subluxation of L7 in relation to L6 (**c**: arrow) and a minimally displaced fracture of the right L6 transverse process (**c**: arrowhead). Images **d–f** are ordered from cranial to caudal, with image **d** at the level of caudal C6 and images **e** and **f** at the level of cranial L7. Ventral and right-sided luxation of the L7 cranial articular facets is seen relative to the caudal articular facets of L6 (**e**,**f**: arrow). Dorsal migration of the cauda equina between the L7 cranial articular facets (**d–f**: arrowhead) has limited compression of the lateral margins of the cauda equina by the ventral articular margins of the L7 facets. The luxation was reduced and stabilized surgically, and neurologic status progressively improved during the perioperative period.

Figure 3.2.14 High-Velocity Penetrating Injury (Canine)   CT

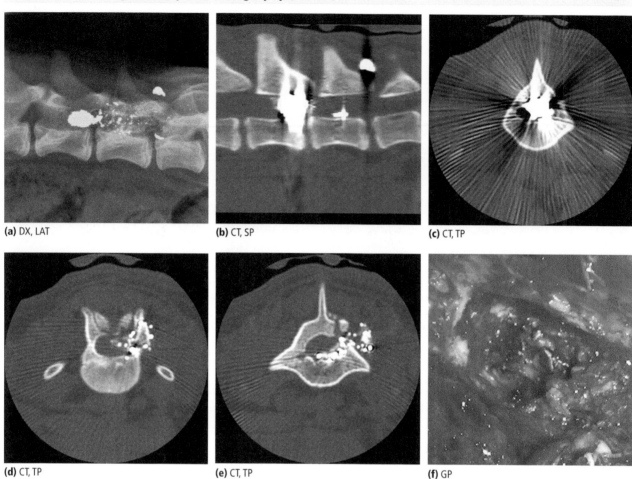

(a) DX, LAT   **(b)** CT, SP   **(c)** CT, TP

(d) CT, TP   **(e)** CT, TP   **(f)** GP

2y MC Beagle with a gunshot injury of the lumbar spine. Neurologic signs were consistent with an L4–caudal functional spinal cord transection. Survey radiographs reveal a highly fragmented lead bullet distributed primarily within and around the fourth and fifth lumbar vertebrae (**a**). This finding is reproduced on a sagittal reformatted CT image of the same anatomic site (**b**). A transverse image through mid L4 documents that a large volume of metal is located centrally within the vertebral canal (**c**). Images acquired at the level of cranial L5 (**d**) and mid L5 (**e**) show the distribution of highly fragmented metal within the ventral spinal canal and adjacent to the left pedicle, which is fractured. Multiple metallic fragments are seen in the surgical site following hemilaminectomy (**f**). A large lead fragment embedded in the spinal cord was removed surgically, but the dog suffered a permanent functional spinal cord transection at this level.

Figure 3.2.15   Sacral Fracture and Sacroiliac Luxation (Canine)   CT

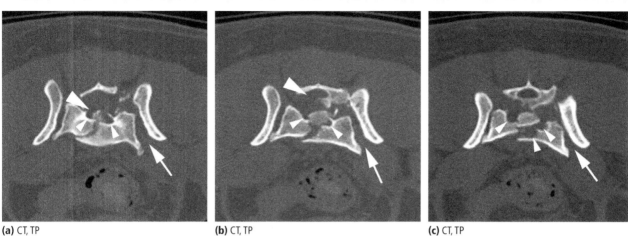

(a) CT, TP   **(b)** CT, TP   **(c)** CT, TP

4y FS Terrier struck by an automobile 1 day previously. The dog currently has left pelvic limb plegia and no deep pain perception, indicative of left sciatic neuropathy. CT images of the sacrum and sacroiliac joints are ordered from cranial to caudal. There is a comminuted fracture of the sacrum with displacement of major fragments (**a–c**). The fracture disrupts the ventral margin of the vertebral canal (**a,b**: large arrowhead), and fracture fissures also involve the dorsal and pelvic sacral foramina (**a–c**: small arrowheads). A mildly displaced left sacroiliac luxation is also evident (**a–c**: arrow). Additional fractures involving the ischia and pubis are not shown. Injuries were managed medically because of the degree of sacral fracture comminution. The dog partially recovered left sacral nerve function.

Figure 3.2.16   Sacroiliac Luxation (Feline)   CT

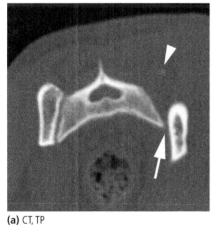
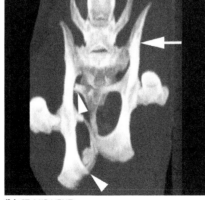
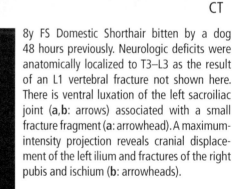

8y FS Domestic Shorthair bitten by a dog 48 hours previously. Neurologic deficits were anatomically localized to T3–L3 as the result of an L1 vertebral fracture not shown here. There is ventral luxation of the left sacroiliac joint (**a,b**: arrows) associated with a small fracture fragment (**a**: arrowhead). A maximum-intensity projection reveals cranial displacement of the left ilium and fractures of the right pubis and ischium (**b**: arrowheads).

(a) CT, TP   **(b)** CT, MIP, VENT

Figure 3.2.17 Presumptive Traumatic Intervertebral Disk Extrusion. (Canine)   CT & MR

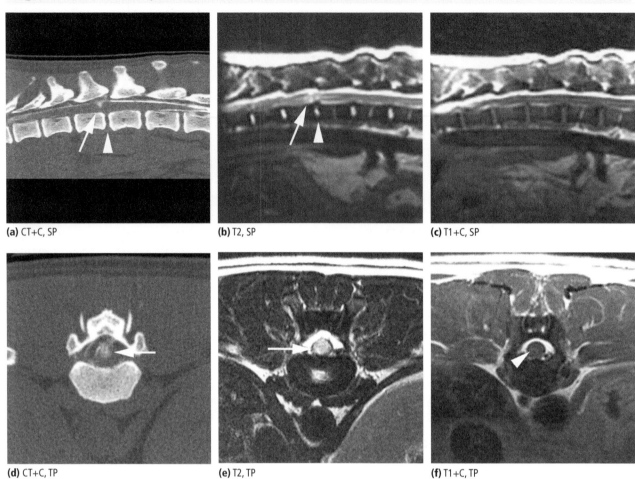

(a) CT+C, SP   **(b)** T2, SP   **(c)** T1+C, SP

(d) CT+C, TP   **(e)** T2, TP   **(f)** T1+C, TP

3y FS Labrador Retriever with acute-onset paraplegia during exercise. There is evidence of noncompressive increased spinal cord diameter and parenchymal uptake of intrathecally administered contrast medium at the level of T13–L1 on a CT myelogram (**a,d:** arrow), indicative of an intrinsic lesion. The T13–L1 intervertebral disk width is also slightly narrower than those of the adjacent disk spaces (**a:** arrowhead). There is T2 hyperintensity of the spinal cord at the same level on MR images (**b,e:** arrow), but the cord minimally contrast enhances (**f:** arrowhead), and the lesion is not compressive. The T13–L1 intervertebral disk intensity is moderately less than that of adjacent disks (**b:** arrowhead). There was no evidence of solid disk material within the spinal canal on any of the images. The dog partially recovered neurologic function with medical management.

Figure 3.2.18   Spinal Cord Contusion (Canine)   MR

(a) T2, SP

(b) T1, SP

(c) T1+C, SP

(d) T2, TP

(e) T1, TP

(f) T1+C, TP

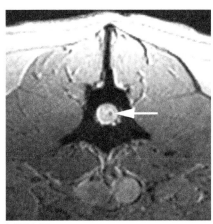

(g) T2*, TP

4y MC Border Collie stepped on by a bull 1 day previously, resulting in injuries to the lumbar spine and abdomen. Current neurologic deficits are referable to an L3–L5 myelopathy. Spinal radiographs were unremarkable. There is moderate diffuse spinal cord T2 hyperintensity centered at the level of L3 and L4 (**a,d**: arrowheads) indicative of an intrinsic lesion. The spinal cord mildly and diffusely enhances following contrast administration (**c,f**: arrowheads). A T2* sequence reveals pinpoint susceptibility artifacts within the spinal cord indicative of multifocal hemorrhage (**g**: arrow).

Figure 3.2.19 Hematomyelia (Canine)

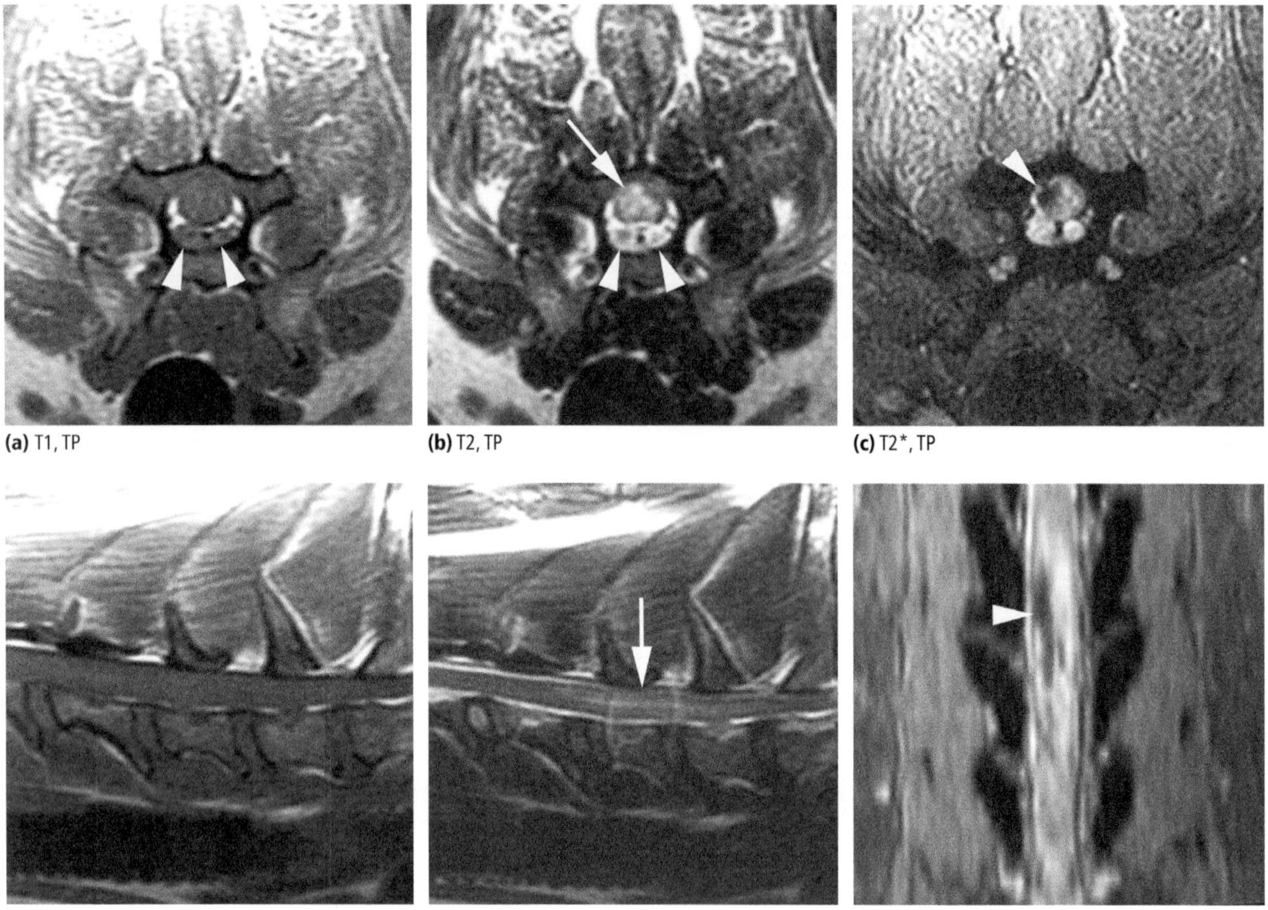

(a) T1, TP

(b) T2, TP

(c) T2*, TP

(d) T1, SP

(e) T2, SP

(f) T2*, DP

12y FS Pit Bull Terrier with acute-onset tetraparesis. The owners have administered aspirin twice weekly for chronic osteoarthrosis. There is T2 hyperintensity of the spinal cord parenchyma and focal central canal dilation centered on C5 (**b,e**: arrow). Cord diameter is enlarged at this level, indicative of intrinsic pathology, but there is no evidence of compression. The internal venous plexus also appears dilated (**a,b**: arrowheads). T2* sequences document hemorrhage within the effected spinal cord segment, as evidenced by prominent susceptibility effect (**c,f**: arrowhead). Postmortem examination confirmed hematomyelia, myelomalacia, and subdural hemorrhage. An underlying cause was not determined, and chronic aspirin administration was thought to have induced a spontaneous hemorrhage. The two vertically oriented curvilinear lines superimposed on the spinal cord in image **e** are artifacts caused by an out-of-field microchip.

Figure 3.2.20 Fibrocartilaginous Embolism (Canine)   CT

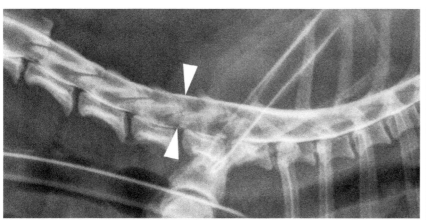

(a) DX+C, LAT

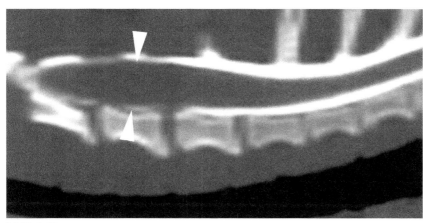

(c) CT+C, SP

(b) CT+C, DP

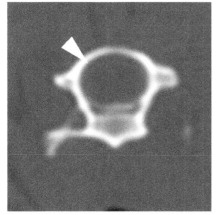

(d) CT+C, TP

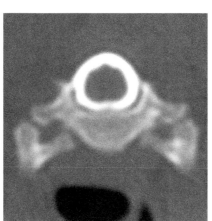

(e) CT+C, TP

4y FS Yorkshire Terrier with peracute onset of tetraparesis shortly after returning from a walk with the owner. A myelographic examination reveals a pronounced increase in spinal cord diameter centered on C6 (**a**: arrowheads). CT myelography further documents a caudal cervical intrinsic lesion (**b–d**: arrowheads). Although there is normally an increase in diameter of the cervical intumescence, the magnitude of the diameter change is abnormal and causes annular attenuation of the subarachnoid contrast column (**d**: arrowhead). A transverse cranial thoracic image acquired caudal to the spinal cord lesion shows a more normal spinal cord diameter and prominent contrast-enhanced subarachnoid space (**e**). Postmortem examination confirmed regional myelomalacia caused by multiple fibrocartilaginous emboli. The degree of spinal cord diameter enlargement in this patient is somewhat unusual and would be less likely to occur in patients with recoverable disease.

Figure 3.2.21   Fibrocartilaginous Embolism (Canine)   MR

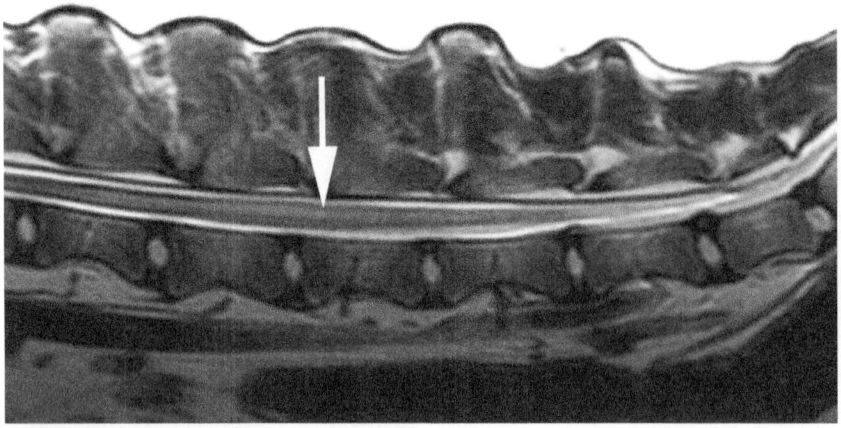

(a) T2, SP

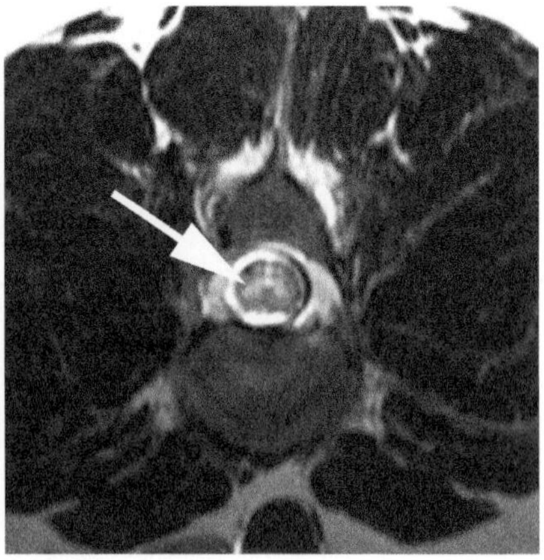

(b) T2, TP

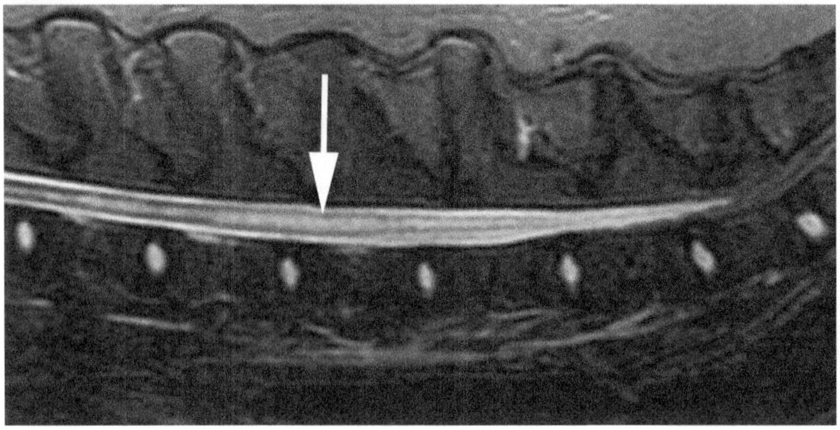

(c) ST, SP

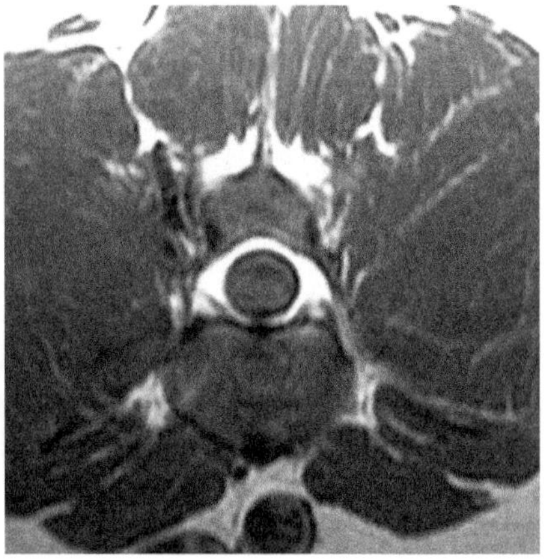

(d) T1, TP

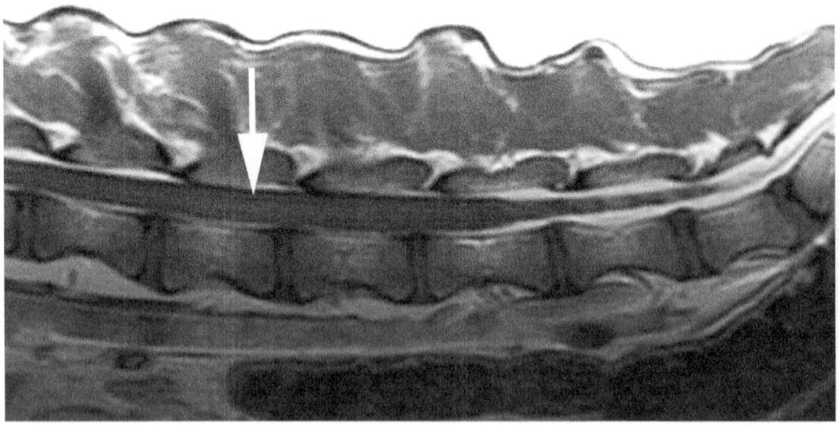

(e) T1+C, SP

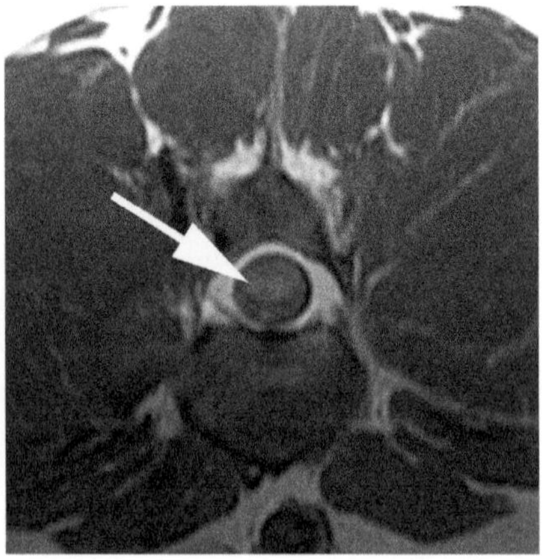

(f) T1+C, TP

4y FS Irish Wolfhound with acute-onset pelvic limb paraparesis with no known initiating cause. There is diffuse T2 hyperintensity in the caudal spinal cord consistent with an intrinsic lesion (a–c: arrow). There is mild, diffuse cord enhancement following contrast administration (e,f: arrow). The central T2 hyperintensity and contrast enhancement suggests predominantly gray matter involvement (b,f: arrow). Neurologic deficits persisted for 14 days with no evidence of improvement. Postmortem examination revealed severe bilateral myelomalacia with hemorrhage from spinal segment L6 caudally. Multiple fibrocartilaginous emboli were present in both the meningeal and spinal vessels.

Figure 3.2.22   Fibrocartilagenous Embolism (Canine)   MR

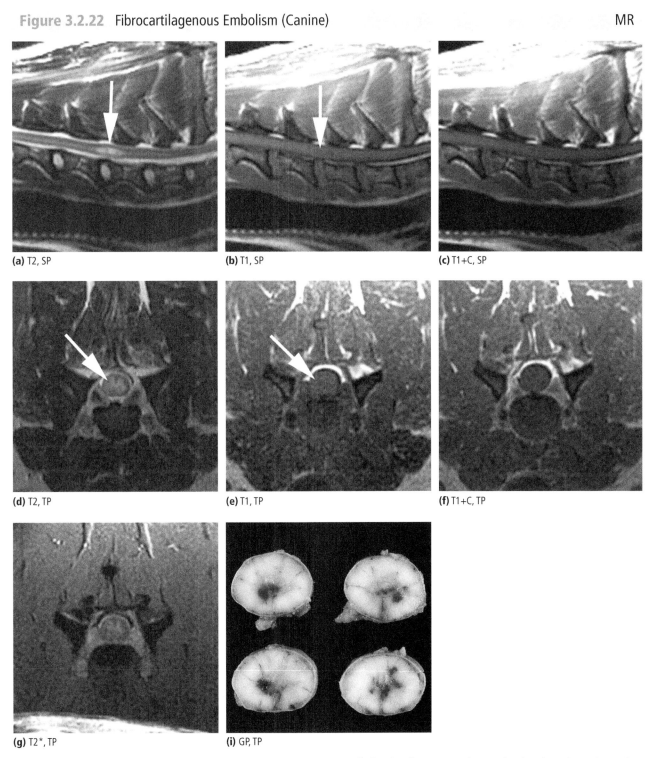

(a) T2, SP

(b) T1, SP

(c) T1+C, SP

(d) T2, TP

(e) T1, TP

(f) T1+C, TP

(g) T2*, TP

(i) GP, TP

8y MC Labrador Retriever with acute-onset neurologic deficits anatomically localized to C6–T2. There is focal T2 hyperintensity and T1 hypointensity of the spinal cord at the level of C5–6 (**a,b,d,e**: arrow) with no evidence of enhancement following contrast administration (**c,f**). The intensity changes are centrally distributed, and spinal cord diameter is focally increased, indicative of an intrinsic lesion. A T2* sequence shows no evidence of hemorrhage within the affected cord parenchyma (**g**). The owners elected to euthanize the dog, and postmortem examination revealed locally extensive, primarily gray matter, myelomalacia, hemorrhage, and neuronal necrosis in the C5–C7 spinal cord segments (**h**). Multiple fibrocartilaginous emboli were evident in meningeal and spinal vessels. It is unclear why the T2* sequence failed to show the intraparenchymal sites of hemorrhage. One possibility is that because of the peracute nature of the disorder, MR imaging was performed early enough after the initial insult that hemoglobin degradation products were not yet present in adequate concentration to yield a susceptibility effect.

References

1. Ross JS. Spine Fracture Classification Models. In: Ross JS, Brant-Zawadzki M, Morre KR, Crim J, Chen MZ, Katzman GL (eds): Diagnostic Imaging: Spine. Salt Lake City: Amirsys, Inc., 2005;II–I–6–9.

2. Kube SA, Olby NJ. Managing acute spinal cord injuries. Compend Contin Educ Vet. 2008;30:496–504; quiz 504, 506.

3. Shores A. Spinal trauma. Pathophysiology and management of traumatic spinal injuries. Vet Clin North Am Small Anim Pract. 1992;22:859–888.

4. Kinns J, Mai W, Seiler G, Zwingenberger A, Johnson V, Caceres A, et al. Radiographic sensitivity and negative predictive value for acute canine spinal trauma. Vet Radiol Ultrasound. 2006;47:563–570.

5. Johnson P, Beltran E, Dennis R, Taeymans O. Magnetic resonance imaging characteristics of suspected vertebral instability associated with fracture or subluxation in eleven dogs. Vet Radiol Ultrasound. 2012;53:552–559.

6. Denis F. The three column spine and its significance in the classification of acute thoracolumbar spinal injuries. Spine. 1983; 8:817–831.

7. Besalti O, Ozak A, Tong S. Management of spinal trauma in 69 cats. Dtsch Tierarztl Wochenschr. 2002;109:315–320.

8. Bruce CW, Brisson BA, Gyselinck K. Spinal fracture and luxation in dogs and cats: a retrospective evaluation of 95 cases. Vet Comp Orthop Traumatol. 2008;21:280–284.

9. Hawthorne JC, Blevins WE, Wallace LJ, Glickman N, Waters DJ. Cervical vertebral fractures in 56 dogs: a retrospective study. J Am Anim Hosp Assoc. 1999;35:135–146.

10. McKee WM. Spinal trauma in dogs and cats: a review of 51 cases. Vet Rec. 1990;126:285–289.

11. Steffen F, Flueckiger M, Montavon PM. Traumatic atlanto-occipital luxation in a dog: associated hypoglossal nerve deficits and use of 3-dimensional computed tomography. Vet Surg. 2003;32:411–415.

12. Middleton G, Hillmann DJ, Trichel J, Bragulla HH, Gaschen L. Magnetic resonance imaging of the ligamentous structures of the occipitoatlantoaxial region in the dog. Vet Radiol Ultrasound. 2012;53:545–551.

13. Bali MS, Lang J, Jaggy A, Spreng D, Doherr MG, Forterre F. Comparative study of vertebral fractures and luxations in dogs and cats. Vet Comp Orthop Traumatol. 2009;22:47–53.

14. Jeffery ND. Vertebral fracture and luxation in small animals. Vet Clin North Am Small Anim Pract. 2010;40:809–828.

15. Anderson A, Coughlan AR. Sacral fractures in dogs and cats: a classification scheme and review of 51 cases. J Small Anim Pract. 1997;38:404–409.

16. Kuntz CA, Waldron D, Martin RA, Shires PK, Moon M, Shell L. Sacral fractures in dogs: a review of 32 cases. J Am Anim Hosp Assoc. 1995;31:142–150.

17. Chang Y, Dennis R, Platt SR, Penderis J. Magnetic resonance imaging of traumatic intervertebral disc extrusion in dogs. Vet Rec. 2007;160:795–799.

18. De Risio L, Adams V, Dennis R, McConnell FJ. Association of clinical and magnetic resonance imaging findings with outcome in dogs with presumptive acute noncompressive nucleus pulposus extrusion: 42 cases (2000–2007). J Am Vet Med Assoc. 2009; 234:495–504.

19. Henke D, Gorgas D, Flegel T, Vandevelde M, Lang J, Doherr MG, et al. Magnetic resonance imaging findings in dogs with traumatic intervertebral disk extrusion with or without spinal cord compression: 31 cases (2006–2010). J Am Vet Med Assoc. 2013;242: 217–222.

20. Park EH, White GA, Tieber LM. Mechanisms of injury and emergency care of acute spinal cord injury in dogs and cats. J Vet Emerg Crit Care (San Antonio). 2012;22:160–178.

21. Griffiths IR. Spinal cord injuries: a pathological study of naturally occurring lesions in the dog and cat. J Comp Pathol. 1978;88: 303–315.

22. Cauzinille L, Kornegay JN. Fibrocartilaginous embolism of the spinal cord in dogs: review of 36 histologically confirmed cases and retrospective study of 26 suspected cases. J Vet Intern Med. 1996;10:241–245.

23. Gandini G, Cizinauskas S, Lang J, Fatzer R, Jaggy A. Fibrocartilaginous embolism in 75 dogs: clinical findings and factors influencing the recovery rate. J Small Anim Pract. 2003; 44:76–80.

24. Nakamoto Y, Ozawa T, Katakabe K, Nishiya K, Yasuda N, Mashita T, et al. Fibrocartilaginous embolism of the spinal cord diagnosed by characteristic clinical findings and magnetic resonance imaging in 26 dogs. J Vet Med Sci. 2009;71:171–176.

25. Marioni-Henry K. Feline spinal cord diseases. Vet Clin North Am Small Anim Pract. 2010;40:1011–1028.

26. De Risio L, Adams V, Dennis R, McConnell FJ, Platt SR. Association of clinical and magnetic resonance imaging findings with outcome in dogs suspected to have ischemic myelopathy: 50 cases (2000–2006). J Am Vet Med Assoc. 2008;233:129–135.

3.3

Inflammatory disorders

Noninfectious inflammatory disorders

Noninfectious inflammatory spinal disorders that have significant CT or MRI imaging abnormalities are relatively uncommon. Diagnosis of such disorders is often made from signalment, clinical presentation, cerebrospinal fluid analysis, and response to therapy. Brief descriptions of two of the most common entities follow.

Spinal granulomatous meningoencephalomyelitis

A description of granulomatous meningoencephalomyelitis (GME) and its intracranial imaging features is included in Chapter 2.6. The disorder involves primarily white matter of the brain, the optic nerves, and spinal cord and can manifest as either focal or disseminated disease.

Descriptions of computed tomography features of spinal GME are lacking, but they would be expected to be subtle or absent. Focal masses could appear as intrinsic lesions with increased cord diameter with or without contrast enhancement. MR features include focal, multifocal, or diffuse parenchymal T1 hypointensity/T2 hyperintensity and variable contrast enhancement (Figures 3.3.1, 3.3.2).

Steroid responsive meningitis–arteritis

Steroid responsive meningitis–arteritis (SRMA) is a systemic immune-mediated disorder that includes inflammatory responses of the leptomeninges and associated blood vessels, which has been reported in young Bernese Mountain Dogs, Beagles, Nova Scotia Duck Tolling Retrievers, Corgis, Boxers, and other breeds.[1-7] The disorder involves the spinal cord primarily and, to a lesser extent, the brain. Although MR features of meningeal thickening and contrast enhancement have been reported, our experience is that imaging studies in dogs with SRMA are often unremarkable.[6]

Infectious inflammatory disorders

Vertebral column

Discospondylitis

Discospondylitis occurs commonly in dogs and is rare in cats. Infection is caused by a wide variety of bacterial and mycotic species. Although the vertebral imaging features of bacterial and fungal discospondylitis can appear similar, the underlying clinical manifestations are quite different.

Bacterial (suppurative) discospondylitis

In a large retrospective study involving over 500 canine patients diagnosed with discospondylitis, two thirds were male, older dogs were more likely to be affected, and Great Danes were overrepresented.[8] *Staphylococcus*, *Brucella*, *Streptococcus*, and *Escherichia* species are most frequently isolated, although many others have been reported.[8-11] Dogs with bacterial discospondylitis most often have an underlying infection of the urinary tract, skin, or other organ system, which leads to bacteremia and embolic seeding of vulnerable disks.

Conventional radiographic examination is an excellent test for diagnosis and monitoring of discospondylitis. CT and MRI are most often employed when neurologic deficits are present or the patient has other clinical signs not explained by radiographic findings or other diagnostic tests.

Atlas of Small Animal CT and MRI, First Edition. Erik R. Wisner and Allison L. Zwingenberger.
© 2015 John Wiley & Sons, Inc. Published 2015 by John Wiley & Sons, Inc.

Imaging features vary widely and depend on the stage of the disease. CT features of early active disease can include vertebral endplate osteolysis and intervertebral joint space widening. In later phases of active disease, more pronounced endplate destruction is seen, which is associated with underlying bone sclerosis, reactive new bone formation, and collapse of the disk space. If there is significant proliferative soft-tissue inflammatory response or intervertebral joint subluxation, spinal cord compression can occur with resultant neurologic signs. In the convalescent or reparative phase, complete collapse of the joint may occur with bridging reactive new bone. Soft tissues within the disk space, medullary bone, and surrounding soft tissues moderately to markedly contrast enhance during the active phases of disease, reflecting the presence of discitis, osteomyelitis, and cellulitis (Figures 3.3.3, 3.3.4).

MR features of bacterial discospondylitis are similar and include mixed T2 intensity within the disk space and T1 hypointensity and T2 and STIR hyperintensity within affected vertebral bodies and adjacent soft tissues during the early active phase of disease. The disk, medullary bone, and adjacent soft tissues intensely contrast enhance during the active phases of disease (Figure 3.3.5).[7,12] MR may be less sensitive than CT for monitoring bone destruction and production in the active and reparative phases, respectively.

Mycotic (granulomatous) discospondylitis

Mycotic discospondylitis is almost always a component of systemic infection with *Aspergillus* or *Paecilomyces* species, although other fungi have also been reported.[13–17] Age of onset is 2–8 years, and German Shepherd Dogs and females are highly overrepresented, accounting for more than two thirds of reported patients.[15,16] Affected dogs are thought to be immunocompromised, resulting in multiorgan involvement.

Imaging features of mycotic discospondylitis are similar to those of bacterial discospondylitis, and often multiple intervertebral disks are affected (Figures 3.3.6, 3.3.7).

Spondylitis

In some geographic areas, inhaled plant awns can migrate through airways and lung parenchyma and exit caudally into the cranial sublumbar region, following the path of the attachment of the *pars lumbalis* of the diaphragm to the ventral margins of the third and fourth lumbar vertebrae. Pyogranulomatous myositis and frank abscess adjacent to the vertebrae lead to spondylitis.[18]

Imaging features of spondylitis include periosteal new bone formation of the ventral and lateral margins of affected vertebral bodies. Underlying bone sclerosis may also be present depending on the duration and severity of infection, resulting in hyperattenuation on CT images and hypointensity on T1 and T2 MR images. Cellulitis or abscess is present with active disease, which will appear as a hypoattenuating sublumbar mass on CT images and a T1 hypointense, T2 hyperintense mass on MR images. Marked, heterogeneous soft-tissue contrast enhancement occurs on images of both modalities (Figure 3.3.8).

Spinal cord, meninges, and epidural space

Spinal epidural empyema

Infections within the spinal epidural space are uncommon and can occur by direct extension of discospondylitis or other local infection or through hematogenous dissemination. Signs include fever and progressive myelopathy, which may have a compressive component.[19,20]

CT findings can be equivocal but include signs of discospondylitis as described above. Subarachnoid and epidural space contrast enhancement can be incomplete or nonuniform on CT myelographic images, and there may be evidence of focal, multifocal, or diffuse spinal cord compression.[20]

MR features include mixed or increased T2 intensity within the epidural space, as well as T2 hyperintensity within the spinal cord at the site of infection. Moderate diffuse or peripheral enhancement is seen following contrast administration with both modalities (Figure 3.3.9).[19]

Meningomyelitis

Infectious meningomyelitis is uncommon in both the dog and cat and can be viral, bacterial, mycotic, protozoal, or parasitic.[7,15,21,22] Because of the spectrum of infectious agents, clinical presentation varies widely, and meningomyelitis may be only part of a systemic or multiorgan disorder. Imaging reports of meningomyelitis in small animals are sparse, but in our experience MR imaging features are also variable. In patients with pyogenic or granulomatous meningomyelitis, fluid and solid-material collections in the subarachnoid space can have variable T1 intensity, T2 heterogeneity, and FLAIR hyperintensity. Meninges can intensely enhance following contrast administration. Depending on the volume and character of inflammatory material in the subarachnoid space, the spinal cord or cauda equina can be displaced and compressed. Spinal cord parenchyma can be T1 hypointense and T2 hyperintense, and cord diameter can be increased because of edema (Figures 3.3.10, 3.3.11).

Figure 3.3.1   Presumptive Spinal Granulomatous Meningoencephalomyelitis (Canine)   MR

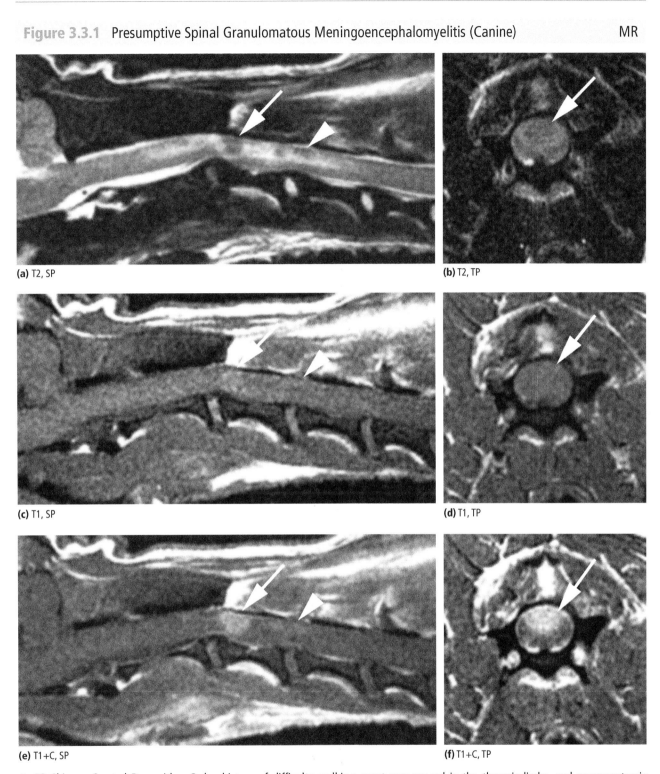

(a) T2, SP

(b) T2, TP

(c) T1, SP

(d) T1, TP

(e) T1+C, SP

(f) T1+C, TP

4y FS Chinese Crested Dog with a 3-day history of difficulty walking, most pronounced in the thoracic limbs, and neuroanatomic localization to C1–T2. There is a T2 hypointense, T1 isointense focus in the dorsal spinal cord at the level of caudal C2 (a–d: arrow). Two smaller intrinsic foci with similar intensity are seen at the level of the C2–3 intervertebral disk space (a,c: arrowhead). There is diffuse T2 hyperintensity in the cranial cervical spinal cord due to surrounding edema (a). A discrete, uniformly enhancing mass is seen following contrast administration (e,f: arrow), and faint enhancement of the two smaller lesions is also evident (e: arrowhead). Diagnosis was made from results of cerebrospinal fluid analysis consistent with granulomatous meningoencephalomyelitis, absence of infectious agents, and response to immunosuppressive doses of steroids.

Figure 3.3.2 Spinal Granulomatous Meningoencephalomyelitis (Canine) MR

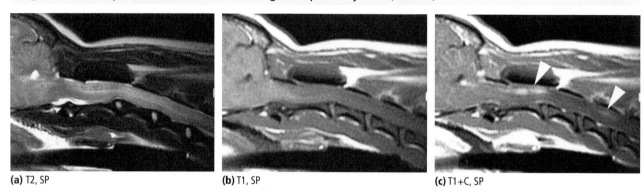

(a) T2, SP   **(b)** T1, SP   **(c)** T1+C, SP

4y FS Jack Russell Terrier with recent onset of nystagmus and circling. There is diffuse moderate T2 hyperintensity of the brainstem and cranial cervical spinal cord associated with parenchymal swelling (**a**). There is mild nonuniform enhancement within the brainstem following contrast administration, and three ill-defined contrast-enhancing intrinsic lesions are seen in the dorsal cervical spinal cord (**c**: arrowheads). Postmortem examination revealed angiocentric inflammatory lesions consistent with granulomatous meningoencephalitis. Multifocal suppurative inflammation with necrosis was also noted.

Figure 3.3.3 Suppurative Discospondylitis (Canine) CT

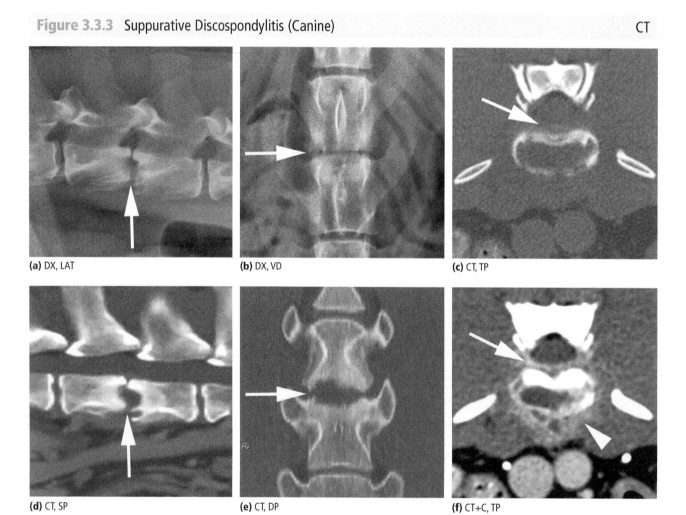

(a) DX, LAT   **(b)** DX, VD   **(c)** CT, TP

(d) CT, SP   **(e)** CT, DP   **(f)** CT+C, TP

5y FS Greyhound with back pain that developed a few weeks following treatment of an inflammatory pulmonary disorder. Vertebral radiographs reveal vertebral endplate osteolysis, surrounding bone sclerosis, and narrowing of the L3–4 intervertebral disk space (**a**,**b**: arrow). These findings are also evident on CT images, and the degree of endplate destruction is more apparent (**d**,**e**: arrow). There is a loss of the normally fat-attenuating ventral epidural space (**c**: arrow), and there is regional enhancement adjacent to the vertebral column (**f**: arrowhead) and within the ventral epidural space (**f**: arrow) following contrast administration, indicative of local extension of the inflammatory response. Fine-needle aspiration cytology revealed suppurative inflammation. Microbial culture failed to yield a causative agent, although the dog had been on antibiotics prior to sampling.

Figure 3.3.4   Inactive Multicentric Discospondylitis (Canine)   CT

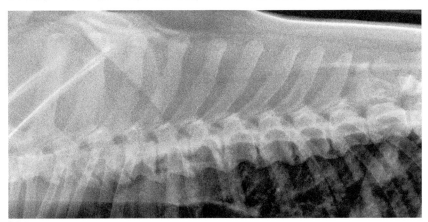

(a) DX, LAT

14y MC Golden Retriever with nasal carcinoma. No clinical signs referable to spinal pain or neurologic deficits. Thoracic radiographs and a thoracic CT examination were obtained for staging purposes. There are multiple sites of vertebral endplate osteolysis, adjacent bone sclerosis, intervertebral disk space narrowing, and spondylotic bridging within the thoracic vertebral column. These features are evident on the radiographic examination but are more clearly delineated on the CT image. The dog was thought to have had multicentric discospondylitis in the past, which had subsequently resolved.

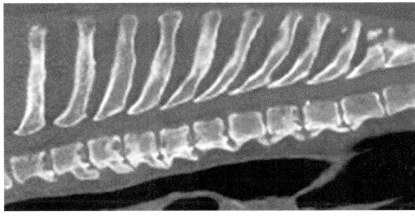

(b) CT, SP

Figure 3.3.5 Suppurative Discospondylitis (Canine)

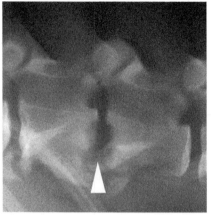

(a) DX, LAT

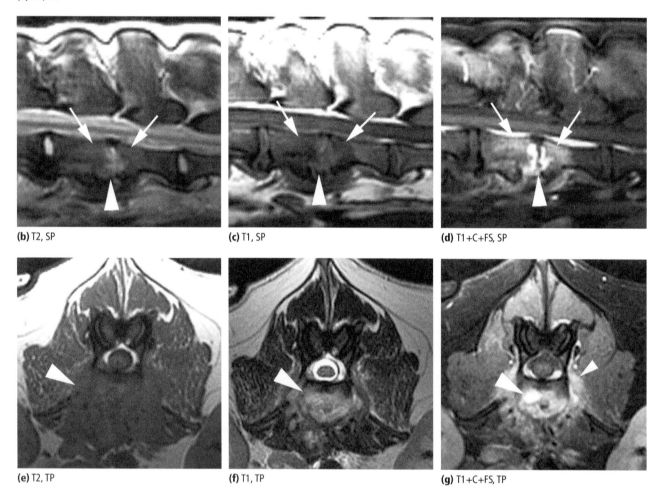

(b) T2, SP

(c) T1, SP

(d) T1+C+FS, SP

(e) T2, TP

(f) T1, TP

(g) T1+C+FS, TP

1.5y MC Boxer with hunched back and stiff pelvic limb gait but minimal neurologic deficits. The radiographic image shows vertebral endplate osteolysis, surrounding bone sclerosis, and mild disk space narrowing of the L2–3 intervertebral disk space (**a**: arrowhead). On MR images, the L2–3 disk space is ill defined with heterogeneous T2 and T1 hyperintensity (**b**,**c**,**e**,**f**: arrowhead). There is also mild T2 hyperintensity and T1 hypointensity of adjacent bone in the vertebral bodies (**b**,**c**: arrows). The affected intervertebral disk (**d**,**g**: large arrowhead), adjacent bone (**d**: arrows), and surrounding soft tissues (**g**: small arrowhead) intensely contrast enhance. Fine-needle aspiration cytology of the lesion revealed suppurative inflammation, and *Staphylococcus intermedius* was cultured.

Figure 3.3.6 Pyogranulomatous (Mycotic) Discospondylitis (Canine)   CT

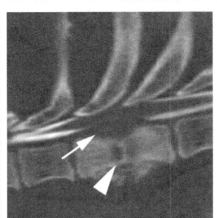

(a) DX, LAT   (b) CT+C, SP

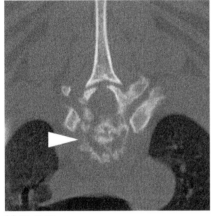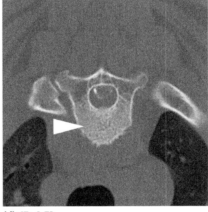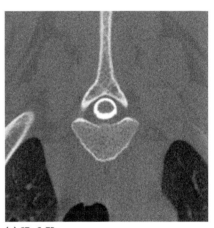

(c) CT+C, TP   (d) CT+C, TP   (e) CT+C, TP

2y F German Shepherd Dog with pelvic limb ataxia and spinal pain response of 2 weeks' duration. The myelographic image shows vertebral endplate osteolysis, surrounding bone sclerosis, disk space narrowing and spondylotic bridging of the T5–6 intervertebral disk space (a: arrowhead), and focal attenuation and elevation of the myelographic contrast columns (a: arrow). Osteolysis (c: arrowhead) and adjacent sclerosis (d: arrowhead) are clearly seen on a CT myelogram, which also reveals evidence of bony bridging across the disk space (b: arrowhead) and a well-delineated cord compressive ventral extradural mass (b: arrow). An image at the level of T4 shows the more normal appearance of the spinal cord and surrounding subarachnoid space (e). The dog was euthanized because of progressive clinical decline. Postmortem examination confirmed pyogranulomatous discospondylitis, and *Aspergillus terreus* was cultured.

Figure 3.3.7 Pyogranulomatous (Mycotic) Discospondylitis (Canine)   MR

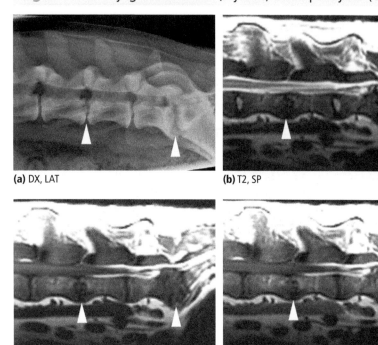

(a) DX, LAT

(b) T2, SP

(c) T1, SP

(d) T1+C, SP

5y MC German Shepherd Dog with progressive pelvic limb paresis of 3 months' duration. The L5–6 and L7–S1 intervertebral disks are ill defined with heterogeneous T2 hypointensity and T1 mixed intensity (**b,c**: arrowheads), reflecting the endplate destruction and adjacent bone sclerosis evident on a survey radiograph (**a**: arrowheads). Heterogeneous enhancement of the affected intervertebral disks, more pronounced at L7–S1, reflects the active inflammatory response (**d**: arrowheads). Many additional intervertebral disks had similar imaging features (not shown). *Sagnomella* (not further characterized) was cultured from a fine-needle aspiration sample harvested from the lumbosacral intervertebral disk space.

Figure 3.3.8 Suppurative Spondylitis (Canine)   CT

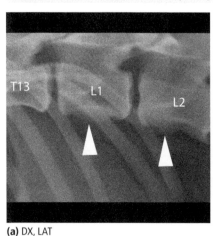

(a) DX, LAT

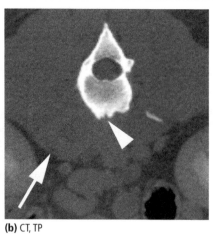

(b) CT, TP

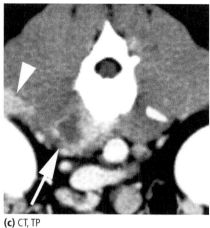

(c) CT, TP

3y F Labrador Retriever with 2-week history of listlessness, weight loss, and lumbar pain. There is ill-defined new bone formation on the ventral aspect of the L1 and L2 vertebral bodies on a survey radiographic examination (**a**: arrowheads). The right sublumbar musculature (quadratus lumborum and psoas minor) is focally enlarged at the level of the first lumbar vertebra (**b**: arrow), which proves to be a peripherally enhancing sublumbar abscess following contrast administration (**c**: arrow). A spiculated periosteal productive response is present on the ventral margin of the first lumbar vertebral body (**b**: arrowhead). An additional tract is seen extending toward the right lateral paraspinal region (**c**: arrowhead). A migrating "foxtail" plant awn was removed at the time of surgical exploration. *Actinomyces*, *Pasteurella*, and multiple anaerobic species were cultured from the abscess site.

Figure 3.3.9 Spinal Epidural Empyema (Canine)   MR

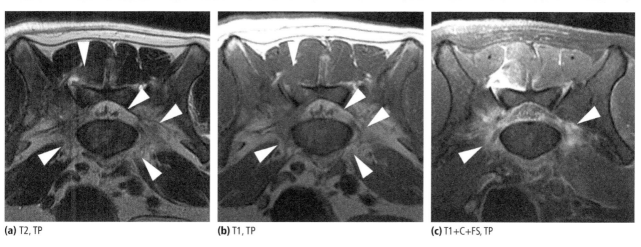

(a) T2, TP   **(b)** T1, TP   **(c)** T1+C+FS, TP

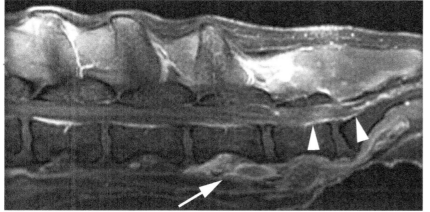

(d) T1+C+FS, SP

8y FS Irish Wolfhound with 2-week history of progressive reluctance to stand and signs referable to lumbar or pelvic pain. Images **a–c** were acquired at the level of the caudal end of the seventh lumbar vertebra. There is mixed T1 and T2 intensity of fat within the vertebral canal, intervertebral foramina, and perivertebral regions (**a,b**: arrowheads). There is marked heterogenous enhancement of these areas following contrast administration (**c,d**: arrowheads), consistent with epidural empyema and surrounding cellulitis. Epidural space enhancement is most pronounced in the L7 to sacral region of the vertebral column and is best appreciated on image **d**. Tissues adjacent to the medial iliac lymph nodes also enhance, indicating regional lymphadenopathy (**d**: arrow). Necrotic fat and collections of purulent material were found at the time of L6–S1 dorsal laminectomy. Biopsy of epidural fat revealed acute fibrinosuppurative steatitis with Gram-positive cocci. There was no growth on microbial cultures, but the dog had been on antibiotics.

Figure 3.3.10 Pyogranulomatous (Mycotic) Meningomyelitis (Canine)   MR

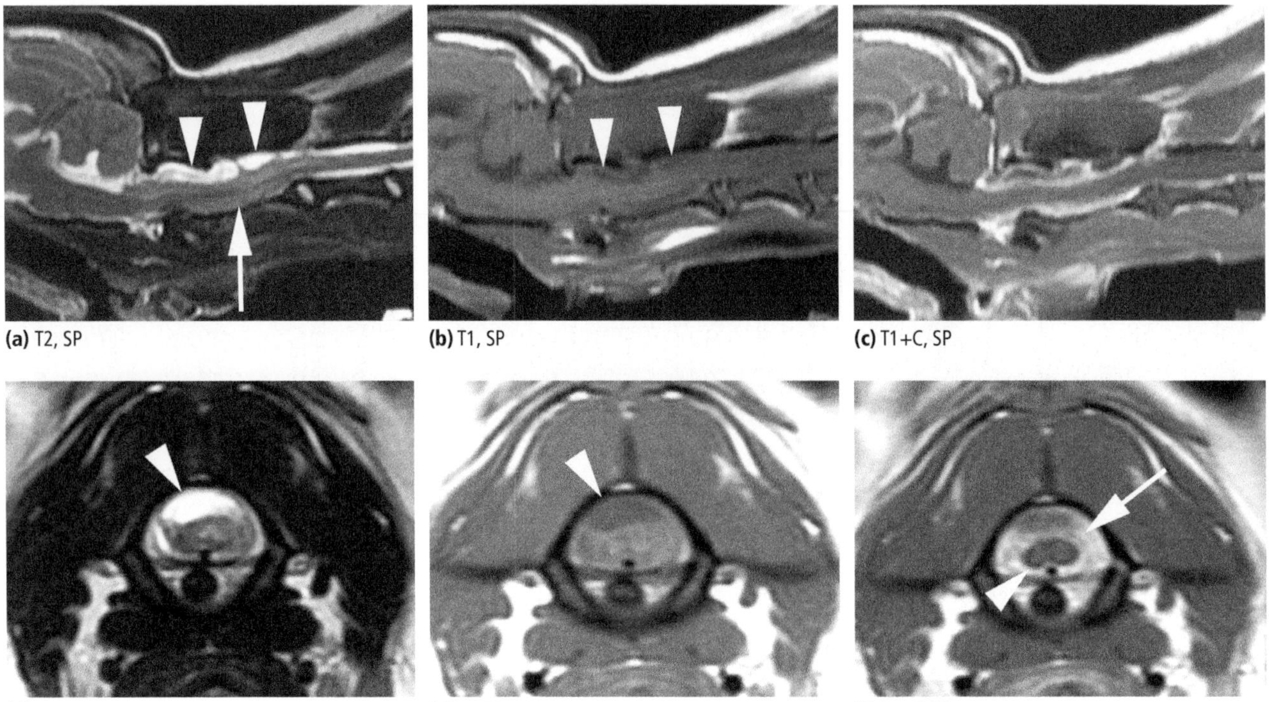

(a) T2, SP

(b) T1, SP

(c) T1+C, SP

(d) T2, TP

(e) T1, TP

(f) T1+C, TP

9y MC Manchester Terrier with mild ataxia and signs referable to cervical pain. Images **d–f** are at the level of C1–2. There is regional T2 hyperintensity and T1 hypointensity surrounding the spinal cord consistent with a fluid collection, which causes cord deformation and compression (**a,b,d,e**: arrowheads). This appears to have an annular component that is both extradural and intradural based on the concentric pattern seen on the transverse T2 image (**d**) and the intense extradural (**f**: arrow) and extramedullary intradural (**f**:arrowhead) enhancement on the transverse contrast-enhanced T1 image. There is also diffuse parenchymal T2 hyperintensity associated with increased spinal cord diameter at the level of C2, indicative of an intrinsic component (**a**: arrow). Cerebrospinal fluid analysis showed marked mixed lymphocytic/neutrophilic inflammation. Decompressive dorsal laminectomy was performed, and biopsy revealed marked pyogranulomatous inflammation of the meninges and extradural tissues. Fungal culture of the surgical biopsy material yielded *Coccidioides immitis.*

Figure 3.3.11   Pyogranulomatous (Amoebic) Meningomyelitis (Canine)   MR

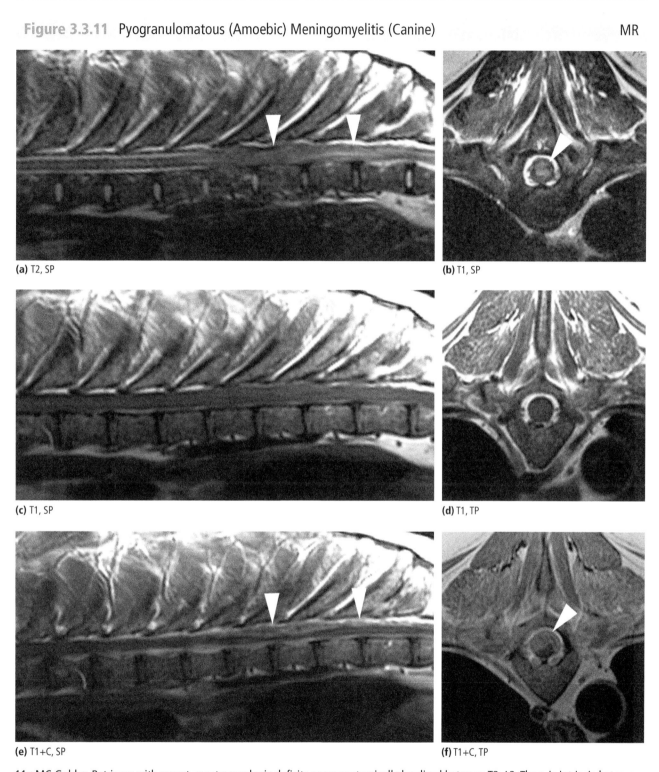

(a) T2, SP

(b) T1, SP

(c) T1, SP

(d) T1, TP

(e) T1+C, SP

(f) T1+C, TP

11y MC Golden Retriever with recent-onset neurologic deficits neuroanatomically localized between T3–L3. There is intrinsic heterogeneous T2 hyperintensity of the midthoracic spinal cord associated with a loss of definition and reducing intensity of the subarachnoid space (**a,b**: arrowheads). There is marked, heterogeneous enhancement in the same region following contrast administration (**e**: arrowheads), and enhancing material fills the subarachnoid space, causing marked spinal cord compression (**f**: arrowhead). Postmortem examination revealed severe, diffuse, chronic necrotizing and pyogranulomatous meningomyelitis with *Acanthamoeba* cysts and trophozoites. Neurologic findings were part of more widespread multisystem infection.

References

1. Behr S, Cauzinille L. Aseptic suppurative meningitis in juvenile boxer dogs: retrospective study of 12 cases. J Am Anim Hosp Assoc. 2006;42:277–282.

2. Cherubini GB. Steroid-responsive meningitis–arteritis in the Pembroke Welsh corgi. Vet Rec. 2008;162:424.

3. Hansson-Hamlin H, Lilliehook I. Steroid-responsive meningitis-arteritis in Nova Scotia duck tolling retrievers. Vet Rec. 2013;173:527.

4. Redman J. Steroid-responsive meningitis-arteritis in the Nova Scotia duck tolling retriever. Vet Rec. 2002;151:712.

5. Rose JH, Harcourt-Brown TR. Screening diagnostics to identify triggers in 21 cases of steroid-responsive meningitis–arteritis. J Small Anim Pract. 2013;54:575–578.

6. Tipold A, Schatzberg SJ. An update on steroid responsive meningitis–arteritis. J Small Anim Pract. 2010;51:150–154.

7. Tipold A, Stein VM. Inflammatory diseases of the spine in small animals. Vet Clin North Am Small Anim Pract. 2010;40:871–879.

8. Burkert BA, Kerwin SC, Hosgood GL, Pechman RD, Fontenelle JP. Signalment and clinical features of diskospondylitis in dogs: 513 cases (1980–2001). J Am Vet Med Assoc. 2005;227:268–275.

9. Hurov L, Troy G, Turnwald G. Diskospondylitis in the dog: 27 cases. J Am Vet Med Assoc. 1978;173:275–281.

10. Kerwin SC, Lewis DD, Hribernik TN, Partington B, Hosgood G, Eilts BE. Diskospondylitis associated with *Brucella canis* infection in dogs: 14 cases (1980–1991). J Am Vet Med Assoc. 1992;201:1253–1257.

11. Thomas WB. Diskospondylitis and other vertebral infections. Vet Clin North Am Small Anim Pract. 2000;30:169–182, vii.

12. Harris JM, Chen AV, Tucker RL, Mattoon JS. Clinical features and magnetic resonance imaging characteristics of diskospondylitis in dogs: 23 cases (1997–2010). J Am Vet Med Assoc. 2013;242:359–365.

13. Armentano RA, Cooke KL, Wickes BL. Disseminated mycotic infection caused by *Westerdykella* species in a German Shepherd dog. J Am Vet Med Assoc. 2013;242:381–387.

14. Foley JE, Norris CR, Jang SS. Paecilomycosis in dogs and horses and a review of the literature. J Vet Intern Med. 2002;16:238–243.

15. Schultz RM, Johnson EG, Wisner ER, Brown NA, Byrne BA, Sykes JE. Clinicopathologic and diagnostic imaging characteristics of systemic aspergillosis in 30 dogs. J Vet Intern Med. 2008;22:851–859.

16. Watt PR, Robins GM, Galloway AM, O'Boyle DA. Disseminated opportunistic fungal disease in dogs: 10 cases (1982–1990). J Am Vet Med Assoc. 1995;207:67–70.

17. Zhang S, Corapi W, Quist E, Griffin S, Zhang M. *Aspergillus versicolor*, a new causative agent of canine disseminated aspergillosis. J Clin Microbiol. 2012;50:187–191.

18. Brennan KE, Ihrke PJ. Grass awn migration in dogs and cats: a retrospective study of 182 cases. J Am Vet Med Assoc. 1983;182:1201–1204.

19. De Stefani A, Garosi LS, McConnell FJ, Diaz FJ, Dennis R, Platt SR. Magnetic resonance imaging features of spinal epidural empyema in five dogs. Vet Radiol Ultrasound. 2008;49:135–140.

20. Lavely JA, Vernau KM, Vernau W, Herrgesell EJ, LeCouteur RA. Spinal epidural empyema in seven dogs. Vet Surg. 2006;35:176–185.

21. Griffin JF, Levine JM, Levine GJ, Fosgate GT. Meningomyelitis in dogs: a retrospective review of 28 cases (1999–2007). J Small Anim Pract. 2008;49:509–517.

22. Tipold A. Diagnosis of inflammatory and infectious diseases of the central nervous system in dogs: a retrospective study. J Vet Intern Med. 1995;9:304–314.

3.4

Neoplasia

Extradural neoplasia

Juxtavertebral neoplasia

Malignant soft-tissue neoplasms that arise adjacent to the vertebral column can invade vertebrae and the vertebral canal. Such neoplasms are often mesenchymal in origin and include hemangiosarcoma, fibrosarcoma, myxosarcoma, liposarcoma, and synovial tumors (Figures 3.4.1, 3.4.2, 3.4.3).

Neoplasia arising from bone

Benign primary bone tumors

The clinical significance of benign bone tumors, such as vertebral osteomas and osteochondromas, often depends on whether they encroach on the spinal cord or disrupt the structural integrity of the vertebral column. Benign bone tumors are usually highly mineralized, smoothly margined, and have CT attenuation and MR intensities similar to those of normal dense bone (Figure 3.4.4).[1]

Malignant primary bone tumors

Primary bone tumors arising from the vertebral column include osteosarcoma, chondrosarcoma, and fibrosarcoma and typically have aggressive imaging features. Those tumors with significant osteoid production will appear predominantly osteoproductive or have osteoproductive/osteolytic components, while others may have a predominantly osteolytic appearance. Tumors arise from a single vertebra, but reactivity or invasion of adjacent vertebrae may occur. Extension into the vertebral canal can cause spinal cord compression, and pathologic fracture can occur because of loss of structural integrity of the vertebral body.

CT features of primary bone tumors include heterogeneous osteolysis of affected bone with periosteal and endosteal reactive bone formation. Amorphous tumor new bone may also be present in osteoblastic tumors (Figures 3.4.5, 3.4.6, 3.4.7).[2,3]

MR features include altered anatomic margins and T1 and T2 hypointensity in regions of reactive and tumor new bone formation. When the tumor mass includes a significant vascular soft-tissue component, that region will have variable T1 and T2 intensity and can heterogeneously contrast enhance (Figure 3.4.7).[4,5]

Plasma cell tumors

Plasma cell neoplasms arise from malignant proliferation of B-lymphocytes, and they may occur as solitary plasmacytomas or multiple myeloma. Multiple myeloma typically affects bone, including vertebrae, ribs, pelvis, skull, and proximal or distal aspects of long bones, while plasmacytomas may occur in the skin, mucosa, gastrointestinal tract, and bone. Plasmacytomas of the vertebral column generally arise from a single vertebra but can involve adjacent segments. Multiple myeloma is multifocal and polyostotic and is usually widely distributed within both axial and appendicular bone.

CT and MR are superior to survey radiography for determining the presence and size of vertebral plasma cell tumors.[6] CT features of plasmacytoma include osteolysis, often associated with preservation of at least part of the cortical margin, and pathologic fractures are common. Tumor mass can also breach the cortical margin and encroach on the vertebral canal, causing extradural spinal cord compression. Plasmacytomas are soft-tissue attenuating and mildly to markedly enhance

Atlas of Small Animal CT and MRI, First Edition. Erik R. Wisner and Allison L. Zwingenberger.
© 2015 John Wiley & Sons, Inc. Published 2015 by John Wiley & Sons, Inc.

following intravenous contrast administration on CT images. CT myelography can be used to assess presence and location of spinal cord compression. On MR images, plasmacytomas are almost purely osteolytic, T1 iso- to hyperintense and T2 hyperintense compared to epaxial musculature, and variably but uniformly enhance following intravenous contrast administration (Figure 3.4.8). Three-dimensional gradient-echo sequences can be used to more accurately assess bone destruction.

CT and MR features of multiple myeloma include multiple poorly margined to well-demarcated foci of osteolysis, which are often most abundant in the vertebral column (Figure 3.4.9).

Metastatic neoplasia

Both carcinomas and soft sarcomas metastasize to the vertebral column, with carcinoma metastasis occurring more often.[7-9] Lesions are predominantly osteodestructive and can include an extravertebral component when cortical margins are breached. CT imaging features vary depending on cell type but generally include focal or multifocal osteolysis and a soft-tissue attenuating mass that variably enhances following intravenous contrast administration. Pathologic fracture can occur when structural integrity of cortical bone is compromised. A periosteal productive reaction is occasionally present with soft-tissue tumor metastases, and osteosarcoma metastases can have a mixed osteoproductive/destructive appearance. MR features include a space-occupying osteolytic soft-tissue mass that is variably T1 intense, T2 hyperintense, and usually intensely enhancing following intravenous contrast administration (Figures 3.4.10, 3.4.11). Three-dimensional gradient-echo sequences can be used for more accurate assessment of the extent of bone destruction.

Lymphoma

Lymphoma associated with the vertebral column and spinal cord can be extradural, intradural–extramedullary, or intramedullary (intrinsic), although the latter is reported to be less common.[4,10-15] Lymphoma is the most common spinal neoplasm in cats and is often a component of multicentric disease.[10,12,15]

On CT images, extradural lymphoma masses are soft-tissue attenuating and minimally to mildly contrast enhancing following intravenous contrast administration.[16] CT myelography can be used to document spinal cord compression and to determine the compartment of origin, with extrinsic masses producing eccentric spinal cord displacement and compression and intrinsic lesions producing a focal increase in cord diameter and annular attenuation of the subarachnoid contrast column.

MR features include T1 hypo- to isointensity, T2 hyperintensity, and moderate homogeneous enhancement (Figure 3.4.12). Diffuse meningeal enhancement has also been reported.[4,17] The compartment of origin can sometimes be determined, particularly by evaluating the distribution of T2 hyperintense cerebrospinal fluid in relation to the tumor, although large masses may be more difficult to localize.

Other neoplasms

Rarely, other tumors can originate within the extradural space as either primary or metastatic neoplasms. Imaging features will vary widely depending on cell type (Figure 3.4.13).

Intradural–extramedullary neoplasia

Features of intracranial nervous system neoplasms have been described in Chapters 2.8 and 2.10 and spinal neoplasms of the same cell type often have similar imaging characteristics. The most common intradural–extramedullary neoplasms include meningioma, peripheral nerve sheath tumor, nephroblastoma, cerebrospinal fluid disseminated metastasis, and round cell tumors, such as lymphoma and histiocytic sarcoma.[4,10,18-22]

Meningioma

Meningioma is the most common central nervous system neoplasm of the spinal cord in dogs. Median age at onset of clinical signs is 9 years, and Golden Retrievers and Boxers appear to be overrepresented.[23] Most canine spinal meningiomas are World Health Organization (WHO) grade I or II, with a small minority being more biologically aggressive grade III. Nearly 70% are located in the cervical region, about 25% are lumbar, and the remainder are thoracic or multifocal.[22] Although less common, spinal meningioma has also been reported in the cat.[24]

On CT images, spinal meningiomas are soft-tissue attenuating space-occupying masses within the vertebral canal that variably displace and compress the spinal cord, depending on tumor size in relation to the vertebral canal diameter. Meningiomas uniformly enhance following intravenous contrast administration and appear as a contrast-filling defect within the subarachnoid space on CT myelography (Figure 3.4.14). On MR images, meningiomas are mildly to moderately T1 hyperintense, mildly to markedly T2 hyperintense, and uniformly and intensely contrast enhancing. A dural tail sign may be present in some instances but is not consistent. Intradural–extramedullary localization is supported by peripheral T2/STIR hyperintensity due to subarachnoid space distension, comparable to the "golf tee" sign described for conventional myelography (Figure 3.4.15).[22,23] Using either imaging modality, localizing a meningioma to the intradural–extramedullary compartment may not be possible when the tumor mass is large.

Peripheral nerve sheath tumor

The term peripheral nerve sheath tumor (PNST) includes neoplasms that originate from Schwann cells, fibroblasts, or perineural cells.[25] Because the terminology for this group of tumors has been inconsistent, we choose to use the all-encompassing term PNST. Age of onset in dogs is reported to be bimodal, peaking at 2–3 years and 7–9 years, with no apparent breed predilection.[26] Small PNSTs arising from nerve roots contained within the meninges and limited to an intradural–extramedullary distribution within the vertebral canal have CT and MR imaging features similar to spinal meningiomas and cannot be reliably differentiated from other intradural–extramedullary neoplasms (Figure 3.4.16). However, PNSTs are more likely to invade spinal cord parenchyma and can also extend along peripheral nerves external to the vertebral canal, taking on a more tubular or lobular shape (Figure 3.4.17 and Chapter 3.6).

Spinal cord nephroblastoma

Spinal cord nephroblastoma (SCN) is an uncommon neoplasm of young dogs (6 months to 4 years) that arises from transformed embryological renal tissue that is entrapped within the spinal dura matter during development.[21,27] German Shepherd Dogs may be overrepresented, although total numbers reported to date are small. Most SCNs are located within the T9–L3 region of the vertebral column and are unencapsulated and intradural–extramedullary, although invasion into spinal cord parenchyma occurs, which has been correlated with a poorer prognosis.[21,27] CT and MR imaging features are similar to those described for other intradural–extramedullary masses. An SCN appears as a soft-tissue attenuating mass on unenhanced CT images and as a contrast-filling defect on CT myelography. Spinal cord nephroblastomas are T1 iso- to mildly hyperintense, T2 hyperintense, and homogeneously enhance following intravenous contrast administration (Figure 3.4.18).

Cerebrospinal fluid disseminated metastasis

Tumors arising within the subarachnoid space or intracranial ventricular system will occasionally exfoliate cells that seed the spinal leptomeninges as metastatic deposits.[28] Imaging features of CSF disseminated metastases are variable, and their appearance depends on characteristics of the primary neoplasm (Figure 3.4.19).

Other neoplasms

Neoplasms, such as lymphoma and histiocytic sarcoma, can be intradural–extramedullary but do not appear to be as constrained by the meninges and can also simultaneously be extradural and/or intramedullary.[17] Round cell tumors range from well defined to amorphous but usually homogeneously contrast enhance. Other imaging features are variable (Figure 3.4.20).

Intramedullary neoplasia

In a report of 53 dogs with intramedullary spinal cord neoplasia, approximately two thirds of the tumors were of neuroepithelial origin. The remainder were metastatic neoplasms, the most common of which were hemangiosarcoma and transitional cell carcinoma.[14] In this study, ependymoma was the most common neuroepithelial tumor, followed by astrocytoma. Dogs with primary neoplasms were significantly younger than dogs with metastatic disease (5.9 years vs. 10.8 years), and primary neoplasms were distributed in the cervical, caudal thoracic, and lumbar regions, while metastasis occurred predominantly in the mid to caudal lumbar region. The imaging appearance of intracranial neuroepithelial neoplasms is described in Chapter 2.8, and imaging features of primary spinal cord neoplasms are similar. Imaging features of metastatic neoplasms is more variable, and, particularly with hemangiosarcoma metastasis, the presence of hemorrhage may add to the complexity of the MR imaging characteristics.[14] A common feature of all intramedullary neoplasms is the presence of an intraparenchymal mass that causes an increase in spinal cord diameter and annular narrowing of the surrounding subarachnoid space. This appears as circumferential attenuation of the subarachnoid space on CT myelographic or T2 and STIR MR images (Figures 3.4.21, 3.4.22, 3.4.23).

Figure 3.4.1   Paravertebral Myxosarcoma (Canine)   CT

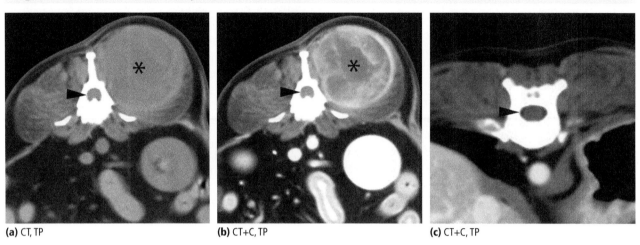

(a) CT, TP   **(b)** CT+C, TP   **(c)** CT+C, TP

13y FS Boston Terrier with a left-sided lumbar mass that was determined to be a myxosarcoma by tissue biopsy. The mass has rapidly increased in size recently, and the dog now has pelvic limb paralysis. There is a large encapsulated soft-tissue attenuating mass adjacent to the third lumbar vertebra (**a**: asterisk). Tissue within the vertebral canal is also uniformly soft-tissue attenuating without evidence of epidural fat (**a**: arrowhead). The paravertebral mass heterogeneously enhances following intravenous contrast administration (**b**: asterisk), and there is an approximately 10 HU incremental increase in attenuation within the vertebral canal at this level (**b**: arrowhead), which does not occur at locations distant to the mass. An enhanced CT image cranial to the mass shows clearly defined spinal cord surrounded by lower-attenuating epidural fat (**c**: arrowhead). Postmortem examination confirmed infiltrative left paralumbar myxosarcoma with invasion of the spinal canal.

Figure 3.4.2   Synovial Cell Sarcoma (Canine)   MR

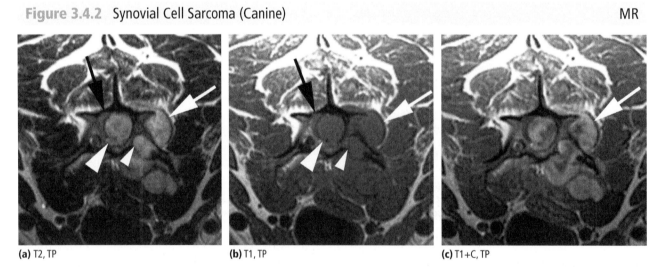

(a) T2, TP   **(b)** T1, TP   **(c)** T1+C, TP

10y FS Rottweiler with neurologic deficits localized to C1–5. There is a large multilobular mass adjacent to the fourth cervical vertebra, which is T1 isointense and T2 hyperintense compared to adjacent muscle (**a,b**: white arrow). The mass has caused osteolysis of the left transverse process and invades the vertebral canal (**a,b**: large arrowhead) and transverse foramen (**a,b**: small arrowhead). There is marked displacement and compression of the cervical spinal cord (**a,b**: black arrow). The mass intensely but nonuniformly enhances following intravenous contrast administration (**c**: white arrow). Microscopic examination of tissue obtained from postmortem examination revealed this to be a poorly differentiated malignancy consistent with synovial cell sarcoma.

Figure 3.4.3   Paravertebral Liposarcoma (Canine)   CT & MR

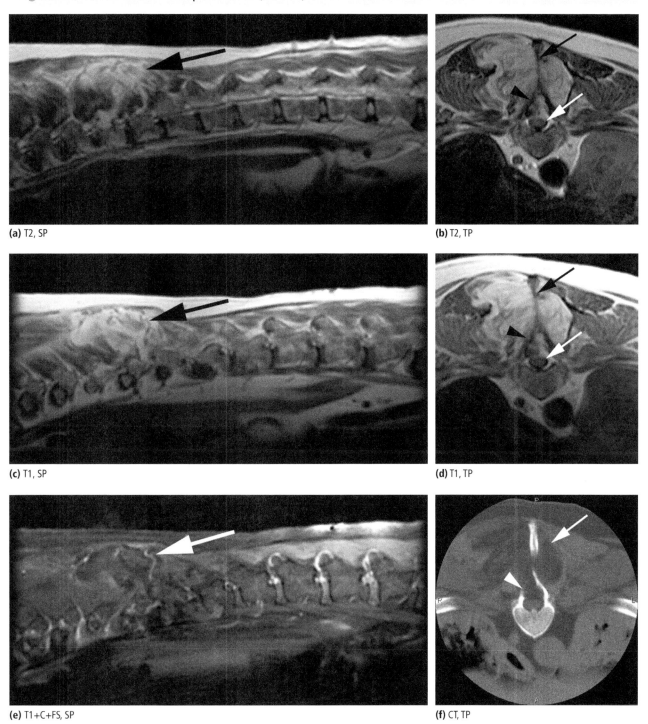

(a) T2, SP

(b) T2, TP

(c) T1, SP

(d) T1, TP

(e) T1+C+FS, SP

(f) CT, TP

14y FS Bearded Collie with a 3-week history of progressive pelvic limb ataxia and paresis. There is an irregularly margined T1 and T2 hyperintense mass dorsal to the caudal thoracic vertebral column (**a–d**: black arrow) that has caused osteolysis of the vertebral lamina and pedicles (**b,d**: black arrowhead). The mass also extends into the vertebral canal producing spinal cord compression (**b,d**: white arrow). The mass is hypointense on a fat-suppressed contrast-enhanced sequence and has minimal peripheral enhancement (**e**: white arrow). On CT images, the mass is predominantly fat attenuating (**f**: white arrow), and the osteolysis and spinal cord compression are again apparent (**f**: white arrowhead). Imaging features are consistent with invasive liposarcoma, which was confirmed on postmortem examination.

Figure 3.4.4 Osteochondroma (Canine)   CT & MR

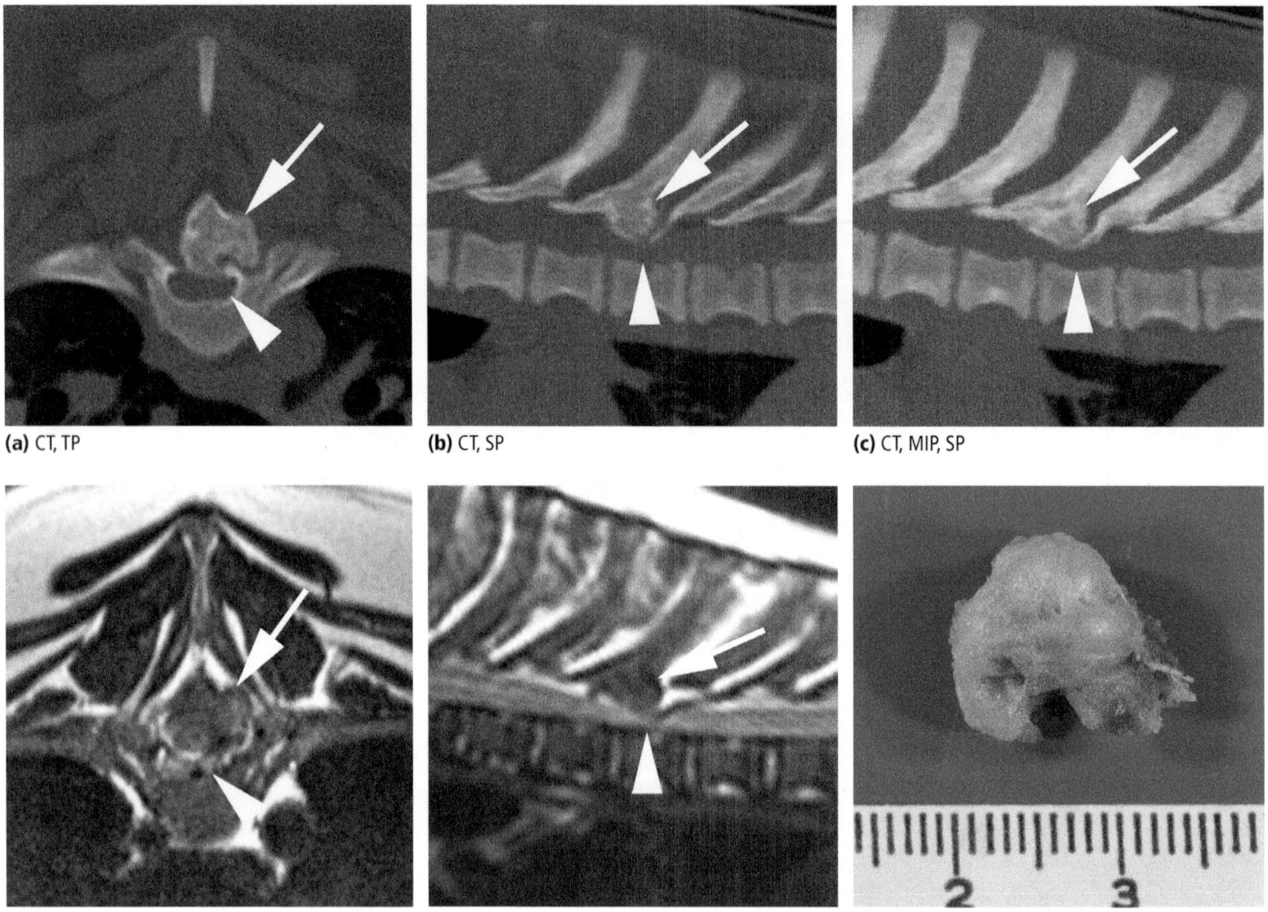

(a) CT, TP

(b) CT, SP

(c) CT, MIP, SP

(d) T2, TP

(e) T2, SP

(f) GP

10mo FS Dachshund with recent onset of paraparesis neuroanatomically localized to T3–L3. There is a well-defined, bone-attenuating mass arising from the caudal lamina of T6 that appears contiguous with more normal adjacent bone of the basilar part of the T6 spinous process (**a–c**: arrow). Encroachment into the vertebral canal implies spinal cord compression (**a–c**: arrowhead), although the cord is not clearly delineated. The mass also has T2 (**d,e**: arrow) and T1 (not shown) intensity similar to adjacent normal bone, and spinal cord compression is documented (**d,e**: arrowhead). Surgical excision biopsy revealed the mass to be a solitary osteochondroma (**f**).

Figure 3.4.5 Osteosarcoma (Canine)

CT

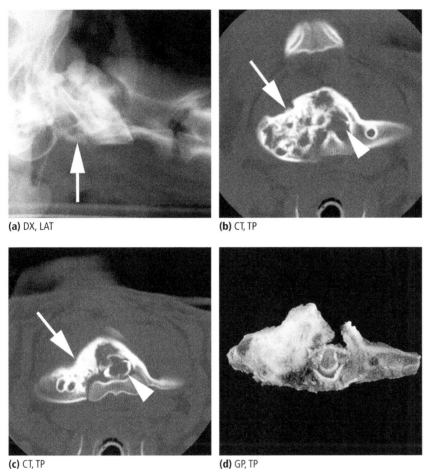

(a) DX, LAT

(b) CT, TP

(c) CT, TP

(d) GP, TP

Adult M American Staffordshire Terrier with recent onset of tetraparesis. Spinal radiographic examination reveals a mixed pattern of osteoproduction and osteolysis of the first cervical vertebra (**a**: arrow). CT myelographic images at the level of the midbody (**b**) and caudal end (**c**) of the atlas confirm a predominantly right-sided osteoproductive and destructive expansile mass (**b,c**: arrow) that extends into the vertebral canal, causing spinal cord compression (**b,c**: arrowhead). Postmortem examination confirmed a diagnosis of poorly differentiated osteosarcoma. The gross pathology specimen (**d**) is at the same level as the transverse CT image depicted in image **b**.

Figure 3.4.6 Osteosarcoma (Canine)   CT

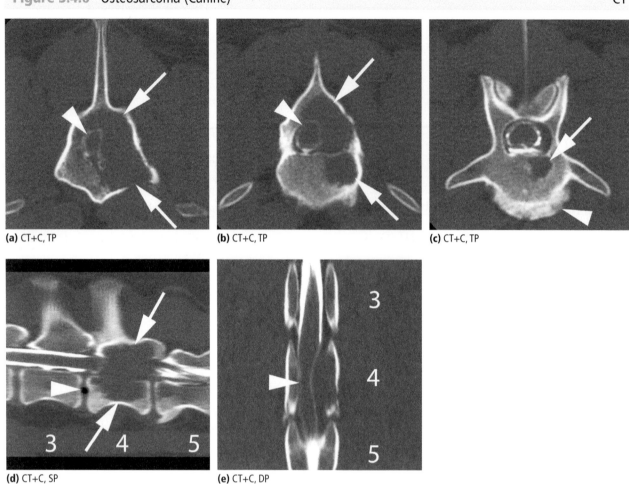

(a) CT+C, TP   **(b)** CT+C, TP   **(c)** CT+C, TP

(d) CT+C, SP   **(e)** CT+C, DP

8y FS Doberman Pinscher with 1-week history of progressive paraparesis. Transverse images are at the midbody (**a**) and caudal end (**b**) of L4 and at the cranial end of L5 (**c**). An osteodestructive mass is seen within the body, left pedicle, lamina, and vertebral canal of L4 (**a,b,d**: arrows) and has extended caudally into the body of L5 (**c**: arrow). CT myelography confirms left-sided spinal cord compression (**a,b,e**: arrowhead). There are also incidental findings of ventral spondylosis (**c**: arrowhead) and an L3–4 vacuum sign (**d**: arrowhead). Postmortem examination revealed osteosarcoma. The imaging features of this neoplasm are somewhat unusual given the purely destructive appearance that suggests an osteoclastic or primitive cell lineage.

Figure 3.4.7   Osteosarcoma (Canine)   CT & MR

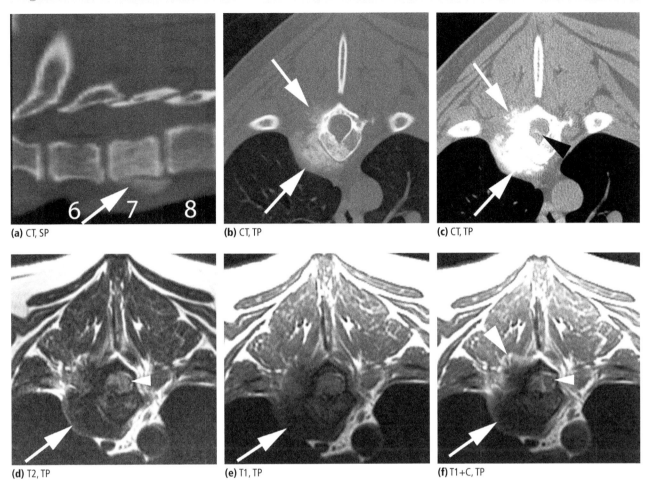

(a) CT, SP   **(b)** CT, TP   **(c)** CT, TP

(d) T2, TP   **(e)** T1, TP   **(f)** T1+C, TP

10y MC Boxer cross with unlocalized pain and neurologic deficits anatomically localized to T3–L3. Images **b–f** are at the level of the midbody of T7. On CT images, an irregularly margined, predominantly osteoproductive mass involves the left side of the seventh thoracic vertebra (**a–c**: arrows). Ill-defined mineral attenuation, best seen in the narrowly windowed image (**c**: arrowhead), suggests encroachment of the mass into the vertebral canal. The mass is predominantly T1 and T2 hypointense on MR images, consistent with its osteoproductive composition (**d–f**: arrow). Spinal cord compression is best documented on T2 and contrast-enhanced T1 images (**d,f**: small arrowhead). There is minimal peripheral enhancement following intravenous contrast administration (**f**: large arrowhead). Biopsy of the mass confirmed a diagnosis of osteosarcoma.

Figure 3.4.8 Plasmacytoma (Canine)   MR

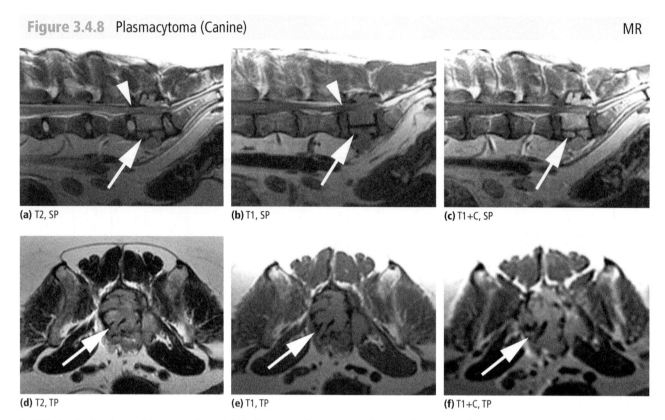

(a) T2, SP   **(b)** T1, SP   **(c)** T1+C, SP

(d) T2, TP   **(e)** T1, TP   **(f)** T1+C, TP

8y FS Labrador Retriever with progressive pelvic limb neuropathy. An expansile mass that is T1 and T2 hyperintense compared to adjacent muscle arises from the body of the seventh lumbar vertebra (**a,b,d,e**: arrow). There is extensive cortical osteolysis, and the mass extends into the vertebral canal, elevating and enveloping the cauda equina (**a,b**: arrowhead). The mass uniformly and intensely enhances following intravenous contrast administration (**c,f**: arrow). Image-guided aspiration biopsy confirmed plasma cell neoplasia.

Figure 3.4.9   Multiple Myeloma (Canine)   CT

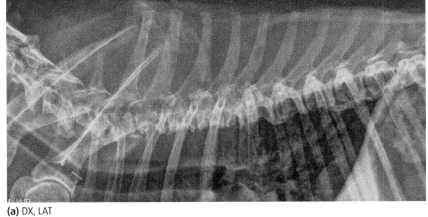

(a) DX, LAT

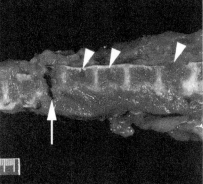

(b) GP, LAT

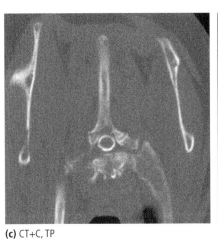

(c) CT+C, TP

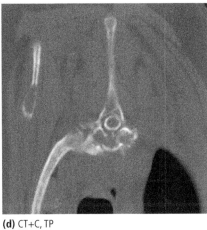

(d) CT+C, TP

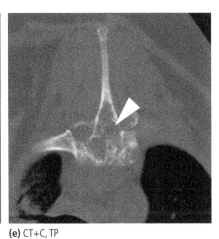

(e) CT+C, TP

12y FS Keeshond with acute paralysis. Survey spinal radiographs show widespread focal and coalescing osteodestructive lesions involving the vertebrae, ribs, and scapulae (**a**). CT myelographic images **c**, **d**, and **e** are at the level of the second, third, and fifth thoracic vertebra, respectively, and further document the multifocal osteolytic lesions in vertebrae, rib heads, and scapular cortices (**c–e**). The subarachnoid contrast column is circumferentially attenuated at the level of T5 (**e**: arrowhead). Postmortem examination confirmed a diagnosis of multiple myeloma and further documented a compression fracture of the fifth thoracic vertebra (**b**: arrow). Medullary and cortical bone destruction is also evident on the gross pathology specimen (**b**: arrowheads).

Figure 3.4.10 Metastatic Prostatic Carcinoma (Canine)

MR

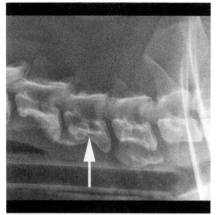

(a) DX, LAT

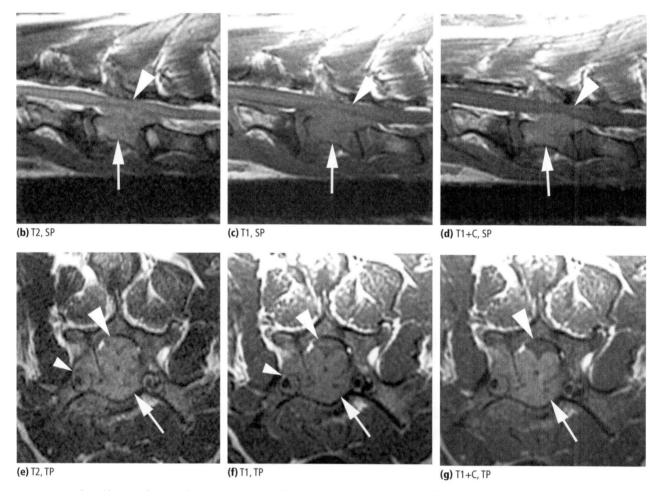

(b) T2, SP

(c) T1, SP

(d) T1+C, SP

(e) T2, TP

(f) T1, TP

(g) T1+C, TP

10y M Rottweiler with cervical pain and progressive paresis of 3–4 weeks' duration. A cytologically confirmed prostatic carcinoma was identified on an abdominal ultrasound examination included as part of the initial diagnostic evaluation. Images **e–g** are through the fifth cervical vertebra. There is reduced opacity of the body of C5 on the survey radiographic examination (**a**: arrow). On MR images, there is an osteodestructive soft-tissue mass arising from the body of C5 that is T2 hyperintense and mildly T1 hyperintense compared to adjacent muscle (**b,c,e,f**: arrow). The mass breaches the dorsal cortex and extends into the floor of the vertebral canal, causing spinal cord compression (**b,c,e,f**: large arrowhead) and also involves the right pedicle and invades the transverse foramen (**e,f**: small arrowhead). The mass is uniformly and intensely enhancing following intravenous contrast administration (**d,g**: arrow), and spinal cord elevation and compression are clearly evident (**d,g**: arrowhead). Postmortem examination confirmed a diagnosis of prostatic carcinoma metastatic to the fifth cervical vertebra.

Figure 3.4.11   Metastatic Hemangiosarcoma (Canine)   MR

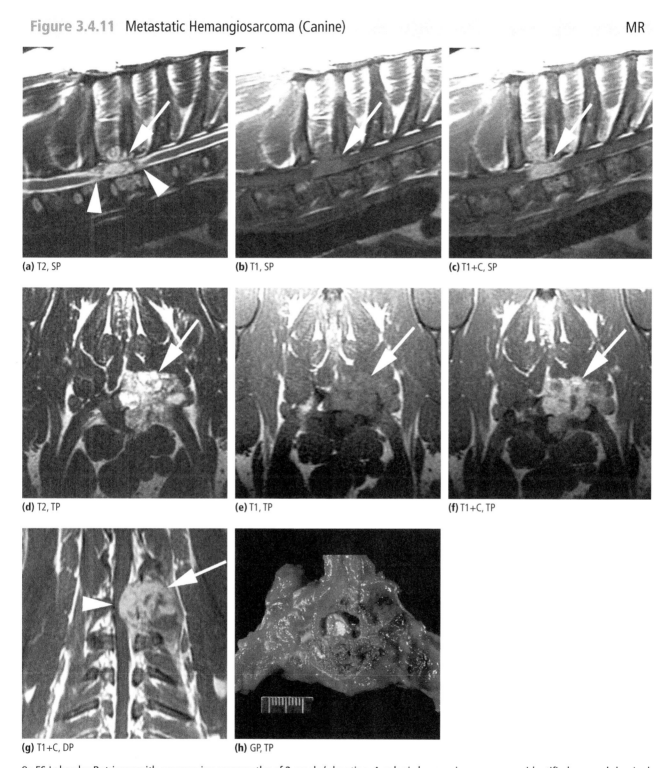

(a) T2, SP

(b) T1, SP

(c) T1+C, SP

(d) T2, TP

(e) T1, TP

(f) T1+C, TP

(g) T1+C, DP

(h) GP, TP

8y FS Labrador Retriever with progressive neuropathy of 2 weeks' duration. A splenic hemangiosarcoma was identified on an abdominal ultrasound examination included as part of the initial diagnostic evaluation. Images **d–f** and **h** are at the level of the second thoracic vertebra. A large, irregularly shaped osteodestructive and expansile mass arises from the left side of the second thoracic vertebra and rib head (**a,b,d,e**: arrow). The mass has heterogeneous T1 and T2 hyperintensity compared to adjacent paraspinal muscle and intensely and nonuniformly enhances following intravenous contrast administration (**c,f,g**: arrow). Axially, it extends into the vertebral canal, causing right-sided spinal cord displacement and compression (**g**: arrowhead). The lateral displacement of the cord without apparent distension of the subarachnoid space suggests an extramedullary localization (**a**: arrowheads). The complex intensity pattern seen in all sequences suggests a hemorrhagic component, which was documented on subsequent gross examination (**h**). Both the splenic mass and the thoracic vertebral mass were histologically confirmed to be hemangiosarcoma.

Figure 3.4.12 Extradural Lymphoma (Canine)   MR

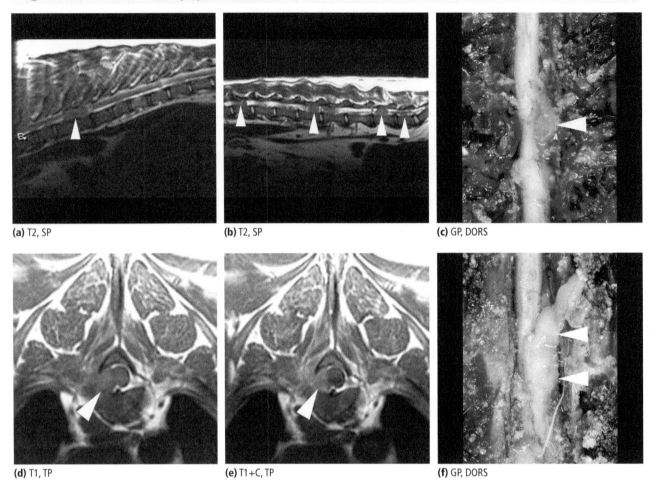

(a) T2, SP

(b) T2, SP

(c) GP, DORS

(d) T1, TP

(e) T1+C, TP

(f) GP, DORS

9y FS Labrador cross with a 2-week history of acute-onset left pelvic limb lameness. Images **d** and **e** are representative transverse images at the level of the fifth thoracic vertebra. Multiple extradural T2 isointense, mildly T1 hyperintense masses are widely distributed within the vertebral canal (**a,b,d**: arrowheads) and uniformly enhance following intravenous contrast administration (**e**: arrowhead). Postmortem examination revealed the extradural masses to be B-cell lymphoma (**c,f**: arrowheads) with widely disseminated multiple organ involvement.

Figure 3.4.13   Extradural Nephroblastoma Metastasis (Canine)   MR

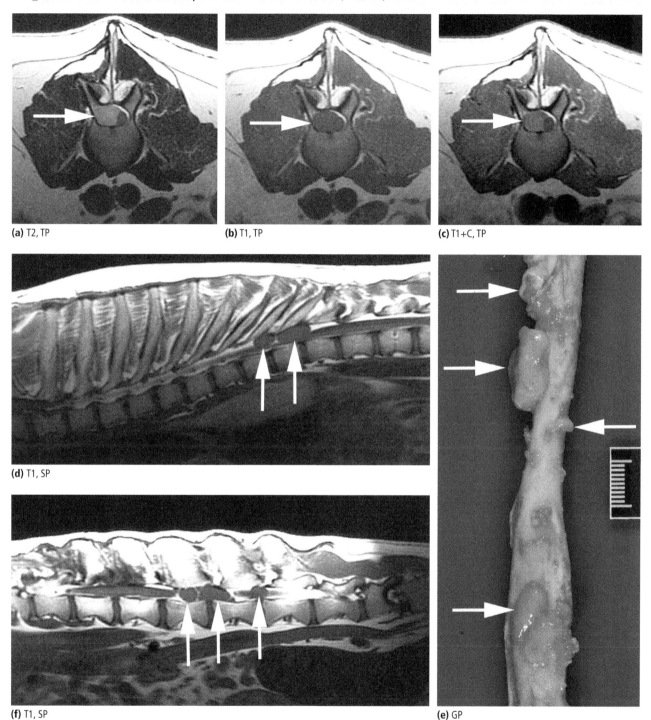

(a) T2, TP

(b) T1, TP

(c) T1+C, TP

(d) T1, SP

(f) T1, SP

(e) GP

2y F Great Dane with history of surgically excised cranial lumbar nephroblastoma 4 months previously. Representative transverse images **a–c** are through the caudal thoracic region. There are multiple T1 isointense, T2 hyperintense, ovoid extradural masses (**a,b,d,f**: arrows) that uniformly enhance following intravenous contrast administration (**c**: arrow). Masses are distributed widely throughout the thoracolumbar vertebral canal and correlate closely with the appearance seen on postmortem examination (**e**: arrows). Masses were confirmed to be extradural nephroblastoma metastases presumably resulting from residual disease or surgical seeding.

Figure 3.4.14   Meningioma (Canine)

CTCT

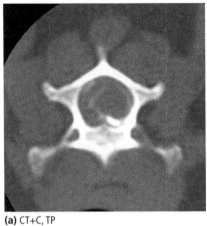

(a) CT+C, TP

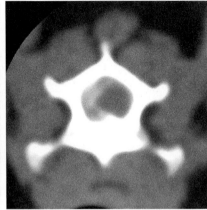

(b) CT+C, TP

12y MC Shih Tzu with progressive neuropathy anatomically localized to C1–C5. A representative CT myelographic image (**a**) at the level of the fifth cervical vertebra shows mild left-sided displacement of the spinal cord and a split contrast column on the right, indicative of an intradural–extramedullary mass. The mass homogeneously enhances following intravenous contrast administration (**b**). Postmortem examination confirmed a crescent-shaped right-sided meningioma extending from C4–C6.

Figure 3.4.15 Meningioma (Canine)

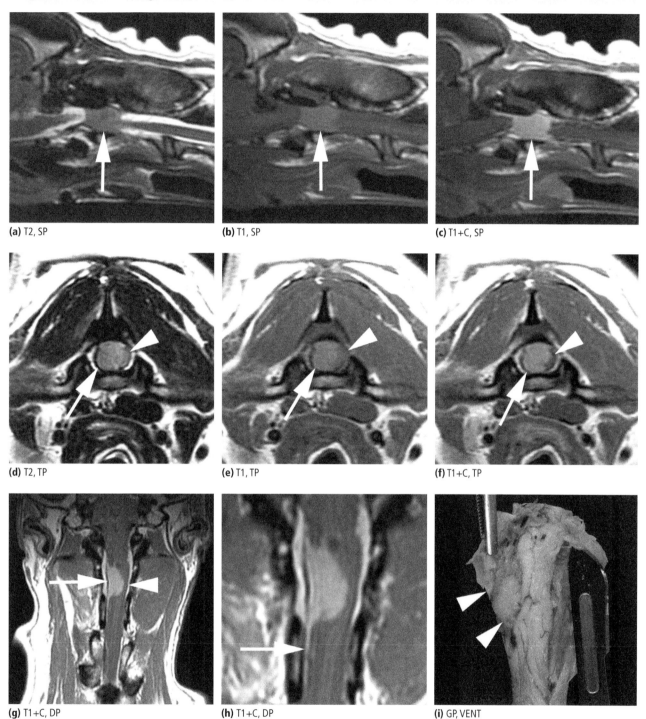

(a) T2, SP

(b) T1, SP

(c) T1+C, SP

(d) T2, TP

(e) T1, TP

(f) T1+C, TP

(g) T1+C, DP

(h) T1+C, DP

(i) GP, VENT

9y FS Boxer with progressive ataxia neuroanatomically localized to C1–C5. Representative transverse images (**d–f**) are at the level of the caudal end of the first cervical vertebra. Image **h** is a magnification of image **g**. There is a large T1 and T2 hyperintense, uniformly contrast-enhancing oval mass within the vertebral canal at the level of C1–C2 (**a–g**: arrow) that results in profound spinal cord compression (**d–g**: arrowhead). A dural tail extends caudally from the mass, indicating meningeal involvement (**h**: arrow). The imaging appearance of the mass mirrors that seen on gross postmortem examination, which establishes its meningeal origin (**i**: arrowheads). The mass was confirmed to be a grade I transitional meningioma.

Figure 3.4.16   Peripheral Nerve Sheath Tumor (Canine)   MR

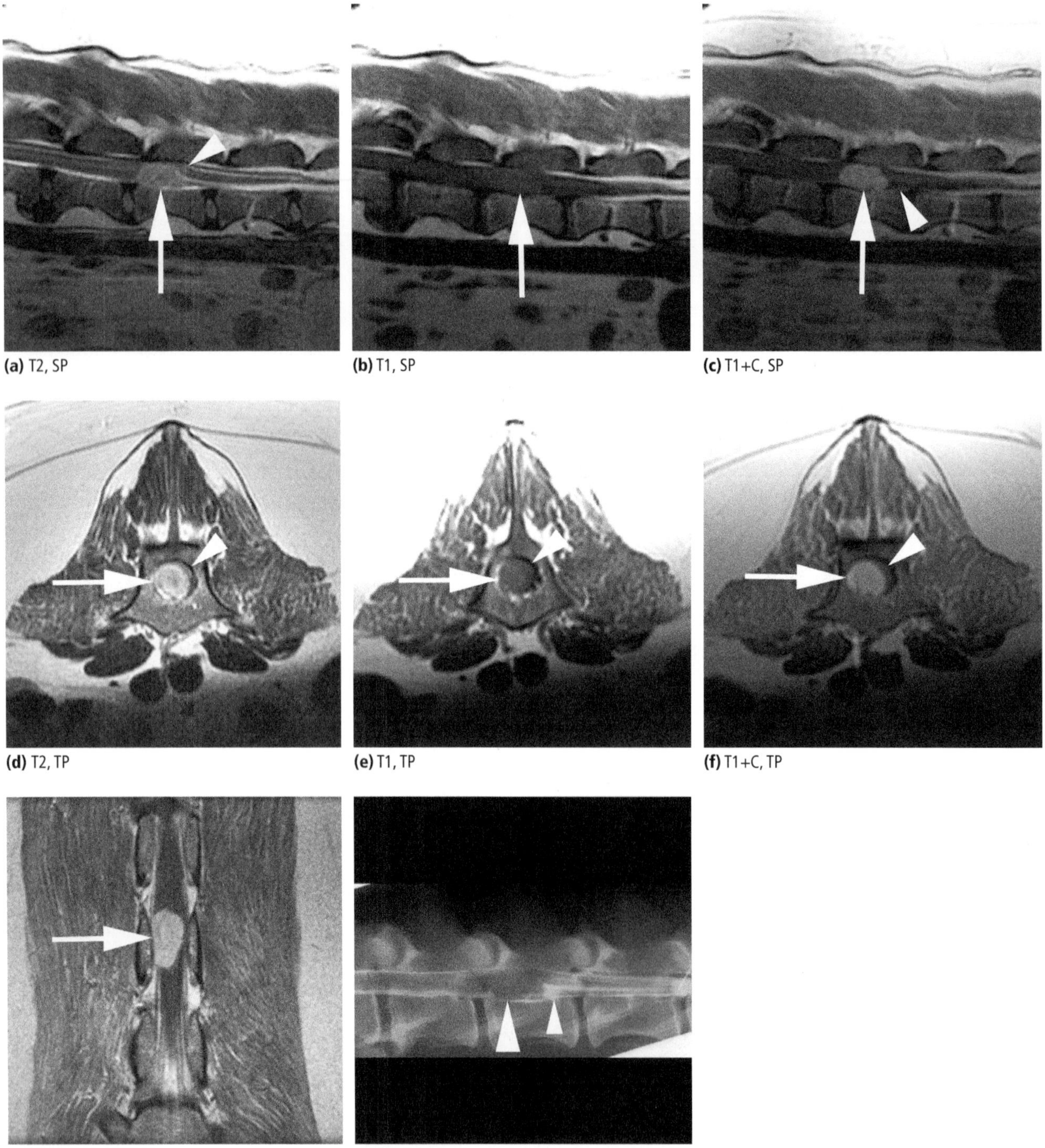

(a) T2, SP

(b) T1, SP

(c) T1+C, SP

(d) T2, TP

(e) T1, TP

(f) T1+C, TP

(g) T1+C, DP

(h) DX+C, LAT

8y FS Siberian Husky cross with slowly progressive pelvic limb gait abnormality. Representative transverse images (d–f) are through the fourth lumbar vertebra. There is a right-sided T2 hyperintense, T1 isointense, uniformly contrast-enhancing mass within the vertebral canal at the level of L4 (a–g: arrow) that results in marked spinal cord compression (d–f: arrowhead). Elevation of the cord (a: arrowhead) and what appears to be focal widening of the subarachnoid space adjacent to the mass (c: arrowhead) suggest it is intradural–extramedullary in location. This is confirmed on conventional myelographic examination, which shows a contrast filling defect (h: large arrowhead) and a "golf tee" sign (h: small arrowhead). Biopsy of the mass confirmed a diagnosis of peripheral nerve sheath tumor.

Figure 3.4.17   Presumptive Peripheral Nerve Sheath Tumor (Canine)   MR

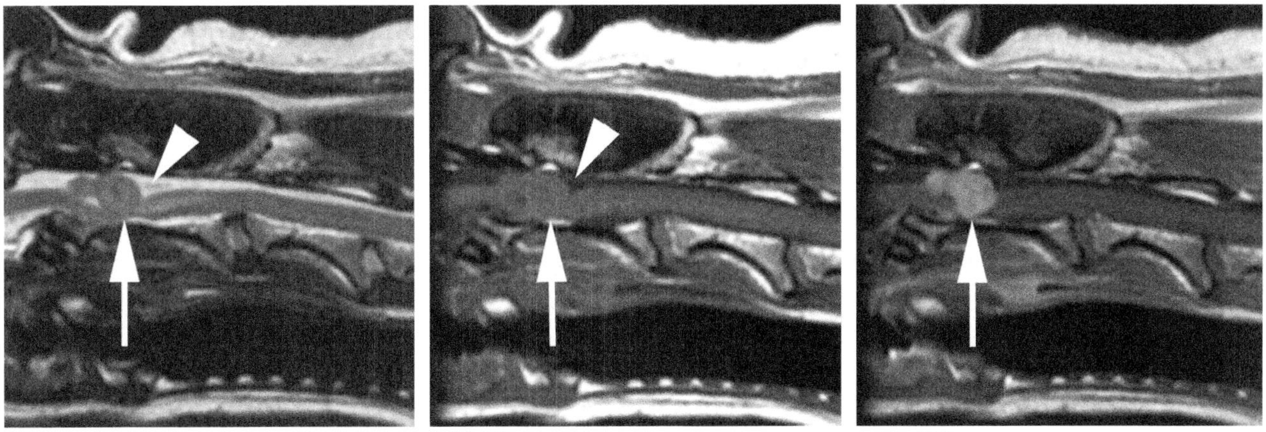

(a) T2, SP

(b) T1, SP

(c) T1+C, SP

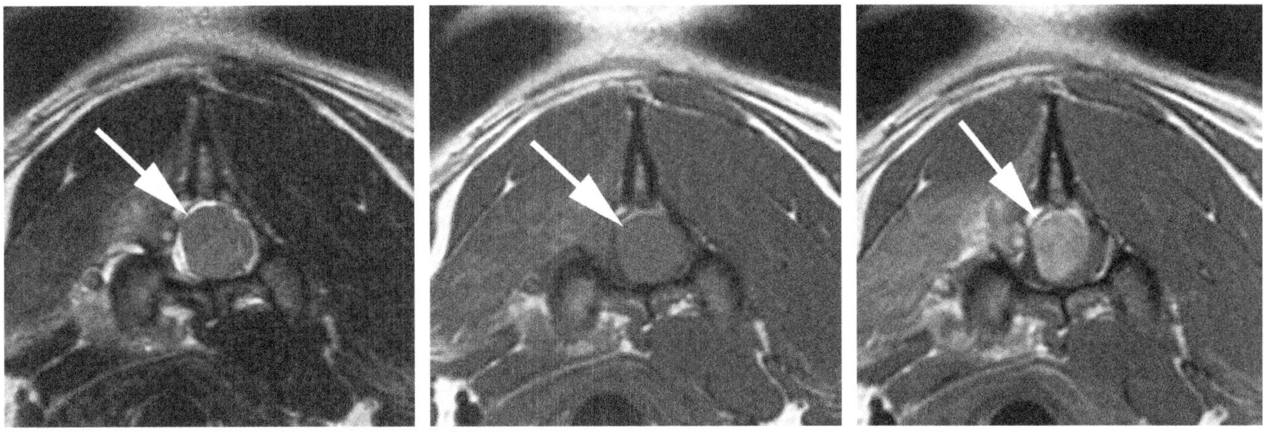

(d) T2, TP

(e) T1, TP

(f) T1+C, TP

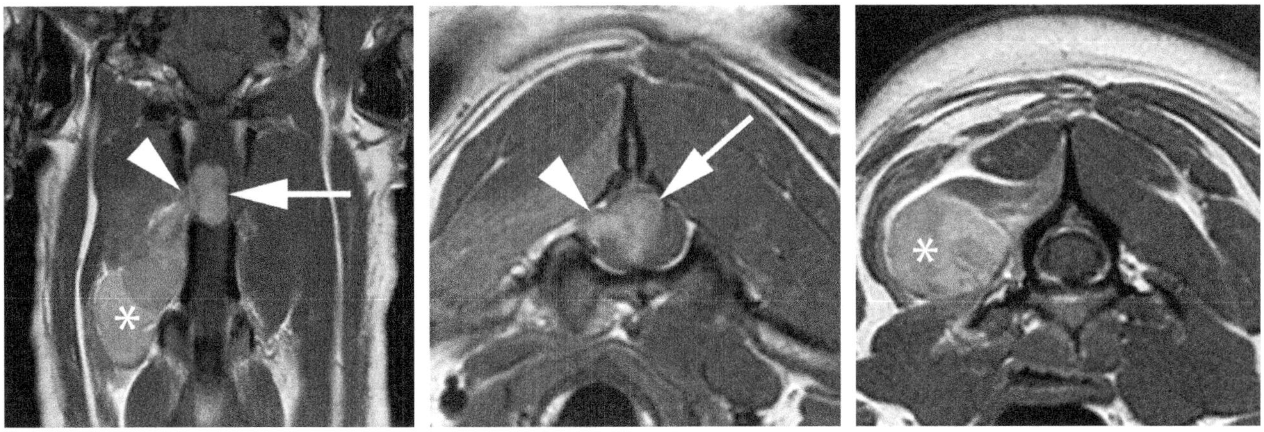

(g) T1+C, DP

(h) T1+C, TP

(i) T1+C, TP

9y FS Border Collie with neck pain and myelopathy neuroanatomically localized to C1–C5. Representative transverse images **d–f** are at the level of the C1–2 articulation. Images **h** and **i** are immediately cranial and caudal, respectively, to images **d–f**. There is a large, lobular, mildly T2 hyperintense, T1 isointense mass within the right dorsal vertebral canal at the level of the C1–2 articulation that intensely enhances following intravenous contrast administration (**a–h**: arrow). The mass has an intradural–extramedullary component, evident from the focal widening of the subarachnoid space adjacent to its caudal margin (**a,b**: arrowhead), and has a narrow extradural stalk that courses through the right intervertebral foramen (**g,h**: arrowheads) before expanding into a larger, lobular juxtavertebral mass (**g,i**: asterisk). Marked spinal cord compression is evident, associated with central T2 hyperintensity immediately caudal to the mass (**a**). A diagnosis of peripheral nerve sheath tumor of the right second spinal nerve was based on imaging features.

Figure 3.4.18 Nephroblastoma (Canine)   MR

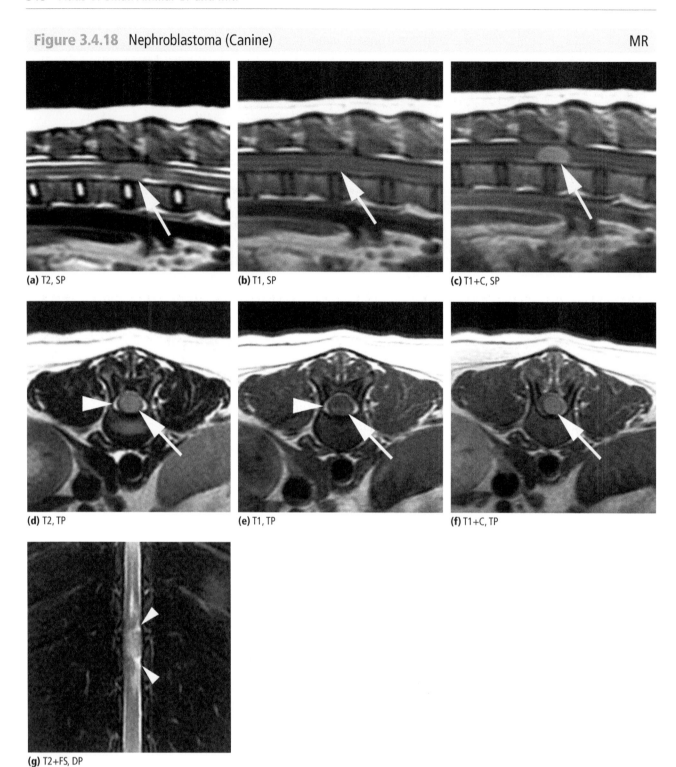

(a) T2, SP

(b) T1, SP

(c) T1+C, SP

(d) T2, TP

(e) T1, TP

(f) T1+C, TP

(g) T2+FS, DP

7mo M West Highland White Terrier with a 2-week history of pelvic limb weakness. Representative transverse images (**d–f**) are at the level of the first lumbar vertebra. MR images show a well-demarcated T2 hyperintense, T1 isointense, uniformly enhancing ovoid mass within the cranial lumbar vertebral canal (**a–f**: arrow). The spinal cord is markedly compressed, but the persistence of epidural fat circumferentially (**d,e**: arrowhead) and flaring of the right cerebrospinal fluid column cranially and caudally (**g**: arrowheads) confirm the mass is intradural–extramedullary. The age of the patient combined with imaging features and the location of the mass make ectopic nephroblastoma the likely diagnosis, which was confirmed on postmortem examination.

Figure 3.4.19 Choroid Plexus Carcinoma Metastasis (Canine)   MR

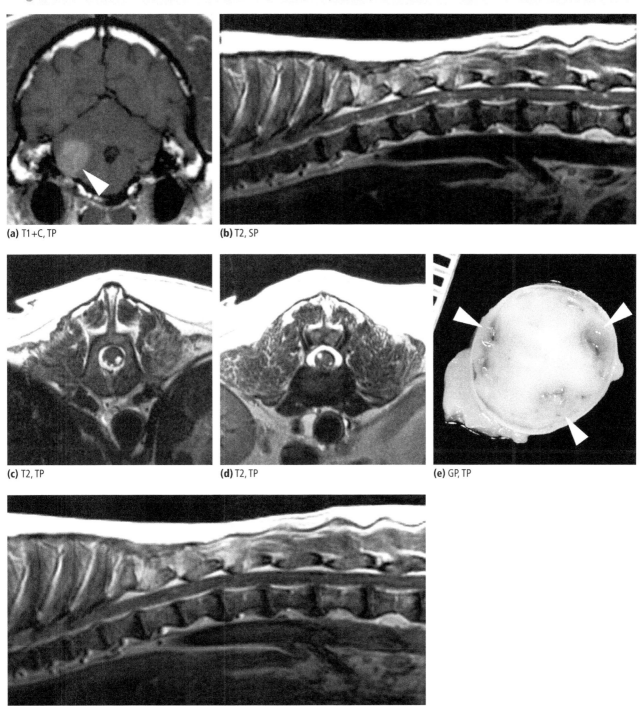

(a) T1+C, TP

(b) T2, SP

(c) T2, TP

(d) T2, TP

(e) GP, TP

(f) T1+C, SP

12y FS English Springer Spaniel with myelopathy neuroanatomically localized to T3–L3. Representative transverse images (**c,d**) are through the lumbar spine. An MR examination of the brain revealed a well-defined, uniformly enhancing caudal fossa mass (**a**: arrowhead). On MR images of the spine, T2 hyperintense (**b–d**), T1 isointense (not shown) military nodules are widely distributed in the periphery of the spinal cord and are intradural in location. Contrast enhancement of the nodules is variable (**f**). Postmortem examination confirmed a choroid plexus carcinoma arising from the right lateral aperture with widespread cerebrospinal fluid disseminated metastasis. Metastatic deposits produced invasive cavitary lesions in the periphery of the spinal cord parenchyma (**e**: arrowheads).

Figure 3.4.20 Intradural Disseminated Histiocytic Sarcoma (Canine)   MR

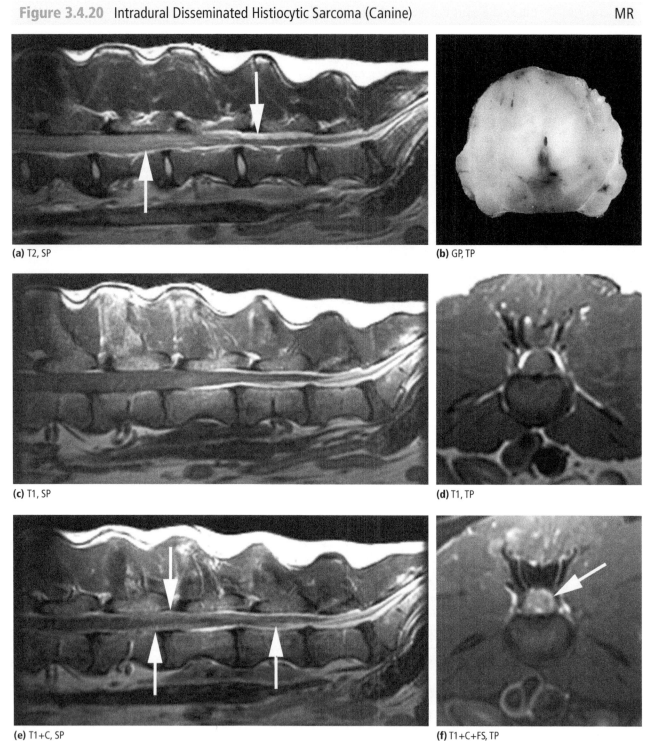

(a) T2, SP

(b) GP, TP

(c) T1, SP

(d) T1, TP

(e) T1+C, SP

(f) T1+C+FS, TP

6y MC Greyhound with myelopathy neuroanatomically localized to L4–caudal. Representative transverse images are at the level of the L4–5 intervertebral disk space. There is diffuse T2 hyperintensity in the caudal lumbar spinal cord and cauda equina (a: arrows) that enhances following intravenous contrast administration (e,f: arrows). The enhancement is plaque-like and appears to be contained by the dura matter. Postmortem examination revealed widely disseminated intradural–extramedullary histiocytic sarcoma. Tumor tissue fills the subarachnoid space circumferentially at the level of the caudal lumbar spinal cord (b). Tzipory et al 2009.[29] Reproduced with permission from Wiley.

Figure 3.4.21 Glioblastoma Multiforme (Feline)   MR

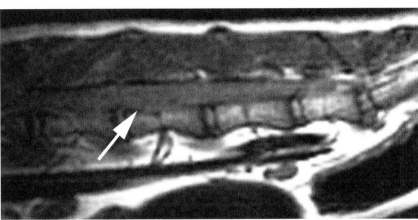

(a) T2, SP

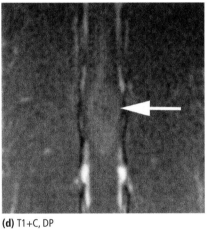

(b) T1+C, TP

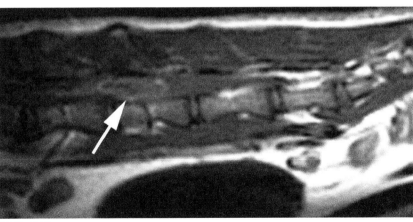

(c) T1, SP

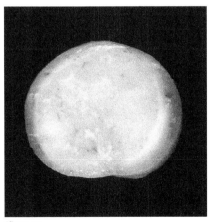

(d) T1+C, DP

(e) T1+C, SP

(f) GP, TP

9y MC Domestic Shorthair with recent-onset progressive pelvic limb paresis. MR images show a T1 isointense, T2 hyperintense, heterogeneously enhancing, ovoid intrinsic spinal cord mass at the level of the fifth lumbar vertebra (**a–e**: arrow). The gross specimen (**f**) shows that the mass displaces neural parenchyma peripherally, resulting in the focal increase in cord diameter seen on MR images (**d**). Microscopic examination confirmed a diagnosis of glioblastoma multiforme (WHO grade IV astrocytoma).

Figure 3.4.22   Grade II Oligodendroglioma (Canine)   MR

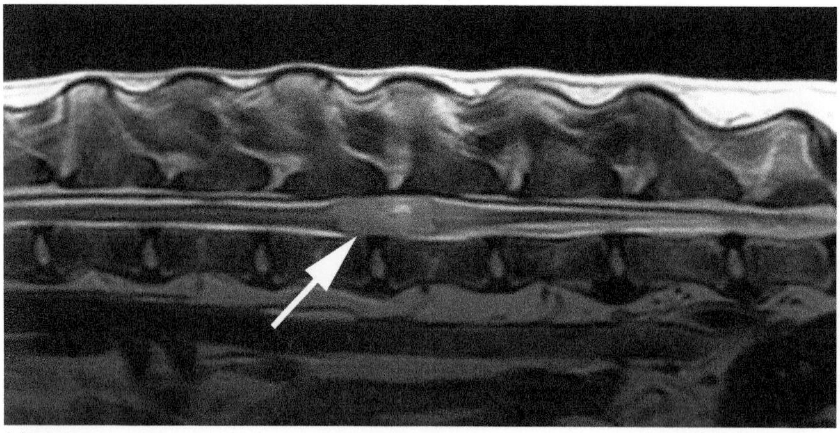

(a) T2, SP

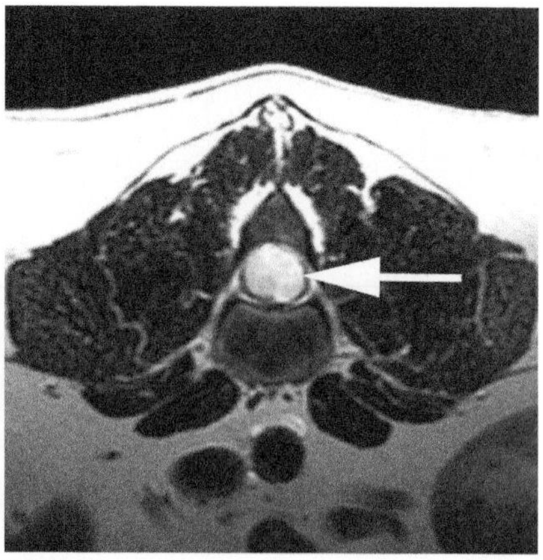

(b) T2, TP

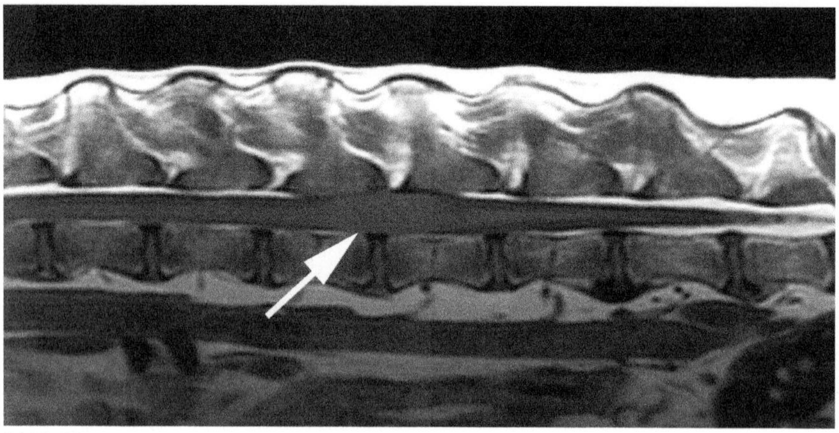

(c) T1, SP

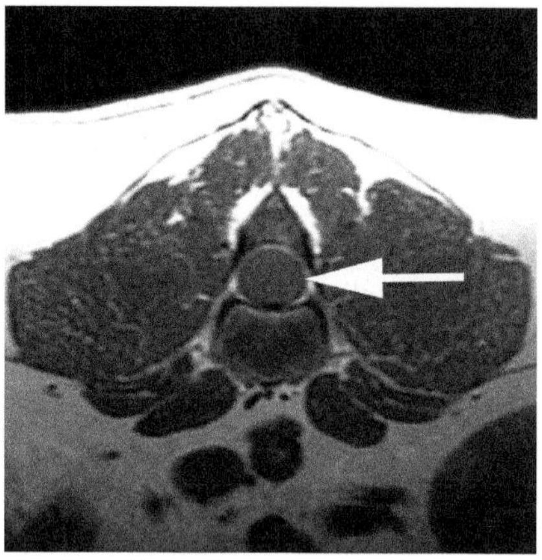

(d) T1, TP

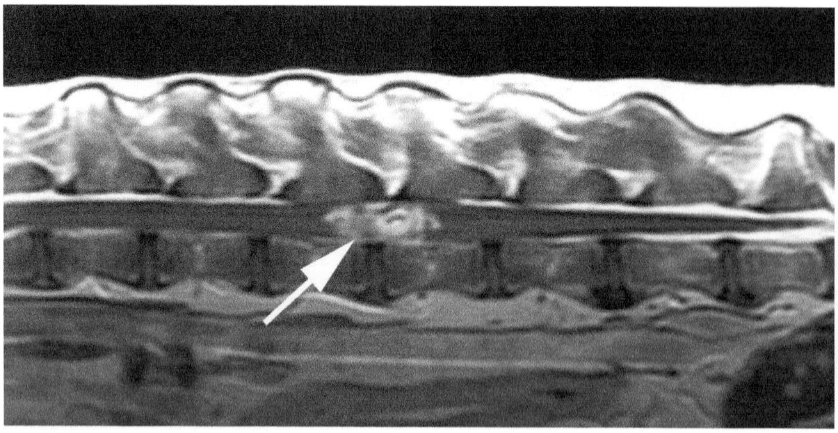

(e) T1+C, SP

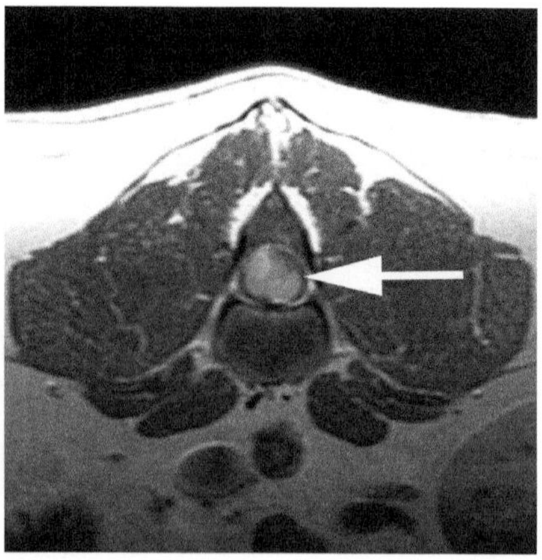

(f) T1+C, TP

8y MC Golden Retriever with 4-month history of progressive pelvic limb paresis. MR images show a T1 isointense, T2 hyperintense, heterogeneously enhancing, ovoid intrinsic spinal cord mass at the level of the L3–4 intervertebral disk space (a–f: arrow). Surgical exposure shows a focal increase in cord diameter consistent with the MR appearance (g: arrowheads). Surgical excisional biopsy confirmed a diagnosis of glioblastoma multiforme WHO grade II oligodendroglioma.

Figure 3.4.22 (*Continued*)   MR

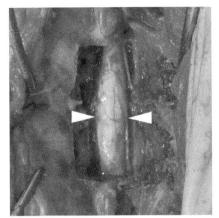

(g) GP, DORS

Figure 3.4.23 Intramedullary Histiocytic Sarcoma (Canine)   MR

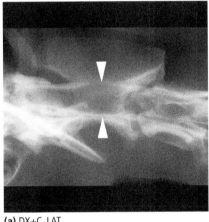 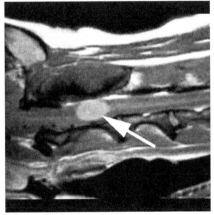 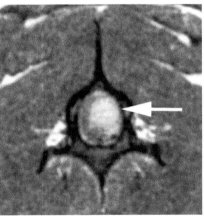

(a) DX+C, LAT   **(b)** T1+C, SP   **(c)** T1+C, TP

11y FS Labrador Retriever with a 3-week history of myelopathy neuroanatomically localized to C1–5. A myelographic examination shows an intrinsic spinal cord mass at the level of the second cervical vertebra causing an increase in cord diameter and attenuation of the subarachnoid contrast columns (a: arrowheads). A well-defined, intensely enhancing intramedullary mass is seen on MR images (b,c: arrow). Postmortem examination revealed a diagnosis of histiocytic sarcoma. The mass was found to have arisen from left of midline within the spinal cord parenchyma, explaining the slightly eccentric appearance on MR images (c).

References

1. Thompson KG, Pool RR. Tumors of Bone. In: Meuten DJ (ed): Tumors in Domestic Animals. Ames, IA: Iowa State Press, 2002;248–255.

2. Davis GJ, Kapatkin AS, Craig LE, Heins GS, Wortman JA. Comparison of radiography, computed tomography, and magnetic resonance imaging for evaluation of appendicular osteosarcoma in dogs. J Am Vet Med Assoc. 2002;220:1171–1176.

3. Karnik KS, Samii VF, Weisbrode SE, London CA, Green EM. Accuracy of computed tomography in determining lesion size in canine appendicular osteosarcoma. Vet Radiol Ultrasound. 2012;53:273–279.

4. Kippenes H, Gavin PR, Bagley RS, Silver GM, Tucker RL, Sande RD. Magnetic resonance imaging features of tumors of the spine and spinal cord in dogs. Vet Radiol Ultrasound. 1999;40:627–633.

5. Wallack ST, Wisner ER, Werner JA, Walsh PJ, Kent MS, Fairley RA, et al. Accuracy of magnetic resonance imaging for estimating intramedullary osteosarcoma extent in pre-operative planning of canine limb-salvage procedures. Vet Radiol Ultrasound. 2002;43:432–441.

6. Healy CF, Murray JG, Eustace SJ, Madewell J, O'Gorman PJ, O'Sullivan P. Multiple myeloma: a review of imaging features and radiological techniques. Bone Marrow Res. 2011;2011:583439.

7. Cooley DM, Waters DJ. Skeletal metastasis as the initial clinical manifestation of metastatic carcinoma in 19 dogs. J Vet Intern Med. 1998;12:288–293.

8. Goedegebuure SA. Secondary bone tumours in the dog. Vet Pathol. 1979;16:520–529.

9. Thompson KG, Pool RR. Tumors of Bone. In: Meuten DJ (ed): Tumors of Domestic Animals. Ames, IA: Iowa State Press, 2002;311–312.

10. Lane SB, Kornegay JN, Duncan JR, Oliver JE, Jr. Feline spinal lymphosarcoma: a retrospective evaluation of 23 cats. J Vet Intern Med. 1994;8:99–104.

11. Marioni-Henry K, Van Winkle TJ, Smith SH, Vite CH. Tumors affecting the spinal cord of cats: 85 cases (1980–2005). J Am Vet Med Assoc. 2008;232:237–243.

12. Marioni-Henry K, Vite CH, Newton AL, Van Winkle TJ. Prevalence of diseases of the spinal cord of cats. J Vet Intern Med. 2004;18:851–858.

13. Northington JW, Juliana MM. Extradural lymphosarcoma in six cats. J Small Anim Pract. 1978;19:409–416.

14. Pancotto TE, Rossmeisl JH, Jr., Zimmerman K, Robertson JL, Werre SR. Intramedullary spinal cord neoplasia in 53 dogs (1990–2010): distribution, clinicopathologic characteristics, and clinical behavior. J Vet Intern Med. 2013;27:1500–1508.

15. Spodnick GJ, Berg J, Moore FM, Cotter SM. Spinal lymphoma in cats: 21 cases (1976–1989). J Am Vet Med Assoc. 1992;200:373–376.

16. Veraa S, Dijkman R, Meij BP, Voorhout G. Comparative imaging of spinal extradural lymphoma in a Bordeaux dog. Can Vet J. 2010;51:519–521.

17. Palus V, Volk HA, Lamb CR, Targett MP, Cherubini GB. MRI features of CNS lymphoma in dogs and cats. Vet Radiol Ultrasound. 2012;53:44–49.

18. Bagley RS. Spinal neoplasms in small animals. Vet Clin North Am Small Anim Pract. 2010;40:915–927.

19. Jose-Lopez R, de la Fuente C, Pumarola M, Anor S. Spinal meningiomas in dogs: description of 8 cases including a novel radiological and histopathological presentation. Can Vet J. 2013;54:948–954.

20. Levy MS, Kapatkin AS, Patnaik AK, Mauldin GN, Mauldin GE. Spinal tumors in 37 dogs: clinical outcome and long-term survival (1987–1994). J Am Anim Hosp Assoc. 1997;33:307–312.

21. Liebel FX, Rossmeisl JH, Jr., Lanz OI, Robertson JL. Canine spinal nephroblastoma: long-term outcomes associated with treatment of 10 cases (1996–2009). Vet Surg. 2011;40:244–252.

22. McDonnell JJ, Tidwell AS, Faissler D, Keating J. Magnetic resonance imaging features of cervical spinal cord meningiomas. Vet Radiol Ultrasound. 2005;46:368–374.

23. Petersen SA, Sturges BK, Dickinson PJ, Pollard RE, Kass PH, Kent M, et al. Canine intraspinal meningiomas: imaging features, histopathologic classification, and long-term outcome in 34 dogs. J Vet Intern Med. 2008;22:946–953.

24. Levy MS, Mauldin G, Kapatkin AS, Patnaik AK. Nonlymphoid vertebral canal tumors in cats: 11 cases (1987–1995). J Am Vet Med Assoc. 1997;210:663–664.

25. Koestner A, Higgins RJ. Tumors of the nervous system. In: Meuten DJ (ed): Tumors of Domestic Animals. Ames, IA: Iowa State Press, 2002;731–735.

26. Hayes HM, Priester WA, Jr., Pendergrass TW. Occurrence of nervous-tissue tumors in cattle, horses, cats and dogs. Int J Cancer. 1975;15:39–47.

27. Brewer DM, Cerda-Gonzalez S, Dewey CW, Diep AN, Van Horne K, McDonough SP. Spinal cord nephroblastoma in dogs: 11 cases (1985–2007). J Am Vet Med Assoc. 2011;238:618–624.

28. Engelhard HH, Corsten LA. Leptomeningeal metastasis of primary central nervous system (CNS) neoplasms. Cancer Treat Res. 2005;125:71–85.

29. Tzipory L, Vernau KM, Sturges BK, Zabka TS, Highland MA, et al. Antemortem diagnosis of localized central nervous system histiocytic sarcoma in 2 dogs. J Vet Intern Med 2009;23:369–74.

3.5

Intervertebral disk disease and other degenerative disorders

Intervertebral disk disease

Intervertebral disk degeneration

The normal intervertebral disk is comprised of four major components: the nucleus pulposus, the annulus fibrosis, a transition zone, and the cartilaginous endplates. The nucleus pulposus is located eccentrically in the disk and has a high mucoprotein and water content. The annulus fibrosis surrounds the nucleus and is composed of multilayered fibrocartilage.[1] The transition zone is located between the mucoid nucleus and the fibrous annulus and appears to be wider and less distinct in chondrodystrophoid breeds.[2] Cartilaginous endplates form the cranial and caudal margins of the disk with fibrous connections to the annulus and the adjacent bony endplates of the vertebrae (Figure 3.5.1). Vascular supply to the intervertebral disk is minimal and limited to outer layers of the annulus.[1] In addition, the dorsal longitudinal ligament courses over the ventral surface of the spinal canal, and intercapital ligaments cross the intervertebral disks from T2–T10.

Deterioration of the extracellular matrix of the intervertebral disk leads to degeneration. As a disk degenerates, the nucleus pulposus and, to a lesser extent, the remainder of the disk dehydrate, causing narrowing of the disk. Nonphysiologic loading of the disk can also lead to annular tears and cartilaginous endplate fissures. Structural changes to the disk lead to herniation or extrusion.[1]

Disk degenerative changes differ between chondrodystrophoid and nonchondrodystrophoid breeds. The nucleus pulposus of chondrodystrophoid breeds undergoes chondroid metaplasia, resulting in a loss of water and hydroelasticity. This process occurs along the entire vertebral column, with dystrophic mineralization a common sequela. Disks of nonchondrodystrophoid breeds tend to undergo fibrous metaplasia, characterized by fibrous collagenization of the nucleus pulposus in concert with annulus fibrosis degeneration.[1-3] Degenerative changes in chondrodystrophoid breeds occur at an earlier age (3–7 years) and in the cervical and thoracolumbar spine, while nonchondrodystrophic degeneration occurs later (6–8 years) and preferentially affects the caudal cervical region and the lumbosacral junction, although thoracolumbar disease also occurs.[2]

Intervertebral disk extrusion and protrusion

Intervertebral disk lesions are classified as type I or type II using a system first introduced by Hansen.[4,5] Hansen's type I disk extrusion occurs when degenerated nucleus pulposus herniates through all layers of a ruptured annulus fibrosis.[2] Type I disease occurs predominately in chondrodystrophic breeds but is also seen in larger nonchondrodystrophic breeds.[2,6,7] Due to the altered physical characteristics of the chondroid metaplastic nucleus pulposus, type I disk extrusion tends to be acute and explosive. Because of the eccentric position of the nucleus within the disk, herniation occurs dorsally into the vertebral canal or dorsolaterally into the intervertebral foramina.

Hansen's type II disk protrusion occurs when fibroid degenerated disk material migrates dorsally or dorsolaterally because of partial tearing or rupture of the annulus. Because the nucleus pulposus is still contained within the remaining annulus fibrosus, disk material is

Atlas of Small Animal CT and MRI, First Edition. Erik R. Wisner and Allison L. Zwingenberger.
© 2015 John Wiley & Sons, Inc. Published 2015 by John Wiley & Sons, Inc.

not extruded, and the dorsal longitudinal ligament remains intact.[2,3] Hansen's type II disk protrusion results from fibrous degeneration and is most common in nonchondrodystrophoid breeds.[2,3]

Extrusion of apparently normal disk material can also occur as a result of physical activity or overt trauma. These are sometimes referred to as high-velocity extrusions because of the force of extrusion and the predominately liquid composition of normal nucleus pulposus. A description of traumatic intervertebral disk disease can be found in Chapter 3.2. Acute spontaneous extrusion of hydrated disk material seemingly unrelated to activity or trauma can also occasionally occur.[8] In one canine study, a variety of nonchondrodystrophic and chondrodystrophic breeds were represented with a median age of 9 years at the time of diagnosis. Clinical signs include acute onset tetraparesis or tetraplegia, and the mid to caudal cervical intervertebral disks are most commonly affected.[8]

Imaging features of Hansen's type I disk extrusion

There are several studies that have compared the accuracy of unenhanced CT, contrast-enhanced CT, MRI, and conventional myelography for detection of Hansen's type I disk herniation.[9–15] Unenhanced CT has been reported to be 89–100% accurate for lesion localization, and CT myelography is slightly better.[7,9,10,15] CT has been shown to be better than conventional myelography for detecting disk herniation in large dogs, but myelography was found to be better in dogs weighing less than 5 kg.[16] Authors of one report found similar detection accuracy for CT myelography and contrast-enhanced CT following intravenous contrast administration.[14] MRI is thought to be the most accurate imaging method, but the degree of improvement compared to CT myelography is minor.[10,13]

CT features of type I disk extrusion include the presence of hyperattenuating disk material in the epidural space, with the density depending on the degree of mineralization. Disk material can migrate horizontally along the floor of the vertebral canal and circumferentially around the spinal cord. Material can also be dorsolaterally extruded into the intervertebral foramina. Depending on the volume and distribution of extruded disk material, the spinal cord is displaced and compressed. Subarachnoid contrast columns are attenuated at the site of compression on CT myelography. Diffuse alterations with mixed attenuation in the epidural space can be seen in acute disease associated with hemorrhage, and edema can cause an increase in cord diameter. The affected intervertebral disk space is often narrowed, and residual mineralized *in situ* disk material is sometimes present (Figures 3.5.2, 3.5.3, 3.5.4, 3.5.5).[10,17]

Similar features are seen on MR images, with disk material appearing T1 and T2 hypointense. Attenuation of the T2 hyperintense cerebrospinal fluid layer occurs at the site of cord compression, and T2 hyperintensity of cord parenchyma may also be seen as a result of edema. When present, hemorrhage appears as variable, mixed T1 and T2 intensity (Figure 3.5.6, 3.5.7, 3.5.8, 3.5.9, 3.5.10).[18] Other uninvolved disks will appear T2 hypointense because of disk dehydration.

Imaging features of Hansen's type II disk protrusion

CT may be less accurate for detecting type II disk protrusions according to one report.[9] CT features include a variable decrease in intervertebral disk space width and a mildly hyperattenuating mass arising from the dorsal aspect of the affected disk and extending into the ventral or ventrolateral vertebral canal. The bulging annulus cannot be distinguished from the overlying dorsal longitudinal ligament. The spinal cord is displaced, and its shape is often distorted by impingement of the disk even when overt compression is absent. Contrast columns are attenuated at the site of impingement or compression on CT myelographic images.

MR features of type II disk protrusions are similar to those seen on CT images. Protruding disk material is T1 and T2 hypointense and appears contiguous with *in situ* disk material and the overlying longitudinal ligament. The spinal cord can be displaced, distorted, and compressed, and the T2 hyperintense cerebrospinal fluid columns are attenuated at the site of protrusion. It is common to see multiple sites of involvement with varying degrees of disk protrusion, and in these patients it can be useful to use a single-shot turbo spin-echo sequence as a "rich man's myelogram" to localize the clinically relevant site (Figure 3.5.11).[19] In patients with chronic disease, the spinal cord can be focally atrophic, with syringohydromyelia and T2 parenchymal intensity suggesting gliosis. Uninvolved disks are often T2 hypointense because of dehydration.

Imaging features of hydrated nucleus pulposus extrusion

MR imaging features include narrowing of the intervertebral disk, T2 hyperintensity of extruded disk material that is difficult to distinguish from epidural fat, and a characteristic "seagull sign" on T2 transverse images representing the dorsal margin of the extruded material. Extrusion results in spinal cord compression, and many dogs have intrinsic T2 hyperintensity at the site of compression (Figure 3.5.12).[8]

Cauda equina and lumbosacral disorders

Static and dynamic lumbosacral abnormalities that cause cauda equina syndrome include intervertebral disk protrusion, lumbosacral subluxation, vertebral canal stenosis, proliferation of soft tissues within or adjacent to the vertebral canal, and spondylotic new bone encroachment on the intervertebral foramina.[20] Large-breed male dogs are most commonly affected, and German Shepherd Dogs are highly overrepresented.[20–22] The lumbosacral angle of inclination, decreased lumbosacral joint mobility, articular process joint angle, and the presence of transitional vertebrae and sacral endplate osteochondrosis have all been postulated as inciting anatomical factors. Dogs with cauda equina syndrome are more likely to have a more sagittally oriented articular facet angle, a greater difference in caudal lumbar and sacral spine angle, and asymmetry of the facet articulations.[23,24] The caudal lumbar and sacral vertebral canal transverse areas, normalized to vertebral body sagittal diameter or transverse vertebral body area, have also been shown to be significantly smaller in dogs with cauda equina syndrome as compared to clinically normal dogs.[25] CT examinations acquired in hindlimb flexion and extension have been used to assess dynamic changes in vertebral canal diameter and intervertebral foraminal area in dogs with lumbosacral disease.[25–28] The L7–S1 intervertebral foraminal area is significantly smaller on extended limb images, suggesting that positional imaging studies may be useful for diagnosis of dynamic foraminal nerve entrapment.[27]

Imaging features of the lumbosacral region of dogs with cauda equina syndrome are highly variable. Although there seems to be excellent agreement between CT and MR for detection of intervertebral disk protrusion or extrusion, dural sac position, quantity of epidural fat, and spinal nerve root swelling, the correlation of these features with surgical findings is only moderate.[22]

CT examinations should include thinly collimated transverse images through the caudal lumbar and sacral region acquired at an angle perpendicular to the vertebral canal. CT features associated with cauda equina syndrome include lumbar spine (LS) subluxation, intervertebral disk degeneration and extrusion, spondylosis, reduction of vertebral canal transverse area (primarily due to reduced canal height) at the level of the LS junction, and loss of distinction of nerve roots at the LS junction due to diminished epidural fat. Extruded intervertebral disk material can migrate into the caudal lumbar and LS intervertebral foramina causing nerve root compression and resulting lateralized clinical signs. Extruded disk material is hyperattenuating and displaces the relatively low attenuating epidural fat in the vertebral canal and intervertebral foramina.

MR imaging features are similar to those seen with CT. Nerve roots of the cauda equina are T1 and T2 hypointense relative to surrounding epidural fat and are therefore well visualized on both sequences in the normal dog. Vertebral canal and intervertebral foraminal T1 and T2 intensity is reduced when epidural fat is displaced because of intervertebral disk extrusion/protrusion, stenosis, or subluxation. In addition to standard sequences, a 3D volume acquisition (e.g. T1 + C SPGR) of the lumbosacral junction provides thinly collimated images that can provide more in-plane anatomical detail and be reformatted in other planes. Neuritis is sometimes detected because of enlargement and increased contrast enhancement compared to the contralateral spinal nerve. A dorsal plane, STIR, or fat-suppressed contrast-enhanced T1 sequence generally provides an excellent symmetrical view of the caudal lumbar spinal cord, the cauda equina, and associated spinal nerves when performed with thin collimation (≤2 mm) (Figures 3.5.13, 3.5.14).

Other degenerative disorders of the spine

Articular facet osteoarthrosis

Osteoarthrosis of the articular facets can occur as a progressive geriatric disorder or as the sequela of an underlying disorder, such as cervical spondylomyelopathy or trauma. General features of osteoarthrosis include periarticular new bone formation, subchondral bone sclerosis, enthesopathy, and synovial hypertrophy. This proliferation can result in dorsolateral spinal cord compression. CT and MR features of degenerative joint disease are addressed in Chapter 6.5.

Spondylosis deformans

Spondylosis deformans is characterized by progressive new bone formation that bridges adjacent vertebral bodies and is usually distributed on the ventral and lateral surfaces of the affected vertebrae. Although spondylosis deformans is generally considered clinically insignificant, encroachment of lateralized new bone on intervertebral foramina can result in nerve root entrapment with subsequent clinical signs. Distribution is most common in the thoracic and lumbar spine and at the lumbosacral junction.[29–31] A study assessing the relationship of spondylosis and intervertebral disk disease (IVDD) found a weak positive association in dogs with type II IVDD but no correlation in dogs with type I IVDD.[32]

CT features of spondylosis deformans include hyperattenuating new bone formation contiguous with the ventral margins of affected vertebrae. New bone may be incompletely or completely bridging depending on the stage of progression and will often have delineated cortical and medullary components. Associated intervertebral disks can be narrowed, and disk material can be mineralized. MR features are structurally similar to those seen with CT. New bone has variable T1 and T2 signal intensity depending on bone density. If degenerate, associated intervertebral disks can be narrowed and have reduced T2 signal intensity.

Disseminated idiopathic skeletal hyperostosis

As the name implies, the underlying cause for disseminated idiopathic skeletal hyperostosis (DISH) is unknown. Diagnosis in people is based on several radiographic criteria:

- the presence of flowing ossification on the anterolateral (ventrolateral) margins of at least four adjacent vertebrae with or without associated localized pointed excrescences at the intervening vertebral body/intervertebral disk junctions;
- relative preservation of intervertebral disk height (width) and absence of degenerative changes;
- absence of other associated signs of spinal degenerative disease.[33]

There are only sporadic reports of DISH in the veterinary literature, and there appears to be no consensus of what imaging features constitute the syndrome in dogs and cats.[34–37] Using the criteria defined in the human literature, new bone formation seen on CT and MR images will appear similar to that described for mature spondylosis but will span a minimum of four adjacent vertebrae (Figure 3.5.15).

Extrinsic cysts

Facet synovial cysts

Synovial cysts occasionally arise from the articular facet joints and can extend into the extradural space of the vertebral canal. Cyst formation appears to be a sequela of degenerative joint disease of the vertebral facet articulations.[38] Although sometimes seen as an incidental finding, synovial cysts have been implicated as a cause or exacerbating factor in spinal cord compression in dogs with cervical spondylomyelopathy.[38–40] They have also been reported as a cause of spinal nerve compression in dogs with cauda equina signs.[41,42]

CT features include a well-defined, usually ovoid, fluid-attenuating mass in the extradural space associated with a vertebral articulation. Synovial cysts appear as T1 hypointense, T2 hyperintense thin-walled cystic masses on MR images (Figure 3.5.16). Cyst walls will variably enhance.[38,41,42]

Spinal meningeal cysts

Meningeal cysts are diverticula of the arachnoid or dura mater or of a spinal nerve root sheath. In people, cysts can occur at any level of the spinal cord but are often located at the level of the lower lumbar cord or sacrum and are classified as type I (an extradural meningeal cyst that does not contain neural tissue), type II (an extradural cyst that contains neural tissue), and type III (an intradural arachnoid cyst).[43,44] Although type I and type II cysts have not been reported in veterinary medicine, type III cysts seem to closely resemble spinal arachnoid diverticula described in dogs.[45] In recent retrospective reports, diverticula typically occur in the dorsal subarachnoid space at the first to third cervical vertebrae of young, large-breed dogs or the caudal thoracic vertebrae of older, small-breed dogs and are most often located dorsal to the spinal cord.[45,46] Although the etiology of arachnoid diverticula is unclear, it appears that some are likely developmental, while others are acquired.[45,46] Regardless of type, meningeal cysts are thin-walled and contain cerebrospinal fluid, and because of their similarity in appearance to other types of spinal cysts, they are included in this chapter.

On CT images in people, type I and II meningeal cysts are well-defined, ovoid, fluid-attenuating masses that are well delineated by surrounding extradural fat. Cysts will uniformly enhance on CT myelographic studies because of direct communication with the subarachnoid space. MR features include a uniform, thin-walled T1 hypointense and T2 hyperintense mass. No enhancement would be expected following intravenous contrast administration with either imaging modality.

Myelography of spinal arachnoid diverticula, similar to type III cysts in people, results in a teardrop-shaped widening of the dorsal contrast column in those cysts that communicate with the subarachnoid space (25/36 in one review).[46] Similar focal fluid collections are seen on CT images associated with varying degrees of spinal cord compression. MR features include focal T1 hypointense, T2 hyperintense fluid collections, most of which signal attenuate on FLAIR sequences (Figure 3.5.17).[46]

Figure 3.5.1 Normal Intervertebral Disks (Canine)   MR

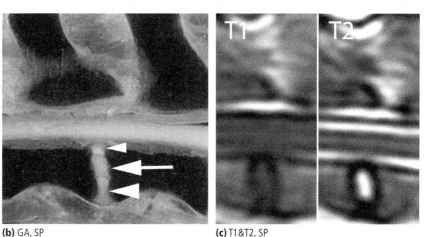

(a) GA, LAT   **(b)** GA, SP   **(c)** T1&T2, SP

The gross appearance of the dorsal annulus fibrosis (**a,b**: small arrowhead), the nucleus pulposus (**a,b**: arrow), and ventral annulus fibrosis (**a,b**: large arrowhead). Compare the appearance of the intervertebral disk in image **b** to the appearance on T1 (**c**: T1) and T2 (**c**: T2) images acquired in the same anatomic plane.

Figure 3.5.2 Mineralized Type I Extrusion (Canine)   CT

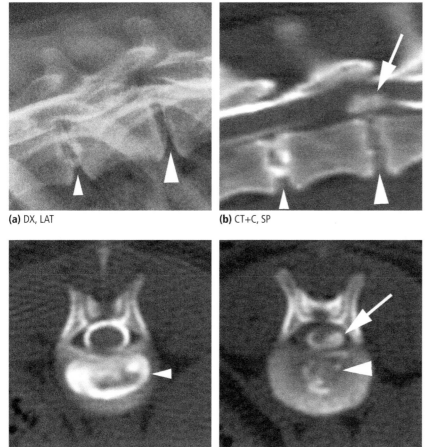

(a) DX, LAT   **(b)** CT+C, SP

(c) CT+C, TP   **(d)** CT+C, TP

5y MC Dachshund found acutely paretic earlier in the day with neuroanatomic localization to T3–L3. Images **a** and **b** include the T11–12 and T12–13 intervertebral disk spaces. Images **c** and **d** are through the T11–12 and T12–13 disks, respectively. CT images were acquired as part of a CT myelogram. An *in situ* mineralized nucleus pulposus is present at the T11–12 intervertebral disk space (**a–c**: small arrowhead). Mineralized disk material from the T12–13 intervertebral disk space has herniated into the ventral subdural space of the vertebral canal, causing focal spinal cord compression with attenuation of the contrast columns (**b,d**: arrow). The T12–13 disk space is narrow and contains residual mineralized disk material (**a,b,d**: large arrowhead).

A hemilaminectomy performed at T12–13 confirmed mineralized disk material within the extradural space. Adjacent disks were fenestrated.

Figure 3.5.3 Mineralized Type I Extrusion (Canine)   CT

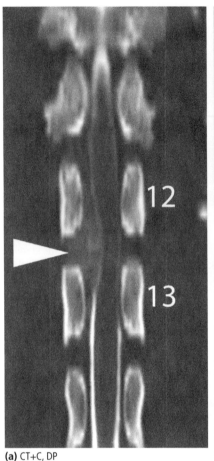

(a) CT+C, DP

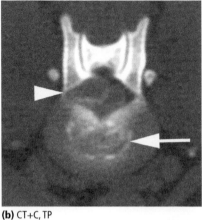

(b) CT+C, TP

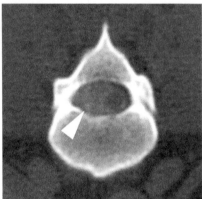

(c) CT+C, TP

9y M Basset Hound with acute onset para-paresis beginning 1 week previously. Neuroanatomic localization is to T3–L3. Image **a** is centered on the T12–13 intervertebral disk space (**a**: 12,13). Image **b** is through the T12–13 disk, and image **c** is through the midbody of T12. Images were acquired as part of a CT myelogram. A large mass of partially mineralized disk material has been extruded into the right side of the vertebral canal extradural space, causing lateralized spinal cord compression (**a,b**: arrowhead). Some disk material has migrated cranially and can be seen within the midbody of T12 (**c**: arrowhead). The T12–13 disk space contains residual mineralized disk material (**b**: arrow).

A double hemilaminectomy performed at T12–L1 revealed a combination of mineralized disk material and old hemorrhage within the extradural space. Adjacent disks were fenestrated.

Figure 3.5.4 Type I Disk Extrusion with a Foraminal Component (Canine)   CT

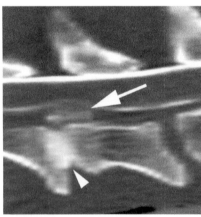

(a) CT+C, SP

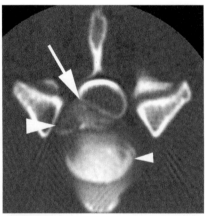

(b) CT+C, TP

11y MC Golden Retriever with acute-onset cervical pain. Initially lame on the right thoracic limb but is now nonambulatory. Image **a** includes the C5–6 and C6–7 intervertebral disk spaces. Image **b** is through the C5–6 disk. Images were acquired as part of a CT myelogram. Mineralized disk material from the C5–6 intervertebral disk space has herniated into the right ventral extradural space of the vertebral canal, causing focal spinal cord impingement with attenuation of the contrast columns (**a,b**: arrow). Part of the herniated disk material also extends into the right intervertebral foramen, potentially compressing the origin of the right sixth cervical spinal nerve (**b**: large arrowhead). The C5–6 disk space contains residual mineralized disk material (**a,b**: small arrowhead). Ventral slot decompression surgery was performed at C5–6, and a large quantity of mineralized disk material was removed.

Figure 3.5.5 Type I Disk Extrusion with Hemorrhage (Canine)

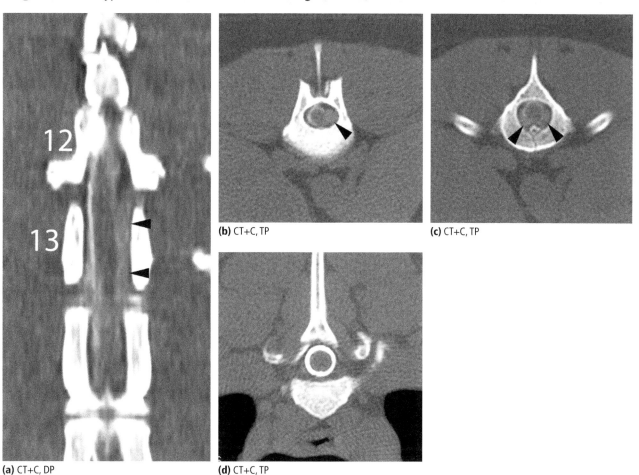

(a) CT+C, DP

(b) CT+C, TP

(c) CT+C, TP

(d) CT+C, TP

2y FS Corgi with acute-onset paraplegia neuroanatomically localized to T3–L3. Image **a** is centered on the T12–13 intervertebral disk space (**a**: 12,13). Images **b** and **c** are at the cranial end and midbody of T13, respectively. Image **d** is at the level of the midthoracic vertebral column. Images were acquired as part of a CT myelogram. There is moderately attenuating material in the caudal thoracic and cranial lumbar extradural space (**a–c**: arrowheads) producing right-sided spinal cord displacement and compression. The subarachnoid contrast column is circumferentially attenuated at this level (**a–c**). The spinal cord and contrast column appear normal more cranially (**d**). A double hemilaminectomy was performed at T11–T13, and disk material that had extruded from the T12–13 disk space and dispersed from T11 to L1 was removed from the extradural space. There was also extensive hemorrhage and regional spinal cord swelling. Neurologic status declined postoperatively, and postmortem examination revealed severe regional myelomalacia and extradural/subdural hemorrhage.

Figure 3.5.6   Mineralized Type I Disk Extrusion (Canine)   MR

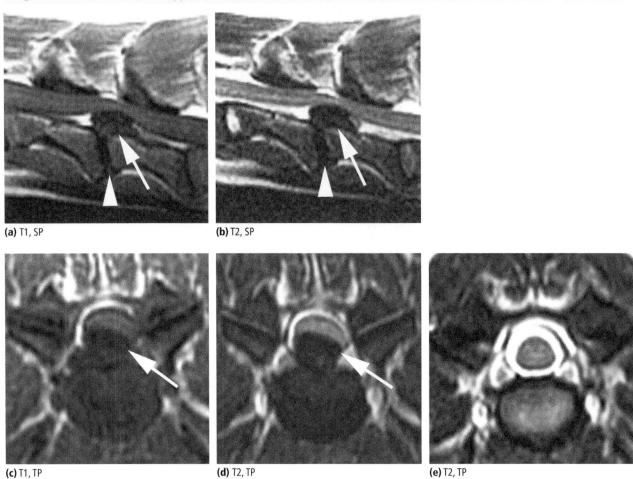

(a) T1, SP

(b) T2, SP

(c) T1, TP

(d) T2, TP

(e) T2, TP

10y MC Alaskan Malamute cross with progressive cervical pain and recent ataxia and paresis neuroanatomically localized to C1–C5. Images **a** and **b** are centered on the C4–5 intervertebral disk space. Images **c** and **d** are through the C4–5 disk, and image **e** is through the C3–4 disk. A large volume of T1 and T2 hypointense disk material has been extruded into the ventral extradural space of the vertebral canal at C4–5, causing dorsal displacement and compression of the spinal cord (**a–d**: arrow). The C4–5 disk space is narrow and hypointense (**a,b**: arrowhead). The normal appearance of the spinal cord and surrounding T2 hyperintense subarachnoid space is shown in image **e**. Ventral slot decompression surgery was performed at C4–5, and a large volume of mineralized disk material was removed.

Figure 3.5.7 Mineralized Type I Disk Extrusion (Canine)   MR

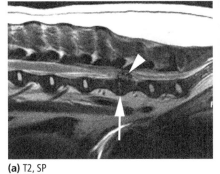

(a) T2, SP

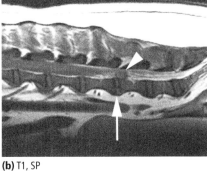

(b) T1, SP

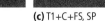

(c) T1+C+FS, SP

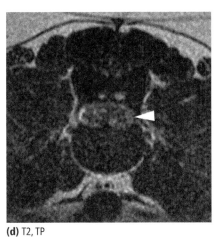

(d) T2, TP

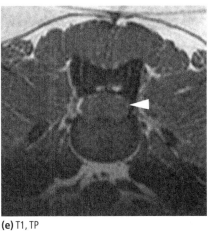

(e) T1, TP

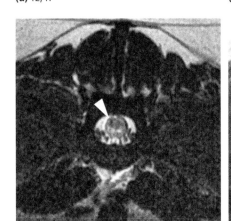

(f) T2, TP

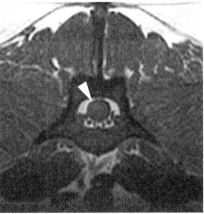

(g) T1, TP

5y Jack Russell Terrier with a 2-week history of progressive pelvic limb ataxia and paraparesis neuroanatomically localized to L6–caudal. Vertebral column radiographs (not shown) revealed the dog had eight lumbar vertebrae. Images **d** and **e** are at the level of the L6–7 intervertebral disk. Images **f** and **g** are at the level of the midbody of the sixth lumbar vertebra. The L6–7 intervertebral disk is T2 hypointense and narrow (**a,b**: arrow). A large mass of T1 and T2 hypointense mineralized disk material has extruded from the L6–7 space, causing elevation and compression of the terminus of the conus medullaris and associated nerves of the cauda equina (**a,b,d,e**: arrowhead). The conus and cauda equina are in a more normal position cranial to the disk extrusion, but mixed signal intensity within the conus on both T1 and T2 images suggests hemorrhage (**f,g**: arrowhead). Local contrast enhancement adjacent to the extruded disk material is indicative of a traumatic inflammatory response (**c**: arrowhead). A hemilaminectomy performed at L6–7 confirmed the presence of extruded disk material within the extradural space.

Figure 3.5.8 Type I Disk Extrusion (Canine)   MR

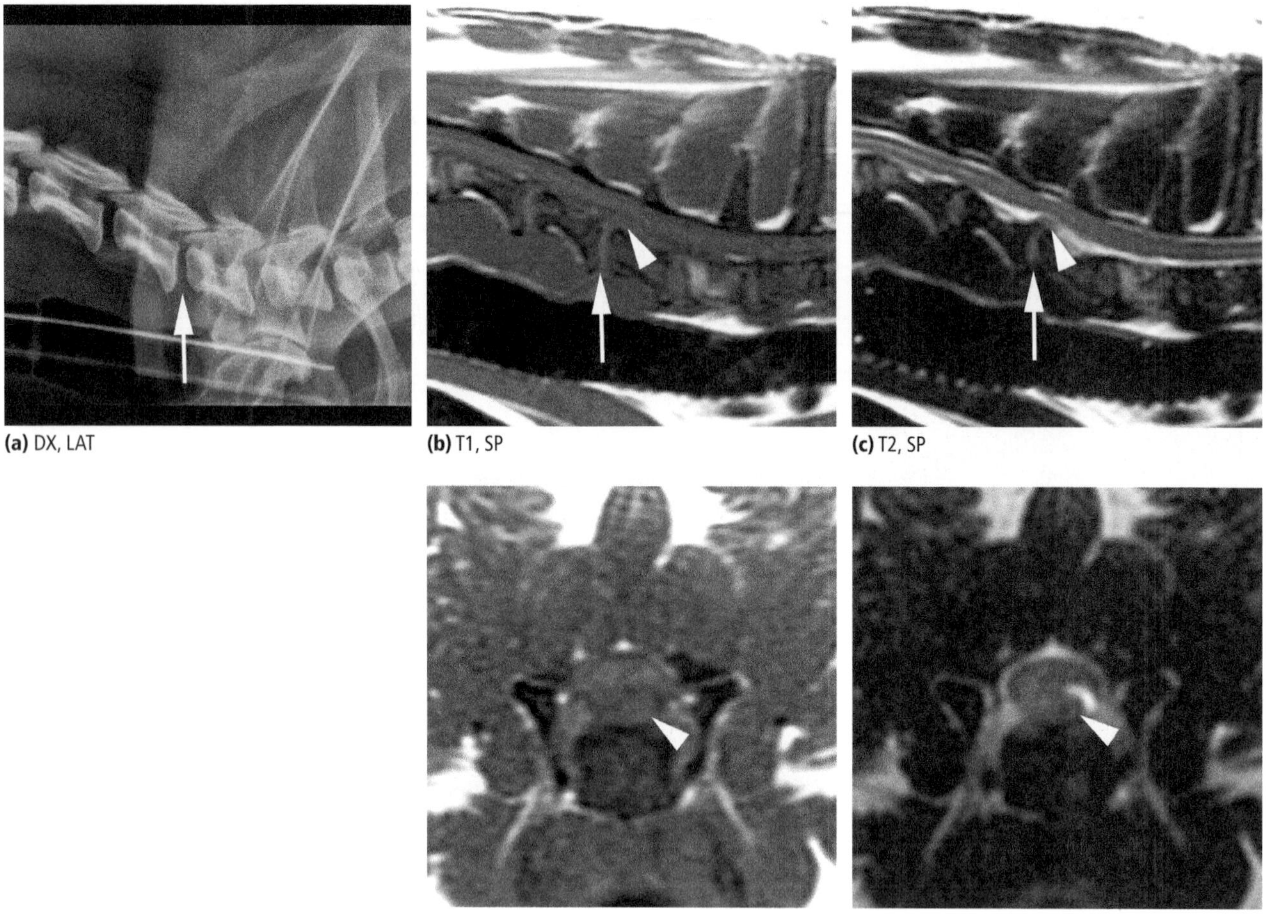

(a) DX, LAT

(b) T1, SP

(c) T2, SP

(d) T1, TP

(e) T2, TP

13y MC Miniature Dachshund with progressive neurologic deficits of 10 days duration. The dog became acutely worse and now has marked tetraparesis. Images **d** and **e** are at the level of the C5–6 intervertebral disk. The C5–6 intervertebral disk space is narrow (**a–c**: arrow). Mildly T1 and T2 hypointense extruded disk material (**b–e**: arrowhead) compresses and displaces the spinal cord dorsally. Ventral slot decompression surgery was performed at C5–6, and partially mineralized disk material was removed from the ventral extradural space.

Figure 3.5.9   Mineralized Type I Disk Extrusion with Foraminal Migration (Canine)   MR

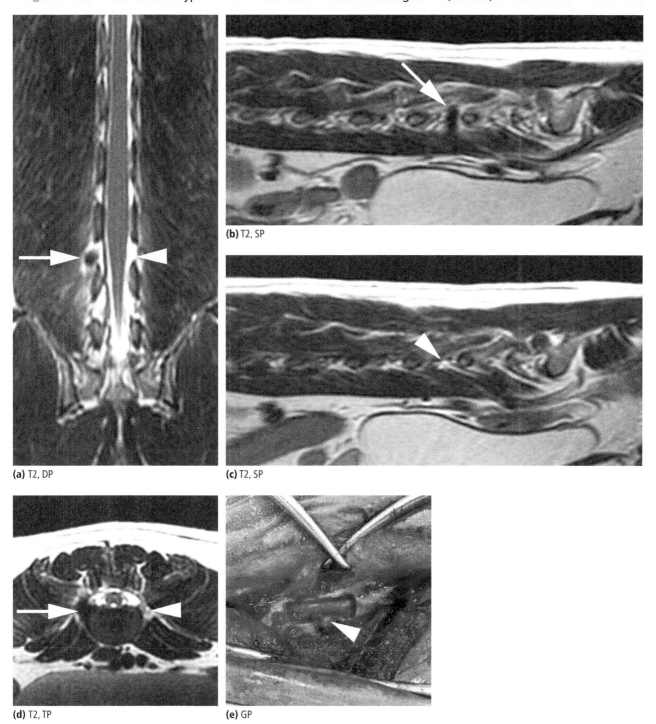

(a) T2, DP

(b) T2, SP

(c) T2, SP

(d) T2, TP

(e) GP

5y FS Miniature Dachshund with acute-onset right pelvic limb lameness following a racing competition. Neuroanatomically localized as a right-sided L4–L6 radiculoneuropathy. Image **a** is a dorsal plane T2 image through the caudal lumbar intervertebral foramina. Images **b** and **c** are parasagittal T2 images through the right and left caudal lumbar intervertebral foramina, respectively. Image **d** is a transverse T2 image at the level of the L5–6 intervertebral disk space. Focal T2 signal void in the right L5–6 intervertebral foramen represents extruded disk material lodged within the foramen (**a**,**b**,**d**: arrow). The contralateral intervertebral foramen has normal signal intensity by comparison (**a**,**c**,**d**: arrowhead). A hemilaminectomy was performed at L5–6, and disk material was removed from the right intervertebral foramen. Impingement of the disk material on the right fifth lumbar spinal nerve root resulted in neuritis and explains the neurologic signs (**e**: arrowhead).

Figure 3.5.10   Type I Disk Extrusion with Hemorrhage (Canine)   MR

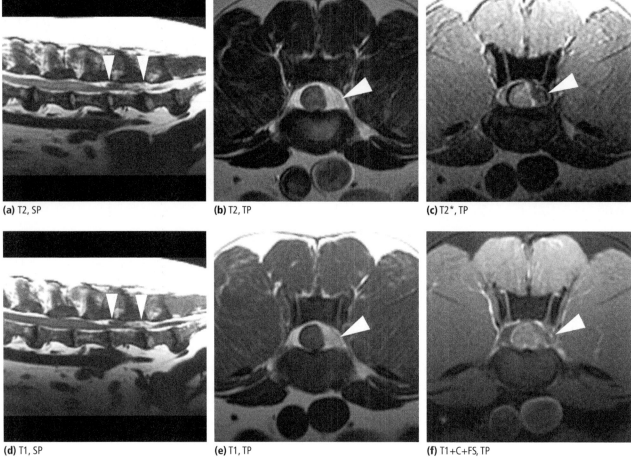

(a) T2, SP

(b) T2, TP

(c) T2*, TP

(d) T1, SP

(e) T1, TP

(f) T1+C+FS, TP

9y MC Australian Shepherd with 48-hour history of progressive back pain and paraparesis. Neuroanatomic localization was an L4–caudal myelopathy. Extradural material of heterogeneous T1 and T2 intensity displaces and compresses the conus medullaris and cauda equina (a,d: arrowheads). Extradural material at the level of the midbody of L6 is predominantly T1 and T2 hyperintense and partially fat suppresses (b,c,e,f: arrowhead). Prominent susceptibility effect in the left epidural space (c: arrowhead) is indicative of hemorrhage. A double hemilaminectomy was performed at L5–7. A large volume of hemorrhage and disk material extruded from L6–7 was removed from the left extradural space.

Figure 3.5.11   Multiple Type II Disk Protrusions (Canine)   MR

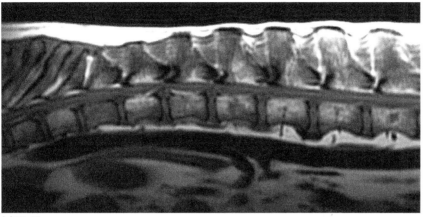
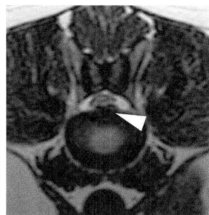

(a) T1, SP   **(b)** T2, TP

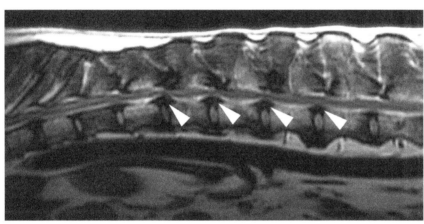
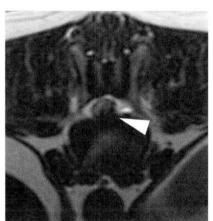

(c) T2, SP   **(d)** T2, TP

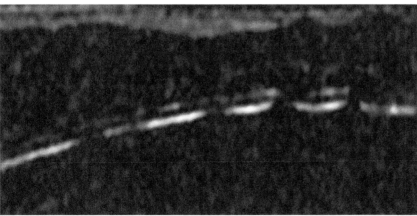

(e) SSTSE, SP

13y MC Labrador Retriever with 4-week history of pelvic limb paraparesis with acute progression of signs. Neuroanatomic localization is to T3–L3 myelopathy. Images **b** and **d** are at the level of T12–13 and T13–L1, respectively. Thoracolumbar intervertebral disk spaces appear to be of normal width and are T1 isointense and heterogeneously T2 hyperintense, indicating variable nuclear dehydration (**a,c**). The dorsal annulus fibrosis/dorsal longitudinal ligament is prominent at multiple levels, elevating and compressing the overlying spinal cord (**b–d**: arrowheads). A single-shot turbo spin-echo image of the thoracolumbar spine documents discontinuity of the subarachnoid cerebrospinal fluid columns at multiple levels, corresponding to sites of Hansen's type II disk protrusion (**e**). Neurologic signs improved with medical management.

Figure 3.5.12 Hydrated Disk Extrusion (Canine) MR

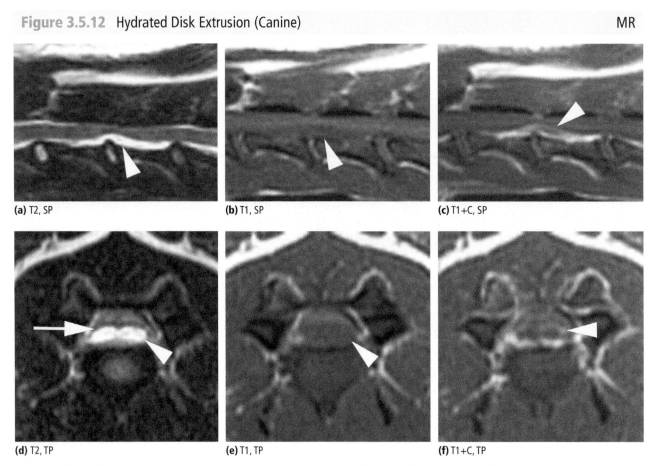

(a) T2, SP

(b) T1, SP

(c) T1+C, SP

(d) T2, TP

(e) T1, TP

(f) T1+C, TP

10y FS Poodle with peracute tetraparesis with no apparent inciting cause. There is T2 hyperintense, T1 hypointense material distributed in the ventral aspect of the vertebral canal at the level of the C3–4 intervertebral disk space, which focally elevates and compresses the spinal cord (**a,b,d,e**: arrowhead). The ventral margin of the spinal cord has a double arching "seagull" wing appearance that has been ascribed to high liquid content disk extrusion (**d**: arrow). Focal linear contrast enhancement likely represents reactive dural enhancement (**c,f**: arrowhead). Ventral slot decompression surgery was performed and a large volume of clear fluid was encountered along with more solid material that was composed of atypical chondroid-like cells and a small amount of matrix.

Figure 3.5.13   Normal Lumbosacral Junction (Canine)   MR

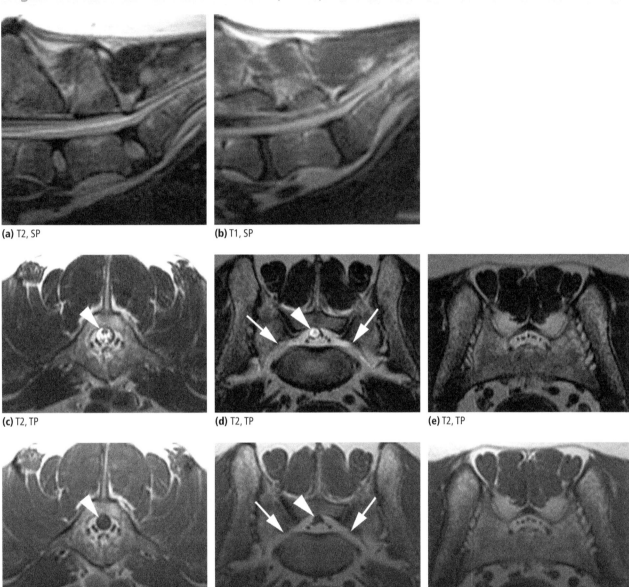

(a) T2, SP

(b) T1, SP

(c) T2, TP

(d) T2, TP

(e) T2, TP

(f) T1, TP

(g) T1, TP

(h) T1, TP

4y FS Doberman Pinscher with hindlimb lameness. The dog was diagnosed with a sensory polyneuromyopathy (dancing Doberman disease) based on lesion localization and electromyography. Images **c** and **f**, **d** and **g**, and **e** and **h** were acquired at the level of the midbody of L7, the cranial edge of the L-S disk space, and the middle of S1, respectively. The L6–7 and L-S disks appear normal anatomically and have normal signal intensity with a T2 hyperintense nucleus pulposus and hypointense annulus fibrosis (**a,b**). The caudal terminus of the lumbar cistern extends to the L-S intervertebral space (**c,d,f,g**: arrowhead) and is bounded on either side by the lumbar spinal nerves (**c,d,f,g**), which are hypointense to surrounding epidural fat. The sacral spinal nerves are also easily identified further caudally (**e,h**). The L-S intervertebral foramina are large and well defined by hyperintense fat (**d,g**: arrows). Radiating intradural lumbar spinal nerve roots and associated dorsal root ganglia are well delineated on dorsal plane STIR and contrast-enhanced, fat-suppressed T1 thin-slab maximum-intensity projection (MIP) images (**i,j**: arrowheads). (Figure continues on next page.)

Figure 3.5.13 (*Continued*) MR

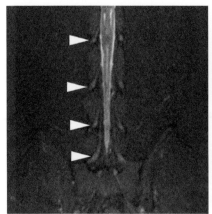

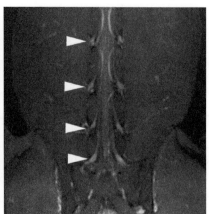

(i) STIR, MIP, DP

(j) T1+C+FS, MIP, DP

Figure 3.5.14 Lumbosacral Type II Disk Protrusion and Neuritis (Canine)   MR

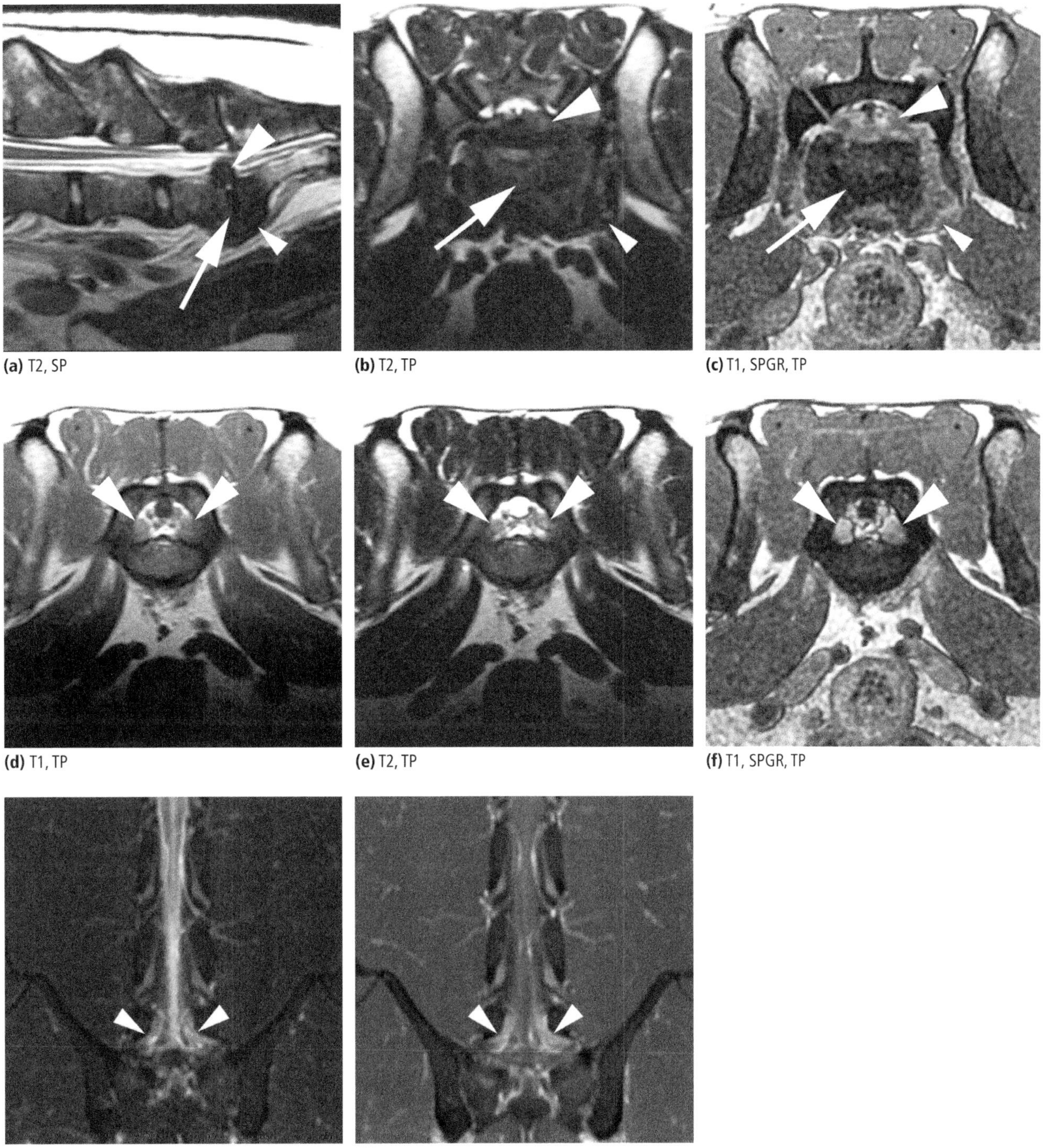

(a) T2, SP

(b) T2, TP

(c) T1, SPGR, TP

(d) T1, TP

(e) T2, TP

(f) T1, SPGR, TP

(g) STIR, MIP, DP

(h) T1+C+FS, MIP, DP

8y MC Bull Terrier with pain referable to the lumbosacral region. Images **b** and **c** are at the level of the lumbosacral intervertebral disk. Images **d–f** are at the level of the midbody of the seventh lumbar vertebra. Images **g** and **h** are thin-slab STIR and contrast-enhanced, fat-suppressed T1 thin-slab maximum-intensity projection (MIP) images, respectively. The lumbosacral intervertebral disk space is narrow, and hydrated nucleus pulposis is nearly absent (**a–c**: arrow). The dorsal annulus fibrosis protrudes into the vertebral canal, causing elevation of the cauda equina (**a–c**: large arrowhead). Marked lumbosacral spondylosis is present, and lateralized new bone encroaches on the lumbosacral intervertebral foramina (**a–c**: small arrowhead). New bone and ligamentous structures are T2 hypointense (**a,b**) but have moderate T1 hyperintensity on the T1-weighted SPGR sequence (**c**). The seventh lumbar spinal nerve roots are enlarged and contrast enhance cranial to their emergence through the intervertebral foramina (**d–h**: arrowheads). An L7–S1 dorsal laminectomy was performed and documented lumbosacral stenosis from annulus fibrosis protrusion and hypertrophy of the interarcuate and dorsal longitudinal ligaments. These changes, in conjunction with the lateral spondylosis, resulted in intervertebral foraminal stenosis and consequent bilateral seventh lumbar spinal neuritis.

Figure 3.5.15   Disseminated Idiopathic Skeletal Hyperostosis (Canine)

MR

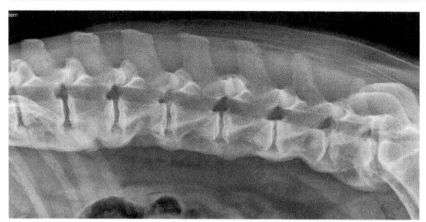

(a) DX, LAT

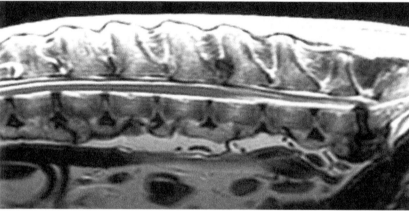

(b) T2, SP

7y M Catahoula Leopard Dog with lumbosacral pain. Spinal radiographs reveal dense flowing new bone formation involving the ventral and lateral surfaces of the lumbar vertebral bodies (a). The L5–6 intervertebral space is slightly narrow, but there are no other signs indicative of degenerative disease. New bone is hyperintense on the T2 MR image (b). There is heterogeneity to nucleus pulposus intensity in the lumbar spine, but disk architecture appears to be preserved, and the dorsal part of the annulus fibrosis appears normal at each lumbar disk space. There are radiographic and MR imaging features consistent with lumbosacral degenerative disease, which was the likely source of clinical signs.

Figure 3.5.16 Synovial Cyst (Canine)

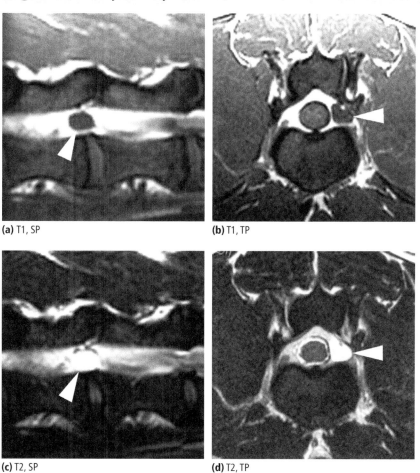

(a) T1, SP

(b) T1, TP

(c) T2, SP

(d) T2, TP

5y MC American Staffordshire Terrier with acute-onset pelvic limb paresis. There is a well-demarcated T1 hypointense, T2 hyperintense, thin-walled cystic mass in the epidural space adjacent to the ventral margin of the left L3–4 facet articulation, consistent with a noncompressive synovial cyst (a–d: arrowhead). Clinical signs in this dog were from a T12–13 intervertebral disk extrusion (not shown).

Figure 3.5.17 Meningeal Cyst with Arachnoid Communication (Canine)

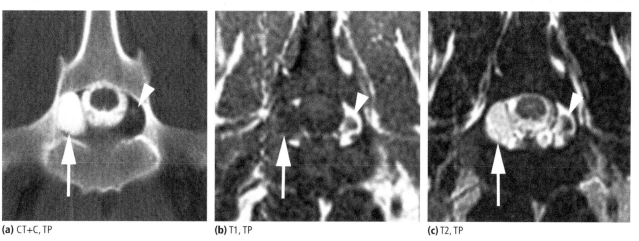

(a) CT+C, TP

(b) T1, TP

(c) T2, TP

9y M Borzoi with 1-year history of pelvic limb paresis. Image **a** was acquired as part of a CT myelogram. There is a large, well-demarcated, thin-walled, ovoid cystic mass in the right epidural space at the level of the first thoracic vertebra (**a**: arrow). Intense and uniform contrast enhancement within the cyst documents direct communication with the subarachnoid space. A faint extradural contrast blush is also evident to the left of the spinal cord (**a**: arrowhead). The large cyst is T1 hypointense and T2 hyperintense, consistent with imaging characteristics of normal cerebrospinal fluid (**b,c**: arrow). The uniform attenuation and intensity of the large cyst is consistent with a type I spinal meningeal cyst that contains no neural tissue. The smaller structure to the left of the spinal cord is hypointense on both T1 and T2 images, which is more consistent with a type II cyst containing neural tissue (**b,c**: arrowhead). This dog had a compressive C4–5 intervertebral disk extrusion (not shown) that was the cause of clinical signs. The meningeal cysts were considered incidental findings.

References

1. Bergknut N, Smolders LA, Grinwis GC, Hagman R, Lagerstedt AS, Hazewinkel HA, et al. Intervertebral disc degeneration in the dog. Part 1: Anatomy and physiology of the intervertebral disc and characteristics of intervertebral disc degeneration. Vet J. 2013;195:282–291.

2. Smolders LA, Bergknut N, Grinwis GC, Hagman R, Lagerstedt AS, Hazewinkel HA, et al. Intervertebral disc degeneration in the dog. Part 2: chondrodystrophic and non-chondrodystrophic breeds. Vet J. 2013;195:292–299.

3. Brisson BA. Intervertebral disc disease in dogs. Vet Clin North Am Small Anim Pract. 2010;40:829–858.

4. Hansen HJ. A pathologic-anatomical interpretation of disc degeneration in dogs. Acta Orthop Scand. 1951;20:280–293.

5. Hansen HJ. A pathologic-anatomical study on disc degeneration in dog, with special reference to the so-called enchondrosis intervertebralis. Acta Orthop Scand Suppl. 1952;11:1–117.

6. Cudia SP, Duval JM. Thoracolumbar intervertebral disk disease in large, nonchondrodystrophic dogs: a retrospective study. J Am Anim Hosp Assoc. 1997;33:456–460.

7. Macias C, McKee WM, May C, Innes JF. Thoracolumbar disc disease in large dogs: a study of 99 cases. J Small Anim Pract. 2002;43:439–446.

8. Beltran E, Dennis R, Doyle V, de Stefani A, Holloway A, de Risio L. Clinical and magnetic resonance imaging features of canine compressive cervical myelopathy with suspected hydrated nucleus pulposus extrusion. J Small Anim Pract. 2012;53:101–107.

9. Bibevski JD, Daye RM, Henrickson TD, Axlund TW. A prospective evaluation of CT in acutely paraparetic chondrodystrophic dogs. J Am Anim Hosp Assoc. 2013;49:363–369.

10. Cooper JJ, Young BD, Griffin JF 4th, Fosgate GT, Levine JM. Comparison between noncontrast computed tomography and magnetic resonance imaging for detection and characterization of thoracolumbar myelopathy caused by intervertebral disk herniation in dogs. Vet Radiol Ultrasound. 2014;55:182–189.

11. Kuroki K, Vitale CL, Essman SC, Pithua P, Coates JR. Computed tomographic and histological findings of Hansen type I intervertebral disc herniation in dogs. Vet Comp Orthop Traumatol. 2013;26:379–384.

12. Newcomb B, Arble J, Rochat M, Pechman R, Payton M. Comparison of computed tomography and myelography to a reference standard of computed tomographic myelography for evaluation of dogs with intervertebral disc disease. Vet Surg. 2012;41:207–214.

13. Robertson I, Thrall DE. Imaging dogs with suspected disc herniation: pros and cons of myelography, computed tomography, and magnetic resonance. Vet Radiol Ultrasound. 2011;52:S81–84.

14. Schroeder R, Pelsue DH, Park RD, Gasso D, Bruecker KA. Contrast-enhanced CT for localizing compressive thoracolumbar intervertebral disc extrusion. J Am Anim Hosp Assoc. 2011; 47:203–209.

15. Shimizu J, Yamada K, Mochida K, Kako T, Muroya N, Teratani Y, et al. Comparison of the diagnosis of intervertebral disc herniation in dogs by CT before and after contrast enhancement of the subarachnoid space. Vet Rec. 2009;165:200–202.

16. Israel SK, Levine JM, Kerwin SC, Levine GJ, Fosgate GT. The relative sensitivity of computed tomography and myelography for identification of thoracolumbar intervertebral disk herniations in dogs. Vet Radiol Ultrasound. 2009;50:247–252.

17. Olby NJ, Munana KR, Sharp NJ, Thrall DE. The computed tomographic appearance of acute thoracolumbar intervertebral disc herniations in dogs. Vet Radiol Ultrasound. 2000;41:396–402.

18. Mateo I, Lorenzo V, Foradada L, Munoz A. Clinical, pathologic, and magnetic resonance imaging characteristics of canine disc extrusion accompanied by epidural hemorrhage or inflammation. Vet Radiol Ultrasound. 2011;52:17–24.

19. Pease A, Sullivan S, Olby N, Galano H, Cerda-Gonzalez S, Robertson ID, et al. Value of a single-shot turbo spin-echo pulse sequence for assessing the architecture of the subarachnoid space and the constitutive nature of cerebrospinal fluid. Vet Radiol Ultrasound. 2006;47:254–259.

20. Meij BP, Bergknut N. Degenerative lumbosacral stenosis in dogs. Vet Clin North Am Small Anim Pract. 2010;40:983–1009.

21. Amort KH, Ondreka N, Rudorf H, Stock KF, Distl O, Tellhelm B, et al. MR-imaging of lumbosacral intervertebral disc degeneration in clinically sound German shepherd dogs compared to other breeds. Vet Radiol Ultrasound. 2012;53:289–295.

22. Suwankong N, Voorhout G, Hazewinkel HA, Meij BP. Agreement between computed tomography, magnetic resonance imaging, and surgical findings in dogs with degenerative lumbosacral stenosis. J Am Vet Med Assoc. 2006;229:1924–1929.

23. Rossi F, Seiler G, Busato A, Wacker C, Lang J. Magnetic resonance imaging of articular process joint geometry and intervertebral disk degeneration in the caudal lumbar spine (L5–S1) of dogs with clinical signs of cauda equina compression. Vet Radiol Ultrasound. 2004;45:381–387.

24. Seiler GS, Hani H, Busato AR, Lang J. Facet joint geometry and intervertebral disk degeneration in the L5–S1 region of the vertebral column in German Shepherd dogs. Am J Vet Res. 2002; 63:86–90.

25. Jones JC, Wright JC, Bartels JE. Computed tomographic morphometry of the lumbosacral spine of dogs. Am J Vet Res. 1995; 56:1125–1132.

26. Higgins BM, Cripps PJ, Baker M, Moore L, Penrose FE, McConnell JF. Effects of body position, imaging plane, and observer on computed tomographic measurements of the lumbosacral intervertebral foraminal area in dogs. Am J Vet Res. 2011;72:905–917.

27. Jones JC, Davies SE, Werre SR, Shackelford KL. Effects of body position and clinical signs on L7–S1 intervertebral foraminal area and lumbosacral angle in dogs with lumbosacral disease as measured via computed tomography. Am J Vet Res. 2008;69:1446–1454.

28. Saunders FC, Cave NJ, Hartman KM, Gee EK, Worth AJ, Bridges JP, et al. Computed tomographic method for measurement of inclination angles and motion of the sacroiliac joints in German Shepherd Dogs and Greyhounds. Am J Vet Res. 2013;74:1172–1182.

29. Morgan JP. Spondylosis derformans in the dog. A morphologic study with some clinical and experimental observations. Acta Orthop Scand. 1967:7–87.

30. Morgan JP, Ljunggren G, Read R. Spondylosis deformans (vertebral osteophytosis) in the dog. A radiographic study from England, Sweden and U.S.A. J Small Anim Pract. 1967;8:57–66.

31. Wright JA. Spondylosis deformans of the lumbo-sacral joint in dogs. J Small Anim Pract. 1980;21:45–58.

32. Levine GJ, Levine JM, Walker MA, Pool RR, Fosgate GT. Evaluation of the association between spondylosis deformans and clinical signs of intervertebral disk disease in dogs: 172 cases (1999–2000). J Am Vet Med Assoc. 2006;228:96–100.

33. Resnick D, Niwayama G. Diffuse Idiopathic Skeletal Hyperostosis (DISH). In: Resnick, D (ed): Bone and Joint Imaging. Philadelphia: W.B. Saunders Company, 1989;440-451.

34. Greatting HH, Young BD, Pool RR, Levine JM. Diffuse idiopathic skeletal hyperostosis (DISH). Vet Radiol Ultrasound. 2011; 52:472-473.

35. Kranenburg HC, Westerveld LA, Verlaan JJ, Oner FC, Dhert WJ, Voorhout G, et al. The dog as an animal model for DISH? Eur Spine J. 2010;19:1325-1329.

36. Ortega M, Goncalves R, Haley A, Wessmann A, Penderis J. Spondylosis deformans and diffuse idiopathic skeletal hyperostosis (DISH) resulting in adjacent segment disease. Vet Radiol Ultrasound. 2012;53:128-134.

37. Woodard JC, Poulos PW, Jr., Parker RB, Jackson RI, Jr., Eurell JC. Canine diffuse idiopathic skeletal hyperostosis. Vet Pathol. 1985;22:317-326.

38. Levitski RE, Chauvet AE, Lipsitz D. Cervical myelopathy associated with extradural synovial cysts in 4 dogs. J Vet Intern Med. 1999;13:181-186.

39. Levitski RE, Lipsitz D, Chauvet AE. Magnetic resonance imaging of the cervical spine in 27 dogs. Vet Radiol Ultrasound. 1999; 40:332-341.

40. Lipsitz D, Levitski RE, Chauvet AE, Berry WL. Magnetic resonance imaging features of cervical stenotic myelopathy in 21 dogs. Vet Radiol Ultrasound. 2001;42:20-27.

41. Forterre F, Kaiser S, Garner M, Stadie B, Matiasek K, Schmahl W, et al. Synovial cysts associated with cauda equina syndrome in two dogs. Vet Surg. 2006;35:30-33.

42. Sale CS, Smith KC. Extradural spinal juxtafacet (synovial) cysts in three dogs. J Small Anim Pract. 2007;48:116-119.

43. Nabors MW, Pait TG, Byrd EB, Karim NO, Davis DO, Kobrine AI, et al. Updated assessment and current classification of spinal meningeal cysts. J Neurosurg. 1988;68:366-377.

44. Tani S, Hata Y, Tochigi S, Ohashi H, Isoshima A, Nagashima H, et al. Prevalence of spinal meningeal cyst in the sacrum. Neurol Med Chir (Tokyo). 2013;53:91-94.

45. Skeen TM, Olby NJ, Munana KR, Sharp NJ. Spinal arachnoid cysts in 17 dogs. J Am Anim Hosp Assoc. 2003;39:271-282.

46. Mauler DA, De Decker S, De Risio L, Volk HA, Dennis R, Gielen I, et al. Signalment, clinical presentation, and diagnostic findings in 122 dogs with spinal arachnoid diverticula. J Vet Intern Med. 2014;28:175-181.

3.6

Brachial and lumbosacral plexus

Normal anatomy of the brachial and lumbosacral plexus

Brachial plexus

Spinal segment dorsal and ventral nerve roots arise separately from the spinal cord before merging to form a spinal nerve. The nerve exits the intervertebral foramen then separates into a dorsal and ventral branch. The brachial plexus is formed by a complex convergence of the ventral branches of the sixth, seventh, and eighth cervical nerves and the first and second thoracic nerves, although contributions are variable, and the fifth cervical nerve is sometimes included (Figure 3.6.1). The ventral spinal nerve branches divide and reorganize deep within the axilla to form the peripheral nerves that supply the forelimb and parts of the cranial thoracic wall. Because of their location relative to their respective ribs, the ventral branches of the first and second thoracic nerves course along the internal aspect of the cranial thoracic wall for a short distance before exiting at the thoracic inlet.[1]

Lumbosacral plexus

The lumbosacral plexus is normally formed by ventral branches of the third through seventh lumbar nerves and the first through third sacral nerves (Figure 3.6.1), although variations do occur. Similar to the brachial plexus, the lumbosacral plexus results from the divergence of the spinal nerves with reorganization proximally along the caudal paraspinal region and within the pelvis to form peripheral nerves that innervate the pelvic limb and parts of the pelvis and pelvic viscera.[1]

Muscle denervation

Although muscle denervation pathology is not limited to plexus disorders, clinical and imaging manifestations of muscle denervation can be striking in these patients.

Acute muscle denervation is rarely recognized in dogs and cats, although it is described in people. Acute denervation results in muscle injury with increased extracellular fluid volume. CT imaging features in people include mild increase in muscle volume and variable, mild contrast enhancement. MR features include mild increase in muscle mass, no change in T1 intensity, increased T2 and STIR intensity, and mild contrast enhancement. Chronic muscle denervation results in marked reduction in muscle mass and fatty replacement. CT features include hypoattenuation of remaining muscle volume due to increased fat content. MR findings include heterogeneous increased T1 and T2 intensity (Figure 3.6.2).[2]

Trauma

Brachial plexus traction injury

Traction injuries of the plexus involve abnormal tensile forces applied to the limb, which cause avulsion of spinal nerve roots or injury to the spinal nerves. In people, a distinction is made between preganglionic brachial plexus injuries, those occurring at or near the spinal roots and proximal to the dorsal root ganglion, and postganglionic injuries, since this can determine the applicable surgical approaches for repair or nerve transfer.[3] Although brachial plexus injury has been described

Atlas of Small Animal CT and MRI, First Edition. Erik R. Wisner and Allison L. Zwingenberger.
© 2015 John Wiley & Sons, Inc. Published 2015 by John Wiley & Sons, Inc.

in the veterinary literature, there are few references to cross-sectional imaging of the disorder.[4–8]

CT myelography has been used in people for diagnosis of preganglionic brachial plexus injury. Intact dorsal and ventral nerve roots are seen as radiating linear filling defects in the contrast-enhanced subarachnoid space, and avulsion is diagnosed based on an absence of this finding. Pseudomeningoceles are also indicative of avulsion and appear as a focal dilation of the enhanced subarachnoid space.[9] CT myelography has been used for diagnosis of nerve root avulsion in a small case series of dogs and cats.[4]

MR features of postganglionic injuries in people include thickened nerves that are T1 hypointense, T2 hyperintense and contrast enhance. Discontinuity of transected nerves may also be evident. Features of preganglionic injuries include direct evidence of nerve root avulsion from the spinal cord (Figure 3.6.3). A pseudomeningocele, a focal dilatation of the arachnoid space, is often also present. Evidence of intrinsic spinal cord disease can also be seen.[10] MR imaging following intrathecal administration of contrast medium has been used to detect traumatic dural tears associated with avulsion injury in a dog.[5]

Inflammatory disorders

Brachial plexus neuritis is rare but has been reported in the veterinary literature.[11] In people, MR features of brachial plexus neuritis include diffuse nerve enlargement, T2 hyperintensity, and variable contrast enhancement.[12]

Neoplasia

Peripheral nerve sheath tumors

Peripheral nerve sheath tumors (PNST) can be either benign or malignant and account for the vast majority of neoplasms of the brachial and lumbosacral plexus in dogs and cats. The veterinary literature and experience suggest that PNST are more common in the brachial plexus.[13–16] Clinical signs of brachial plexus PNST include unilateral forelimb lameness and muscle atrophy. Affected animals may also show signs of pain on limb manipulation and may lick or chew the extremity because of abnormal sensation. Those PNST that involve the spinal nerves proximal to their arborization into the plexus can extend to the spinal nerve roots and invade the spinal cord. Those PNST that include the T1 and T2 spinal nerves will have an intrathoracic or thoracic inlet component.

In a study describing CT features of brachial plexus neoplasms in dogs, consistent findings included periscapular muscle atrophy, well-defined axillary mass margins, and contrast enhancement of most masses, with peripheral distribution in about half. Over 25% of masses extended proximally to the vertebral canal, and approximately 25% extended into the thoracic cavity (Figure 3.6.4).[17] Although these features are consistent with our experience with brachial plexus PNST, only one third of dogs had histologic confirmation of tumor type in this study. In an investigation of MR features of brachial plexus PNST, findings included diffuse brachial plexus nerve thickening or discrete axillary mass, T1 isointensity and T2 hyperintensity compared to muscle, and variable and often heterogeneous contrast enhancement (Figures 3.6.5, 3.6.6).[16] Muscle atrophy and signal changes associated with muscle denervation (described above) are also often present. It can be helpful to begin an MR imaging study of suspected brachial plexus neoplasia with a dorsal plane, large field-of-view STIR sequence to localize the lesion as focal or regional hyperintensity.

Imaging features of lumbosacral plexus PNST are similar to those of brachial plexus tumors (Figures 3.6.7, 3.6.8).

Other neoplasms

Other neoplasms affecting the brachial and lumbar plexus are rare but include lymphoma, hemangiosarcoma, other sarcomas, and a variety of other tumors. Although CT and MR imaging descriptions are lacking, our experience is that lymphoma can appear similar to and is not reliably distinguishable from PNST (Figure 3.6.9). Lipomas frequently arise in the axillary region and can displace or incorporate nerves of the brachial plexus (Figure 3.6.10).

Figure 3.6.1   Brachial and Lumbosacral Plexus Anatomy (Canine)

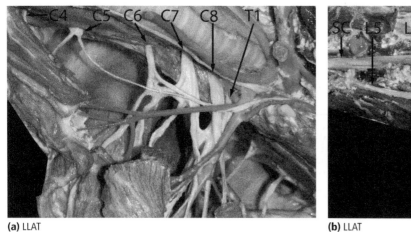

(a) LLAT

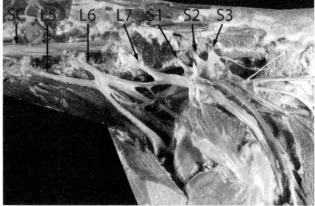

(b) LLAT

Gross appearance of the brachial (**a**) and lumbosacral (**b**) plexus. Spinal nerves (**a**,**b**) and the spinal cord (**b**: SC) are labeled in abbreviated form. The authors acknowledge Mr. Ken Taylor, University of California, Davis, for dissections.

Figure 3.6.2   Chronic Muscle Denervation (Canine)   MR

(a) T1, TP   **(b)** T2, TP   **(c)** T1+C+FS, TP

7y MC Boston Terrier with progressive left thoracic limb lameness of 4 months' duration. Transverse images were acquired at the level of the midbody of the first thoracic vertebra and immediately caudal to the scapular spines. There is marked volume reduction of the left serratus ventralis (**a–c**: single asterisk), subscapularis (**a–c**: arrowhead), and infraspinatus (**a–c**: double asterisks) muscles, with mild increased T1 and T2 hyperintensity that is most pronounced in the serratus ventralis. The fat-suppressed T1 image nullifies much of the increased signal intensity, documenting the cause as fatty infiltration (**b**). A contrast-enhancing mass at the bottom of the images represents a peripheral nerve sheath tumor (**a–c**: arrow).

Figure 3.6.3 Brachial Plexus Traction Injury (Canine)   MR

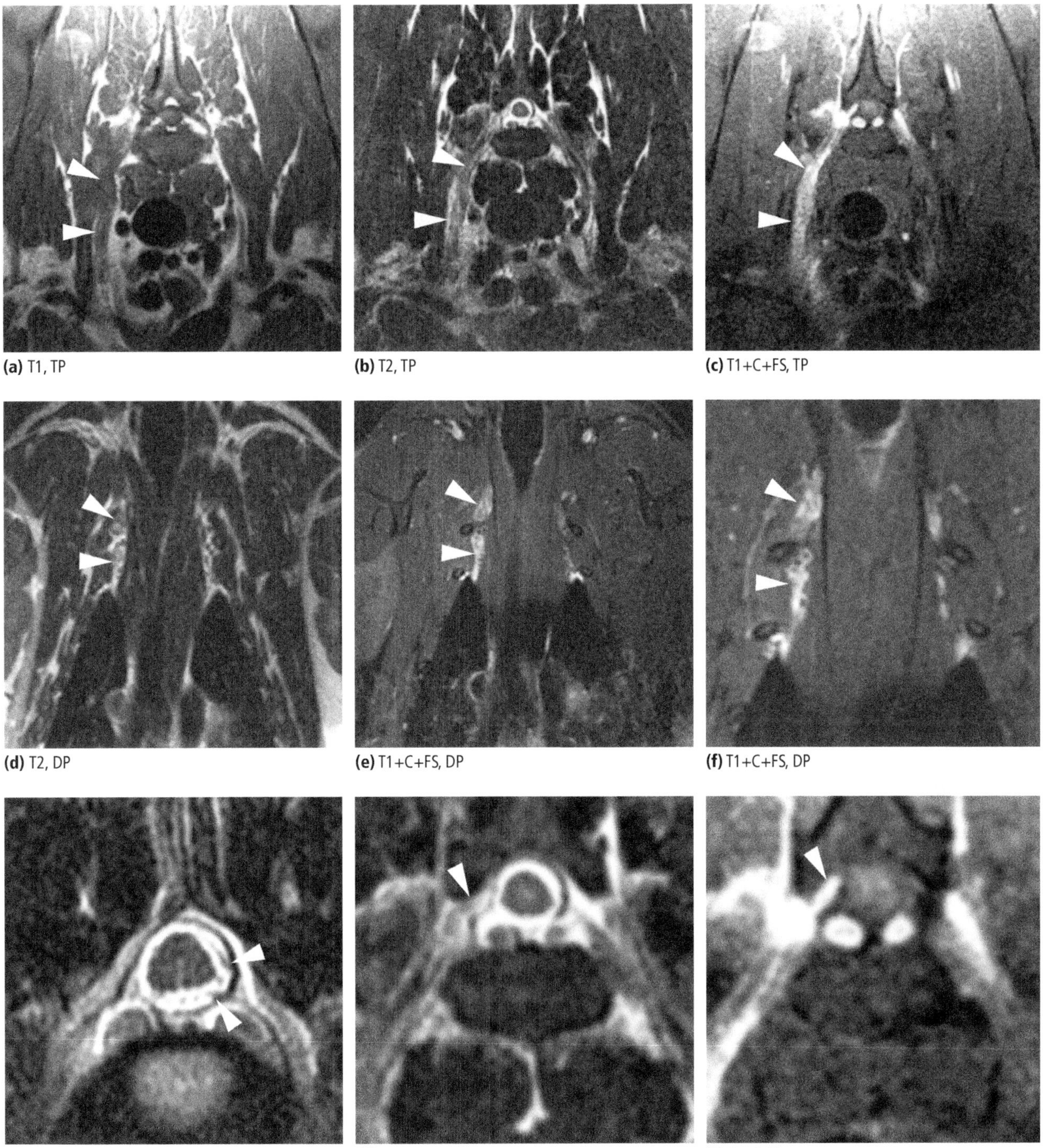

(a) T1, TP

(b) T2, TP

(c) T1+C+FS, TP

(d) T2, DP

(e) T1+C+FS, DP

(f) T1+C+FS, DP

(g) T2, TP

(h) T2, TP

(i) T1+C, TP

1y MC Labrador Retriever with acute right thoracic limb lameness after falling off a table 3 weeks previously. Currently has neurologic deficits involving right spinal nerves C7, C8, and T1. Images **a–c** were acquired at the level of the caudal body of the first thoracic vertebra. Images **d** and **e** are dorsal plane images acquired immediately ventral to the cervicothoracic spinal column, and image **f** is ventral to images **d** and **e**. Image **g** was acquired at the level of the C7–T1 intervertebral space. Images **h** and **i** are magnifications of images **b** and **c**, respectively. The right first thoracic spinal nerve is diffusely enlarged, T2 hyperintense and contrast enhances (**a–c**: arrowheads). Dorsal plane images reveal multiple postganglionic nerves of the brachial plexus with similar imaging abnormalities (**d–f**: arrowheads). The left dorsal and ventral nerve roots of the eighth cervical spinal nerve are readily apparent (**g**: arrowheads), although the right nerve roots are not seen, suggesting avulsion on the right. The right first thoracic spinal nerve dorsal root is seen within the vertebral canal and appears thickened, is T2 hyperintense, and contrast enhances (**h,i**: arrowheads), also suggesting preganglionic injury. The dog showed little neurologic improvement on subsequent recheck examinations.

Figure 3.6.4   Presumptive Brachial Plexus Peripheral Nerve Sheath Tumor (Canine)   CT

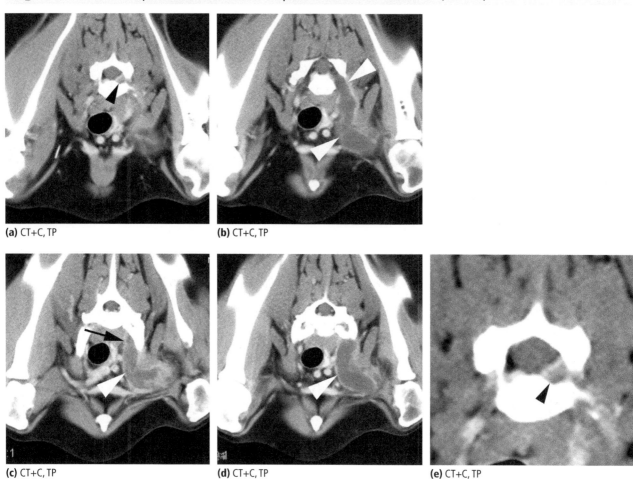

(a) CT+C, TP

(b) CT+C, TP

(c) CT+C, TP

(d) CT+C, TP

(e) CT+C, TP

6y FS Australian Shepherd with a left axillary mass. The dog is currently nonweightbearing on the left thoracic limb. Images **a–d** were acquired from the midbody of the seventh cervical vertebra through the midbody of the first thoracic vertebra and arranged from cranial to caudal. Image **e** is a magnification of image **a**. There is an extrinsic contrast-enhancing mass within the vertebral canal at the level of the seventh cervical vertebra (**a,e**: arrowhead), which exits the left C7–T1 intervertebral foramen as a grossly enlarged eighth cranial nerve mass (**b–d**: arrowheads). The left first thoracic spinal nerve also appeared abnormal (not shown), and the subcostal location of part of the mass is indicative of a first thoracic nerve component (**c**: arrow). Fine-needle aspiration biopsy confirmed sarcoma.

Figure 3.6.5 Brachial Plexus Peripheral Nerve Sheath Tumor (Canine) MR

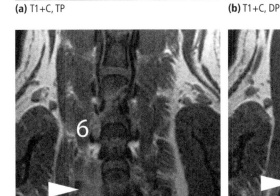

(a) T1+C, TP

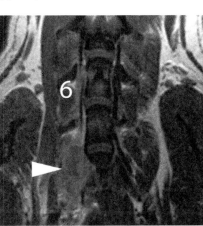

(b) T1+C, DP

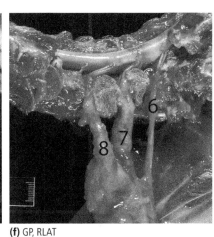

(c) T1+C, DP

(d) T1+C, DP

(e) T1+C, DP

(f) GP, RLAT

4y FS Labrador Retriever with right thoracic limb lameness. Image **a** was acquired at the level of the seventh cervical vertebra. Images **b–e** are consecutive dorsal plane images with image **b** through the caudal cervical spinal cord, and images ordered from dorsal to ventral. There is a large contrast-enhancing mass with an intrinsic component at the level of the seventh cervical spinal segment (**a**,**b**: arrows). The seventh and eighth cervical spinal nerves are grossly enlarged as they exit the intervertebral foramina (**b**,**c**: 7,8). The left sixth cervical spinal nerve is smaller but also pathologically enlarged (**d**,**e**: 6). The nerves converge to form a large irregularly shaped axillary mass (**d**,**e**: arrowhead). Imaging features of the spinal nerves and mass closely match the postmortem appearance (**f**: 6,7,8). A diagnosis of peripheral nerve sheath tumor involving spinal nerves C6-C8 was confirmed histologically.

Figure 3.6.6 Brachial Plexus Peripheral Nerve Sheath Tumor (Canine)   MR

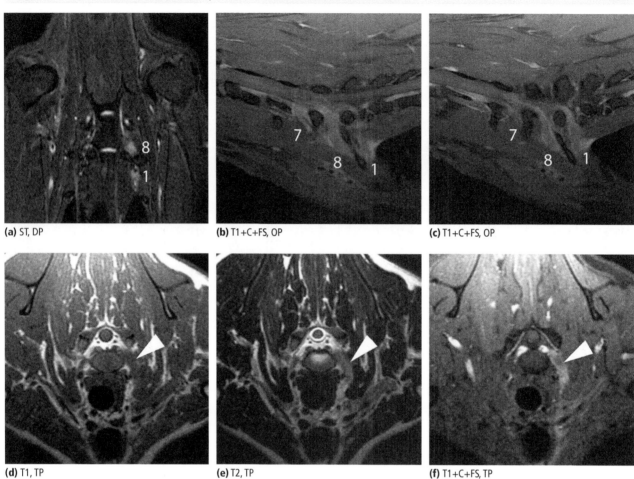

(a) ST, DP   **(b)** T1+C+FS, OP   **(c)** T1+C+FS, OP

(d) T1, TP   **(e)** T2, TP   **(f)** T1+C+FS, TP

Adult M Husky with progressive left thoracic limb lameness of 7 weeks' duration. Multiple focal areas of high signal intensity are seen in the region of the origins of left eighth cervical and first thoracic spinal nerves (**a**: 8,1) on a dorsal plane STIR image. Marked enlargement and contrast enhancement of the seventh and eighth cervical and first thoracic spinal nerves is seen on consecutive contrast-enhanced fat-suppressed images acquired at two slightly different oblique angles approximating the plane of the proximal brachial plexus (**b,c**: 7,8,1). The left eighth cervical spinal nerve is enlarged, T2 hyperintense, and moderately contrast enhancing near its origin on transverse images (**d–f**: arrowheads).

Figure 3.6.7   Presumptive Lumbosacral Plexus Peripheral Nerve Sheath Tumor (Canine)   CT

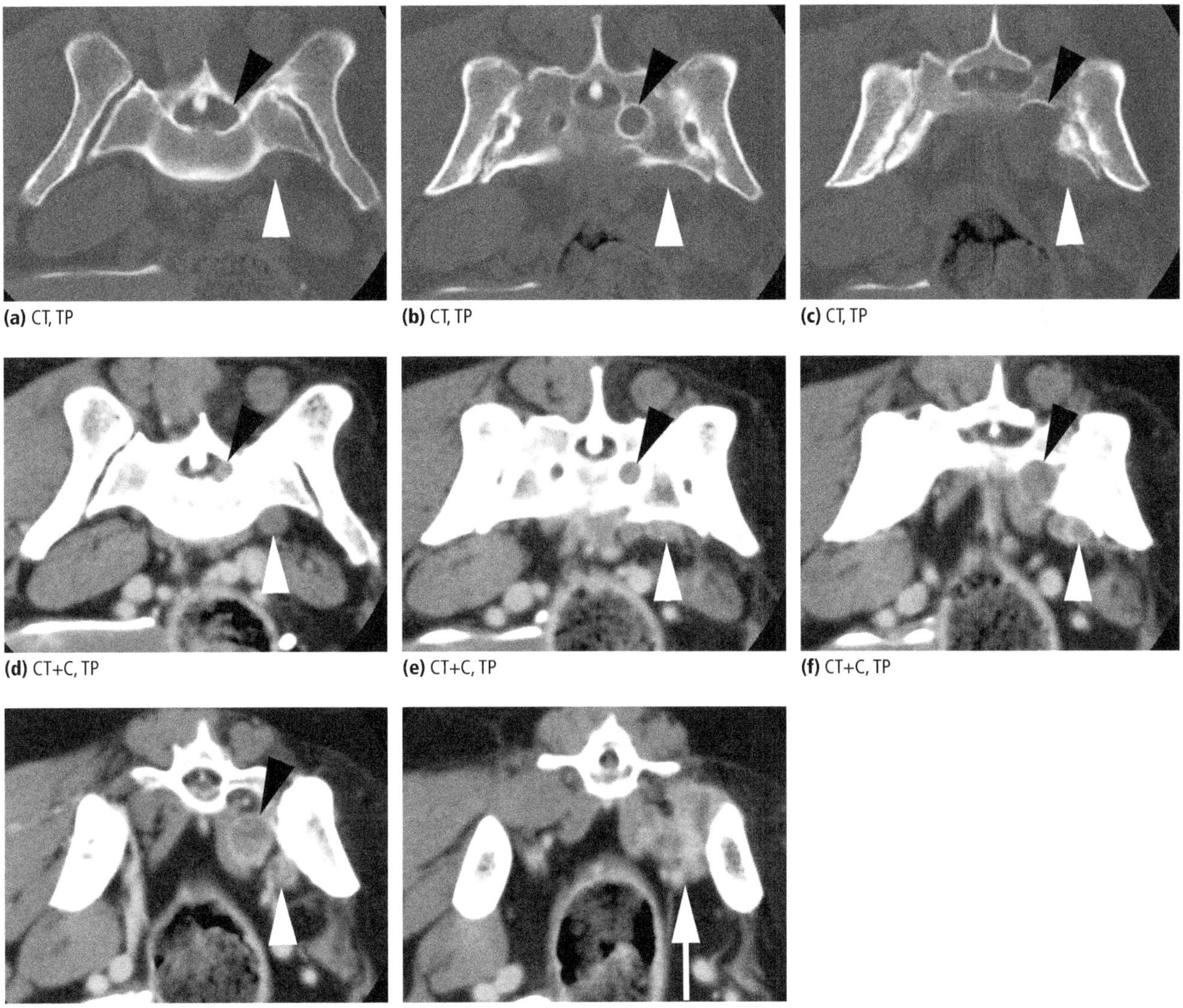

(a) CT, TP

(b) CT, TP

(c) CT, TP

(d) CT+C, TP

(e) CT+C, TP

(f) CT+C, TP

(g) CT+C, TP

(h) CT+C, TP

6y MC Labrador Retriever with progressive left pelvic limb lameness of 6 months' duration. Images **a–c** were acquired at the level of the sacrum and are ordered from cranial to caudal. Images **d–f** are at the same level as images **a–c**, and images **g** and **h** are further caudal. An enlarged nerve is identified ventral to the left side of the sacrum, which represents a coalescence of components of the left fifth through seventh lumbar spinal nerves (**a–g**: white arrowhead). A second mass representing an enlarged left first sacral nerve originates within the spinal canal (**a,d**: black arrowhead) and exits into the left first sacral foramen (**b,c,e–g**: black arrowhead), which is grossly dilated as the result of chronic bone resorption. The two nerves merge to form a single mass in the sacral network of the lumbosacral plexus (**h**: arrow). Marked left-sided pelvic muscle atrophy is also present (**d–h**). The diagnosis of peripheral nerve sheath tumor was based on the CT imaging appearance, clinical signs, and the long and progressive clinical history.

Figure 3.6.8 Lumbosacral Plexus Peripheral Nerve Sheath Tumor (Canine)   MR

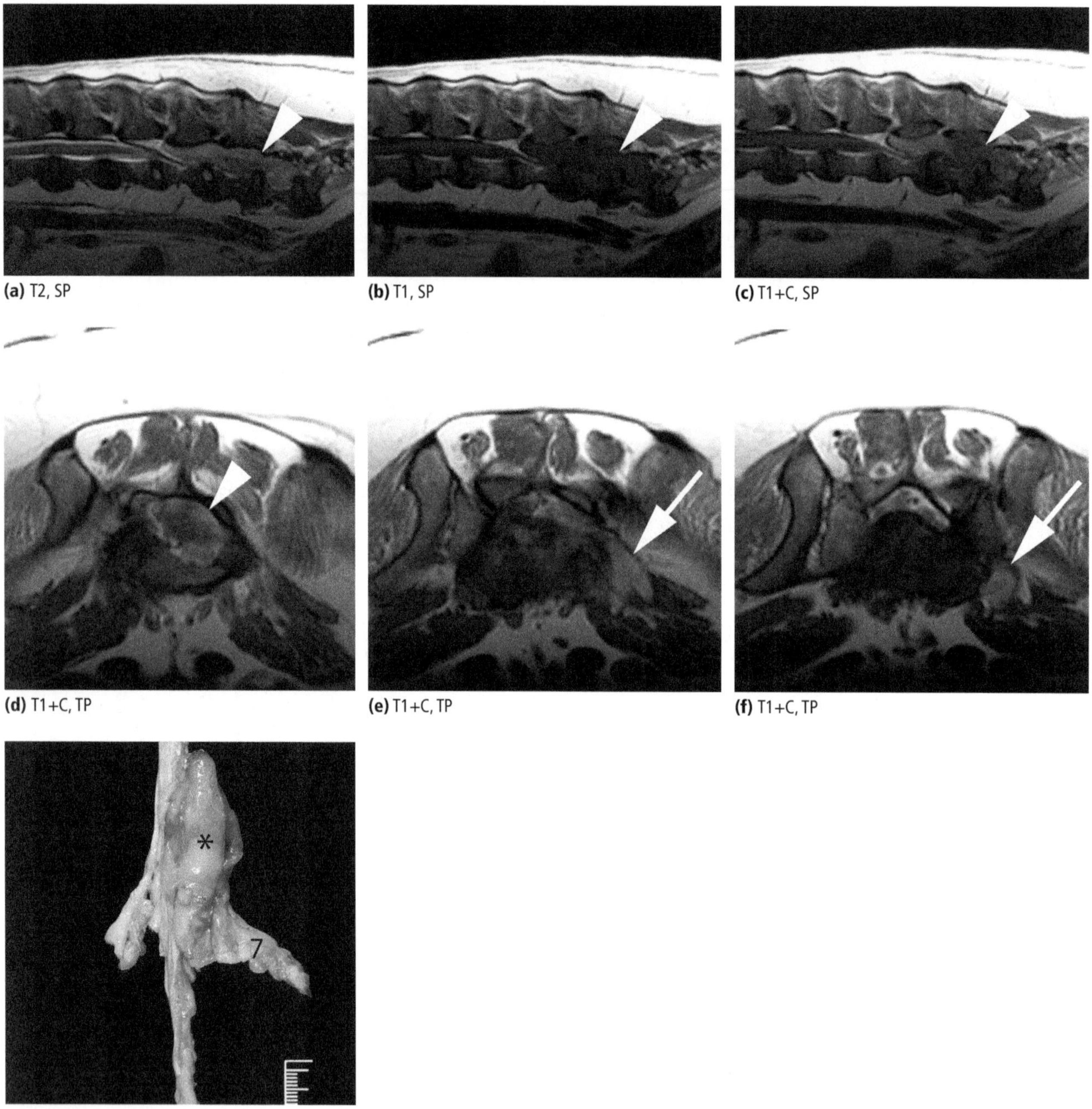

(a) T2, SP

(b) T1, SP

(c) T1+C, SP

(d) T1+C, TP

(e) T1+C, TP

(f) T1+C, TP

(g) GP, DORS

7y English Bulldog with a 2-week history of difficulty walking. Neuroanatomic localization of the lameness was L4–caudal. Images a–c were acquired through the caudal lumbar vertebral column. Images d, e, and f are at the level of the midbody of L7, the LS junction, and S1, respectively. There is a large, tubular extradural mass in the caudal vertebral canal that extends from the fifth through seventh lumbar vertebrae, which is T1 isointense and T2 hyperintense compared to normal spinal cord and heterogeneously contrast enhancing (a–d: arrowhead). The mass exits the left L7–S1 intervertebral foramen and extends peripherally (e,f: arrow). Postmortem examination confirmed a malignant peripheral nerve sheath tumor arising from the left L7 spinal nerve (g: 7), which incorporated the left spinal nerves L4 through S1 (g: asterisk).

Figure 3.6.9 Brachial Plexus Lymphoma (Feline)   MR

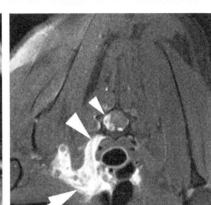
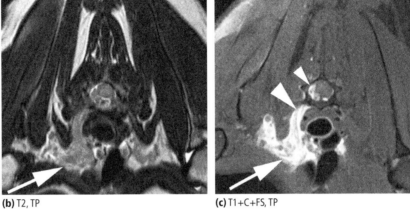

(a) T1, TP

(b) T2, TP

(c) T1+C+FS, TP

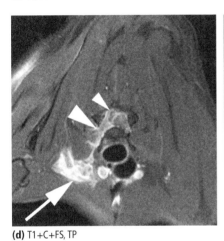
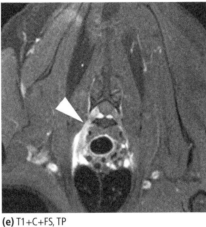
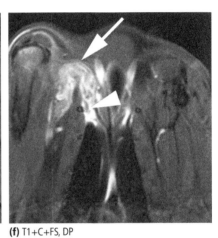

(d) T1+C+FS, TP

(e) T1+C+FS, TP

(f) T1+C+FS, DP

10y MC Domestic Shorthair with progressive right thoracic limb lameness of 2 months' duration. Images **a–c** were acquired at the level of the midbody of the fifth cervical vertebra. Images **d** and **e** are at the level of the C4–5 and C6–7 intervertebral disk spaces, respectively. Image **f** is a dorsal plane image centered on the thoracic inlet. A T1 isointense, T2 hyperintense highly contrast-enhancing mass is present in the right axilla and thoracic inlet (**a–d,f**: arrow) Multiple cervical and cranial thoracic spinal nerves are involved, as depicted by diffuse enlargement and contrast enhancement (**c–f**: large arrowhead) and encroachment into the vertebral canal (**c,d**: small arrowhead). Although not all affected spinal nerves are shown, C5–C8 and T1–T2 were abnormal. Involvement of the thoracic spinal nerves results in extension of the mass into the thoracic inlet (**f**). Ultrasound-guided aspiration biopsy confirmed high-grade large-cell lymphoma.

Figure 3.6.10   Axillary Lipoma (Canine)   CT

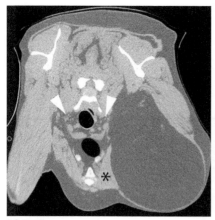
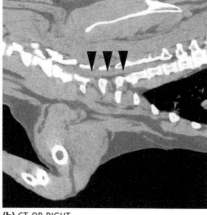
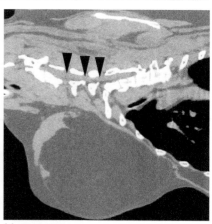

(a) CT, TP   **(b)** CT, OP, RIGHT   **(c)** CT, OP, LEFT

9y MC Coonhound with 4-year history of progressively enlarging left axillary mass. Image **a** was acquired at the level of the caudal body of the sixth cervical vertebra. Images **b** and **c** are long-axis oblique reformatted images approximating the plane of the caudal cervical spinal nerves near their origin. There is a large lipoma in the left axilla that distorts and displaces the left sternocephalicus muscle medially (**a**: asterisk). The soft-tissue attenuating stippling on either side of the trachea (**a**: arrowheads) represents components of the brachial plexus viewed out of plane. Evaluation of adjacent images (not shown) documented the linear interconnected matrix of nerves that comprise the plexus. Images **b** and **c** show the path of the spinal nerves as they exit the caudal cervical intervertebral foramina (**b**,**c**: arrowheads). The lipoma in this dog did not incorporate nerves of the brachial plexus but does encroach on them and illustrates the potential of such masses to displace or infiltrate the plexus and the radiating peripheral nerves.

References

1. Kitchell RL, Evans HE. The Spinal Nerves. In: Evans HE (ed): Miller's Anatomy of the Dog. Philadelphia: W.B. Saunders Company, 1993;829–893.
2. Kamath S, Venkatanarasimha N, Walsh MA, Hughes PM. MRI appearance of muscle denervation. Skeletal Radiol. 2008;37: 397–404.
3. Yang LJ, Chang KW, Chung KC. A systematic review of nerve transfer and nerve repair for the treatment of adult upper brachial plexus injury. Neurosurgery. 2012;71:417–429; discussion 429.
4. Forterre F, Gutmannsbauer B, Schmahl W, Matis U. [CT myelography for diagnosis of brachial plexus avulsion in small animals]. Tierarztl Prax Ausg K Kleintiere Heimtiere. 1998;26: 322–329.
5. Munoz A, Mateo I, Lorenzo V, Martinez J. Imaging diagnosis: traumatic dural tear diagnosed using intrathecal gadopentate dimeglumine. Vet Radiol Ultrasound. 2009;50:502–505.
6. Steinberg HS. Brachial plexus injuries and dysfunctions. Vet Clin North Am Small Anim Pract. 1988;18:565–580.
7. Van Soens I, Struys MM, Polis IE, Bhatti SF, Van Meervenne SA, Martle VA, et al. Magnetic stimulation of the radial nerve in dogs and cats with brachial plexus trauma: a report of 53 cases. Vet J. 2009;182:108–113.
8. Welch JA. Peripheral nerve injury. Semin Vet Med Surg (Small Anim). 1996;11:273–284.
9. Carvalho GA, Nikkhah G, Matthies C, Penkert G, Samii M. Diagnosis of root avulsions in traumatic brachial plexus injuries: value of computerized tomography myelography and magnetic resonance imaging. J Neurosurg. 1997;86:69–76.
10. van Es HW, Bollen TL, van Heesewijk HP. MRI of the brachial plexus: a pictorial review. Eur J Radiol. 2010;74:391–402.
11. Cummings JF, Lorenz MD, De Lahunta A, Washington LD. Canine brachial plexus neuritis: a syndrome resembling serum neuritis in man. Cornell Vet. 1973;63:589–617.
12. Sureka J, Cherian RA, Alexander M, Thomas BP. MRI of brachial plexopathies. Clin Radiol. 2009;64:208–218.
13. Brehm DM, Vite CH, Steinberg HS, Haviland J, van Winkle T. A retrospective evaluation of 51 cases of peripheral nerve sheath tumors in the dog. J Am Anim Hosp Assoc. 1995;31:349–359.
14. Hanna FY. Primary brachial plexus neoplasia in cats. J Feline Med Surg. 2013;15:338–344.
15. Jones BR, Alley MR, Johnstone AC, Jones JM, Cahill JI, McPherson C. Nerve sheath tumours in the dog and cat. N Z Vet J. 1995;43:190–196.
16. Kraft S, Ehrhart EJ, Gall D, Klopp L, Gavin P, Tucker R, et al. Magnetic resonance imaging characteristics of peripheral nerve sheath tumors of the canine brachial plexus in 18 dogs. Vet Radiol Ultrasound. 2007;48:1–7.
17. Rudich SR, Feeney DA, Anderson KL, Walter PA. Computed tomography of masses of the brachial plexus and contributing nerve roots in dogs. Vet Radiol Ultrasound. 2004;45:46–50.

Section 4
Thorax

4.1

Thoracic wall and diaphragm

Thoracic wall

Developmental disorders

Clinically significant developmental anomalies of the thoracic wall and sternum are uncommon and can usually be adequately characterized by clinical evaluation, survey radiographs, and ultrasound examination. CT is sometimes useful for definitive diagnosis or treatment planning.

Trauma

Fractures of the ribs and sternum are a common sequela to thoracic trauma. Rib fractures can also occur from cyclic stress injury in patients with respiratory disorders that lead to increased respiratory effort. This is more often seen in cats.[1] Acute fractures have sharply demarcated fracture margins on CT images and may be displaced depending on the type and severity of injury (Figure 4.1.1). Chronic or healed fractures usually have a productive bridging or nonbridging bony callus (Figure 4.1.2). Callus can be exuberant with displaced fractures or fracture site motion.

Penetrating thoracic wall injuries from bite wounds or foreign bodies are also common but usually manifest with pleural or pulmonary clinical signs (Figure 4.1.3).

Inflammatory disorders

Thoracic wall cellulitis or abscess can be seen as a sequela to regional infectious inflammatory disease. Cellulitis manifests as thoracic wall thickening, associated with a loss of fascial plane definition on unenhanced CT images. Affected regions moderately to markedly enhance following contrast administration, and lesion margins are poorly defined. Abscesses typically have a fluid-attenuating center as well as a thick surrounding soft-tissue rim on unenhanced CT images and peripherally enhance following contrast administration (Figure 4.1.4).

Osteomyelitis of the ribs or sternum usually appears as a mixed destructive and productive lesion on CT images, with moderate to marked, ill-defined contrast enhancement (Figure 4.1.5).

Neoplasia

Neoplasms of the thoracic wall can be benign or malignant and of either soft-tissue or bone origin. Soft-tissue tumors include lipomas, benign mesenchymal neoplasms, sarcomas, and round cell tumors.

Lipomas have a homogeneous fat-attenuating appearance on CT images, do not significantly enhance, and usually have encapsulated margins. Some lipomas can be invasive, dissecting along fascial planes or infiltrating muscle (Figure 4.1.6). Lipomas are T1 and T2 hyperintense on MR images.

Malignant soft-tissue neoplasms can be uniformly or heterogeneously attenuating on unenhanced CT images and can run the spectrum from well encapsulated to poorly defined (Figure 4.1.7). Vaccine-associated fibrosarcomas are particularly invasive. The degree and homogeneity of contrast enhancement is variable and depends on tumor type.

Benign bone tumors, such as osteomas and chondromas, are rare. These neoplasms alter normal bone anatomy but typically have a nonaggressive appearance, showing no evidence of active bone destruction or rapid rate of change.

Atlas of Small Animal CT and MRI, First Edition. Erik R. Wisner and Allison L. Zwingenberger.
© 2015 John Wiley & Sons, Inc. Published 2015 by John Wiley & Sons, Inc.

Primary malignant bone tumors commonly involve the ribs and rarely arise from the sternum. Osteosarcoma is the most common of the primary bone tumors to affect the ribs, followed by chondrosarcoma, and they frequently arise at or near the costochondral junction.[2-5] These masses have an expansile appearance on CT images, with mixed destructive and productive components (Figure 4.1.8). Depending on size, masses can encroach on, displace, or envelop adjacent ribs. Masses can enhance on CT images following contrast administration, although enhancement may appear to be limited if the mass margins do not extend beyond the bone proliferative response.

Rib metastasis occurs frequently enough that close inspection of the ribs should be a part of every thoracic (pulmonary) metastasis CT examination. Rib metastases usually have an aggressive mixed destructive and productive appearance on CT images, with destruction often being the predominating component (Figure 4.1.9).

Diaphragm

The normal diaphragm is not well delineated from adjacent liver on unenhanced CT images, except for the dorsal diaphragmatic crura near their insertion on the ventral aspect of the cranial lumbar vertebral bodies.

Diaphragmatic hernia

Congenital diaphragmatic hernia is uncommon and is characterized by discontinuity of the diaphragm due to incomplete fusion of its components, which can lead to abdominal visceral migration into the thoracic cavity. A similar abnormality may occur with the loss of structural integrity of the central tendon of the diaphragm, which results in a thin distensible membrane within which abdominal viscera can be displaced. Traumatic diaphragmatic hernia results from muscle or tendinous tears.

The CT appearance of traumatic diaphragmatic hernia depends primarily on the size of the defect and the specific abdominal viscera displaced into the pleural space. Imaging features include the presence of solid and hollow viscera in the thoracic cavity, pulmonary atelectasis, and cardiac displacement. The liver is frequently herniated because of its position relative to the central tendon (Figure 4.1.10). The omentum, stomach, small bowel, and spleen may also herniate, resulting in a more complex pattern of attenuation of the herniated contents

(Figure 4.1.11). Visceral enhancement occurs following contrast medium administration unless strangulation inhibits blood flow.

Peritoneopericardial diaphragmatic hernia

A description of peritoneopericardial diaphragmatic hernia can be found in Chapter 4.4.

Hiatal hernia

Hiatal hernias include simple sliding hernias as well as less common paraesophageal hernias.[6] Both dogs and cats are affected, and English Bulldogs and Chinese Shar-Pei dogs are predisposed.[7-9] Although hiatal hernias are routinely diagnosed using other imaging techniques, such as fluoroscopy, they are occasionally seen in patients undergoing thoracic or abdominal CT for other reasons. The cranial displacement of the cardiac region of the stomach through the esophageal hiatus leads to a characteristic stellate pattern produced by the gastric rugal folds on transverse CT images (Figure 4.1.12). On long-axis images, the gastroesophageal junction is displaced cranially.

Gastroesophageal intussusception

Hiatal hernias must be distinguished from caudal esophageal masses and another rare disorder, gastroesophageal intussusception. In these patients, the stomach everts as it migrates through the gastroesophageal junction into the esophageal lumen (Figure 4.1.13).

Inflammatory disorders

Phrenitis (diaphragmitis) can occur by extension of pleuritis or peritonitis. Cross-sectional imaging features of phrenitis and phrenic abscess have not been reported. Rigid linear gastric foreign bodies occasionally penetrate the stomach wall and diaphragm (see Figure 5.4.4). Clinical signs in these patients are usually referable to the thorax, liver, stomach, or peritoneal cavity.

Neoplasia

Primary neoplasms of the diaphragm are rare, and cross-sectional imaging features have not been reported. Malignant neoplasms do metastasize to the diaphragm, but in our review of CT imaging studies of patients with confirmed diaphragmatic metastatic disease, imaging findings are ambiguous or unremarkable.

Figure 4.1.1 Acute Rib Fractures (Canine) CT

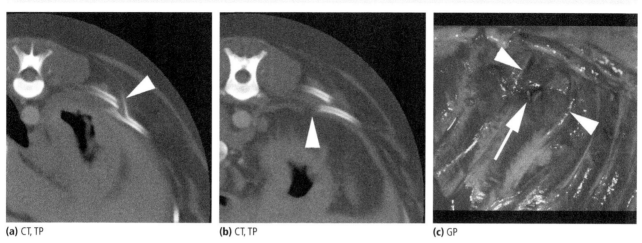

(a) CT, TP   (b) CT, TP   (c) GP

2y MC Shetland Sheepdog hit by a car earlier in the same day. Transverse CT images centered on two consecutive ribs and ordered from cranial to caudal show displaced proximal fractures (a,b). The fracture of the cranial rib is comminuted (a: arrowhead), and the distal fracture fragment of the caudal rib impinges on the parietal pleura (b: arrowhead). Postmortem examination viewed from the internal surface of the left thoracic wall reveals fracture displacement (c: arrowheads) as well as a puncture through the parietal pleura (c: arrow).

Figure 4.1.2 Chronic Rib Fractures (Feline) CT

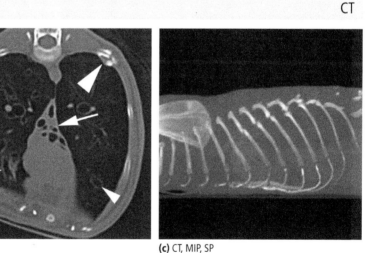

(a) CT, TP   (b) CT, TP   (c) CT, MIP, SP

Adult MC Domestic Shorthair with cough and weight loss of a few months' duration. More recently has had progressive respiratory distress. Transverse CT images centered on two consecutive ribs and ordered from cranial to caudal show displaced proximal left-sided fractures (a,b: large arrowheads). Both fractures are minimally displaced and have nonbridging, proliferative responses at the fracture margins. Fractures are evident involving six consecutive ribs on the left (c). Pulmonary findings included a marked, diffuse bronchial pattern (a,b), accessory lobe atelectasis and consolidation (b: arrow), and bronchiectasis (a,b: small arrowheads). A bronchoalveolar lavage showed purulent inflammation, and *Mycoplasma* was cultured. The fractures were thought to have resulted from cyclical stress from prolonged increased respiratory effort.

Figure 4.1.3 Thoracic Wall Penetrating Foreign Body (Canine)   CT

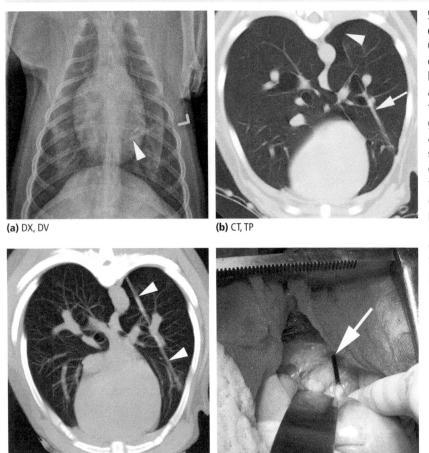

(a) DX, DV

(b) CT, TP

(c) CT, MIP, TP

(d) GP

5y FS Pointer cross with abrupt coughing episode while outside 5 months previously. Owners noted a small open wound on the chest wall at that time. Currently has a 5-day history of dyspnea. A short, linear, soft-tissue attenuating opacity is seen in the region of the left caudal lung lobe on survey radiographs (**a**: arrowhead). A soft-tissue attenuating, linear foreign body (**b**: arrow) and a small pneumothorax (**b**: arrowhead) are seen on transverse CT images. The full length of the foreign body is best appreciated on a MIP image oriented in the transverse plane (**c**: arrowheads). The foreign body was removed via thoracotomy (**d**: arrow) and was determined to be a carbon fiber or plastic rod that the dog had impaled itself on 5 months previously.

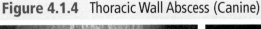

Figure 4.1.4 Thoracic Wall Abscess (Canine)   CT

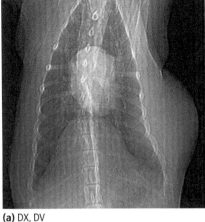

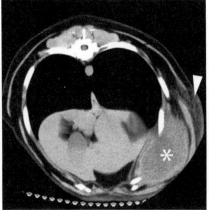

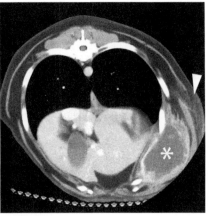

(a) DX, DV

(b) CT, TP

(c) CT+C, TP

6y MC Golden Retriever with a fluctuant mass of the left ventral body wall. The dorsoventral scout view of the thorax shows a large soft-tissue mass arising from the left thoracic wall (**a**). A large, ovoid mass is present on the left ventral body wall, deep to the external abdominal oblique muscles and with encroachment internal to the costal margins (**b,c**: asterisk). The central part measures approximately 15 HU on both unenhanced and enhanced CT images (**b,c**), and the mass has a thick, peripherally enhancing rim (**c**). There is also evidence of diffuse cellulitis more superficially (**b,c**: arrowhead). The mass was surgically drained and found to contain purulent material.

Figure 4.1.5   Sternal Osteomyelitis (Canine)

CT

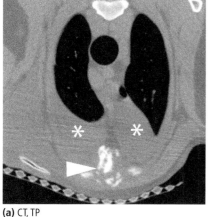

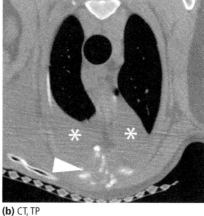

18mo MC Doberman Pinscher. Images **a** and **b** represent consecutive transverse images of the cranial thorax ordered from cranial to caudal. Unorganized bone destruction involving the second sternabral segment (**a–d**: arrowhead) is evident. A pathologic fracture is also present (**c**: arrowhead). A moderate volume of pleural fluid has collected bilaterally in the dependent pleural space (**a,b**: asterisks). Bone biopsy confirmed chronic neutrophilic osteomyelitis, and cytology of the pleural fluid revealed suppurative inflammation.

(a) CT, TP

(b) CT, TP

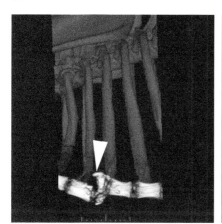

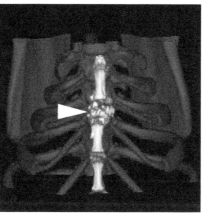

(c) CT, 3D, LLAT

(d) CT, 3D, VENT

Figure 4.1.6   Thoracic Wall Lipoma (Canine)

CT

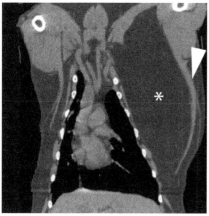

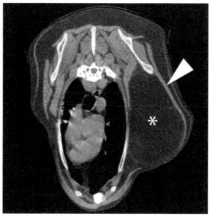

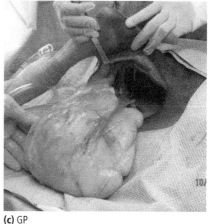

(a) CT, DP

(b) CT, TP

(c) GP

9y MC Coonhound with a left thoracic wall and axillary mass. A large, fat-attenuating mass is present in the left lateral body wall and axilla (**a,b**: asterisk). The mass is bounded by the latissimus dorsi muscle laterally (**a,b**: arrowhead) and appears homogeneous and encapsulated. The mass was removed en bloc (**c**), and biopsy confirmed it to be a lipoma.

Figure 4.1.7 Thoracic Wall Histiocytic Sarcoma (Canine)   CT

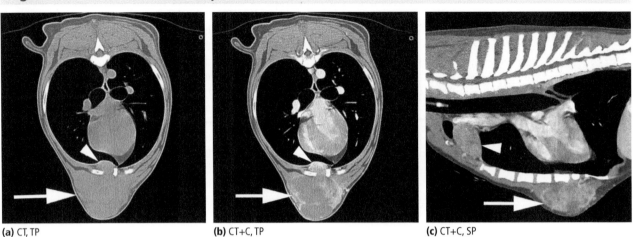

(a) CT, TP   **(b)** CT+C, TP   **(c)** CT+C, SP

4y FS Golden Retriever with a substernal thoracic wall mass. The dog was imaged in dorsal recumbency, and images have been reoriented. A large, superficial, irregularly margined, soft-tissue attenuating mass is present ventral to the sternum (**a**,**b**: arrow). The internal margin extends into the ventral thoracic cavity (**a**,**b**: arrowhead). The mass heterogeneously contrast enhances (**b**,**c**: arrow). A large, ovoid mass dorsal to the cranial sternum represents marked sternal lymphadenopathy (**c**: arrowhead). Postmortem examination confirmed thoracic wall histiocytic sarcoma with sternal lymph node metastasis. Other sites of distal metastasis were also found.

Figure 4.1.8 Rib Chondrosarcoma (Canine)   CT

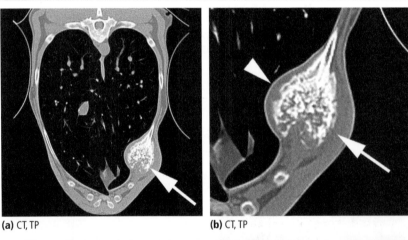

(a) CT, TP   **(b)** CT, TP

9y FS Greyhound with a left rib mass. Image **b** represents a magnification of image **a**. There is a moderately well circumscribed destructive and productive mass involving the ventral aspect of the left seventh rib near the costochondral junction (**a–c**: arrow). The mass causes a focal extrapleural sign at its interface with the left parietal pleural and lung margins (**b**: arrowhead). There is minimal enhancement beyond the bone proliferative margin following contrast administration (**d**). Excisional biopsy confirmed high-grade chondrosarcoma.

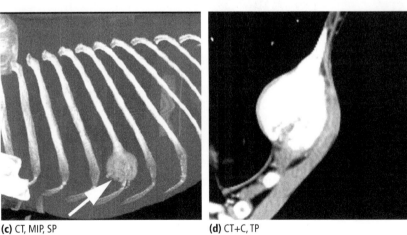

(c) CT, MIP, SP   **(d)** CT+C, TP

Figure 4.1.9 Rib Metastasis (Canine) CT

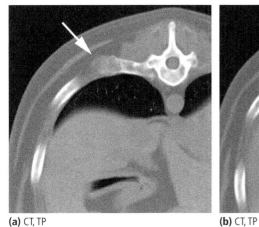 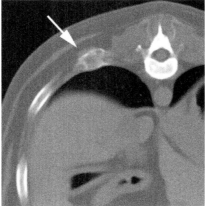

11y M Rottweiler with a primary osteosarcoma involving the right scapula. Two consecutive CT images of the caudal thorax ordered from cranial to caudal reveal an expansile destructive and productive mass in the proximal end of the right eleventh rib, representative of a bone metastasis from the primary neoplasm (a,b: arrow).

(a) CT, TP

(b) CT, TP

Figure 4.1.10 Diaphragmatic Hernia (Feline) CT

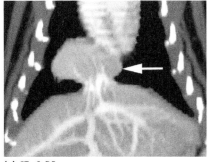 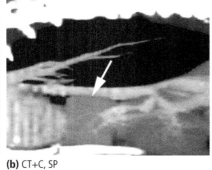

10y MC Domestic Longhair referred for a caudal thoracic mass. An ovoid mass is seen in the caudoventral thorax (a,b: arrow), and continuity of liver vasculature across a small window in the diaphragm verifies hepatic origin. Transverse images show the appearance of the abdominal (c) and herniated thoracic (d) components of the liver. The left medial lobe was determined to be herniated through the diaphragm on surgical exploration.

(a) CT+C, DP

(b) CT+C, SP

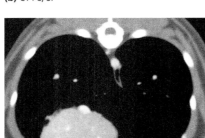 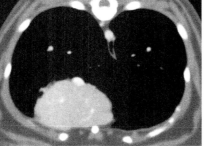

(c) CT+C, TP

(d) CT+C, TP

Figure 4.1.11 Diaphragmatic Hernia (Feline)   CT

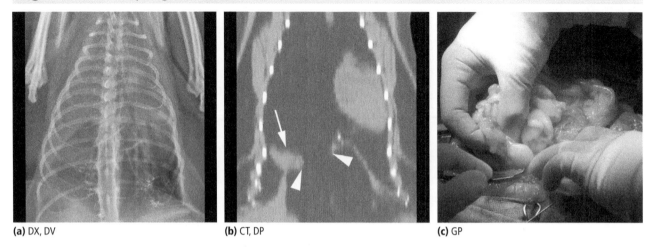

(a) DX, DV   **(b)** CT, DP   **(c)** GP

7y FS Domestic Shorthair with dyspnea and a possible thoracic mass. A traumatic diaphragmatic hernia was surgically repaired 5 years previously. A large volume of fat attenuating tissue is seen throughout the thorax on survey radiographs (**a**). Surgical wire is present in the caudal thorax and is presumably associated with the previous hernia repair. The fat-attenuating tissue is also seen on CT images (**b**), and a large defect is present within the diaphragm (**b**: arrowheads). The ovoid, soft-tissue attenuating mass at the right edge of the defect represents contracted and scarified muscle (**b**: arrow). A large volume of herniated omentum and falciform fat was reduced back into the abdomen during surgical repair (**c**).

Figure 4.1.12 Hiatal Hernia (Feline)   CT

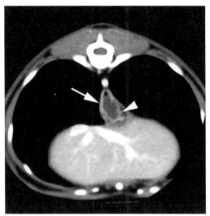

1.5y MC Domestic Shorthair with an esophageal stricture at the level of the heart base. A hiatal hernia (arrow) was seen on a thoracic CT examination acquired to evaluate the stricture. Gastric rugal folds are clearly delineated on this contrast-enhanced image (arrowhead).

(a) CT+C, TP

Figure 4.1.13   Gastroesophageal Intussusception (Canine)   CT

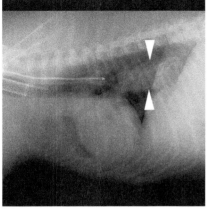

(a) DX, LLAT

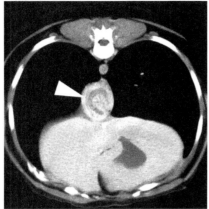

(b) CT+C, TP

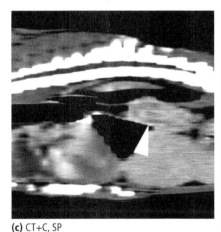

(c) CT+C, SP

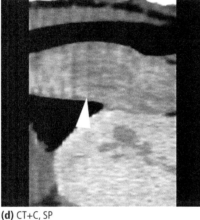

(d) CT+C, SP

5y FS Keeshond with a 7-month history of coughing and a left cranial lung lobe mass. A tubular soft-tissue mass is present in the region of the caudal esophagus on survey radiographs (**a**: arrowheads). Although the left cranial lung lobe mass is not clearly delineated, there is increased opacity in the cranioventral thorax. The leading edge of a gastric intussusceptum is seen on a transverse CT image (**b**: arrowhead) and has a striated appearance when viewed in long axis (**c,d**: arrowheads). Image **d** represents a sagittal plane reformation from more thinly collimated images than image **c**. The gastroesophageal intussusception was documented and reduced at the time of left cranial lung lobectomy.

References

1. Hardie EM, Ramirez O 3rd, Clary EM, Kornegay JN, Correa MT, Feimster RA, et al. Abnormalities of the thoracic bellows: stress fractures of the ribs and hiatal hernia. J Vet Intern Med. 1998;12:279–287.
2. Feeney DA, Johnston GR, Grindem CB, Toombs JP, Caywood DD, Hanlon GF. Malignant neoplasia of canine ribs: clinical, radiographic, and pathologic findings. J Am Vet Med Assoc. 1982;180:927–933.
3. Liptak JM, Kamstock DA, Dernell WS, Monteith GJ, Rizzo SA, Withrow SJ. Oncologic outcome after curative-intent treatment in 39 dogs with primary chest wall tumors (1992–2005). Vet Surg. 2008;37:488–496.
4. Matthiesen DT, Clark GN, Orsher RJ, Pardo AO, Glennon J, Patnaik AK. En bloc resection of primary rib tumors in 40 dogs. Vet Surg. 1992;21:201–204.
5. Pirkey-Ehrhart N, Withrow SJ, Straw RC, Ehrhart EJ, Page RL, Hottinger HL, et al. Primary rib tumors in 54 dogs. J Am Anim Hosp Assoc. 1995;31:65–69.
6. Dean C, Etienne D, Carpentier B, Gielecki J, Tubbs RS, Loukas M. Hiatal hernias. Surg Radiol Anat. 2012;34:291–299.
7. Guiot LP, Lansdowne JL, Rouppert P, Stanley BJ. Hiatal hernia in the dog: a clinical report of four Chinese shar peis. J Am Anim Hosp Assoc. 2008;44:335–341.
8. Lorinson D, Bright RM. Long-term outcome of medical and surgical treatment of hiatal hernias in dogs and cats: 27 cases (1978–1996). J Am Vet Med Assoc. 1998;213:381–384.
9. Stickle R, Sparschu G, Love N, Walshaw R. Radiographic evaluation of esophageal function in Chinese Shar Pei pups. J Am Vet Med Assoc. 1992;201:81–84.

4.2

Pleural space

Normal pleural space

Because normal pleura measure less than 1–2 mm in thickness, and because except for the small volume of normal lubricating pleural fluid, the pleural cavity is anatomically a potential space, characteristic imaging features of the normal pleural space are conspicuously absent. Fine lines corresponding to pleural margins can be identified on CT images of the normal thorax, but they are typically subtle and generally not confused with pleural pathology.

Pneumothorax

Pneumothorax most often results from penetrating injury of the chest wall or from disruption of the visceral pleura. Pulmonary causes of pneumothorax include rupture of peripheral pulmonary bulla or subpleural blebs, shear injuries of the lung parenchyma, penetrating and migrating foreign bodies, and necrotizing inflammatory and neoplastic lung lesions. Occasionally, injury to the trachea or esophagus with concurrent involvement of adjacent mediastinal parietal pleura can result in pneumothorax and pneumomediastinum.

Although thoracic radiography is recognized as an excellent screening tool for detecting and quantifying pneumothorax, small volumes of free pleural air can be missed. In general, CT is performed after a diagnosis of pneumothorax has been made and the patient appropriately stabilized. In many patients, thoracostomy catheters have been placed to evacuate free pleural gas and re-expand the lungs, which can improve imaging detection of underlying lesions of pulmonary origin.

A prominent CT feature of uncomplicated pneumothorax is collection of free gas in nondependent regions of the pleural space (Figure 4.2.1). Lung lobe volume will be variably reduced depending on the severity of the pneumothorax, resulting in an increase in pulmonary attenuation. This may be relatively uniform, although dependent lung is usually more affected and may be overtly atelectatic. Lateral shift of the heart and mediastinum may also be seen as a result of passive displacement, with unilateral or asymmetrical effusions. In patients with concurrent pleural disease, the pleural membrane may be thickened and can be readily recognized by evaluating the lung margins at their interface with the free pleural air.[1,2]

Pleural effusion

Pleural effusions result from a variety of disorders and are classified as transudative, modified transudative (e.g. chylous), exudative, or hemorrhagic. The volume of effusion is variable and may be diffusely distributed, unilateral, or regionally compartmentalized (Figure 4.2.2).

Transudative effusion

Transudative pleural effusions are most commonly caused by right-sided heart failure or marked hypoproteinemia. Because the macromolecular concentration and cellularity of transudates are low, the attenuation of the fluid approaches that of water, and these effusions

Atlas of Small Animal CT and MRI, First Edition. Erik R. Wisner and Allison L. Zwingenberger.
© 2015 John Wiley & Sons, Inc. Published 2015 by John Wiley & Sons, Inc.

typically range from 0–30 HU. Large fluid volumes cause partial or complete atelectasis with the greatest effect on the right middle lobe, followed by the two cranial lobes.[3]

As normal lung collapses, its attenuation increases in proportion with the degree of volume loss. Completely atelectatic lung has attenuation of approximately 50–60 HU on unenhanced CT images. Large volumes of effusion also cause significant displacement of the lungs from their normal location (Figure 4.2.2). Pleural fluid tends to distribute to the dependent part of the pleural space, and aerated lung, although tethered at the hilus, is buoyed toward the nondependent regions. Moderate to large volumes of effusion, regardless of fluid characteristics, cause lung lobes to "float", altering the course of affected airways and distortion of lung contours. Effusion also leads to lung lobe torsion (Figure 4.2.3) (see Chapter 4.6).[3]

Hemorrhagic effusion and hemothorax

Hemorrhagic effusion may be caused by trauma, bleeding masses, anticoagulant poisoning and other bleeding diatheses, or increased vascular permeability of compromised tissue. Frank blood has attenuation of 40–50 HU on CT images, although mixed hemorrhagic effusions may be less dense than this. Depending on the initiating cause, hemorrhagic effusions and hemothorax may be asymmetrical or compartmentalized (Figure 4.2.3). Active hemorrhage may result in hematoma formation, and cellular elements may settle to the dependent regions, resulting in a denser dependent effusion layer.

Chylous effusion

Chylous effusions are usually caused by thoracic duct trauma or a disruption of the hydrostatic gradient between the thoracic duct and cranial vena cava, leading to lymphangiectasia and increased lymphatic permeability. Mediastinal masses may also occasionally result in a chylous effusion by obstructing lymphatic return through the duct. While the fluid volume is often marked in patients with chylous effusion, clinical progression of the disease may be relatively slow and insidious. The composition of the effusion and its chronic contact with pleural surfaces typically results in a low-grade sterile pleuritis that in turn leads to pleural thickening that is easily detected on CT images (Figure 4.2.4). Pleural thickening and loss of compliance result in lung volume reduction and rounding of the lobar margins. In severe cases, removal of effusion may result in incomplete reinflation of the lungs and the presence of an *ex vacuo* pneumothorax because of the restrictive pleuritis.

CT lymphangiography

CT lymphangiography is performed to visualize thoracic duct anatomy, to define location and character of chyle leakage, and to preoperatively plan for thoracic duct ligation. Iodinated contrast medium is injected either directly into a popliteal lymph node or into a mesenteric lymph node using ultrasound guidance, and thoracic CT is performed after the thoracic duct is fully opacified. The normal lymphangiogram reveals one or more thoracic duct branches coursing next to the thoracic aorta and entering the cranial vena cava (Figure 4.2.5). Near this junction, a variable number of smaller lymphatic branches are seen that connect with the cranial mediastinal lymph nodes.[4,5]

In patients with thoracic duct injury or obstruction, extravasated contrast medium may be seen dispersing within the mediastinum (Figure 4.2.6). In other patients, a proliferation of many small lymphatic vessels in the cranial mediastinum is indicative of lymphangiectasia from lymphatic flow obstruction. The transverse view of the thoracic duct on CT images provides a means of accurately determining the number of parallel branches and their location relative to the aorta in anticipation of surgical ligation.[4,5]

Pleuritis/pyothorax

Infectious pleuritis or pyothorax may be due to direct penetrating injury or be a sequela of systemic disease. For the sake of this discussion, pleuritis is a general term defined as any inflammatory condition of the pleural membranes, whereas pyothorax describes an effusive, infectious, suppurative inflammatory condition of the pleural space and pleura. In addition to the CT features descriptive of other effusions described above, infectious pleuritis/pyothorax sometimes has a characteristically sedimentary component of relatively high attenuation due to the settling of solids, exudate inspissation, and inflammatory pleural proliferation.[6] Pleural membranes are often markedly thickened and may be highly contrast enhancing (Figures 4.2.7, 4.2.8). Small volumes of free gas may be seen because of the presence of gas-forming organisms or penetrating injury.[6,7] Rarely, foreign bodies initiating a pyothorax can be seen within the effusion (Figure 4.2.9).

Pleural masses

Most clinically significant pleural masses are malignant and include primary pleural tumors, such as mesothelioma, or other neoplasms that arise from the thoracic wall, mediastinum, or diaphragm and invade or encroach on the pleura. Mesotheliomas may appear as a discrete mass on CT images but can go undetected in patients in which the tumor invades the pleura diffusely (Figure 4.2.10).[8,9] CT imaging features of other masses depend on anatomic location and tumor type (Figure 4.2.11).[9]

Pleural thickening/fibrosis

Pleural thickening is sometimes evident without other associated radiographic abnormalities or clinical signs and is thought to be due to previous pleural inflammatory disease with resulting pleural fibrosis (Figure 4.2.12).[9]

Figure 4.2.1 Pneumothorax (Canine)   CT

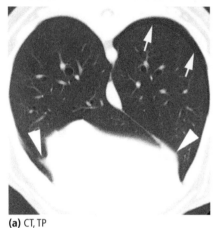 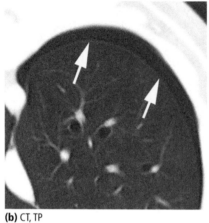

(a) CT, TP   **(b)** CT, TP

12y Doberman Pinscher with an axillary mass. Image **b** represents a magnified view of the left dorsal thorax. A mild left-sided pneumothorax is present, causing retraction of the visceral pleura away from the thoracic wall (**a,b**: arrows). A small volume of pleural fluid is also present, causing separation of visceral pleural surfaces (**a**: arrowheads).

Figure 4.2.2 Positional Lung Changes with Transudative Pleural Effusion (Canine)   CT

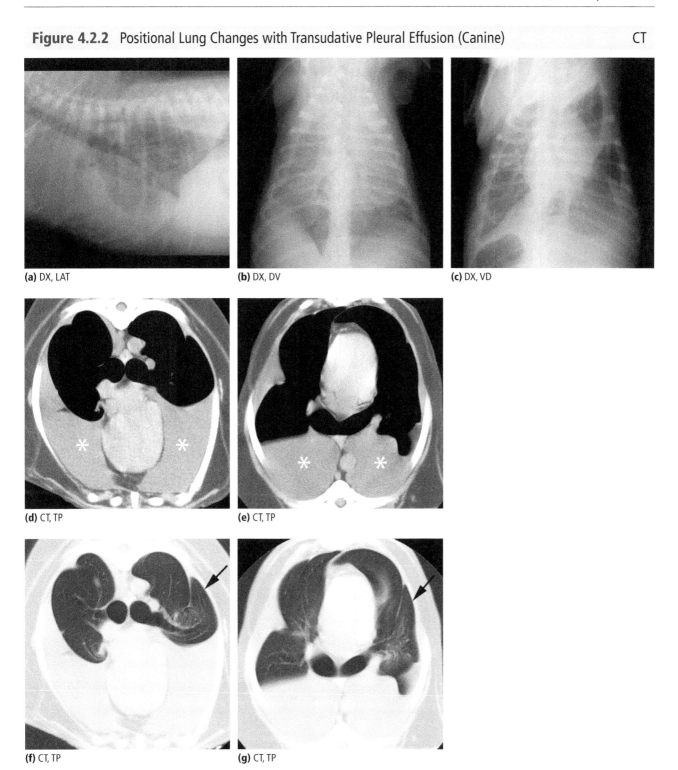

(a) DX, LAT   **(b)** DX, DV   **(c)** DX, VD

(d) CT, TP   **(e)** CT, TP

(f) CT, TP   **(g)** CT, TP

10y FS Golden Retriever in respiratory distress for 1 month. The radiographic study (**a–c**) reveals a large volume of pleural fluid that obscures the aerated lungs and cardiac silhouette. CT images were acquired with the patient in sternal (**d,f**) and dorsal (**e,g**) recumbency at the level of the midthorax, immediately caudal to the carina. A moderate volume of dependent fluid is seen in both positions (**d,e**: asterisks), indicating the effusion is not compartmentalized. Aerated lungs are displaced by the effusion and migrate depending on position. In particular, note the marked displacement of the apical region of the left cranial lung lobe when the dog is in sternal recumbency (**f**: arrow), which migrates back to a more normal orientation when the dog is placed in dorsal recumbency (**g**: arrow). Effusion cytology revealed a transudate. Pleural biopsy material was interpreted as either mesothelioma or reactive pleuritis.

Figure 4.2.3 Pleural Effusion with Lung Lobe Torsion (Canine)   CT

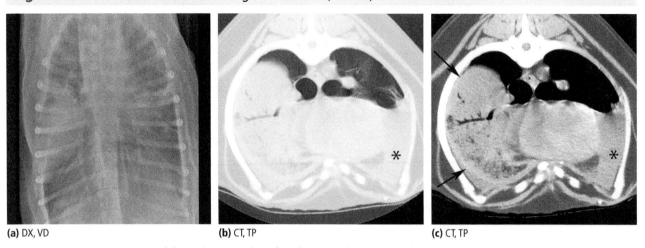

(a) DX, VD   **(b)** CT, TP   **(c)** CT, TP

9y MC Bernese Mountain Dog with hemothorax resulting from heparin administration for an unrelated medical problem. The ventrodorsal radiograph reveals pleural effusion and an ill-defined mass in the region of the right middle lung lobe (**a**). Images **b** and **c** are the same images optimized for viewing aerated lung and soft tissues, respectively. There is moderate pleural effusion distributed in the dependent part of the pleural space (**b,c**: asterisk) and an enlarged, malpositioned right middle lung lobe with CT features consistent with lobar torsion (**c**: arrows). A right middle lung lobe torsion was confirmed surgically.

Figure 4.2.4 Chronic Chylous Pleural Effusion (Feline)   CT

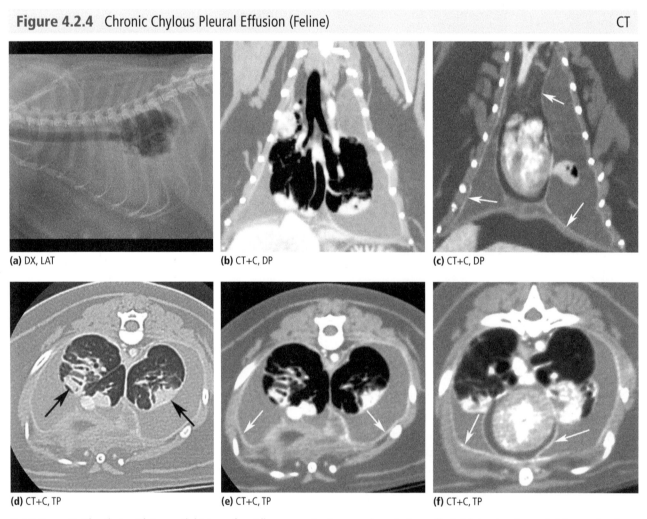

(a) DX, LAT   **(b)** CT+C, DP   **(c)** CT+C, DP

(d) CT+C, TP   **(e)** CT+C, TP   **(f)** CT+C, TP

8y FS Domestic Shorthair with 1-month history of rapidly progressive increased respiratory effort. A lateral radiograph (**a**) reveals a large volume of pleural effusion and rounding of the lung margins consistent with chronic pleural thickening and reduced compliance. CT images also document the pleural effusion and restricted pulmonary inflation (**b,d–f**). A CT image optimized for viewing aerated lung reveals multiple focal regions of atelectasis (**d**: arrows). Contrast-enhanced images also highlight uniform visceral and parietal pleural thickening and enhancement, all of which are consistent with pleuritis (**c,e,f**: arrows). Analysis of fluid from thoracocentesis confirmed chylous effusion. Clinical diagnosis was chronic chylothorax with restrictive pleuritis.

Figure 4.2.5 Normal Thoracic Duct Lymphangiogram (Canine)   CT

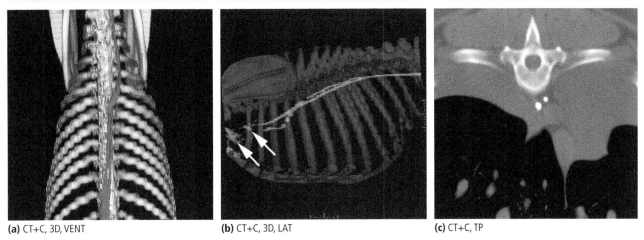

(a) CT+C, 3D, VENT   **(b)** CT+C, 3D, LAT   **(c)** CT+C, TP

Adult dog of unknown breed or gender with documented chylothorax. Three-dimensional CT renderings acquired following injection of iodinated contrast medium directly into a mesenteric lymph node reveal a redundant thoracic duct (**a,b**: red coloration). Also contrast enhancing is a plexus of smaller lymphatic vessels and cranial mediastinal lymph nodes (**b**: arrows). A conventional transverse CT image acquired following lymph node injection shows two redundant branches of the lymphatic duct adjacent and dorsal to the aorta in the caudal thorax (**c**). Johnson EJ, et al. 2009.[4] Reproduced with permission from Wiley.

Figure 4.2.6 Abnormal Thoracic Duct Lymphangiogram (Canine)   CT

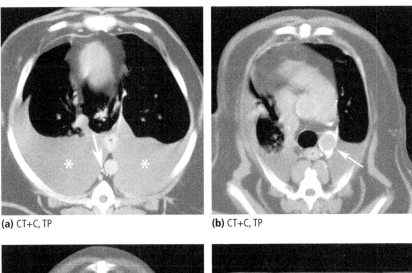

(a) CT+C, TP   **(b)** CT+C, TP

11y Australian Cattle Dog with thyroid carcinoma and associated thrombi involving the left jugular and brachiocephalic veins and cranial vena cava. Images **a–c** are oriented with the dog in dorsal recumbency. Moderate dependent pleural effusion (**a**: asterisks) and multiple small parallel branches of the caudal thoracic duct are seen (**a**: arrow) following ultrasound-guided contrast medium injection into a jejunal lymph node. More cranially, extravasated contrast medium surrounds the descending aorta (**b**: arrow), the brachiocephalic trunk, and the left subclavian artery (**c**: arrows). A sagittally oriented maximum intensity projection (MIP) image (**d**) reveals widespread extralymphatic dispersal of contrast medium in the cranial mediastinum. Thrombi were confirmed surgically as the source of lymphatic duct obstruction.

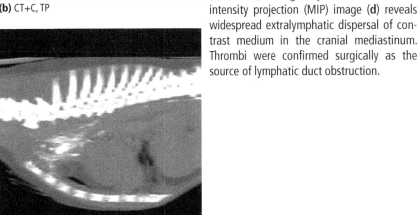

(C) CT+C, TP   **(d)** CT+C, MIP, SP

Figure 4.2.7 Pleuritis and Pleural Foreign Body (Canine)

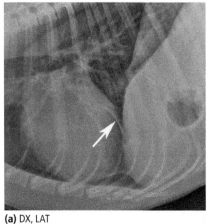

(a) DX, LAT

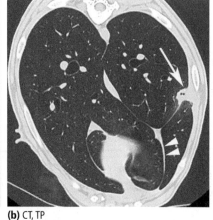

(b) CT, TP

2y MC Belgian Malinois. Thoracic radiographs revealed a focal left caudal pulmonary infiltrate and pleural fissure lines (**a**: arrow). Thoracic CT confirmed the presence of a small pleural fluid volume (**b**: arrowheads) and a focal lesion consisting of a peripheral consolidating pulmonary component and an adjacent pleural component (**b**: arrow). Presumptive diagnosis was focal foreign-body pneumonia and pleuritis from migrating plant awn. The diagnosis was confirmed by bronchoscopy and partial lung lobectomy performed 3 days following the CT scan.

Figure 4.2.8 Pyothorax (Canine)

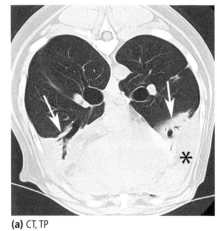

(a) CT, TP

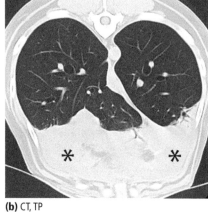

(b) CT, TP

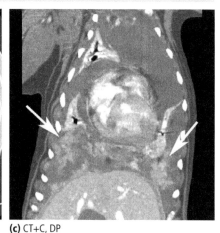

(c) CT+C, DP

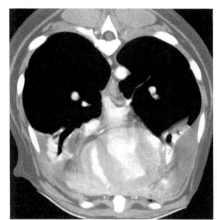

(d) CT+C, TP

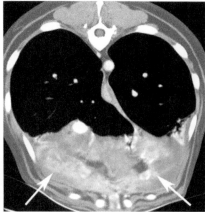

(e) CT+C, TP

8y MC Labrador Retriever with recent-onset increased respiratory effort. Representative CT images include unenhanced (**a,b**) and corresponding contrast-enhanced (**d,e**) transverse images and a dorsal plane reformatted image (**c**) of the ventral thorax. Moderate bilateral pleural effusion is present with fluid distributed primarily in the dependent thorax (**a,b**: asterisks). The ventral lungs are atelectatic (**a**: arrows) with nondependent regions better aerated. Following contrast medium administration, there is ill-defined but marked heterogeneous contrast enhancement in the ventral paramediastinal and ventral pleural space regions (**c,e**: arrows). Surgical exploration with biopsy revealed chronic fibrinosuppurative pleuritis with villonodular mesothelial proliferation and multifocal abscessation. A plant awn foreign body was found in the suppurative effusion.

Figure 4.2.9 Pyothorax and Pleural Foreign Body (Canine)   CT

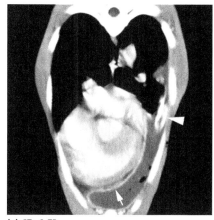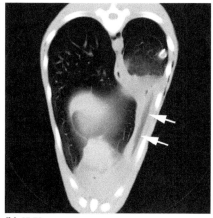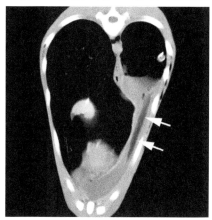

(a) CT+C, TP   **(b)** CT, TP   **(c)** CT, TP

Young adult M Saluki with pyrexia and dyspnea. A thoracostomy catheter was placed in the left pleural space prior to the CT examination. Moderate, predominantly left-sided pleural effusion is present. The parietal pleura in the midthorax is markedly thickened and contrast enhances (**a**: arrow), consistent with active pleuritis. The fragmented gas pattern in the effusion was thought to be iatrogenic. A portion of the thoracostomy catheter can also be seen (**a**: arrowhead). A large, linear, low-attenuation defect is seen within the pleural effusion in the caudal thorax (**b**,**c**: arrows). The effusion was suppurative and cultured positive for multiple bacteria. A thoracotomy was performed and a 6 cm × 1 cm wooden stick was removed from the left pleural space.

Figure 4.2.10 Mesothelioma (Canine)   CT

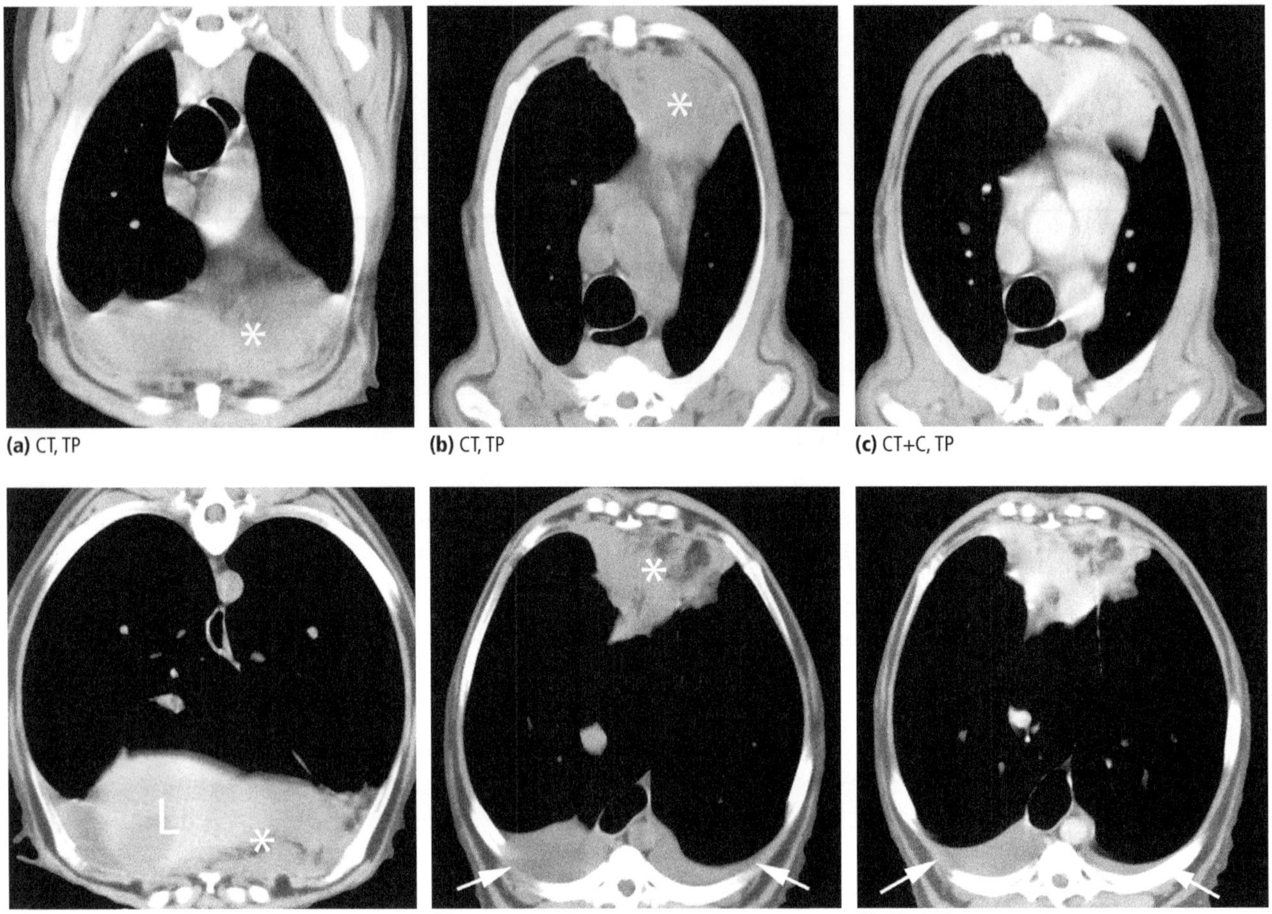

(a) CT, TP

(b) CT, TP

(c) CT+C, TP

(d) CT, TP

(e) CT, TP

(f) CT+C, TP

11y FS Golden Retriever with coughing, dyspnea, and weight loss. Representative images include ventral and dorsal recumbent images acquired cranial (**a–c**) and caudal (**d–f**) to the heart. An ill-defined mass extends the length of the ventral thorax on the sternal recumbent unenhanced images (**a,d**: asterisk; **d**: L = liver). A small volume of dependent pleural fluid is also present, which partially obscures the mass. The mass is more clearly seen on the dorsal recumbent unenhanced images (**b,e**: asterisk), and incorporation of adipose tissue contributes to a heterogeneous attenuation caudally (**e**). Comparable contrast-enhanced images reveal uniform enhancement of the soft-tissue component of the mass (**c,f**). Dependent pleural fluid is again seen (**e,f**: arrows). Cytologic evaluation of the pleural effusion was interpreted as mild mesothelial proliferation. Tissue biopsy of the mass revealed mesothelioma.

Figure 4.2.11 Metastatic Mammary Carcinoma (Feline)   CT

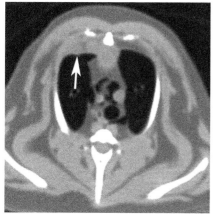 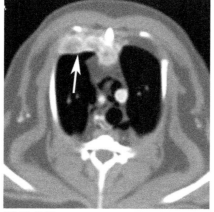 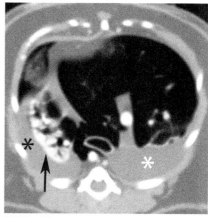

(a) CT, TP   **(b)** CT+C, TP   **(c)** CT+C, TP

12y FS Domestic Longhair with progressive respiratory distress. Representative CT images include an unenhanced (**a**) and corresponding contrast-enhanced (**b**) transverse image of the cranial thorax and an additional transverse image at the level of the midthorax (**c**). The patient is positioned in dorsal recumbency, and images are displayed in that orientation. A heterogeneous contrast-enhancing mass is present in the right ventral thoracic wall and extends into the ventral mediastinum (**a,b**: arrow). Moderate bilateral pleural effusion is present with fluid distributed primarily in the dependent thorax (**c**: asterisks). The ventral lung is atelectatic (**c**: arrow) with nondependent regions better aerated. The mass was confirmed to be a subpleural metastatic mammary carcinoma with pleural effusion.

Figure 4.2.12 Pleural Fibrosis (Canine)   CT

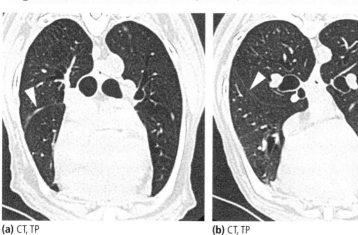

(a) CT, TP   **(b)** CT, TP

8y FS Shiba Inu with a retrobulbar mass. CT was performed as a metastasis-screening test. Heterogeneous pleural thickening is present involving visceral pleura of multiple lung lobes bilaterally (**a,b**: arrowheads). There is no suggestion of a pleural effusion component, which suggests pleural changes are inactive. Pleural thickening was thought to represent residual pleural fibrosis from previous inflammatory disease.

References

1. Au JJ, Weisman DL, Stefanacci JD, Palmisano MP. Use of computed tomography for evaluation of lung lesions associated with spontaneous pneumothorax in dogs: 12 cases (1999–2002). J Am Vet Med Assoc. 2006;228: 733–737.

2. Lipscomb V, Brockman D, Gregory S, Baines S, Lamb CR. CT scanning of dogs with spontaneous pneumothorax. Vet Rec. 2004;154: 344.

3. Dechman G, Mishima M, Bates JH. Assessment of acute pleural effusion in dogs by computed tomography. J Appl Physiol. 1994;76: 1993–1998.

4. Johnson EG, Wisner ER, Kyles A, Koehler C, Marks SL. Computed tomographic lymphography of the thoracic duct by mesenteric lymph node injection. Vet Surg. 2009;38: 361–367.

5. Lee N, Won S, Choi M, Kim J, Yi K, Chang D, et al. CT thoracic duct lymphography in cats by popliteal lymph node iohexol injection. Vet Radiol Ultrasound. 2012;53: 174–180.

6. Swinbourne F, Baines EA, Baines SJ, Halfacree ZJ. Computed tomographic findings in canine pyothorax and correlation with findings at exploratory thoracotomy. J Small Anim Pract. 2011;52: 203–208.

7. Schultz RM, Zwingenberger A. Radiographic, computed tomographic, and ultrasonographic findings with migrating intrathoracic grass awns in dogs and cats. Vet Radiol Ultrasound. 2008;49: 249–255.

8. Echandi RL, Morandi F, Newman SJ, Holford A. Imaging diagnosis – canine thoracic mesothelioma. Vet Radiol Ultrasound. 2007;48: 243–245.

9. Reetz JA, Buza EL, Krick EL. CT features of pleural masses and nodules. Vet Radiol Ultrasound. 2012;53: 121–127.

4.3

Mediastinum and esophagus

Normal mediastinum and variants

The margins of the mediastinum are formed by the internal parietal pleura of the two hemithoraces. The cranial mediastinum contains mediastinal and sternal lymph nodes, the thymus or thymic remnants, major blood vessels, the esophagus, and a variable amount of fat (Figure 4.3.1). The middle, hilar, and caudal regions of the mediastinum contain the heart, aorta, thoracic duct, esophagus, and tracheobronchial lymph nodes. The normal thymus has a mildly striated, glandular appearance with soft-tissue attenuation on unenhanced CT images and a homogeneous appearance on MR images with T1 isointensity and T2 hyperintensity as compared to skeletal musculature.

Developmental disorders

Cranial mediastinal cyst

Cranial mediastinal cysts are uncommon and most often arise from branchial cleft remnants that contribute to the formation of the thymus.[1-3] Uncomplicated mediastinal cysts are generally well-delineated, thin-walled, fluid-filled masses that may displace other cranial mediastinal structures when large. Mediastinal cysts are fluid attenuating on unenhanced CT images and do not contrast enhance, although thymic remnants adherent to the margins of the cyst may enhance (Figure 4.3.2). Pleural effusion may also be present in some patients.

Trauma

Pneumomediastinum

Pneumomediastinum can occur as the result of thoracic or cervical trauma or incidentally as a sequela to jugular phlebotomy. Mediastinal gas distributes along fascial planes and surrounds organs and tissues contained within the mediastinal space. On CT images, mediastinal gas is low attenuating, may have a fragmented distribution, and accentuates margins of the soft-tissue structures, around which the gas collects (Figure 4.3.3). Gas can migrate into the cervical region in patients with large active leaks, leading to pronounced subcutaneous emphysema.

Hemomediastinum

Hemomediastinum can result from thoracic trauma or bleeding diatheses, such as those induced by anticoagulant toxicity. Depending on the volume of blood in the mediastinum, uniform or nonuniform mediastinal widening may occur. Hemorrhage will appear mildly hypo- to hyperattenuating compared to soft tissues on unenhanced CT images and may be amorphous or organized depending on the age of the bleeding episode (Figure 4.3.4).

Inflammatory disorders

Reactive lymphadenopathy and lymphadenitis

Sternal, cranial mediastinal, and tracheobronchial lymph nodes can enlarge as a result of reactivity from a regional or systemic inflammatory disorder or from overt infection within the nodes. Bacterial and mycotic agents are

Atlas of Small Animal CT and MRI, First Edition. Erik R. Wisner and Allison L. Zwingenberger.
© 2015 John Wiley & Sons, Inc. Published 2015 by John Wiley & Sons, Inc.

most commonly involved. Generalized lymph node enlargement occurs in response to an inflammatory insult and may progress to abscessation (bacterial or fungal) or granuloma formation (fungal) (Figures 4.3.5, 4.3.6, 4.3.7). Lymph nodes are soft-tissue attenuating on unenhanced CT images and are moderately and uniformly contrast enhancing. Abscessed or granulomatous nodes may peripherally contrast enhance with variable or no central enhancement.

Mediastinitis

Mediastinitis may result from contamination through direct penetrating injury, such as occurs with penetrating esophageal foreign bodies, or from systemic infection. The mediastinum is often widened by the presence of inflammatory fluid and associated lymphadenopathy (Figure 4.3.8).

Mediastinal neoplasia

Thymoma and other solid mediastinal neoplasms

Thymomas are variable in size but can be quite large, occupying a significant volume in the cranial thorax and causing cranial lung lobe displacement and atelectasis as well as displacement of the heart, mediastinal blood vessels, and the cranial thoracic esophagus and trachea. Because of the orientation of the ventral recess of the cranial mediastinum, which is often positioned to the left of midline, large thymomas often extend caudally primarily along the left hemithorax.[1,4,5] Thymomas can have a cystic center with a thick and internally irregular parenchymal margin on CT images, and solid components have a moderate to intense heterogeneous pattern of contrast enhancement (Figures 4.3.9, 4.3.10, 4.3.11). Thymomas can also be associated with development of megaesophagus in some patients.

A number of other mediastinal neoplasms have been reported, including thyroid carcinoma, carcinomas of other origin, sarcomas, and round cell tumors.[6] Imaging features of these neoplasms may be similar to those described for thymomas but vary depending on cell type (Figure 4.3.12).

An important reason for imaging cranial mediastinal neoplasms is to determine the presence and extent of vascular invasion, which can determine operability and prognosis. With CT imaging, vascular luminal defects representing local tumor extension are best seen on images acquired shortly after contrast administration while intravascular contrast medium concentration is high.[4] However, if images are acquired too quickly, intravascular contrast concentration may be nonuniform because of inadequate recirculation,

which can create pseudo-filling defects. Intraluminal tumors appear as relatively hypoattenuating masses surrounded by hyperattenuating blood (Figures 4.3.10, 4.3.11). Filling defects can also result from tumor-associated thrombi, which usually cannot be distinguished from tumor invasion.

Lymphoma

Lymphoma in the mediastinum may involve the thymus or the mediastinal lymph nodes, the latter often resulting in marked nodal enlargement with affected lymph nodes retaining their normal shape.[6,7] Lymph nodes are normally soft-tissue attenuating on unenhanced CT images and may have a uniform or mildly heterogeneous pattern of moderate contrast enhancement (Figure 4.3.13).

Esophagus

The entire length of the normal esophagus can be seen on CT images, and detection is made easier with the presence of luminal gas or fluid that defines the esophageal lumen and outlines the characteristic rosette pattern of the esophageal mucosal folds when viewed in cross-section.

Megasophagus

Generalized or regional esophageal distension is easily recognized on CT images, and the appearance depends on the extent of dilation and the presence of luminal gas or fluid (Figure 4.3.14).

Esophageal stricture and entrapment

Although esophageal strictures can be detected using CT or MR, these are typically not the preferred imaging modalities for diagnosis, unless an associated mass is present. A stricture may not be detected directly on CT images, but its presence may be implied by gas or fluid distension cranial to the stricture (Figure 4.3.15).

Esophagitis

Esophagitis would typically not be detected with CT imaging but may occasionally appear as a focal or regional thickening of the esophageal wall, perhaps associated with an irregular mucosal margin when gas is present in the lumen (Figure 4.3.17).

Paraesophageal abscess

Paraesophageal abscesses preferentially involve the caudal thoracic esophagus, intimately involve the esophageal wall, and are presumably caused by penetrating foreign bodies. Paraesophageal abscesses are generally well-delineated, fluid-filled, spheroid to ellipsoid masses arising in the mediastinum. The esophagus appears as a thin soft-tissue attenuating crescent associated with part of the abscess margin on transverse CT images (Figure 4.3.16). Abscesses are fluid attenuating on unenhanced CT images and peripherally contrast enhance. The flattened esophageal mucosa has a characteristic curvilinear pattern of contrast enhancement conforming to the curvature of the abscess. Additional imaging features associated with mediastinitis may also be present. The adjacent lung lobes can sometimes be atelectatic as a result of encroachment by the mass.[8]

Esophageal neoplasia

Neoplasia of the esophagus is rare and includes carcinoma, sarcoma (associated with *Spirocerca lupi* infection), leiomyoma, leiomyosarcoma, and lymphoma. Imaging features depend on the size and location of the mass. Obstruction may be a sequela with resulting esophageal dilation cranial to site of the neoplasm. Neoplasms may be solid or heterogeneous on CT and MR images and typically appear as an eccentric or circumferential mass. The intensity and pattern of contrast enhancement are variable (Figure 4.3.17).

Figure 4.3.1 Normal Cranial Mediastinum (Canine)   CT

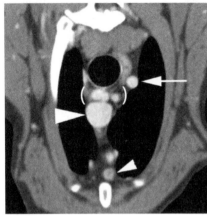 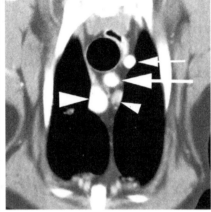 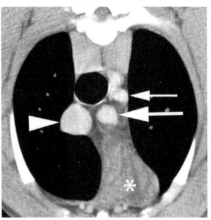

(a) CT+C, TP   **(b)** CT+C, TP   **(c)** CT+C, TP

CT images are of three different dogs. The cranial mediastinum contains major arteries and veins, sternal and mediastinal lymph nodes, and a variable amount of fat. Normal features include the cranial vena cava (**a–c**: large arrowhead), left subclavian artery (**a–c**: small arrows), brachiocephalic trunk (**b,c**: large arrow), common carotid and right subclavian arteries (**a**: brackets), and sternal and cranial mediastinal lymph nodes (**a,b**: small arrowhead). The thymus may also be visible in young animals (**c**: asterisk).

Figure 4.3.2 Cranial Mediastinal Cyst (Feline)   CT

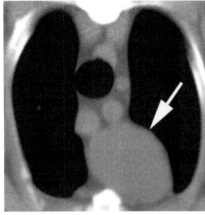 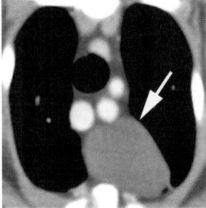 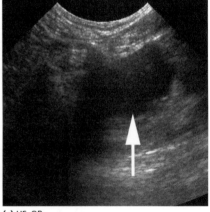

(a) CT, TP   **(b)** CT+C, TP   **(c)** US, OP

17y MC Domestic Shorthair with pelvic mass. The thoracic CT examination was performed for cancer staging. There is a well-defined ovoid mass in the cranial mediastinum (**a**: arrow). The mass is of uniform fluid density, has an average attenuation of approximately 5 HU, and does not enhance following contrast administration (**b**: arrow). Mediastinal ultrasonography further documented the presence of a thin-walled, anechoic cyst (**c**: arrow).

Figure 4.3.3 Pneumomediastinum (Canine)

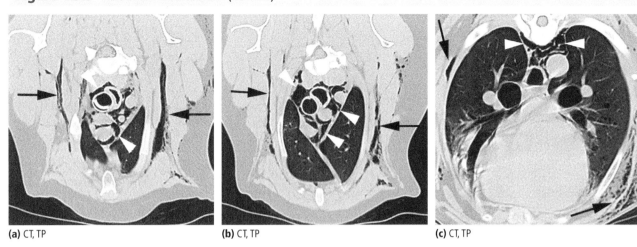

(a) CT, TP　　　　　**(b)** CT, TP　　　　　**(c)** CT, TP

6y FS Golden Retriever with previously diagnosed pneumothorax. The dorsal aspect of the mediastinum is gas distended, resulting in increased definition of the external margins of the trachea, esophagus, and major blood vessels (**a–c**: white arrowheads). Subcutaneous and fascial emphysema is also present (**a–c**: black arrows). The specific source of the pneumomediastinum and subcutaneous emphysema was not determined.

Figure 4.3.4 Mediastinal Hematoma (Canine)

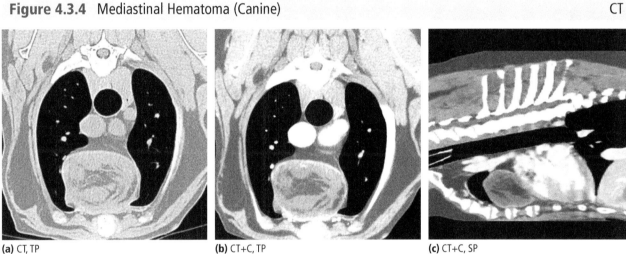

(a) CT, TP　　　　　**(b)** CT+C, TP　　　　　**(c)** CT+C, SP

10y MC Golden Retriever with a cranial mediastinal mass discovered on a recent thoracic radiographic examination. There is a large, well-defined, ovoid mass in the cranial mediastinum. The mass is heterogeneously attenuating and has a thin peripheral rim of enhancement following contrast administration. Excisional biopsy revealed a chronic organizing hematoma with necrosis of entrapped adipose tissue. This latter finding explains the heterogeneity of the mass on CT images.

Figure 4.3.5 Mediastinal Mycotic Granulomatous Lymphadenopathy (Canine)

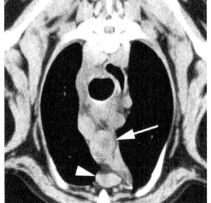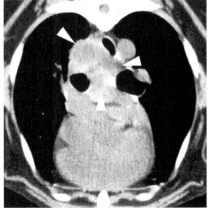

4y FS Labrador Retriever with a 1-week history of coughing and fever and a rapid decline in clinical condition. The sternal (**a**: arrowhead), cranial mediastinal (**a**: arrow), and tracheobronchial (**b**: arrowheads) lymph nodes are markedly enlarged and heterogeneously attenuate. The dog was confirmed to have a systemic *Aspergillus deflectus* infection.

(a) CT, TP　　　　　**(b)** CT, TP

Figure 4.3.6 Tracheobronchial Lymphadenopathy (Canine) CT

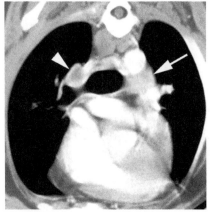

(a) CT+C, TP

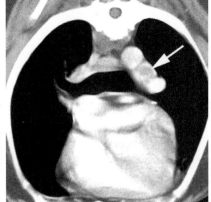

(b) CT+C, TP

7y MC Border Collie with cough and previously diagnosed hilar lymphadenopathy. The right (**a,d**: arrowhead), left (**a,b,d**: small arrow), and central (**c,d**: large arrow) tracheobronchial lymph nodes are enlarged and moderately contrast enhance. The lymph nodes were large enough to cause bronchial compression, which is best seen at the origin of the right mainstem bronchus in image **d**. A bronchoalveolar lavage revealed marked inflammation with chronic hemorrhage, but a definitive cause for the tracheobronchial lymphadenopathy was not determined.

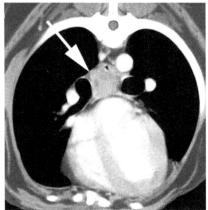

(c) CT+C, TP

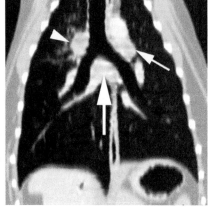

(d) CT+C, DP

Figure 4.3.7 Cryptococcal Mediastinal Granuloma (Feline)   MR

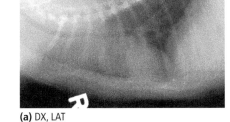 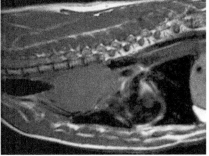 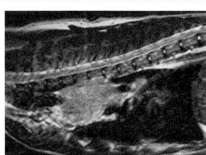

(a) DX, LAT   **(b)** T1, SP   **(c)** T2, SP

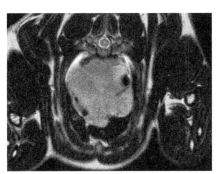 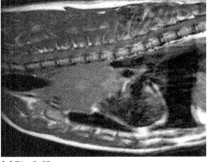

(d) T2, TP   **(e)** T1+C, SP

3y FS Siamese with a recent history of vomiting, anorexia, and abdominal distension. Pelvic limb paresis has developed within the past 24 hours. A cranial mediastinal mass is detected on survey thoracic radiographs (**a**). There is a large, irregularly margined cranial medias-tinal mass that is moderately T1 intense and T2 hyperintense (**b–d**). The mass mildly and nonuniformly enhances following contrast administration (**e**). Large numbers of cryptococcal organisms were detected on a fine-needle aspiration biopsy sample collected from the mediastinal mass. A diagnosis of systemic cryptococcosis was confirmed from fungal titers.

Figure 4.3.8 Mycotic Mediastinitis (Canine)   CT

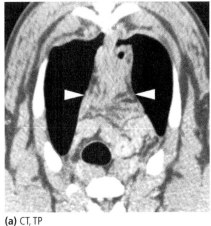 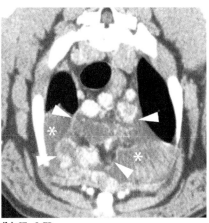 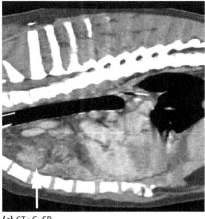

(a) CT, TP   **(b)** CT+C, TP   **(c)** CT+C, SP

4y M Rottweiler with a 3-week history of lethargy, inappetence, and pleural effusion. The dog was initially imaged in dorsal recumbency (**a**) to redistribute pleural fluid. The mediastinum is widened and has a heterogeneous pattern of attenuation (**a**: arrowheads). A contrast-enhanced examination performed with the dog in sternal recumbency reveals a widened and irregularly margined cranial mediastinum with a heterogeneous pattern of enhancement (**b**: arrowheads). Mediastinal lymphadenopathy is also evident (**c**: arrow). Pleural fluid is present in the dependent regions of the pleural space (**b**: asterisks). Surgical biopsy revealed pyogranulomatous mediastinitis, lymphadenitis, and pleuropneumonia that were subsequently confirmed to be due to *Coccidioides immitis*.

Figure 4.3.9 Large Thymoma (Canine) CT

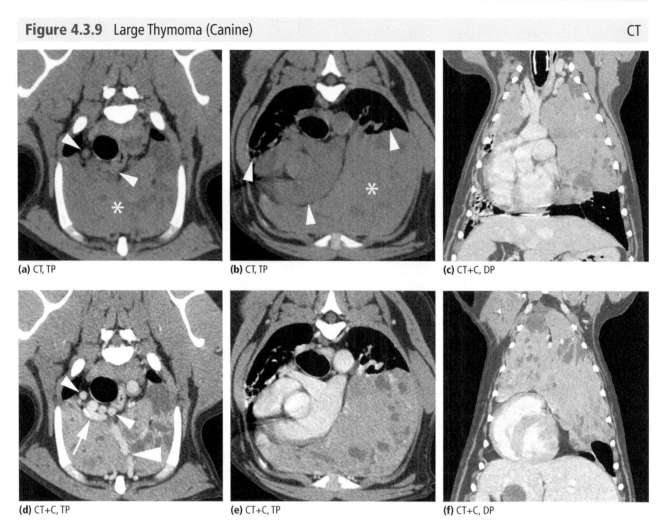

(a) CT, TP

(b) CT, TP

(c) CT+C, DP

(d) CT+C, TP

(e) CT+C, TP

(f) CT+C, DP

9y FS Labrador Retriever with a large mediastinal mass detected on thoracic radiographs obtained as part of a diagnostic evaluation for hypercalcemia. A large, predominantly soft-tissue attenuating mediastinal mass fills the cranioventral thoracic cavity (**a,b**: asterisk), displacing the mediastinal vasculature dorsally (**a**: arrowheads) and the heart and lungs caudally and dorsally (**b**: arrowheads). The parenchymal part of the mass moderately and uniformly enhances following contrast administration (**c–f**). Multiple small fluid-attenuating cysts are distributed throughout the mass (**c–f**). Although major cranial mediastinal blood vessels are markedly displaced (**d**: small arrowheads), there is no evidence of vascular invasion, although the cranial vena cava is compressed (**d**: arrow). The right internal thoracic vein is prominent because of increased venous return from mass perfusion (**d**: large arrowhead). The ventral reflection of the cranial mediastinum often causes large mediastinal masses such as this to preferentially expand into the left hemithorax, resulting in asymmetry that can sometimes mimic a left cranial lung lobe mass. Thymoma without vascular invasion was confirmed by excisional biopsy.

Figure 4.3.10 Mediastinal Mass with Cranial Vena Cava Invasion (Feline)   CT

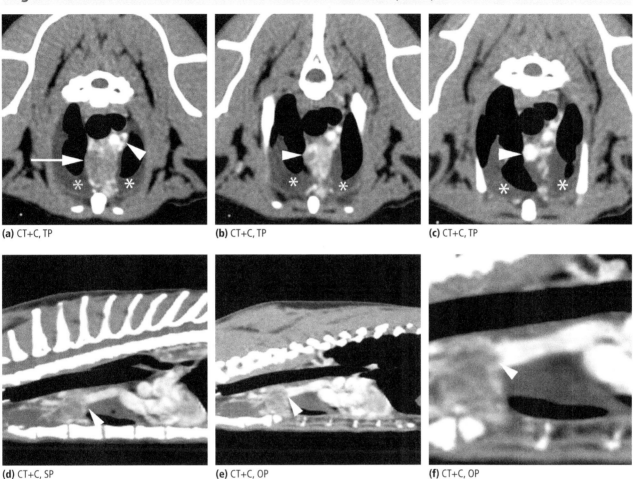

(a) CT+C, TP   **(b)** CT+C, TP   **(c)** CT+C, TP

(d) CT+C, SP   **(e)** CT+C, OP   **(f)** CT+C, OP

12y FS Himalayan with recent increased respiratory effort. An irregularly margined but well-defined, heterogeneously contrast-enhancing mass is present in the cranial mediastinum. On an image acquired at the level of the center of the mass (**a**: arrow), the left subclavian artery and brachiocephalic trunk are clearly identified (**a**: arrowhead), but the cranial vena cava is not seen. On an image at the caudal margin of the mass, the cranial vena cava is seen but contains a central contrast filling defect (**b**: arrowhead). A third transverse image caudal to the mass shows a normal appearance to the contrast-enhanced cranial vena cava (**c**: arrowhead). The relationship of the mass to the vena cava is clearly depicted on the sagittal reformatted image (**d**: arrowhead). A long-axis oblique image reveals the convex luminal filling defect induced by invasion of the mass into the vena cava (**e,f**: arrowhead). Image **f** represents a magnification of image **e**. Bilateral pleural effusion is present in the dependent part of the pleural space (**a–c**: asterisks). Fine-needle aspiration biopsy of the mass revealed epithelial neoplasia, likely thymoma. The cat also had a chylous effusion that was thought to be due to obstruction of the terminal thoracic duct by the mass.

Figure 4.3.11   Thrombus of the Jugular Vein (Canine)   CT

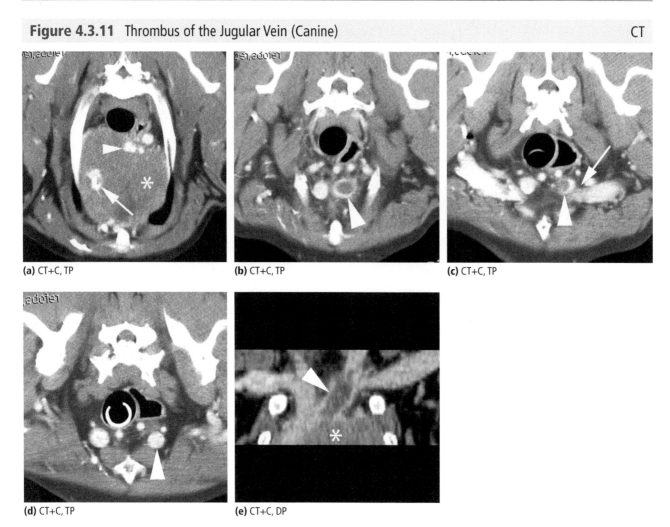

(a) CT+C, TP   **(b)** CT+C, TP   **(c)** CT+C, TP

(d) CT+C, TP   **(e)** CT+C, DP

7y FS Labrador Retriever with thoracic limb lameness and lethargy. Transverse images **a–d** were acquired through the cranial thorax and thoracic inlet and are ordered from caudal to cranial. A cranial mediastinal mass was detected on thoracic radiographs. There is a large, well-defined soft-tissue attenuating mass in the cranial mediastinum (**a**: asterisk). The mass engulfs the cranial vena cava (**a**: arrow) and the branches of the brachiocephalic trunk (**a**: arrowhead). Cranial to the mass, the paired brachiocephalic veins are seen, and a large central contrast filling defect is present in the left vein (**b**: arrowhead). Further cranial, the filling defect persists (**c**: arrowhead) at the level of the convergence of the jugular and subclavian vein (**c**: arrow). Further cranial, the jugular veins appear normal (**d**: arrowhead). The thymoma (**e**: asterisk) and the intraluminal filling defect (**e**: arrowhead) are clearly depicted on a dorsal reformatted image. Fine-needle aspiration biopsy confirmed a diagnosis of thymoma. The composition of the filling defect was not determined, but it was thought to represent either thrombus or caval invasion by the thymoma.

Figure 4.3.12 Invasive Ectopic Thyroid Carcinoma (Canine)   CT

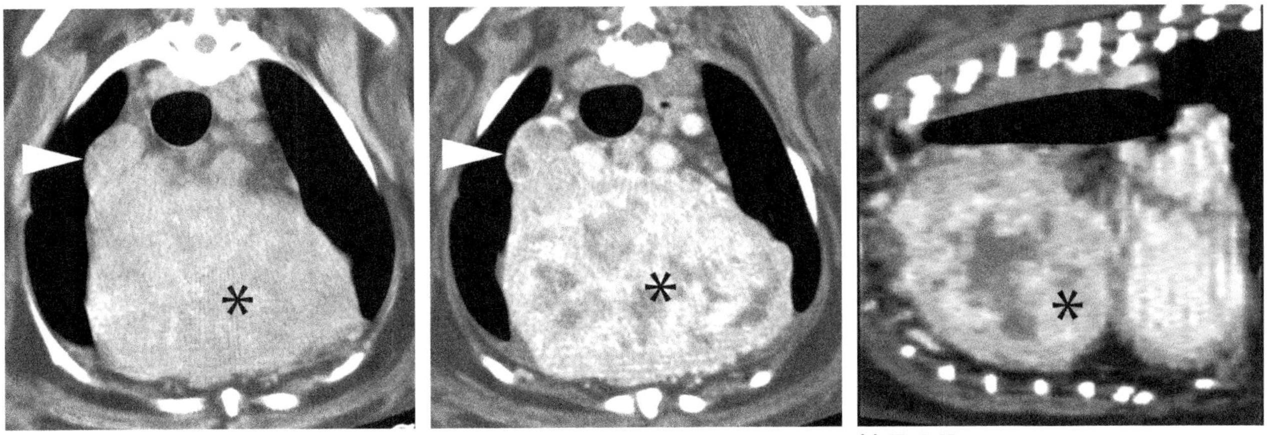

(a) CT, TP   **(b)** CT+C, TP   **(c)** CT+C, SP

10y F Shetland Sheepdog with recent onset facial and cervical edema. There is a large, irregularly contoured, heterogeneous but predomi-nately soft-tissue attenuating, mass in the cranial mediastinum (**a**: asterisk). The cranial vena cava is displaced dorsally by the mass (**a**: arrowhead). The mass intensely and heterogeneously enhances following contrast administration (**b,c**: asterisk). There is a lobulated filling defect within the cranial vena cava that nearly completely occludes the lumen (**b**: arrowhead). Postmortem examination confirmed an aggressive ectopic mediastinal thyroid carcinoma. The filling defect in the cranial vena cava consisted of both local tumor extension and thrombus.

Figure 4.3.13   Lymphoma (Feline)   CT

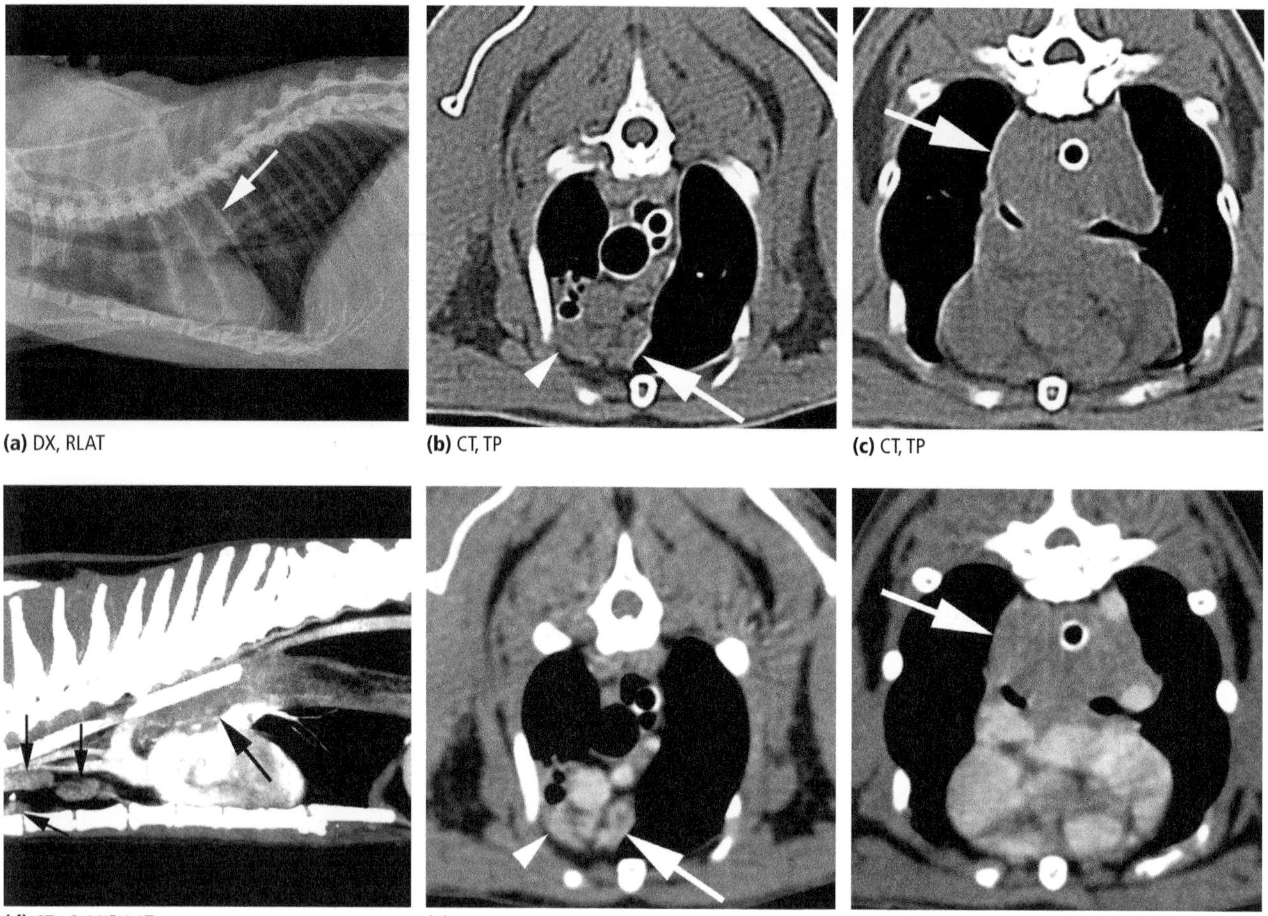

(a) DX, RLAT

(b) CT, TP

(c) CT, TP

(d) CT+C, MIP, LAT

(e) CT+C, TP

(f) CT+C, TP

10y MC Domestic Shorthair with increasing respiratory effort of 4-day duration. There is an ill-defined soft-tissue hilar mass causing depression of the trachea and mainstem bronchi (**a**: arrow). There is enlargement of cranial mediastinal lymph nodes (**b**,**e**: arrow; **d**: small black arrows) and a hilar mass that engulfs the esophagus and compresses and displaces the mainstem bronchi (**c**,**f**: arrow; **d**: large black arrow). Mediastinal lymph nodes moderately enhance following contrast administration. The hilar mass uniformly and mildly enhances (approximately 30 HU increase). The ventral aspect of the right cranial lung lobe is atelectatic (**b**,**e**: arrowhead). Postmortem examination revealed large B-cell lymphoma of the mediastinum. The hilar mass incorporated the esophagus, trachea and large airways, and pulmonary vasculature.

Figure 4.3.14 Megaesophagus (Canine)   CT

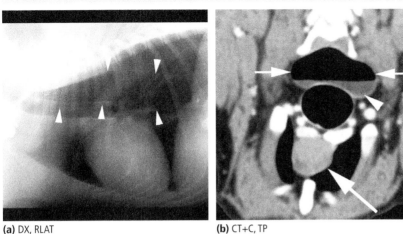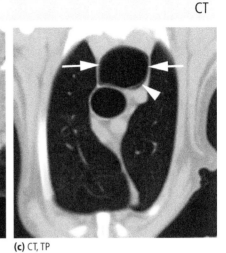

(a) DX, RLAT   **(b)** CT+C, TP   **(c)** CT, TP

9y MC Labrador Retriever cross with an initial presentation for frequent regurgitation. The dog was subsequently diagnosed with a thymoma and myasthenia gravis. The thoracic esophagus is markedly gas distended on survey thoracic radiographs of the unanesthetized patient (**a**: arrowheads). A small, uniformly and moderately enhancing mass is present in the cranial mediastinum, consistent with the presumptive diagnosis of thymoma (**b**: large arrow). The esophagus is markedly gas distended (**b,c**: small arrows) and contains fluid in the dependent part of the lumen (**b,c**: arrowhead). The mass was confirmed to be a thymoma based on excisional biopsy, and acetylcholine titers confirmed the diagnosis of myasthenia gravis. Although it is common for esophageal dilation to occur as an incidental finding in the anesthetized patient, in this instance, the distension resulted from myasthenia gravis likely associated with the thymoma.

Figure 4.3.15 Esophageal Stricture (Canine)

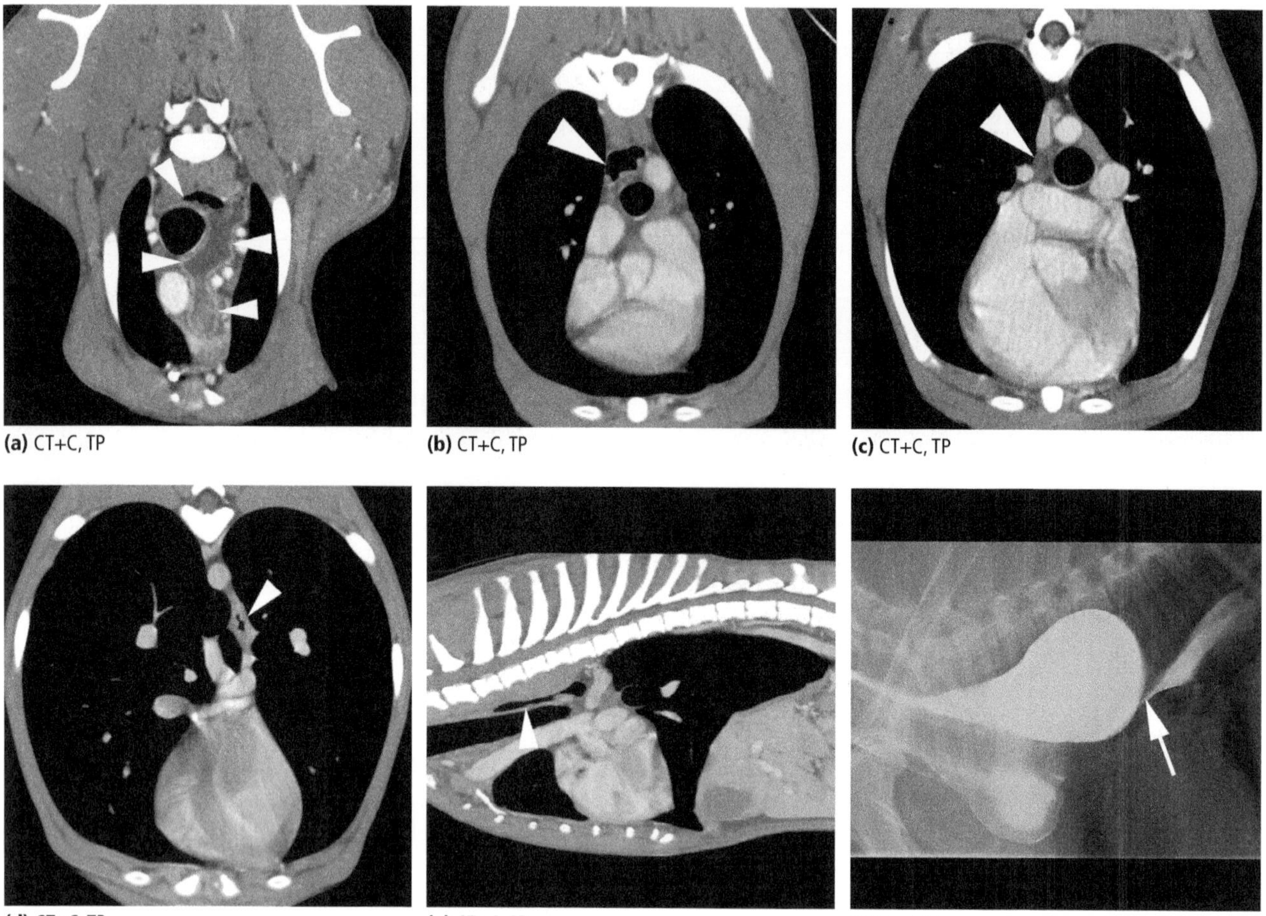

(a) CT+C, TP

(b) CT+C, TP

(c) CT+C, TP

(d) CT+C, TP

(e) CT+C, SP

(f) DX, LAT

2y FS Border Collie with regional megaesophagus. Images **a–d** are ordered from cranial to caudal. The cranial thoracic esophagus is markedly enlarged, appears flaccid, and contains a mix of fluid and gas (**a,b,e**: arrowheads). The esophagus contracts and appears smaller in diameter than expected in the midthorax (**c**: arrowhead). The caudal thoracic esophagus appears normal (**d**: arrowhead). No extramural cause for the obstruction was identified on the remainder of the CT examination. An esophagram and endoscopic examination confirmed an esophageal stricture at the level of esophageal contraction seen on CT (**f**: arrow).

Figure 4.3.16 Paresophageal Abscess (Canine)   CT

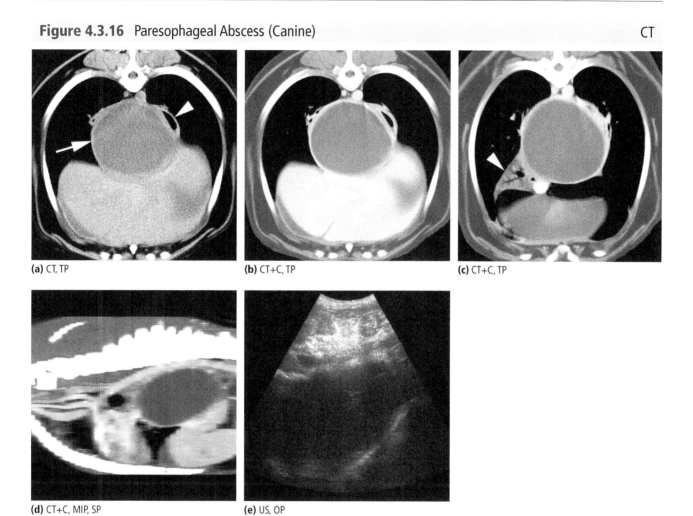

(a) CT, TP   **(b)** CT+C, TP   **(c)** CT+C, TP

(d) CT+C, MIP, SP   **(e)** US, OP

5y FS Dalmation with lethargy, vomiting, and respiratory distress. Thoracic radiographs revealed a caudal thoracic mass. There is a well-defined, encapsulated, fluid-attenuating (approx. 35 HU), ovoid mass within the caudodorsal mediastinum (**a**: arrow). The gas-containing esophagus is seen as an eccentrically located crescent-shaped structure adjacent to the mass (**a**: arrowhead). The thick peripheral capsule of the mass moderately enhances following contrast administration, but the central part of the mass remains unchanged (**b–d**). The right middle lung lobe is volume depleted with associated increased attenuation (**c**: arrowhead). The mass is fluid filled and thick walled on ultrasound examination (**e**). A definitive diagnosis of chronic encapsulated paraesophageal bacterial abscess was based on excisional biopsy.

Figure 4.3.17 Esophageal Spindle Cell Sarcoma (Canine)   CT

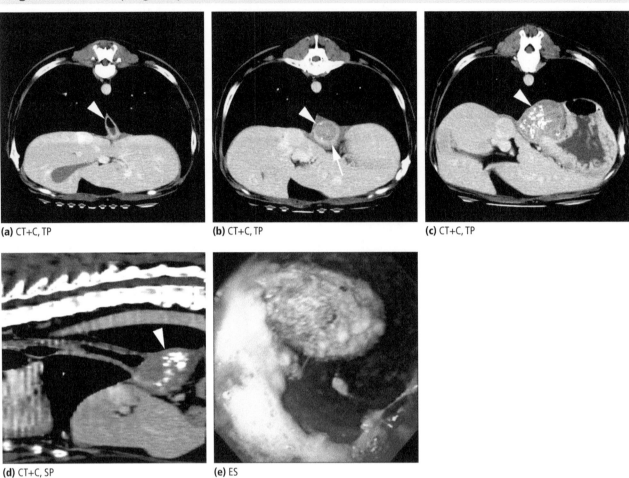

(a) CT+C, TP   **(b)** CT+C, TP   **(c)** CT+C, TP

(d) CT+C, SP   **(e)** ES

12y FS Golden Retriever with a 1-month history of vomiting or regurgitation. Images **a–c** include the caudal thorax and are ordered from cranial to caudal. The caudal thoracic esophagus is mildly gas and fluid distended (**a**: arrowhead). Further caudally, a partially mineralized soft-tissue attenuating mass fills the esophageal lumen near the gastroesophageal junction (**b–d**: arrowhead). The mass is visualized as an eccentrically positioned mural lesion on an endoscopic examination (**e**). Excisional biopsy revealed the mass to be a spindle cell sarcoma arising from the esophageal wall near the gastroesophageal junction. The relatively thicker esophageal wall seen in image **b** (arrow) was likely due to esophagitis that was also documented microscopically.

References

1. Day MJ. Review of thymic pathology in 30 cats and 36 dogs. J Small Anim Pract. 1997;38: 393–403.
2. Liu S, Patnaik AK, Burk RL. Thymic branchial cysts in the dog and cat. J Am Vet Med Assoc. 1983;182: 1095–1098.
3. Nelson LL, Coelho JC, Mietelka K, Langohr IM. Pharyngeal pouch and cleft remnants in the dog and cat: a case series and review. J Am Anim Hosp Assoc. 2012;48: 105–112.
4. Scherrer W, Kyles A, Samii V, Hardie E, Kass P, Gregory C. Computed tomographic assessment of vascular invasion and resectability of mediastinal masses in dogs and a cat. N Z Vet J. 2008;56: 330–333.
5. Zitz JC, Birchard SJ, Couto GC, Samii VF, Weisbrode SE, Young GS. Results of excision of thymoma in cats and dogs: 20 cases (1984–2005). J Am Vet Med Assoc. 2008;232: 1186–1192.
6. Yoon J, Feeney DA, Cronk DE, Anderson KL, Ziegler LE. Computed tomographic evaluation of canine and feline mediastinal masses in 14 patients. Vet Radiol Ultrasound. 2004;45: 542–546.
7. Gabor LJ, Malik R, Canfield PJ. Clinical and anatomical features of lymphosarcoma in 118 cats. Aust Vet J. 1998;76: 725–732.
8. Brissot HN, Burton CA, Doyle RS, Bray JP. Caudal mediastinal paraesophageal abscesses in 7 dogs. Vet Surg. 2012;41: 286–291.

4.4

Heart, pulmonary vasculature, and great vessels

Pericardium

The normal parietal pericardium is thin (1–2 mm) and is therefore inconsistently seen on CT images. The pericardial sac holds only a small volume of fluid but can contain a significant amount of fat that accentuates both the parietal pericardial and the epicardial margins.

Peritoneopericardial diaphragmatic hernia

Peritoneopericardial diaphragmatic hernia is the result of incomplete development of the diaphragm, leading to the formation of a window between the pericardial sac and the peritoneal cavity. The disorder appears to be more common in cats than in dogs, and Himalayan, Maine Coon, and other longhaired cats as well as Weimaraner dogs are predisposed.[1,2] The CT appearance of peritoneopericardial diaphragmatic hernia depends on the specific viscera and visceral volume that has migrated into the pericardial sac. Displaced omentum will appear primarily fat attenuating unless it is strangulated and edematous. Liver lobes often herniate, and liver parenchyma and hepatic veins have a characteristic appearance on contrast-enhanced CT images (Figure 4.4.1). Small intestinal herniation appears as a tubular, fluid- and gas-attenuating collection. Peritoneopericardial diaphragmatic hernias are often associated with anomalies of the sternum.

Pericardial effusion

Pericardial fluid may be transudative, exudative, or hemorrhagic, and the underlying causes of pericardial effusion are idiopathic, inflammatory, neoplastic, traumatic, or cardiovascular in origin (Figure 4.4.2).[3–5] Simple transudative pericardial effusions are fluid attenuating on CT images. The pericardium may be well defined on unenhanced images and will mildly enhance following contrast medium administration.

Pericarditis

Pericarditis can include an exudative pericardial effusion that is fluid attenuating on unenhanced CT images, although density may be greater with high cellularity. The pericardium can be markedly thickened, and the pericardium and epicardium moderately to intensely enhance following contrast administration (Figure 4.4.3).[6]

Neoplasia

Neoplasms that can cause a pericardial mass or hemorrhagic/malignant pericardial effusion include cardiac hemangiosarcoma, chemodectoma, mesothelioma, lymphoma, rhabdomyosarcoma, and fibrosarcoma.[4] Hemorrhagic pericardial effusion from erosive right atrial hemangiosarcoma is reported to be the most common cause of pericardial effusion in dogs.[7] As with exudative effusions, hemorrhagic and malignant effusions can be highly cellular and will therefore have a density somewhat greater than a transudative effusion on CT images. The CT imaging appearance of neoplastic pericardial masses will vary depending on cell type, complexity, and vascularity, but they often appear as mural and/or intraluminal masses that are isoattenuating compared to myocardium and enhance following contrast administration (Figure 4.4.4). Cardiac MR has been compared to transthoracic and transesophageal echocardiography for evaluation of pericardial effusion caused by cardiac neoplasia.[8] Cardiac MR did not improve diagnostic accuracy but did yield additional anatomical information. Imaging

Atlas of Small Animal CT and MRI, First Edition. Erik R. Wisner and Allison L. Zwingenberger.
© 2015 John Wiley & Sons, Inc. Published 2015 by John Wiley & Sons, Inc.

technique consisted of dark blood, steady-state free procession cine, unenhanced and contrast-enhanced T1-weighted imaging, and delayed inversion recovery prepped imaging. MR features included mixed T1 intensity, T2 hyperintense mural masses that variably enhanced following contrast administration.

Heart

Although cardiac CT and MRI are frequently used in people for diagnosis of coronary artery, myocardial viability, and cardiac function disorders, there are only sporadic reports of their use in clinical veterinary medicine.[9–16] This may be in large part due to the relative paucity of coronary artery disease in domestic animals and to the utility of ultrasound for diagnosis and monitoring of the common cardiac disorders of dogs and cats. Rapid multislice CT scanning with prospective or retrospective cardiac gating is necessary to accurately depict cardiac anatomy with minimal motion artifact. Cardiac MR imaging requires specific imaging software and also employs cardiac gating techniques. An in-depth discussion of cardiac MR imaging pulse sequences is beyond the scope of this text, but studies typically include "dark blood" fast spin-echo sequences, "bright blood" gradient-recalled echo (GRE) or steady-state free procession sequences, and inversion recovery (IR) and phase-contrast sequences in both short and long-axis imaging planes.[17]

Normal heart

The complex internal and external anatomy of the heart and great vessels is depicted in Figure 4.4.5.

Developmental disorders

The imaging appearance of the various developmental cardiac disorders depends on the specific anomaly. From a combination of two-dimensional CT images and 3D renderings, one can assess for chamber enlargement, presence of stenosis, poststenotic dilatation, intracardiac or extracardiac shunting lesions, and other anatomic defects (Figures 4.4.6, 4.4.7).[18] CT is also useful for identifying cardiac vascular ring anomalies (Figure 4.4.8).

Acquired disorders

Acquired cardiac disorders in veterinary patients are typically not evaluated using CT or MR since other diagnostic tests yield satisfactory results. However, changes in cardiac chamber volume and myocardial wall thickness are frequently seen in patients undergoing thoracic imaging for other disorders. Coronary artery angiography, another common use for CT in human medicine, is likewise rarely used in veterinary medicine because of the lack of significant coronary arterial disease.

Cardiac chamber enlargement

Left and right atrial/ventricular enlargement results from mitral or tricuspid insufficiency, respectively, and may be seen in patients imaged for reasons other than cardiac disease. On unenhanced CT images, the dilated chamber is hypoattenuating compared to adjacent myocardium. The presence of intravascular contrast media results in enhancement within the cardiac chambers, which are well delineated by surrounding myocardium (Figure 4.4.9). Pulmonary CT features of left ventricular failure are described in Chapter 4.6.

Myocardium

CT and MR are not routinely used for evaluation of cardiomyopathy since these disorders are well characterized using conventional radiography and echocardiography. However, ventricular chamber dilatation (dilated cardiomyopathy) or myocardial thickening associated with reduced ventricular chamber volume (hypertrophic cardiomyopathy) may occasionally be seen in patients with clinically silent or controlled cardiomyopathy imaged for other reasons (Figure 4.4.10). Characterization of myocardial perfusion deficits in cats with hypertrophic cardiomyopathy using contrast-enhanced MR has been reported, although results were inconsistent (Figure 4.4.11).[19] The use of MR for anatomic and functional myocardial imaging in veterinary medicine is otherwise limited.[20–23]

Neoplasia

Hemangiosarcoma is the most common cardiac neoplasm of dogs and usually arises from the right atrium. Cardiac hemangiosarcoma can be either primary or metastatic, and hemopericardium is a frequent sequela to erosion through the myocardium. Cardiac hemangiosarcoma appears as a space-occupying luminal mass that may be isoattenuating to adjacent myocardium and enhances following contrast medium administration (Figure 4.4.12). Pericardial effusion may be evident in those patients with active pericardial hemorrhage. Other cardiac-associated neoplasms occasionally encountered include aortic body tumors (chemodectoma), lymphoma, and rhabdomyosarcoma (Figure 4.4.13). Other than hemangiosarcoma, cardiac metastasis is rare.[24,25]

Pulmonary vasculature

Oligemia

Generalized pulmonary oligemia can occur from hypovolemia, resulting in reduced pulmonary perfusion volume, or may be regional, multifocal, or solitary and result from pulmonary artery branch occlusion or pulmonary arterial hypertension (Figure 4.4.14). Nonuniform pulmonary perfusion results in regions of lower than expected attenuation on CT images, referred to as a mosaic pattern in the human literature.

Pulmonary hypertension

Pulmonary hypertension is the sequela to either increased flow resistance in the pulmonary arteries from vasoconstriction, stenosis, pulmonary disease, or obstruction or from pulmonary venous congestion due to left heart failure or other causes of disrupted venous return. Typical CT features of pulmonary arterial hypertension in people include right heart, pulmonary trunk, and proximal lobar artery enlargement, with arterial narrowing or truncation peripherally, depending on the underlying cause. Lung parenchyma may also have a nonuniform density (mosaic pattern) associated with variable perfusion. CT features of pulmonary venous hypertension include increased interstitial to alveolar pulmonary attenuation due to pulmonary edema and hemorrhage associated with small vessel obstruction.[26] We have observed similar imaging features in dogs and cats with pulmonary arterial and venous hypertension (Figure 4.4.15).

Pulmonary thromboembolism

Pulmonary thromboembolism is often seen as a sequela of a hypercoagulable state or in patients with inflammatory pulmonary vascular disorders, such as heartworm disease. In people, CT angiography is considered the imaging study of choice for diagnosis of pulmonary thromboembolism, and characteristic imaging features of acute and chronic forms have been described. In the acute phase, blood clots are rarely seen on unenhanced CT images but are clearly seen as well-defined filling defects on contrast-enhanced images, with arterial enlargement sometimes present proximal to the site of obstruction and an abrupt termination of the enhancing vessel distally with complete obstruction. Partial obstruction results in eccentric filling defects. Widespread or large artery thromboembolism can result in right ventricular failure with associated distension of the right ventricle, vena cava, and hepatic veins. Small artery embolism may result in focal pulmonary infarction in the periphery of the lung. These often have a wedge shape corresponding to the geographic perfusion distribution of the affected vessel.

CT features of chronic pulmonary thromboembolism in people are characterized by filling defects on contrast-enhanced images. Chronic thrombi are approximately 90 HU, so they will appear hyperattenuating compared to patent vessels on unenhanced CT images. Affected vessels are of smaller diameter than unaffected vessels. Development of collateral bronchial circulation may occur with chronic disease. Pulmonary arterial hypertension

leads to main pulmonary artery enlargement and mosaic perfusion pattern (low-attenuation areas due to oligemia). Although CT features of pulmonary thromboembolism have not been well described in domestic animals, clinical experience suggests features are similar to those described in people (Figure 4.4.16).[27]

Heartworm disease

Canine heartworm disease is endemic in many geographic areas and can cause profound cardiovascular and pulmonary abnormalities associated with arteritis, pulmonary hypertension, vascular obstruction by adult filariae, and thromboembolism. These changes can be amplified during adulticide treatment as a result of pulmonary arterial showering of dying adult filariae. CT features of heartworm infestation include mild but progressive enlargement of the lobar pulmonary arteries and intermittent periarterial interstitial infiltrates in the prepatent phase of infection.[28] Adult filariae have been detected in pulmonary arteries on contrast-enhanced CT images.[28] In dogs followed with serial CT examinations before and during adulticide therapy, peripheral arteries increased in diameter in the first month following initiation of treatment then subsided over a 15-month period, although size did not reduce to pretreatment diameter. Periarterial pulmonary infiltrates accompanied the arterial changes in some instances. The increase in arterial diameter was found to be due to arteritis and intraluminal dead adult filariae lodged in the peripheral vessels, and the eventual reduction in arterial diameter was thought to be associated with recanalization of affected vessels. Pulmonary infiltrates were found to be due to pneumonia, thought to be an extension of the arteritis.[29]

Great vessels

Aortic mineralization

Radiographic and CT features of aortic mineralization have been reported to involve primarily the aortic root and arch. Mineralization is thought to represent dystrophic calcification associated with degeneration in the tunica media in older dogs and was thought to be a clinically silent finding.[30] Aortic mineralization is occasionally seen as an incidental finding on thoracic CT images in dogs and cats and will appear as focal or curvilinear regions of high attenuation that follow the contour of the vascular wall on transverse images (Figure 4.4.17).

Large vessel thrombosis

Thrombosis of the aorta or vena cava is uncommon and is usually a sequela of an underlying primary disorder leading to hypercoagulability or vascular stasis (Figures 4.4.18, 4.4.19).[31]

Figure 4.4.1 Peritoneopericardial Diaphragmatic Hernia (Feline)   CT

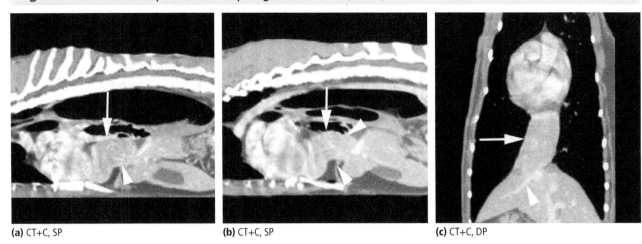

(a) CT+C, SP   **(b)** CT+C, SP   **(c)** CT+C, DP

Adult MC Maine Coon with chronic cough and suspected peritoneopericardial diaphragmatic hernia based on previous thoracic radiographs. Images **a** and **b** are at slightly different levels in the sagittal plane. Part of the liver is cranially displaced into the pericardial sac, causing encroachment on, and cranial displacement of, the heart (**a–c**: arrow). The defect in the diaphragm (**b**: arrowheads) and characteristic branching hepatic vasculature can be seen (**a,c**: arrowhead). Echocardiography confirmed the presence of herniated liver in the pericardial sac.

Figure 4.4.2 Pericardial Effusion (Canine)   CT

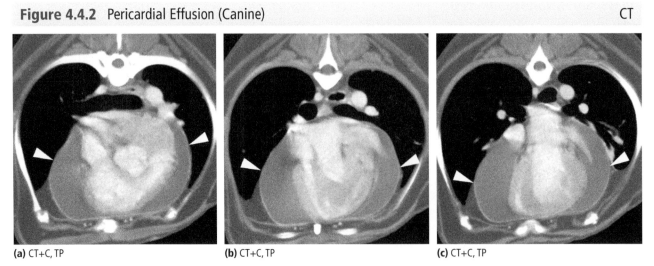

(a) CT+C, TP   **(b)** CT+C, TP   **(c)** CT+C, TP

11y FS Terrier cross with previously diagnosed pericardial effusion. A moderate volume of pericardial effusion is present, surrounded by the uniformly thin, mildly contrast-enhancing parietal pericardium (**a–c**: arrowheads). The heterogeneity of the heart is due to contrast-enhanced blood in the cardiac chambers. The average attenuation of pericardial fluid was approximately 12 HU both before and after contrast administration. Cytologic analysis revealed the fluid to be a modified transudate.

Figure 4.4.3   Pericarditis (Canine)   CT

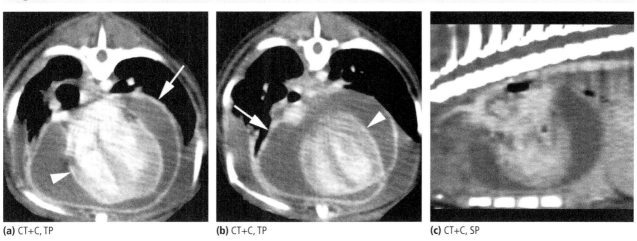

(a) CT+C, TP   **(b)** CT+C, TP   **(c)** CT+C, SP

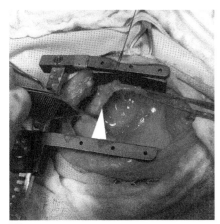

(d) GP

1.5y FS Chihuahua with acute respiratory distress. A moderate pericardial effusion is present, associated with uniform thickening and contrast enhancement of the epicardium (**a**,**b**: arrowhead) and pericardium (**a**,**b**: arrow). The average attenuation of pericardial fluid was approximately 15 HU both before and after contrast administration. Cytologic analysis revealed marked suppurative inflammation with a mixed population of bacteria. A clinical diagnosis of pericarditis was made, and a partial pericardiectomy was performed. The marked thickening of the pericardium is appreciated in the intraoperative image (**d**: arrowhead).

Figure 4.4.4 Pericardial Hamartoma (Canine)   CT

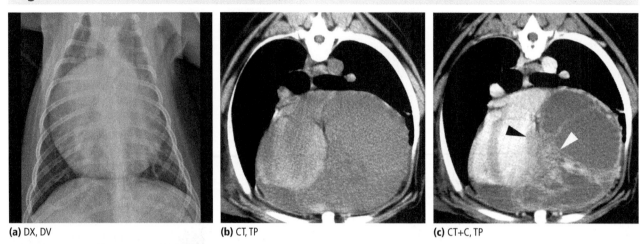

(a) DX, DV   **(b)** CT, TP   **(c)** CT+C, TP

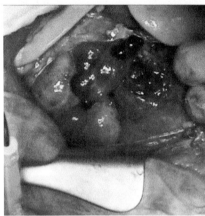

(d) GP

2y FS Australian Shepherd with hypoproteinemia and abdominal effusion. Survey radiographs show a globoid cardiac silhouette consistent with pericardial effusion (**a**). Marked, eccentrically distributed pericardial effusion is present on CT images, and the contrast-enhanced image reveals irregular septations within the pericardial sac and an ill-defined enhancing mass (**c**: white arrowhead) adjacent to the left ventricular free wall (**c**: black arrowhead). Cytology of the pericardial fluid was described as hemorrhagic with mixed inflammation. A cystic, multilobular mass was incompletely excised from the surface of the left ventricle (**d**) and determined to be a mesenchymal hamartoma.

Legend for Figures 4.4.5–4.4.15

Ao	Aorta		LSA	Left subclavian artery
AoV	Aortic valve		LV	Left ventricle
AA	Ascending aorta		MV	Mitral valve
AAr	Aortic arch		PT	Pulmonary trunk
AzV	Azygous vein		RA	Right atrium
CaV	Caudal vena cava		RAA	Right auricular appendage
CCA	Common carotid artery		RPA	Right pulmonary artery
CrV	Cranial vena cava		RPV	Right pulmonary vein
DA	Descending aorta		RSA	Right subclavian artery
Es	Esophagus		RV	Right ventricle
LA	Left atrium		RVM	Right ventricular myocardium
LAu	Left auricle		Tr	Trachea
LPA	Left pulmonary artery		TV	Tricuspid valve
LPV	Left pulmonary vein			

Figure 4.4.5 Cardiac Anatomy (Canine)   CT

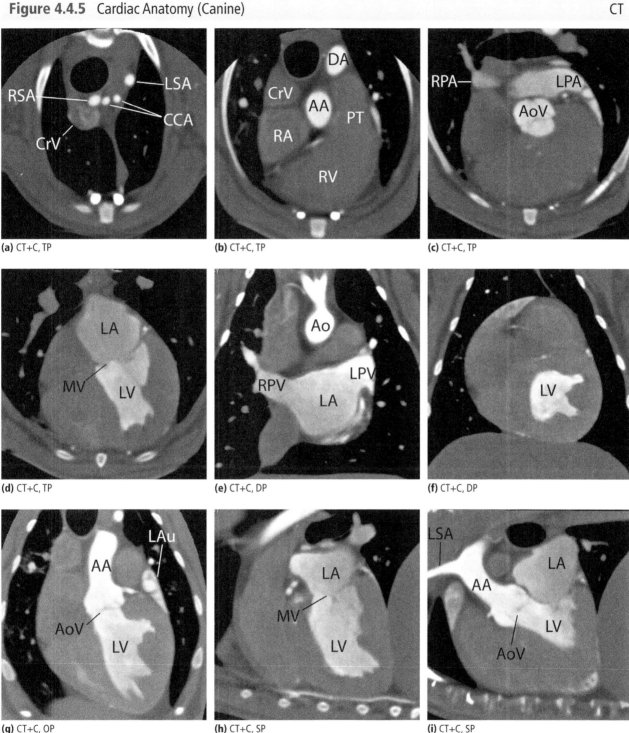

(a) CT+C, TP

(b) CT+C, TP

(c) CT+C, TP

(d) CT+C, TP

(e) CT+C, DP

(f) CT+C, DP

(g) CT+C, OP

(h) CT+C, SP

(i) CT+C, SP

3y F clinically normal Beagle. Images **a–i** were acquired with contrast primarily in the chambers and vessels of the left side of the heart. Images **k–q** (next page) were acquired following a delay in which contrast material enhances structures of both the left and right side of the heart. Images **a–d** and **j–l** were acquired in the transverse plane and are ordered from cranial to caudal. Images **e–f** and **m–n** were acquired in the dorsal plane and are ordered from dorsal to ventral. Image **g** was acquired in a long oblique plane approximating the long axis of the heart. Images **h–i** and **p–q** were acquired in the sagittal plane and are ordered from left to right. The left atrium and right ventricle in image **q** appear to be contiguous as a result of partial volume effect from image collimation and the tangential orientation of the image plane in relation to the myocardial wall. See page 428 for Legend for Figures 4.4.5–4.4.15. (Figure continues on next page.) Susanne Stieger-Vanegas, Oregon State University, Corvallis, OR, 2014. Reproduced with permission from S Stieger-Vanegas.

Figure 4.4.5 (*Continued*) CT

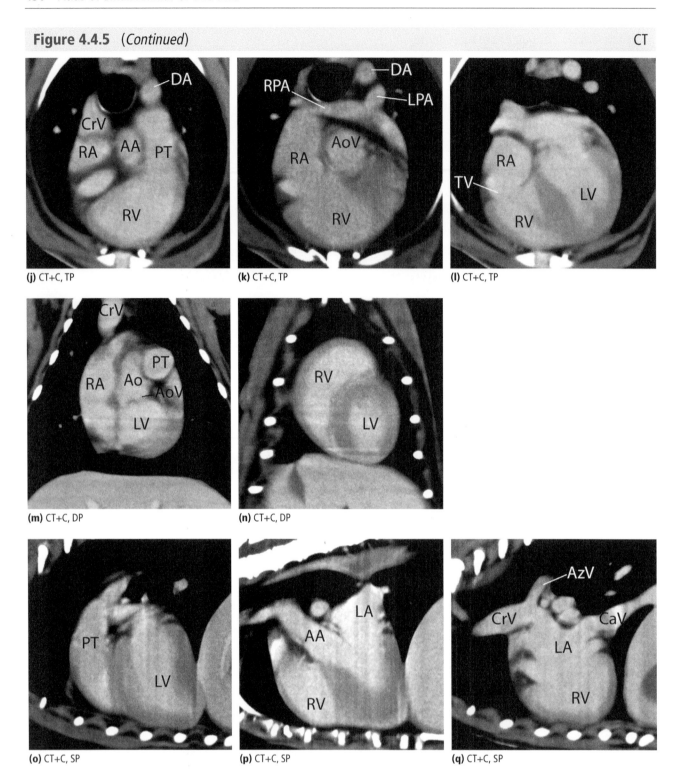

(**j**) CT+C, TP

(**k**) CT+C, TP

(**l**) CT+C, TP

(**m**) CT+C, DP

(**n**) CT+C, DP

(**o**) CT+C, SP

(**p**) CT+C, SP

(**q**) CT+C, SP

Figure 4.4.6 Pulmonic Stenosis (Canine)

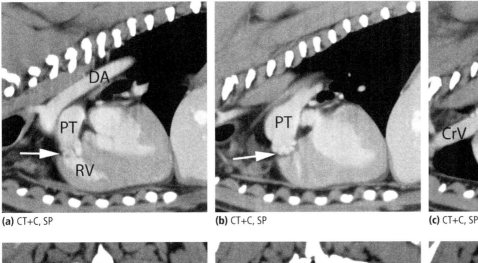
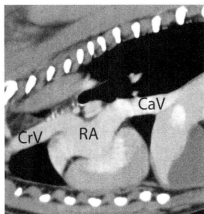

(**a**) CT+C, SP

(**b**) CT+C, SP

(**c**) CT+C, SP

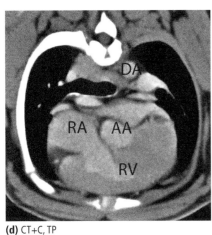
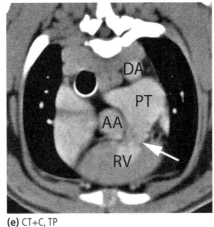
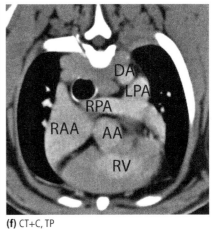

(**d**) CT+C, TP

(**e**) CT+C, TP

(**f**) CT+C, TP

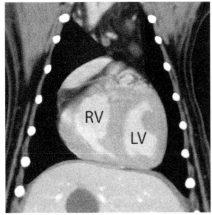

(**g**) CT+C, DP

2y M English Bulldog. Sequential sagittal images show the right ventricle (**a**: RV), the pulmonic valve (**a,b**: arrow), and main pulmonary trunk (**a,b**: PT). A marked poststenotic pulmonary arterial dilatation is best seen in image B. Also seen are the descending aorta (**a**: DA), cranial (**c**: CrV) and caudal (**c**: CaV) vena cava, and the right atrium (**c**: RA). Transverse and dorsal plane images highlight the right ventricle (**d–g**: RV), pulmonary trunk (**e**: PT), the right (**f**: RPA) and left (**f**: LPA) pulmonary arteries, the ascending (**d–f**: AA) and descending (**d–f**: DA) aorta, the right atrium (**d**: RA), the right auricular appendage (**f**: RAA), and the left ventricle (**g**: LV). The pulmonic valve appears stenotic (**e**: arrow), and a poststenotic dilatation of the pulmonary trunk is evident immediately dorsal to the valve. Marked right ventricular myocardial hypertrophy is seen in all images. See page 428 for Legend for Figures 4.4.5–4.4.15. Susanne Stieger-Vanegas, Oregon State University, Corvallis, OR, 2014. Reproduced with permission from S Stieger-Vanegas.

Figure 4.4.7 Right-to-left Patent Ductus Arteriosis (Canine)

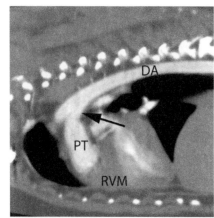

(a) CT+C, SP

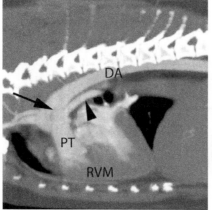

(b) CT+C, SP

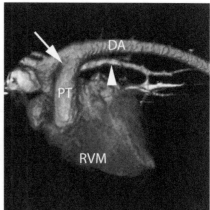

(c) CT+C, 3D, LLAT

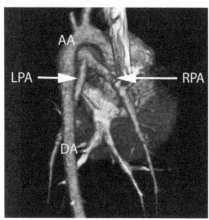

(d) CT+C, 3D, DORS

11mo M Pomeranian with chronic, nonprogressive exercise intolerance. A large patent ductus (**a–c**: arrow) is seen arising from the pulmonary trunk (**a–c**: PT) and merging with the origin of the descending aorta (**a–d**: DA). The proximal segment of the left pulmonary artery (**b,c**: arrowhead) can also be seen at its origin from the pulmonary trunk on sagittally oriented images. Although the ductus is not seen in image **d** because of superimposition from the origin of the descending aorta, the division of the pulmonary trunk into the left (**d**: LPA) and right (**d**: RPA) pulmonary arteries is clearly seen. Right ventricular myocardium (**a–c**: RVM) is also hypertrophic. See page 428 for Legend for Figures 4.4.5–4.4.15. Susanne Stieger-Vanegas, Oregon State University, Corvallis, OR, 2014. Reproduced with permission from S Stieger-Vanegas.

Figure 4.4.8 Persistent Right Aortic Arch (Canine)   CT

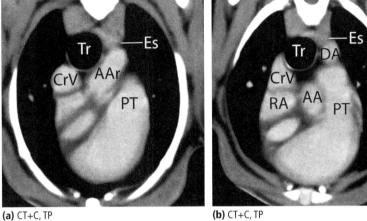

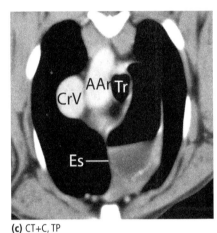
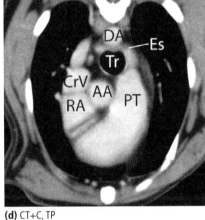

(a) CT+C, TP   **(b)** CT+C, TP

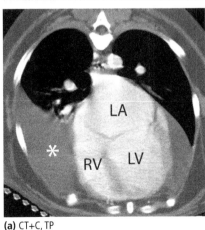
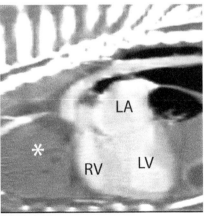

(c) CT+C, TP   **(d)** CT+C, TP

14mo Cocker Spaniel with chronic regurgitation. Images **a** and **b** are from a normal dog and are ordered from cranial to caudal. Images **c** and **d** are from the dog with the persistent right aortic arch and are at approximately the same anatomic level as **a** and **b**, respectively. The cranial thoracic esophagus is markedly dilated with fluid and gas (**c**: Es) The aortic arch (**c**: AAr) is located to the right of the trachea, causing tracheal displacement and luminal narrowing (**c,d**: Tr). Although the ligamentum arteriosum is not directly identified, its presence is implied by the location of the esophagus (**c,d**: Es) relative to the aorta (**c,d**: AAr,AA,DA) and the pulmonary trunk (**d**: PT) and the presence of megaesophagus cranial to the obstruction. See page 428 for Legend for Figures 4.4.5–4.4.15. Susanne Stieger-Vanegas, Oregon State University, Corvallis, OR, 2014. Reproduced with permission from S Stieger-Vanegas.

Figure 4.4.9 Left Cardiac Chamber Enlargement from Mitral Valve Insufficiency (Canine)   CT

(a) CT+C, TP   **(b)** CT+C, SP

10y MC German Shepherd cross with lethargy and pleural effusion. Left atrial (**a,b**: LA) and ventricular (**a,b**: LV) chamber enlargement is evident on enhanced transverse and long-axis images of the heart. Moderate pleural effusion is also present (**a,b**: asterisk). Echocardiographic examination confirmed moderate left atrial and ventricular enlargement and mitral valve regurgitation. Although the right atrium and ventricle (**a,b**: RV) were deemed to be of normal size, tricuspid valvular degeneration was also evident. The cause for pleural effusion was thought to be right ventricular failure. See page 428 for Legend for Figures 4.4.5–4.4.15.

Figure 4.4.10 Hypertrophic Cardiomyopathy (Feline)

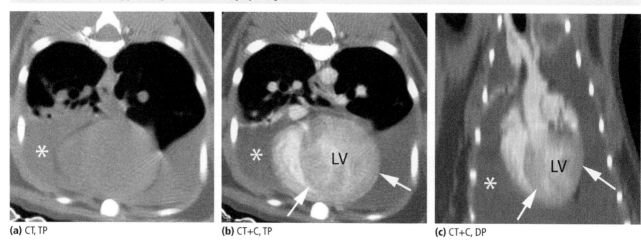

(a) CT, TP   **(b)** CT+C, TP   **(c)** CT+C, DP

8y FS Domestic Shorthair. A computed tomography examination was performed on this cat to evaluate a mediastinal mass and pleural effusion. Hypertrophic cardiomyopathy was previously diagnosed by echocardiography. There is moderate generalized cardiomegaly (a–c). On contrast-enhanced images, the left ventricular chamber is small (**b,c:** LV), and there is marked myocardial hypertrophy of the left ventricular septal and free walls (**b,c:** arrows), which are hypoattenuating relative to the ventricular chamber. A pleural effusion is also present (**a–c:** asterisk). Cardiac ultrasound findings were summarized as marked concentric hypertrophy of the left ventricular and papillary muscles. See page 428 for Legend for Figures 4.4.5–4.4.15.

Figure 4.4.11 Myocardial Perfusion Deficit (Feline)

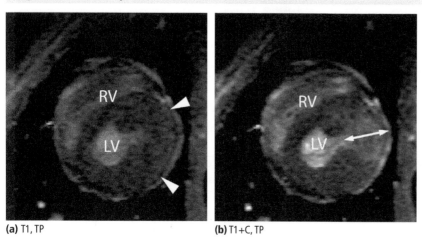

(a) T1, TP   **(b)** T1+C, TP

Adult cat diagnosed with severe hypertrophic cardiomyopathy with asymmetrical hypertrophy. The unenhanced image shows marked left ventricular myocardial hypertrophy, which is most pronounced in the free wall (**a:** arrowheads). The contrast-enhanced image reveals a large, discrete region of delayed enhancement (**b:** two-headed arrow) in the anterior left ventricular free wall, which represents a region of fibrosis. The delayed enhancement in this cat is unusual in that most perfusion defects don't appear to enhance in cats with cardiomyopathy. See page 428 for Legend for Figures 4.4.5–4.4.15. MacDonald et al 2005.[19] Reproduced with permission from AVMA.

Figure 4.4.12 Presumptive Right Atrial Hemangiosarcoma (Canine) CT

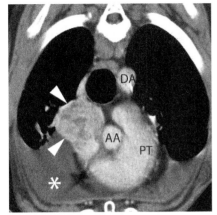

(a) CT+C, TP

10y MC German Shepherd cross with 3-month history of exercise intolerance. There is a heterogeneously enhancing mass filling the lumen of the right atrium (arrowheads). Echocardiography confirmed the presence of a right atrial mass with extension into the cranial and caudal vena cava. Pleural effusion is also present in the dependent thorax (asterisk). The mass was thought to represent a right atrial hemangiosarcoma based on imaging appearance and location. See page 428 for Legend for Figures 4.4.5–4.4.15.

Figure 4.4.13 Chemodectoma (Canine) CT

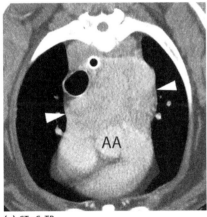 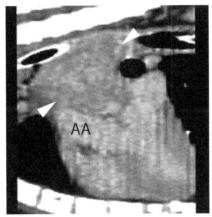

(a) CT+C, TP   (b) CT+C, SP

9y M Rottweiler with recent onset frequent regurgitation. There is a large, irregularly margined and mildly contrast-enhancing mass (a,b: arrowheads) immediately dorsal to the ascending aorta (a,b: AA). Surgical biopsy of the mass confirmed a diagnosis of malignant carotid body tumor (chemodectoma). See page 428 for Legend for Figures 4.4.5–4.4.15.

Figure 4.4.14 Regional Pulmonary Oligemia (Canine)   CT

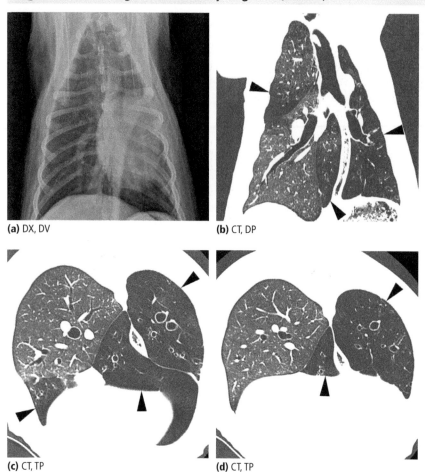

(a) DX, DV

(b) CT, DP

(c) CT, TP

(d) CT, TP

9y MC Belgian Tervuren with chronic cough. There is a midline shift to the left on the survey radiographic image, and the left lung appears hyperlucent (**a**). On CT images, the left lung, accessory lobe, and part of the right cranial lobe are hypoattenuating (**b–d**: arrowheads). Pulmonary volume appears to be partially preserved in these affected lobes, but pulmonary vascular diameter is markedly reduced. Average attenuation of oligemic lung is approximately −960 HU, while that of more normally perfused lung is approximately −850 HU. A diagnosis of chronic bronchial disease with eosinophilic and neutrophilic inflammation was made from bronchoalveolar lavage cytology. The underlying cause for the regional oligemia was not determined and may have been unrelated to the clinical diagnosis.

Figure 4.4.15 Pulmonary Hypertension (Canine)   CT

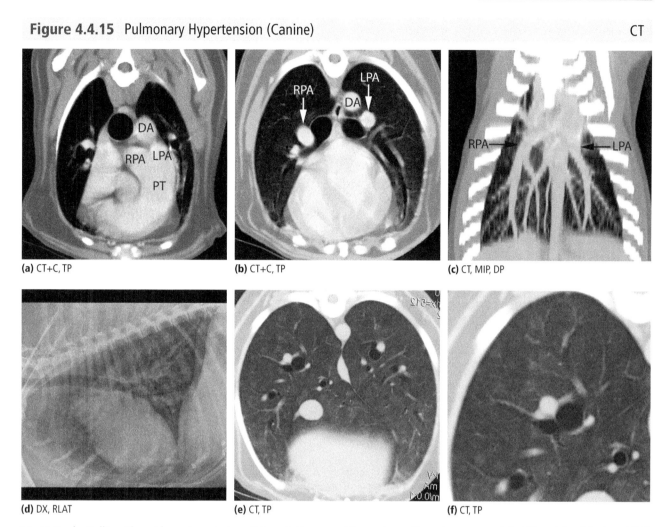

(a) CT+C, TP   **(b)** CT+C, TP   **(c)** CT, MIP, DP

(d) DX, RLAT   **(e)** CT, TP   **(f)** CT, TP

11y FS Border Collie with rapid-onset respiratory distress, lethargy, and inappetence. The pulmonary trunk (**a**: PT) and the right (**a–c**: RPA) and left (**a–c**: LPA) pulmonary arteries are prominent. Descending aorta (**a,b**: DA). There is a diffuse unstructured interstitial pattern on thoracic radiographs (**d**). The interstitial pattern is also present on CT images and is characterized by a patchy ground-glass appearance (**e,f**) that is somewhat more pronounced in the dependent regions of the lung. Echocardiographic examination showed a mildly enlarged pulmonary trunk and increased tricuspid regurgitant velocity, indicative of pulmonary hypertension. Lung biopsy revealed moderate vascular hypertrophy and proliferation with acute to subacute multifocal alveolar degeneration, fibrin exudation, and hemorrhage, consistent with primary pulmonary hypertension. See page 428 for Legend for Figures 4.4.5–4.4.15.

Figure 4.4.16 Pulmonary Thromboembolism (Canine)   CT

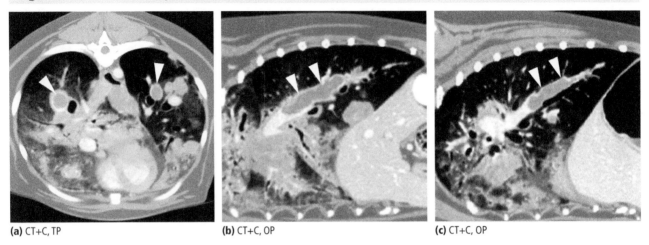

(a) CT+C, TP   **(b)** CT+C, OP   **(c)** CT+C, OP

5y FS Cattle Dog cross with progressive cough following heartworm disease treatment. Images **b** and **c** have been reformatted in oblique planes paralleling the path of the right and left pulmonary artery, respectively. Contrast-enhanced CT images acquired during the vascular phase reveal discrete hypoattenuating filling defects within the right (**b**) and left (**c**) pulmonary arteries, consistent with chronic pulmonary thromboembolism (**a–c**: arrowheads). The dog also had concurrent metastatic carcinoma resulting in multiple pulmonary masses and nodules and thoracic lymphadenopathy (**a–c**).

Figure 4.4.17 Aortic Mineralization (Canine)   CT

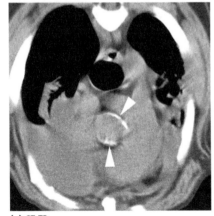

8y MC Border Collie. A thoracic CT examination was performed to evaluate the cause of recent-onset pleural effusion. Circumferential mural mineralization of the ascending aorta was seen as an incidental finding (arrowheads).

(a) CT, TP

Figure 4.4.18 Aortic Thrombosis (Canine)   MR

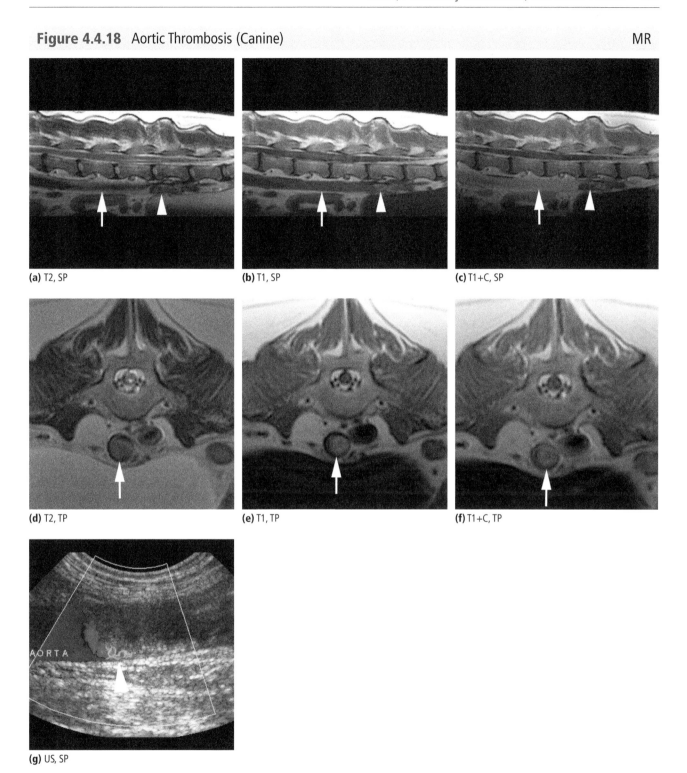

(a) T2, SP

(b) T1, SP

(c) T1+C, SP

(d) T2, TP

(e) T1, TP

(f) T1+C, TP

(g) US, SP

11y FS German Shepherd cross with rapidly progressive L4–S2 myelopathy. The midabdominal aortic lumen is T1 and T2 hyperintense and markedly and uniformly contrast enhances, indicating blood pooling due to flow obstruction (**a–f**: arrow). Immediately caudally, there is an irregularly shaped intraluminal mass that is of mixed T1 and T2 intensity representing an aortic thrombus (**a–c**: arrowhead). Ultrasound confirmed a caudal abdominal aortic flow obstruction that extended to, and included, the trifurcation (**g**: arrowhead).

Figure 4.4.19 Vena Cava Atresia with Aneurism and Thrombosis (Canine) CT

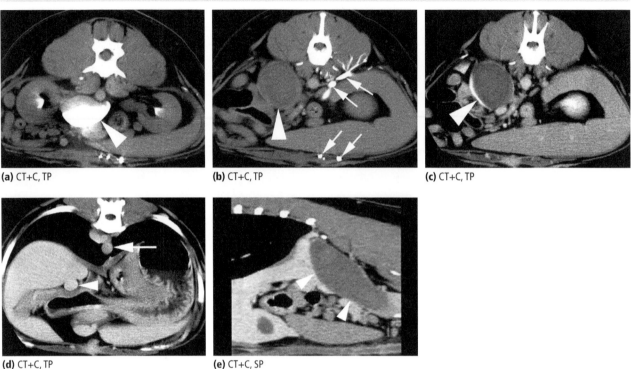

(a) CT+C, TP

(b) CT+C, TP

(c) CT+C, TP

(d) CT+C, TP

(e) CT+C, SP

10mo F English Bulldog with history of collapsing episodes following physical exertion. Following contrast administration through a catheter placed in the saphenous vein, contrast medium pools in the caudal abdominal vena cava (**a**: arrowhead). In the mid abdomen, the vena cava diameter is markedly enlarged, and the lumen remains unenhanced (**b**: arrowhead). A large number of distended veins result from venous recruitment as an alternate venous return path (**b**: arrows). Following a short delay, image **c** was acquired at the same anatomic level as image **b**, revealing nearly complete obstruction of the vena cava at this level, with only a thin rim of contrast medium visible (**c**: arrowhead). Image **d** was acquired cranial to images **b** and **c** and reveals no demonstrative vena cava at this level. Descending aorta (**d**: arrow), portal vein (**d**: arrowhead). The size of the caval thrombus is best appreciated in image **e** (arrowheads). Given the age of the patient and duration of clinical signs, this was thought to represent atresia of the vena cava with secondary thrombosis.

References

1. Banz AC, Gottfried SD. Peritoneopericardial diaphragmatic hernia: a retrospective study of 31 cats and eight dogs. J Am Anim Hosp Assoc. 2010;46:398–404.

2. Reimer SB, Kyles AE, Filipowicz DE, Gregory CR. Long-term outcome of cats treated conservatively or surgically for peritoneopericardial diaphragmatic hernia: 66 cases (1987–2002). J Am Vet Med Assoc. 2004;224:728–732.

3. Alleman AR. Abdominal, thoracic, and pericardial effusions. Vet Clin North Am Small Anim Pract. 2003;33:89–118.

4. Berg J. Pericardial disease and cardiac neoplasia. Semin Vet Med Surg (Small Anim). 1994;9:185–191.

5. Shaw SP, Rush JE. Canine pericardial effusion: pathophysiology and cause. Compend Contin Educ Vet. 2007;29:400–403; quiz 404.

6. Hackney D, Slutsky RA, Mattrey R, Peck WW, Abraham JL, Shabetai R, et al. Experimental pericardial inflammation evaluated by computed tomography. Radiology. 1984;151:145–148.

7. Gidlewski J, Petrie JP. Pericardiocentesis and principles of echocardiographic imaging in the patient with cardiac neoplasia. Clin Tech Small Anim Pract. 2003;18:131–134.

8. Boddy KN, Sleeper MM, Sammarco CD, Weisse C, Ghods S, Litt HI. Cardiac magnetic resonance in the differentiation of neoplastic and nonneoplastic pericardial effusion. J Vet Intern Med. 2011;25:1003–1009.

9. Hoey E, Ganeshan A, Nader K, Randhawa K, Watkin R. Cardiac neoplasms and pseudotumors: imaging findings on multidetector CT angiography. Diagn Interv Radiol. 2012;18:67–77.

10. Hoey ET, Mankad K, Puppala S, Gopalan D, Sivananthan MU. MRI and CT appearances of cardiac tumours in adults. Clin Radiol. 2009;64:1214–1230.

11. Krishnamurthy R. The role of MRI and CT in congenital heart disease. Pediatr Radiol. 2009;39 Suppl 2:S196–204.

12. Marcus RP, Nikolaou K, Theisen D, Reiser MF, Bamberg F. Myocardial perfusion imaging by computed tomography: today and tomorrow. Int J Clin Pract Suppl. 2011:14-22.

13. Morris MF, Maleszewski JJ, Suri RM, Burkhart HM, Foley TA, Bonnichsen CR, et al. CT and MR imaging of the mitral valve: radiologic–pathologic correlation. Radiographics. 2010;30:1603–1620.

14. Perazzolo Marra M, Lima JA, Iliceto S. MRI in acute myocardial infarction. Eur Heart J. 2011;32:284–293.

15. Taylor AJ, Cerqueira M, Hodgson JM, Mark D, Min J, O'Gara P, et al. ACCF/SCCT/ACR/AHA/ASE/ASNC/NASCI/SCAI/SCMR 2010 Appropriate Use Criteria for Cardiac Computed Tomography. J Cardiovasc Comput Tomogr. 2010;4:407.e401–433.

16. Williams MC, Reid JH, McKillop G, Weir NW, van Beek EJ, Uren NG, et al. Cardiac and coronary CT comprehensive imaging approach in the assessment of coronary heart disease. Heart. 2011;97:1198–1205.

17. Ginat DT, Fong MW, Tuttle DJ, Hobbs SK, Vyas RC. Cardiac imaging: Part 1, MR pulse sequences, imaging planes, and basic anatomy. AJR Am J Roentgenol. 2011;197:808–815.

18. Watts JR, Jr., Sonavane SK, Singh SP, Nath PH. Pictorial review of multidetector CT imaging of the preoperative evaluation of congenital heart disease. Curr Probl Diagn Radiol. 2013;42:40–56.

19. MacDonald KA, Wisner ER, Larson RF, Klose T, Kass PH, Kittleson MD. Comparison of myocardial contrast enhancement via cardiac magnetic resonance imaging in healthy cats and cats with hypertrophic cardiomyopathy. Am J Vet Res. 2005;66:1891–1894.

20. Gilbert SH, McConnell FJ, Holden AV, Sivananthan MU, Dukes-McEwan J. The potential role of MRI in veterinary clinical cardiology. Vet J. 2010;183:124–134.

21. MacDonald KA, Kittleson MD, Garcia-Nolen T, Larson RF, Wisner ER. Tissue Doppler imaging and gradient echo cardiac magnetic resonance imaging in normal cats and cats with hypertrophic cardiomyopathy. J Vet Intern Med. 2006;20:627–634.

22. MacDonald KA, Kittleson MD, Larson RF, Kass P, Klose T, Wisner ER. The effect of ramipril on left ventricular mass, myocardial fibrosis, diastolic function, and plasma neurohormones in Maine Coon cats with familial hypertrophic cardiomyopathy without heart failure. J Vet Intern Med. 2006;20:1093–1105.

23. MacDonald KA, Kittleson MD, Reed T, Larson R, Kass P, Wisner ER. Quantification of left ventricular mass using cardiac magnetic resonance imaging compared with echocardiography in domestic cats. Vet Radiol Ultrasound. 2005;46:192–199.

24. Gamlem H, Nordstoga K, Arnesen K. Canine vascular neoplasia – a population-based clinicopathologic study of 439 tumours and tumour-like lesions in 420 dogs. APMIS Suppl. 2008:41-54.

25. Rajagopalan V, Jesty SA, Craig LE, Gompf R. Comparison of presumptive echocardiographic and definitive diagnoses of cardiac tumors in dogs. J Vet Intern Med. 2013;27:1092–1096.

26. Grosse C, Grosse A. CT findings in diseases associated with pulmonary hypertension: a current review. Radiographics. 2010;30:1753–1777.

27. Cronin P, Weg JG, Kazerooni EA. The role of multidetector computed tomography angiography for the diagnosis of pulmonary embolism. Semin Nucl Med. 2008;38:418–431.

28. Seiler GS, Nolan TJ, Withnall E, Reynolds C, Lok JB, Sleeper MM. Computed tomographic changes associated with the prepatent and early patent phase of dirofilariasis in an experimentally infected dog. Vet Radiol Ultrasound. 2010;51:136–140.

29. Takahashi A, Yamada K, Kishimoto M, Shimizu J, Maeda R. Computed tomography (CT) observation of pulmonary emboli caused by long-term administration of ivermectin in dogs experimentally infected with heartworms. Vet Parasitol. 2008;155:242–248.

30. Schwarz T, Sullivan M, Stork CK, Willis R, Harley R, Mellor DJ. Aortic and cardiac mineralization in the dog. Vet Radiol Ultrasound. 2002;43:419–427.

31. Lake-Bakaar GA, Johnson EG, Griffiths LG. Aortic thrombosis in dogs: 31 cases (2000–2010). J Am Vet Med Assoc. 2012;241:910–915.

4.5

Airways

Normal airways

The large airways are well delineated on CT images since the soft-tissue attenuating airway walls are defined both internally and externally by a gas-attenuating interface. CT quantification of tracheal diameter has been performed in anesthetized German Shepherd Dogs and revealed a consistent horizontal to vertical ratio of approximately 1.0, with luminal cross-sectional area progressively decreasing from the cranial cervical region to the thoracic cavity.[1] A CT evaluation of the trachea in normal dogs during respiration revealed a decrease in tracheal cross-sectional area during inspiration, with the change in area being primarily attributable to a decrease in vertical tracheal diameter. Many of these dogs had invagination of the dorsal tracheal membrane at expiration.[2] Ratios of lobar bronchi diameters to corresponding pulmonary arterial diameters in normal dogs have been reported to average 1.45 with an upper limit of 2.0 (Figure 4.5.1).[3] Bronchial/arterial ratio measurements obtained in anesthetized normal cats yielded a mean value of 0.71 with an estimated upper limit of 0.91.[4]

CT is not routinely used to evaluate dynamic changes of the major airways since patients are often intubated, anesthetized, and mechanically ventilated. However, one report describes dynamic tracheal and bronchial collapse due to airway wall malacia on CT images in sedated and nonintubated dogs. Bronchial collapse was defined as a width to height ratio of greater than 2.[5]

Tracheal and bronchial developmental disorders

A single CT report describes tracheal hypoplasia in two English Bulldog puppies but does not include quantitative data.[5] Computed tomography features of other tracheal and bronchial dysplasia have not been previously reported in the dog or cat. Common imaging features in people include bronchi originating from an abnormal location and segmental or complete atresia or hypoplasia with resulting narrowing of the airway lumen (Figure 4.5.2).[6]

Trauma

Tracheal trauma with mural disruption can result in respiratory compromise as well as pneumomediastinum, subcutaneous emphysema, and pneumothorax. CT features include discontinuity of the tracheal wall and a variable volume of extraluminal gas (Figure 4.5.3).

Iatrogenic pulmonary barotrauma from positive-pressure ventilation of anesthetized patients can occasionally lead to alveolar or small airway rupture in people, with resulting perivascular gas dissection.[7] We have seen a similar phenomenon in dogs, which appears as a thin gas-attenuating layer surrounding pulmonary blood vessels on CT images (Figure 4.5.4).

Inflammatory disorders

Tracheobronchitis

Chronic bronchitis is common in dogs and is typically associated with an underlying neutrophilic/eosinophilic

Atlas of Small Animal CT and MRI, First Edition. Erik R. Wisner and Allison L. Zwingenberger.
© 2015 John Wiley & Sons, Inc. Published 2015 by John Wiley & Sons, Inc.

inflammatory response of the airway mucosa. The disorder is more prevalent in small-breed dogs because of the association with tracheobronchial collapse and left atrial enlargement, but may be present in dogs of any breed.

CT imaging features are similar to those present on conventional radiographs, with bronchial wall thickening appearing as "doughnuts" when viewed in cross-section and as "tramtracks" when viewed in long axis. Pulmonary parenchyma may also appear diffusely more attenuating than normal because of small airway involvement. Focal or regional peripheral lung consolidation may be present in more severe cases.

Feline bronchial disease

Feline eosinophilic pulmonary disease is a complex disorder that may take on many forms depending on chronicity and severity. It is thought to be the result of type I hypersensitivity reaction causing airway inflammatory response and smooth muscle contraction. With chronicity and increasing severity, airway walls become thicker, resulting in a typical bronchial pattern. In some patients, inspissated bronchial secretions accumulate within airway lumina, resulting in obstruction and characteristic hyperattenuating branching concretions. In people, the "tree-in-bud" sign describes the characteristic peripheral soft-tissue attenuating branching pattern associated with the accumulation of exudates in the respiratory bronchioles and alveolar ducts (the buds) and the peripheral bronchioles (tree branches).[8] The subgross anatomy in dogs and cats is somewhat different from that in people; however, the tree-in-bud pattern is similar. Although airway concretions are easily recognized as being airway oriented and intraluminal on CT images, they can sometimes be misdiagnosed as hyperattenuating pulmonary masses on conventional radiographic images. In the acute phase of feline bronchial disease, imaging findings may be minimal and limited to reduced airway diameter and increased lung volume due to lower airway obstruction. Routine radiographic imaging would be most commonly employed as part of the diagnostic evaluation at this stage. CT is employed in patients refractory to treatment or when radiographic findings are unclear. CT features include evidence of bronchial thickening; diffusely increased pulmonary density, likely due to terminal airway involvement; exudative airway collections; and sometimes hyperinflation due to lower airway obstruction. This latter feature may be difficult to assess because of assisted ventilation in patients under general anesthesia (Figures 4.5.5, 4.5.6, 4.5.7).

Canine eosinophilic bronchopneumopathy
CT imaging features of eosinophilic bronchopneumopathy are described in Chapter 4.6.[9]

Bronchiectasis

Bronchiectasis is an irreversible dilatation of the bronchi resulting from chronic airway inflammation that damages elastic components of the bronchi leading to bronchial wall destruction and impaired clearance of respiratory secretions. CT features of bronchiectasis in people and domestic animals include abnormal bronchial dilation, lack of peripheral bronchial tapering, and identification of distinct airways more peripherally than expected.[10-13] Secondary features of bronchiectasis include bronchial wall thickening, mucus plugging within the bronchial lumen, and peripheral air trapping, as reflected by measurable reduced pulmonary density in affected regions (Figures 4.5.8, 4.5.9, 4.5.10). In people, a bronchoarterial ratio of greater than 1.0 is an important CT criterion for the diagnosis of bronchiectasis.[10,12] However, in dogs the normal upper threshold has been reported to be approximately 2.0, although bronchiectatic airways can fall below this value.[11]

Bronchial foreign bodies

The most common bronchial foreign bodies are migrating plant awns, which are prevalent in some parts of the world. Pulmonary plant awn foreign bodies most commonly enter the body through nasal inhalation. They then migrate through the trachea and into the lobar and more peripheral bronchi. Multiple awns involving multiple lung lobes are common. Migrating foreign bodies result in multifocal bronchitis that rapidly progresses to consolidating focal or lobar pneumonia. Typical CT features include multifocal mixed alveolar and interstitial pulmonary infiltrates. The proportion of lung involved depends on number and location of plant awns and the chronicity of the pneumonia. Although often masked by bronchial exudates, the awns can sometimes be detected when surrounded by intraluminal gas (Figure 4.5.11).[14]

Neoplasia

Malignant neoplasia originating from the upper airways is rare, with carcinoma being most common in dogs and carcinoma and lymphoma in cats. Rhabdomyosarcomas of the canine larynx have also been reported. Chondromas and osteochondromas may also arise from the tracheal or bronchial wall.[15] Clinical signs depend on location and invasiveness of the neoplasm. Tumors arising from or near the larynx may result in voice change, and neoplasms extending into the airway lumen may lead to clinical signs of upper airway obstruction.

CT features of large-airway neoplasia include focal, regional, or circumferential thickening of the tracheal wall, and large tumors may appear overtly mass-like. The airway patency can be compromised because of intraluminal tumor invasion or mural/extramural compression. Obstructive bronchial tumors may lead to lobar atelectasis. Tumors usually moderately enhance following contrast medium administration (Figures 4.5.12, 4.5.13, 4.5.14, 4.5.15).

Degenerative disorders

Tracheobronchial malacia, a softening of the tracheal cartilages and loss of integrity of the airway walls, is a common cause of large-airway collapse in people and has been documented in dogs. Diagnosis is based on a greater than 50% collapse of the airway, as observed on bronchoscopic examination. Although most veterinary patients are anesthetized or sedated for CT examination and respiration is often assisted, large-airway collapse is sometimes seen (Figure 4.5.16).[16]

Figure 4.5.1   Normal Trachea and Bronchi (Canine)   CT

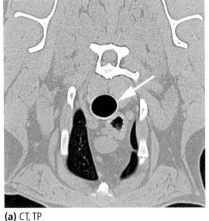

(a) CT, TP

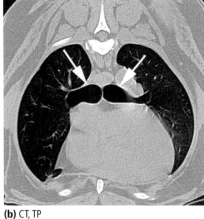

(b) CT, TP

The normal canine trachea should have a height:width ratio close to 1.0 (**a**: arrow). Mainstem bronchi should originate symmetrically at the carina (**b**: arrows). The origin of the lobar bronchi in the normal, well-inflated lung are easily detected (**c**: arrowheads), and bronchi can be followed through five or six generations, depending on image resolution and image collimation. The normal thoracic trachea can sometimes deviate to the right as a result of displacement by the aorta (**c**: arrow) or other cranial mediastinal structures. The average normal canine bronchial:arterial ratio is approximately 1.45 and should not exceed 2.0 (**d**: a = artery; b = bronchus; v = vein).

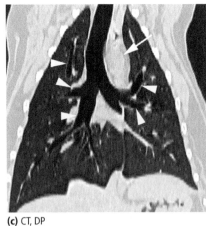

(c) CT, DP

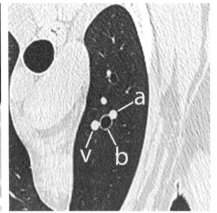

(d) CT, TP

Figure 4.5.2   Bronchial Dysplasia (Canine)   CT

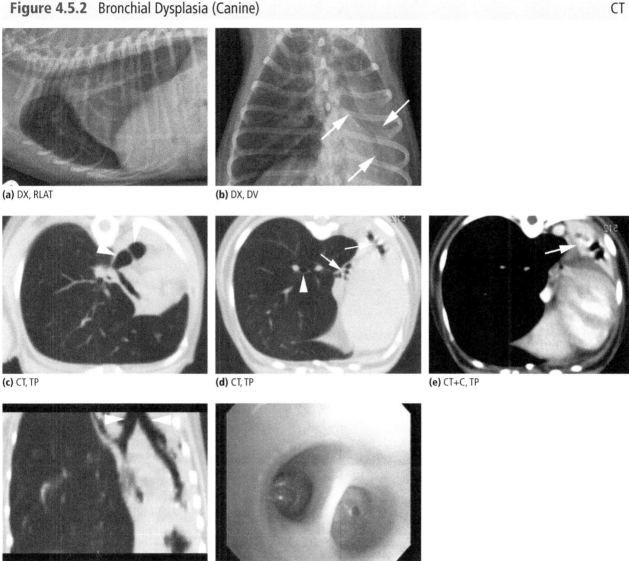

(a) DX, RLAT

(b) DX, DV

(c) CT, TP

(d) CT, TP

(e) CT+C, TP

(f) CT, DP

(g) ES

6mo F Miniature Pinscher with chronic cough, exercise intolerance, and recent onset of dyspnea. Images **c–e** are representative CT images in the cranial (**c**) and middle (**d,e**) thorax. Images **d** and **e** are at the same level and are lung and soft-tissue windowed, respectively. The left lung is atelectatic (**a,b**), but primary and lobar bronchi are air-filled and clearly delineated (**b**: arrows). Compensatory right lung hyperinflation results in a left-sided mediastinal shift (**b**). Mainstem bronchi are displaced dorsally and to the left in the cranial thorax (**c,f**: arrowheads). Smaller air bronchograms are present further caudally (**d**: arrows), and atelectatic lung contrast enhances (**e**: arrow) indicating unimpeded parenchymal perfusion. Evaluation of the entire CT examination revealed that only the right middle lung lobe was inflated. The right middle lobar bronchus can be seen (**d**: arrowhead). The mainstem bronchial lumina are malformed and partially occluded (**g**). Microscopic evaluation of surgically excised lung revealed malformation of large and small airways consistent with congenital bronchial dysplasia.

Figure 4.5.3 Tracheal Rupture (Feline)   CT

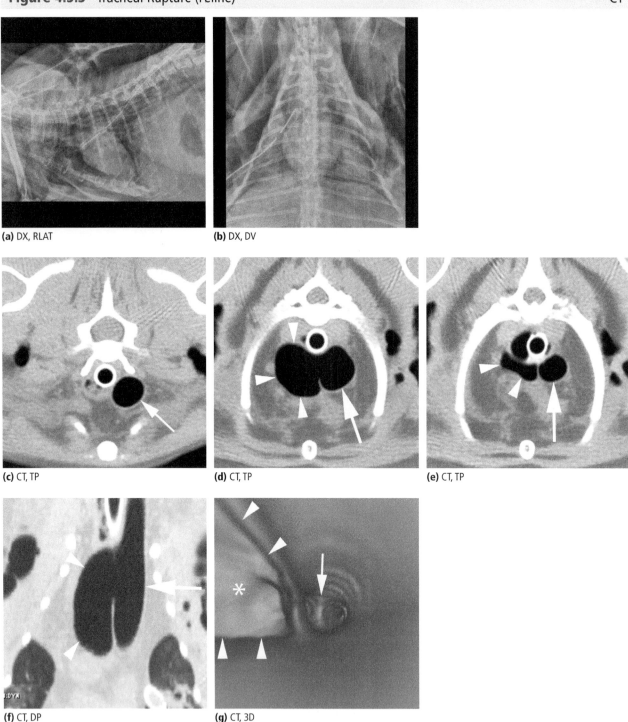

(a) DX, RLAT

(b) DX, DV

(c) CT, TP

(d) CT, TP

(e) CT, TP

(f) CT, DP

(g) CT, 3D

11y FS Domestic Longhair in respiratory distress. The cat was anesthetized 1 week previously for a dentistry procedure. The radiographic study (**a,b**) reveals extensive pneumomediastinum, pneumothorax, subcutaneous emphysema, and caudal lobar alveolar infiltrates. Near the thoracic inlet, the trachea is intact (**c**: arrow). A communicating diverticulum (**d**: arrowheads) arises from the right side of the trachea (**d**: arrow) in the cranial thorax and is well defined during forced inspiration. The diameter of both the tracheal lumen (**e**: arrow) and the diverticulum (**e**: arrowheads) are markedly reduced during expiration. A CT image reformatted in the dorsal plane reveals the size of the diverticulum and tracheal wall defect (**f**: arrowheads). The trachea (**f**: arrow) appears truncated caudally in this image because of the reformatting angle. The intraluminal view on the virtual bronchoscopic image is from cranial to caudal, and the tracheal bifurcation is seen (**g**: arrow), as are the lumen of the diverticulum (**g**: asterisk) and the margins of the tracheal wall defect (**g**: arrowheads). Findings on postmortem examination were consistent with tracheal rupture due to pressure necrosis from an overinflated endotracheal catheter cuff.

Figure 4.5.4   Barotrauma (Canine)   CT

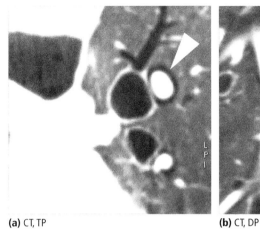

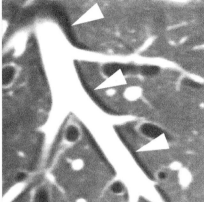

Adult dog with immune-mediated mega-esophagus and pneumonia. There is a uniform cuff of perivascular gas surrounding the pulmonary arteries. (**a,b**: arrowheads). The dog had been under positive-pressure ventilation while under anesthesia, which was thought to have caused alveolar or small airway rupture leading to the perivascular gas dissection. Dr. Giovanna Bertolini, San Marco Veterinary Clinic, Padova, Italy, 2014. Reproduced with permission from G Bertolini.

(a) CT, TP   **(b)** CT, DP

Figure 4.5.5   Feline Bronchial Disease (Feline)   CT

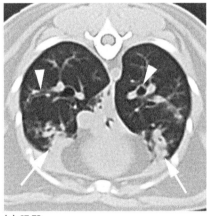

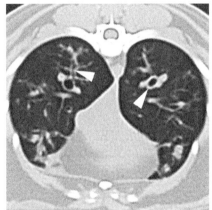

6y FS Domestic Shorthair with chronic cough. Representative CT images of the middle and caudal thorax are ordered from cranial to caudal and reveal widespread airway thickening (**a–c**: arrowheads). There is also regional consolidation or atelectasis of dependent lung (**a**: arrows). Bronchoscopy documented bronchial wall edema, bronchospasm, and copious mucus within lobar bronchi (**d**). Bronchoalveolar lavage cytology interpretation was eosinophilic inflammation with moderate epithelial hyperplasia.

(a) CT, TP   **(b)** CT, TP

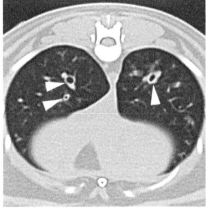

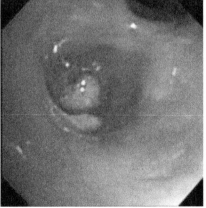

(c) CT, TP   **(d)** ES

Figure 4.5.6 Feline Bronchial Disease (Feline)

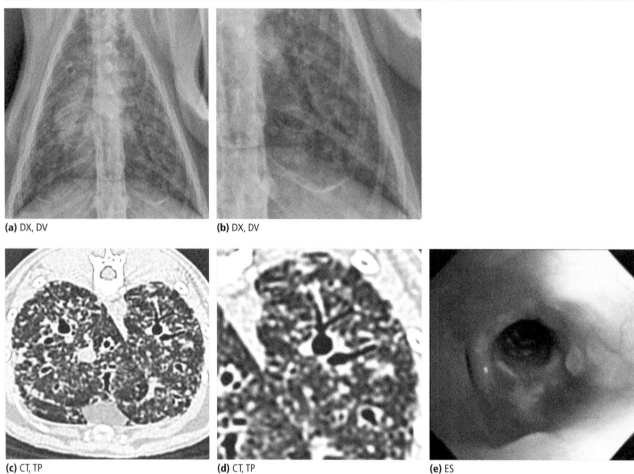

(a) DX, DV

(b) DX, DV

(c) CT, TP

(d) CT, TP

(e) ES

6y MC Domestic Shorthair with increased respiratory rate and effort. Images **b** and **d** are magnified views from images **a** and **c**, respectively. Thoracic radiographs reveal a marked bronchial pattern with a heavy interstitial component (**a,b**). Findings are similar on thoracic CT images, which show generalized bronchial wall thickening with an underlying interstitial infiltrate (**c,d**). The trachea and bronchi were edematous and friable, and there was evidence of bronchiectasis and inspissated mucus on bronchoscopic examination (**e**). Bronchoalveolar lavage cytology interpretation was moderate neutrophilic and eosinophilic inflammation with no microbes cultured.

Figure 4.5.7 Feline Bronchial Disease with Luminal Obstruction (Feline)   CT

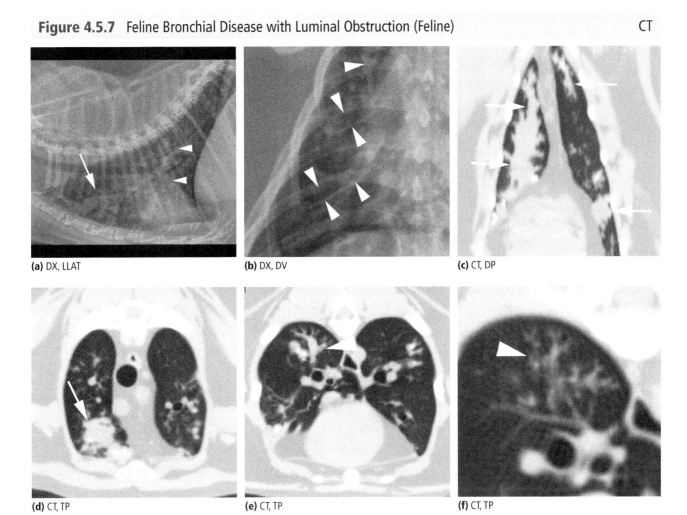

(a) DX, LLAT   **(b)** DX, DV   **(c)** CT, DP

(d) CT, TP   **(e)** CT, TP   **(f)** CT, TP

11y MC Domestic Shorthair with chronic cough. Thoracic radiographs show a heavy generalized bronchial pattern (**a,b**: arrowheads). There are also multiple pulmonary masses or regions of consolidation, best seen in the right cranial lung lobe (**a**: arrow). On CT images, in addition to documenting bronchial wall thickening, the masses are revealed to be large bronchial luminal concretions of inspissated airway exudates (**c,d**: arrows), the largest of which involves the right cranial lobe bronchus. An arborizing concretion in the right caudal lung lobe typifies the "tree-in-bud" pattern (**e**: arrowhead). The bronchial branching pattern is clearly defined on a thinly collimated image (**f**: arrowhead). Bronchoscopy findings included mucosal hyperemia and stenosis and occlusion of multiple bronchi. Bronchoalveolar lavage cytology was suppurative inflammation with mild chronic hemorrhage.

Figure 4.5.8   Focal Bronchiectasis (Canine)

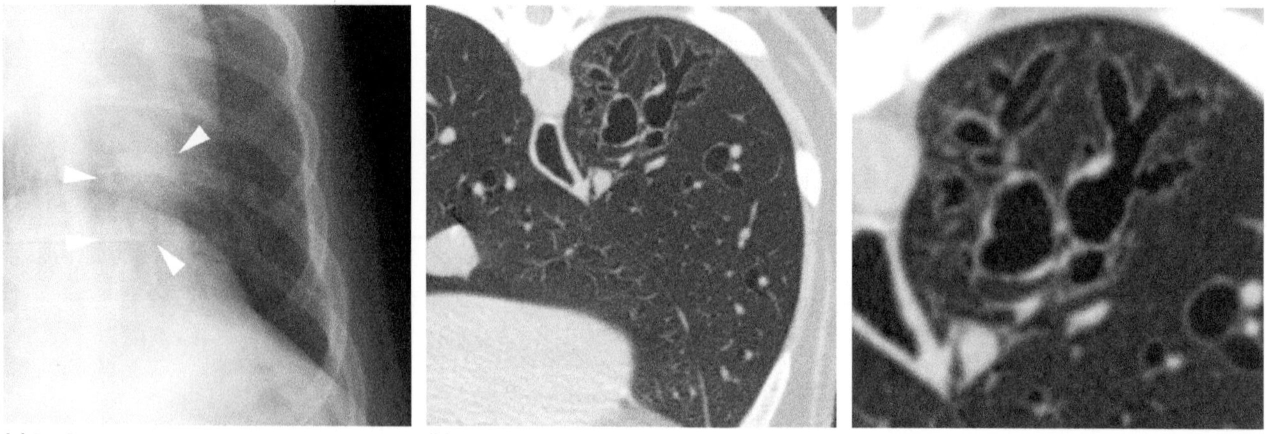

(a) DX, DV   (b) CT, TP   (c) CT, TP

8y FS Labrador Retriever with prior history of plant awn foreign body pneumonia and a recent history of cough. Ill-defined alveolar infiltrates are present in the left caudal lung lobe on an initial radiographic examination (a: arrowheads). The CT examination was performed 12 days following the radiographic study, and the dog was on antibiotic therapy during that interval. Image b is a representative 1 mm collimated CT image of the caudal thorax, and image c is a magnified view of image b. Regional arborizing bronchial dilation is evident in the periphery of the left caudal lung lobe (b,c). Bronchial lumen enlargement is accompanied by bronchial wall thickening, but no significant pulmonary infiltrates or luminal exudates are evident. Microscopic evaluation following lung lobectomy revealed interstitial fibrosis consistent with resolution of pneumonia. The bronchiectasis was presumed to be an end-stage result of the previous bronchopneumonia.

Figure 4.5.9 Bronchiectasis (Canine)   CT

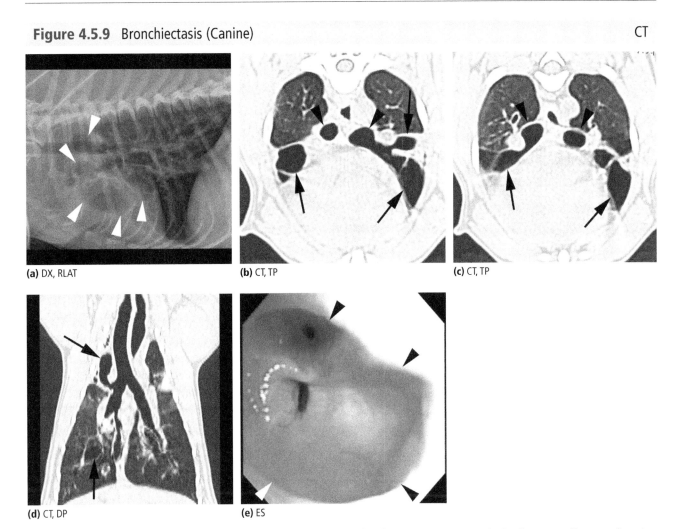

(a) DX, RLAT

(b) CT, TP

(c) CT, TP

(d) CT, DP

(e) ES

4y MC Miniature Schnauzer cross. Chronic respiratory signs since 3 months of age. Progressive exercise intolerance and increased respiratory effort over the past 8 months. Marked saccular bronchiectasis is seen on radiographs and is most pronounced in the right middle and cranial lung lobes (**a**: arrowheads). On CT images acquired caudal to the carina, the mainstem bronchi are seen (**b,c**: arrowheads) as are markedly sacculated and dilated cranial lung lobe bronchi (**b,c**: arrows). Right cranial and caudal lung lobe bronchiectasis is also seen on dorsally reformatted images (**d**: arrows). Bronchoscopic examination further documented severe, sacculated bronchiectasis, as represented by the marked bronchial luminal dilatation (**e**: arrowheads). Bronchoalveolar lavage cytology documented mixed neutrophilic and eosinophilic inflammation and epithelial hyperplasia.

Figure 4.5.10 Severe Bronchiectasis (Canine)

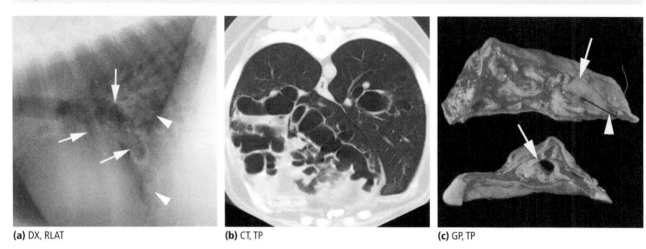

(a) DX, RLAT   **(b)** CT, TP   **(c)** GP, TP

4y MC Rottweiler with previous history of eosinophilic granulomatosis that has clinically responded to treatment. Current clinical signs are consistent with bronchopneumonia. Pronounced dilation of the accessory, middle, and caudal lobe bronchi is evident on thoracic radiographs (a: arrows), and increased peripheral opacity in the dependent regions is consistent with consolidating infiltrates (a: arrowheads). A representative CT image at the level of the accessory and caudal lung lobes reveals marked saccular bronchial dilation involving all visible lung lobes, fluid accumulation in the most dependent airways, and ventral alveolar infiltrates (b). Transverse sections of an excised lung lobe document the presence of dilated thick-walled bronchi filled with exudates (c: arrows). A black thread delineates the path of the bronchial lumen in the upper specimen (c: arrowhead). Microscopic evaluation confirmed suppurative bronchopneumonia and marked bronchiectasis. In this dog, bronchiectasis was a sequela of previously diagnosed chronic eosinophilic granulomatosis. Cannon et al 2013.[11] Reproduced with permission from Wiley.

Figure 4.5.11 Bronchial Foreign Body (Canine)

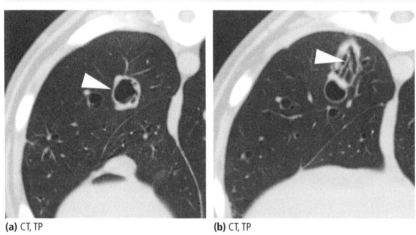

(a) CT, TP   **(b)** CT, TP

4y F Bearded Collie with cough and recent-onset lethargy and fever due to pyothorax. The dog was treated and improved but cough persists. Sequential CT images of the right caudal lung lobe show thickening of the caudal lobar bronchus (a: arrowhead) and a complex linear foreign body more peripherally (b: arrowhead). The foreign body is soft-tissue attenuating and is well defined because of surrounding gas. Surgery revealed an approximately 7 cm long plant fragment, thought to be an evergreen frond that originated in the distal right caudal lobar bronchus, penetrated the pulmonary parenchyma, and terminated in the pleural space. Excisional lung biopsy confirmed chronic catarrhal, suppurative bronchitis, and pleuropneumonia.

Figure 4.5.12 Tracheal Osteochondroma (Canine)   CT

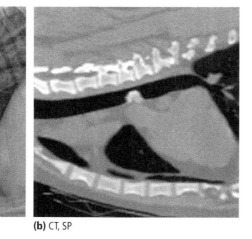

(a) DX, RLAT

(b) CT, SP

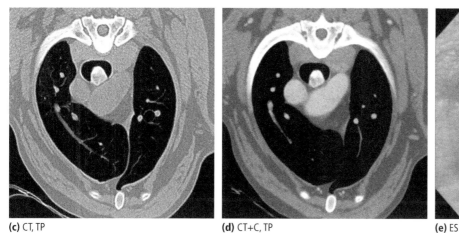

(c) CT, TP

(d) CT+C, TP

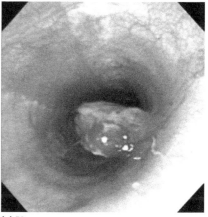

(e) ES

2y FS Bernese Mountain Dog with stridor. There is a sessile soft-tissue mass that arises from the ventral tracheal wall and appears to be primarily intraluminal (**a**: arrow). The mass proves to be of mixed soft-tissue and mineral opacity on unenhanced CT images (**b,c**) and mildly enhances following contrast administration (**d**). CT imaging confirms the mass is well defined and is restricted to the ventral tracheal wall. Bronchoscopic evaluation supports the radiographic and CT imaging findings (**e**). Biopsy confirmed the mass to be an osteochondroma.

Figure 4.5.13 Tracheal Adenocarcinoma (Feline)

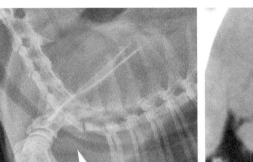

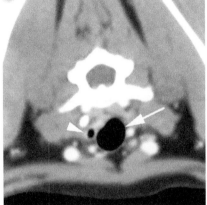

6y FS Egyptian Mau with increased respiratory effort and stridor. A mural mass is seen involving the caudal cervical trachea, resulting in partial luminal occlusion (**a**: arrow). A CT image cranial to the mass shows the normal trachea (**b**: arrow) and the adjacent contrast-enhancing cervical esophagus (**b**: arrowhead). Further caudally, an intensely enhancing tracheal mass is confirmed to be mural (**c,d**: arrows). Mass margins are clearly defined, and the tracheal lumen is narrowed at this level. Excisional biopsy revealed the mass to be a tracheal adenocarcinoma.

(a) DX, RLAT

(b) CT+C, TP

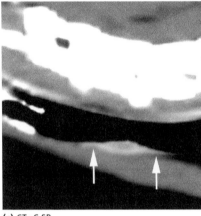

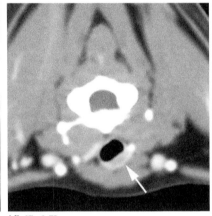

(c) CT+C SP

(d) CT+C, TP

Figure 4.5.14 Tracheobronchial Carcinoma (Feline)   CT

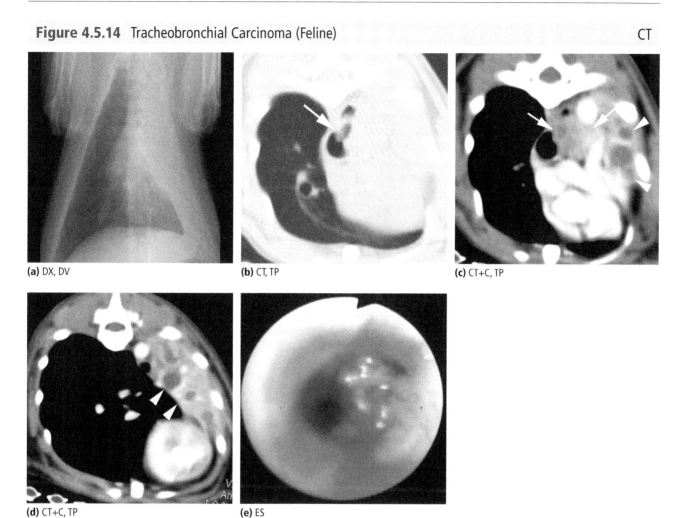

(a) DX, DV   **(b)** CT, TP   **(c)** CT+C, TP

(d) CT+C, TP   **(e)** ES

11y MC Domestic Shorthair with 2-month history of weight loss, lethargy, and coughing. Volume depletion of the left lung is associated with compensatory hyperinflation of the right lung (**a**). A moderately enhancing soft-tissue attenuating mass is present at the level of the origin of the left mainstem bronchus (**c**: arrows) and extends into the right mainstem bronchial lumen (**b**: arrow). The heterogeneous appearance of the atelectatic left lung is due to contrast-enhanced lung parenchyma surrounding fluid-filled airways or fluid bronchograms (**c,d**: arrowheads). The intraluminal component of the mass is clearly identified bronchoscopically (**e**). The microscopic diagnosis from excisional biopsy was bronchial carcinoma.

Figure 4.5.15 Tracheal Lymphoma (Feline)   CT

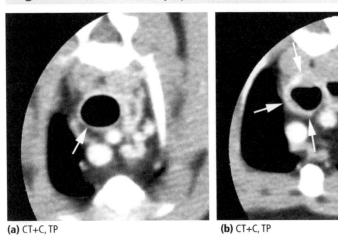

8y FS Domestic Shorthair with 1-month history of stridor. On a CT image cranial to the mass, the trachea has a normal ovoid appearance and is thin walled (**a**: arrow). Caudally, a poorly defined, moderately enhancing mural mass encompasses approximately 75% of the tracheal wall circumference and distorts the tracheal lumen (**b,c**: arrows; **c** is a magnification of **b**). A comparable bronchoscopic view of the mass (**d**) is consistent with the CT findings. Cytologic diagnosis was lymphoma.

(a) CT+C, TP   **(b)** CT+C, TP

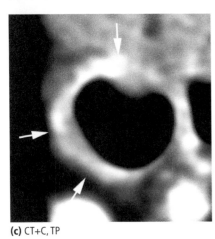
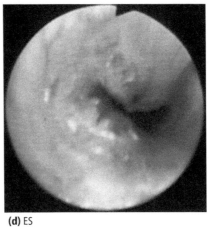

(c) CT+C, TP   **(d)** ES

Figure 4.5.16 Tracheal Malacia (Canine)

CT

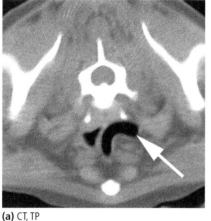

(a) CT, TP

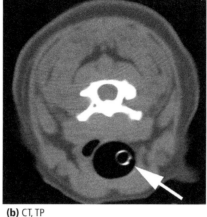

(b) CT, TP

9y FS Yorkshire Terrier with previously documented tracheal collapse. The caudal cervical tracheal lumen (**a**: arrow) is flattened and less than 50% of the cross-sectional area of the midcervical (**b**: arrow) and intrathoracic (**c**: arrow) trachea. Endoscopic examination confirmed dynamic bronchial (**d**: arrowheads) and tracheal (not shown) collapse.

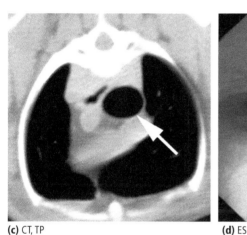

(c) CT, TP

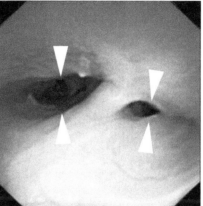

(d) ES

References

1. Kara ME, Turan E, Dabanoglu I, Ocal MK. Computed tomographic assessment of the trachea in the German shepherd dog. Ann Anat. 2004;186:317–321.

2. Leonard CD, Johnson LR, Bonadio CM, Pollard RE. Changes in tracheal dimensions during inspiration and expiration in healthy dogs as detected via computed tomography. Am J Vet Res. 2009;70:986–991.

3. Cannon MS, Wisner ER, Johnson LR, Kass PH. Computed tomography bronchial lumen to pulmonary artery diameter ratio in dogs without clinical pulmonary disease. Vet Radiol Ultrasound. 2009;50:622–624.

4. Reid LE, Dillon AR, Hathcock JT, Brown LA, Tillson M, Wooldridge AA. High-resolution computed tomography bronchial lumen to pulmonary artery diameter ratio in anesthetized ventilated cats with normal lungs. Vet Radiol Ultrasound. 2012;53:34–37.

5. Stadler K, Hartman S, Matheson J, O'Brien R. Computed tomographic imaging of dogs with primary laryngeal or tracheal airway obstruction. Vet Radiol Ultrasound. 2011;52:377–384.

6. Gurney JW. Diagnostic Imaging: Chest. Salt Lake City: Amirsys Inc., 2007.

7. Anzueto A, Frutos-Vivar F, Esteban A, Alia I, Brochard L, Stewart T, et al. Incidence, risk factors and outcome of barotrauma in mechanically ventilated patients. Intensive Care Med. 2004;30:612–619.

8. Eisenhuber E. The tree-in-bud sign. Radiology. 2002;222:771–772.

9. Clercx C, Peeters D. Canine eosinophilic bronchopneumopathy. Vet Clin North Am Small Anim Pract. 2007;37:917–935.

10. Bonavita J, Naidich DP. Imaging of bronchiectasis. Clin Chest Med. 2012;33:233–248.

11. Cannon MS, Johnson LR, Pesavento PA, Kass PH, Wisner ER. Quantitative and qualitative computed tomographic characteristics of bronchiectasis in 12 dogs. Vet Radiol Ultrasound. 2013;54:351–357.

12. Cantin L, Bankier AA, Eisenberg RL. Bronchiectasis. AJR Am J Roentgenol. 2009;193:W158–171.

13. Javidan-Nejad C, Bhalla S. Bronchiectasis. Radiol Clin North Am. 2009;47:289–306.

14. Schultz RM, Zwingenberger A. Radiographic, computed tomographic, and ultrasonographic findings with migrating intrathoracic grass awns in dogs and cats. Vet Radiol Ultrasound. 2008;49:249–255.

15. Lopez A. Respiratory System. In: McGavin MD, Zachary JF (ed): Pathologic Basis of Veterinary Disease, 2007;492.

16. Johnson LR, Pollard RE. Tracheal collapse and bronchomalacia in dogs: 58 cases (7/2001–1/2008). J Vet Intern Med. 2010;24:298–305.

4.6

Small airways and parenchyma

Introduction

Dogs and cats have six well-defined lung lobes that correspond to the anatomic organization of the principal, or lobar, bronchi. Bronchovascular bundles are composed of the bronchi, corresponding pulmonary vessels, and the adjacent interstitial framework. Some pulmonary disorders arise from or are distributed along the bronchovascular bundle.

Tertiary, or segmental, bronchi arise from the lobar bronchi, and the region of lung ventilated by each segmental bronchus is referred to as a bronchopulmonary segment. Bronchopulmonary segments are further subdivided into secondary pulmonary lobules that are small subdivisions of the lung encompassed by interlobular connective tissue septa and composed of a central bronchiole, accompanying arteriole and lymphatic vessel, and a few pulmonary acini.

The acinus is the largest anatomic unit within which gas exchange occurs and includes one or more first order respiratory bronchioles and two to three generations of smaller respiratory bronchioles in the dog. Each branching respiratory bronchiole and its associated alveolar ducts, alveolar sacs, alveoli, and capillaries form a primary pulmonary lobule. Therefore, secondary pulmonary lobules are composed of multiple acini, and acini are composed of multiple primary pulmonary lobules.[1]

Although there are a number of computed tomographic descriptive terms characterizing regional or diffuse pulmonary patterns in people (crazy paving, mosaic, etc.) based on the origin or distribution of pathology in relation to the subgross anatomic architecture of the lung, care should be used in adopting these terms to characterize CT patterns in small animal veterinary medicine. Specific subgross anatomic differences include more limited interlobular septal connective tissue and much more collateral ventilation in exchange regions of the lung in dogs and cats as compared to people.

Atelectasis

Because normal aerated lung volume is comprised predominantly of gas, atelectasis can result in profound volume loss with associated visceral shift and redistribution of remaining aerated lung. Positional atelectasis frequently occurs as a consequence of recumbency and may be exacerbated by general anesthesia when assisted ventilation is not used. For this reason, patients scheduled to undergo thoracic CT should be maintained in sternal recumbency following anesthetic induction and prior to imaging. Atelectasis may also occur because of lung compression by masses and pleural fluid or from airway obstruction. CT features of atelectasis include volume loss and increased lung attenuation that is inversely proportional to the degree of lung collapse. Peripheral lung parenchyma is most often affected when lobar atelectasis is incomplete. Complete collapse of one or more lobes can occur as a sequela to underlying pulmonary disease or pleural effusion (Figure 4.6.1). In uncomplicated atelectasis, the lobar and segmental bronchi remain aerated, producing an air bronchogram sign. A mediastinal shift toward the affected lung is characteristic and helpful in differentiating atelectasis from pulmonary consolidation. The remaining aerated lung may be hyperinflated and can redistribute to compensate for atelectatic volume loss.

Atlas of Small Animal CT and MRI, First Edition. Erik R. Wisner and Allison L. Zwingenberger.
© 2015 John Wiley & Sons, Inc. Published 2015 by John Wiley & Sons, Inc.

Developmental disorders

Emphysema

There is a small number of reports of dogs with emphysema that is associated with underlying bronchial hypoplasia and bronchiectasis.[2–5] A proposed mechanism is dynamic expiratory bronchial collapse leading to increased intrapulmonary pressure and subsequent development of emphysema.[3] Imaging reports are sporadic but include pulmonary hyperlucency, regional lobar collapse, and pneumothorax (Figure 4.6.2).

Pulmonary bulla

Pulmonary bullae are often developmental and may have a similar underlying pathophysiologic mechanism as described above for emphysema. Bullae are generally clinically silent unless less they rupture leading to pneumothorax.[6,7] Pulmonary bullae can also result from shearing trauma of lung parenchyma, arise as a sequela to underlying pulmonary parenchymal disease, or be idiopathic.

Bullae are thin-walled, well demarcated, and hypoattenuating to adjacent normal pulmonary parenchyma on CT images (Figure 4.6.3). Clinically silent bullae are easily detected on routine CT imaging but are often obscured in the presence of pneumothorax. The clinical value of CT for bulla detection is reported to be low in dogs with spontaneous pneumothorax. Detection rate improves with increasing bulla size but does not seem to correlate with the severity of pneumothorax.[8]

Pulmonary edema

Cardiogenic edema

Cardiogenic edema due to left ventricular failure results from increased intravascular hydrostatic pressure at the level of the pulmonary capillaries, causing extravasation of transudative edema fluid into adjacent lung interstitium. CT features of cardiogenic pulmonary edema include interstitial to alveolar infiltrates that may be multifocal or coalescing. Mild to moderate infiltrates have a ground-glass appearance, representing interstitial and partial alveolar edema (Figure 4.6.4). Left atrial and ventricular enlargement can also be seen, and pulmonary venous enlargement, though often present, is inconsistent. Cardiogenic edema typically has a perihilar distribution in dogs but no characteristic distribution in cats.

Noncardiogenic edema

Noncardiogenic pulmonary edema is caused by increased pulmonary capillary permeability, resulting in extravasation of high-protein fluid into the interstitial space. The most common initiators of noncardiogenic edema are acute respiratory distress syndrome (ARDS), which has many underlying causes: neurogenic causes; pulmonary embolic disorders; and occasionally an adverse response to drugs or toxins. CT features of noncardiogenic edema include mixed interstitial to alveolar infiltrates with a random multifocal or coalescing distribution (Figure 4.6.5). In patients with ARDS, the severity of pulmonary infiltrates may be profound, and the imaging appearance may be altered by superimposition of underlying inflammatory lung disease.

Pulmonary contusion and hemorrhage

Pulmonary contusion from trauma and overt pulmonary hemorrhage due to trauma, bleeding diatheses, or other underlying lung pathology varies in appearance depending on the initiating cause and severity. CT features consist of regional interstitial to alveolar infiltrates that are typically asymmetrical and may be unilateral (Figure 4.6.6). Fulminant bleeding may flood airways and alveoli, mimicking lobar consolidation from other causes. In trauma patients, the CT diagnosis of pulmonary contusion is sometimes confounded by the presence of positional atelectasis that results in increased pulmonary attenuation from volume loss.

Lung lobe torsion

Lung lobe torsion has been reported in both dogs and cats, and Pugs are predisposed to the disorder.[9–11] Lobar torsion is frequently a sequela of chronic pleural effusion, with the left cranial and right middle lobes most often involved and rarely more than one lung lobe. CT features include pleural effusion and abrupt termination of the affected lung lobe bronchus. Additional findings are lobar enlargement, peripheral parenchymal collapse/consolidation, and central vesicular emphysema (Figures 4.6.7, 4.6.8).[10,11] Emphysematous lobes have mild or absent enhancement following intravenous contrast administration because of torsional vascular occlusion and necrosis. Lung lobes that have undergone torsion and are small in size are less affected by necrosis, possibly due to hyperacute or chronic time course or partial torsion. These atelectatic lobes are contrast enhancing as they retain blood supply. Virtual CT bronchoscopy has also been reported to aid in diagnosis.[10] Partial lobar torsion can occasionally occur and is more challenging to diagnose since characteristic features associated with complete torsion may be absent.

Inflammatory lung disorders

Idiopathic interstitial pneumonia

A number of inflammatory interstitial lung disorders in people fall under the broad category of idiopathic interstitial pneumonia.[12] Although the array of speculated causes vary, these disorders have characteristic constellations of CT features that are adequate for specific diagnosis, and most eventually lead to end-stage pulmonary fibrosis.[12] These entities have not been well described in dogs and cats, but we do occasionally encounter patients with histologically confirmed interstitial pneumonitis without an apparent underlying infectious or other noninfectious exogenous cause (Figure 4.6.9).

Eosinophilic bronchopneumopathy

Canine eosinophilic bronchopneumopathy is thought to be immune-mediated and the result of a hypersensitivity to aeroallergens, although infectious and other immune-mediated causes have also been proposed as initiators in some instances. Average age of onset is 4–6 years, and both large- and small-breed dogs are affected. Females are at over twice the risk for developing the disease.[13] Although there is not a clear consensus regarding features, our experience suggests three clinical manifestations. Some dogs present with a predominantly bronchitic manifestation, with CT features of bronchial wall thickening and evidence of intraluminal bronchial exudates (Figure 4.6.10). Other dogs have findings more similar to bronchopneumonia with mixed interstitial and alveolar infiltrates. Less commonly, the disorder manifests as pulmonary granulomas that appear as focal, multifocal, or regional irregularly margined nodules or masses (Figure 4.6.11).

Lipid pneumonia

Endogenous and exogenous lipid pneumonia has been reported in both dogs and cats.[14–18] Endogenous lipid pneumonia results from pneumocyte injury with a wide array of proposed toxic, metabolic, and nutritional causes. Radiographic features of endogenous lipid pneumonia in a report of 24 cats included pleural effusion, diffuse interstitial or bronchointerstitial infiltrates, multifocal pulmonary infiltrates with confluence near the hilus, and discrete pulmonary nodules.[17] CT features of endogenous lipid pneumonia have not been reported in dogs or cats (Figure 4.6.12).

Exogenous lipid pneumonia is most often linked to aspiration of lipid-based medications. In people, CT features include diffuse ground-glass interstitial opacities, consolidation, or mass lesions.[19,20] A single case report describing CT findings in a dog with exogenous lipid pneumonia characterized the lesions as lung consolidation with air bronchograms. The affected region mildly and diffusely contrast enhanced.[14]

Viral pneumonia

Although CT appearance of viral pneumonias has been described in people and include ground-glass, unstructured interstitial, and centrilobular nodular interstitial patterns, CT features have not been characterized in companion animals because conventional radiography would likely be used as an initial imaging diagnostic test. Based on reported radiographic features of viral pneumonia in dogs and cats, one might expect to see interstitial, ground-glass opacities regionally or diffusely distributed, with a predilection for the caudodorsal lung fields.

Aspiration pneumonia

Aspiration pneumonia, as the name implies, results from aspiration of gastric or other fluids that cause a chemical pneumonitis. Gastric fluid is acidic and is therefore particularly damaging. Swallowing and esophageal disorders and gastric reflux are common predisposing factors leading to aspiration. Aspiration pneumonia typically occurs in the dependent regions of affected lobes but may have an atypical distribution if aspiration occurs with the patient in lateral or dorsal recumbency, as can occur while under anesthesia. Bacterial contamination will lead to lobar pneumonia.

Bacterial bronchopneumonia and related disorders

In people, bacterial pneumonia is subdivided into bronchopneumonia and lobar pneumonia, reflecting the initial location and subsequent progression of the inflammatory process. Bronchopneumonia arises through accumulation of exudates in terminal bronchioles and respects septal boundaries. Lobar pneumonia results from alveolar flooding of inflammatory exudates and has a greater propensity to spread.[21] Given the differences in subgross anatomy between people and companion animals, this distinction may not be relevant in cats and dogs. CT features of bacterial bronchopneumonia include mixed interstitial and alveolar infiltrates in dependent regions of involved lung lobes. In many instances, complete lobar consolidation occurs with air bronchograms surrounded by uniformly soft-tissue attenuating alveolar infiltrates. Lung volume loss can occur but is usually mild and insufficient to explain the increased lung attenuation (Figure 4.6.13). *Mycoplasma* pneumonia has been reported in both cats and dogs and appears to include airway collapse and bronchitis as part of the clinical manifestation in addition to consolidating pneumonia (Figure 4.6.14).[22,23] Pleuropneumonia can lead to pleural thickening and regional pleural effusion, and necrotizing bronchopneumonia can result in pneumothorax (Figure 4.6.15).

Foreign-body-induced bronchopneumonia is common in some parts of the world where ingested or inhaled plant awns migrate down the bronchial tree, lodging in small-caliber distal airways and initiating a bacterial bronchopneumonia. CT features depend on acuity and severity of pneumonia but often appear as a multifocal consolidating pneumonia (Figure 4.6.16). Alveolar infiltrates are often not in the dependent regions of the lung, and middle and caudal lobes are preferentially affected, presumably because of the migratory path of the awns.[24] Foreign bodies often seed bacteria that can also lead to more fulminant granulomatous pneumonia.

Pulmonary abscess

Pulmonary abscesses are usually bacterial but are occasionally sterile or fungal. Bacterial abscesses can occur as a solitary lesion or in association with more widespread inflammatory disease. On unenhanced CT images, they appear as thick-walled spheroid or ellipsoid cavitary masses that contain fluid-attenuating material and often have a gas component that distributes to the nondependent part of the cavity. Depending on size and location, abscesses can cause bronchial obstruction and lobar atelectasis (Figure 4.6.17). The abscess capsule moderately to intensely contrast enhances, but attenuation of abscess contents remains unchanged.

Infectious granulomatous pneumonia and related disorders

Although infectious granulomatous pneumonias are often mycotic, pyogranulomatous pneumonia can also result from other microbial infections, such as feline coronavirus and *Nocardia* and *Actinomyces* species. The latter two organisms often invade the chest cavity as a sequela to plant awn migration (Figure 4.6.18). Fungal pneumonias occur following inhalation exposure to causative agents, the most common of which are *Coccidioides immitis*, *Blastomyces dermatitidis* and *Histoplasma capsulatum* in North America.

Pulmonary CT features of mycotic pneumonia range from unstructured and nodular interstitial infiltrates to complete lobar consolidation. Large nodules are typically solid and soft-tissue attenuating and are irregularly margined reflecting the inflammatory nature of the disease. Tracheobronchial lymph nodes can be profoundly enlarged, causing depression of the terminus of the trachea and abaxial separation of the mainstem bronchi (Figure 4.6.19). Affected lungs and lymph nodes enhance following contrast medium administration, and a heterogeneous pattern of enhancement may reveal lymph node abscessation.

Pneumocystis carinii, once classified as a protozoan but more recently reclassified as a yeast-like fungus, is a common cause of pneumonia in immunocompromised people and can induce pneumonia in dogs as well. Miniature Dachshunds and Cavalier King Charles Spaniels seem to be predisposed, and there is some suggestion that immune incompetence also plays a role in dogs. Infection results in an accumulation of *P. carinii* cysts within alveolar exudates and an eosinophilic inflammatory response.[25] CT features of *P. carinii* pneumonia include a nonuniform, diffuse increase in pulmonary parenchyma attenuation, which may represent greater or lesser degrees of alveolar flooding in adjacent secondary lobules (Figure 4.6.20).

Parasitic pneumonia

A number of parasites can cause bronchitis and pneumonia in dogs and cats and include migrating larval roundworms (*Toxocara*) and hookworms (*Ancylostoma*), feline lungworm (*Aelurostrongylus*), *Filaroides* species, and lung flukes (*Paragonimus*). Pulmonary manifestations of these disorders in dogs and cats have not been widely reported and will vary depending on the specific parasite involved (Figure 4.6.21). Pulmonary CT features of these parasitic infestations would be expected to parallel the radiographic features that have been described.

Cardiovascular CT features of heartworm (*Dirofilaria*) infestation are described in Chapter 4.4. Embolic pneumonia can occur with heartworm disease, particularly during therapy, when dead heartworms lodge in the peripheral pulmonary arteries. CT manifestations include midzonal and peripheral interstitial to alveolar infiltrates with coalescence in more severely affected patients. Pulmonary eosinophilic granulomatosis can also occur as an immune response to heartworm infestation.

Neoplasia

The vast majority of primary lung tumors are malignant, and most are epithelial in origin, although primary mesenchymal tumors occasionally occur. Older animals are predisposed, and tumors most often arise in the caudal lung lobes. Other neoplasms involving the lungs include malignant histiocytosis, lymphoma, sarcomas, and pulmonary metastasis.[26]

Pulmonary carcinoma

Epithelial tumors are categorized by site of origin (bronchogenic, bronchoalveolar, alveolar) and by cell characteristics (squamous cell, undifferentiated, adenocarcinoma).[26]

To date, CT features of the various types of primary epithelial lung tumors have not been found to be sufficiently unique to distinguish one type from another (Figures 4.6.22, 4.6.23, 4.6.24). However, a recent report on the CT characteristics of 17 primary pulmonary carcinomas found they are solitary, well circumscribed, and located either centrally or in the periphery of the lung. Tumors were bronchocentric in origin and contained air bronchograms. Bronchial lumina are often narrowed and displaced. Most tumors have mild to moderate heterogeneous contrast enhancement, and pulmonary metastatic disease was seen in a few dogs in this report.[27] Bronchial metastases from primary lung tumors can be extensive and occasionally involve lobes in the contralateral hemithorax, making them surgically unresectable. These tumors can be cavitary and will occasionally mineralize.

CT has been shown to be more sensitive and accurate than survey radiography for diagnosis of tracheobronchial lymphadenopathy in dogs with primary lung tumors.[28] CT features included node enlargement and irregular margination with or without contrast enhancement.

Tumors of mesenchymal origin

Mesenchymal tumors include osteosarcoma, chondrosarcoma, malignant histiocytosis, and lymphomatoid granulomatosis. Of these, histiocytic sarcoma is most common, often affecting primarily Bernese Mountain Dogs and Rottweilers, although the disorder has been reported in other breeds as well.

Reported CT features of malignant histiocytic sarcoma in dogs include intrathoracic lymphadenopathy (tracheobronchial and sternal lymphadenopathy predominately) and the presence of pulmonary masses preferentially located within the right middle lung lobe (Figure 4.6.25). Masses are typically multiple, bronchogenic in origin, poorly margined, and mildly to moderately contrast enhancing. Other CT features include pulmonary nodules, pleural effusion, and regional pulmonary patterns.[29]

Lymphoma

Radiographic features of pulmonary lymphoma in dogs and cats have been reported, but as might be expected with this disorder, imaging characteristics are quite variable and include bronchial, interstitial or alveolar infiltrates, nodules or masses, pleural effusion, and lymphadenopathy. CT features would be expected to parallel the radiographic findings (Figure 4.6.26).[30]

Pulmonary metastasis

Computed tomography has been shown to be more sensitive than radiography for pulmonary metastasis detection.[31,32] In one study, only about 10% of nodules seen on CT studies were detected on radiographs, with nodules less than about 8 mm most frequently missed.[32] Metastases usually arise from tumor emboli from a distant neoplasm lodging in the pulmonary capillaries, leading to development of interstitial nodules and masses. On CT images, metastases run the spectrum from widespread and miliary to few and mass-like and can be poorly to well demarcated. Associated hemorrhage or inflammation can cause nodules to be less defined. Most metastases are soft-tissue attenuating,

although those from malignant primary bone tumors, and occasionally other neoplasms, can be mineralized. Nodules mildly to intensely contrast enhance (Figures 4.6.27, 4.6.28, 4.6.29, 4.6.30, 4.6.31, 4.6.32). A minority of lung metastases in people distribute through the pulmonary lymphatic vessels, producing a branching linear pattern rather than nodules, but this has not been described in companion animals.

Degenerative disorders

Pulmonary osseous metaplasia

Pulmonary osseous metaplasia manifests on CT images as multiple widely dispersed mineralized lung nodules usually 3 mm or less in diameter. These have a tendency for subpleural and ventral lung field distribution (Figure 4.6.33). Although these nodules are usually inherently highly attenuating because of mineral content, partial volume averaging in widely collimated CT images can yield apparent HU values lower than expected. Thinly collimated images through the nodule can yield more accurate HU measurements. We have also seen patients with osseous metaplasia nodules with minimal mineralization that can reduce one's confidence in diagnosis.

Pulmonary fibrosis

Pulmonary fibrosis is often the sequela to a variety of disorders and represents the degenerative endpoint of such insults as pneumonia, pulmonary toxins, radiation pneumonitis, and trauma. Depending on the initial cause, pulmonary fibrosis may be focal, regional, or diffuse. On CT images, fibrosis can appear as a reticular interstitial pattern or as a dense linear "scar" (Figures 4.6.34, 4.6.35, 4.6.36). Lungs of older dogs without clinical signs of pulmonary disease may also appear denser on radiographs and CT images because of mild interstitial fibrosis, and anecdotally, this seems to occur primarily in dogs with mitral insufficiency.

A specific entity, idiopathic pulmonary fibrosis, has been described in West Highland White Terriers and has similarities to usual and nonspecific interstitial pneumonias in people.[33] These entities are part of a larger group of pulmonary disorders that fall under the heading of interstitial lung disease, a related group of inflammatory disorders that lead to progressive and irreversible lung scarring. Clinically, dogs with idiopathic pulmonary fibrosis suffer from restrictive lung disease and compromised gas exchange. Histologically, there is interstitial fibrosis, increased alveolar macrophages, and emphysematous change.[34] CT features include linear and reticular opacities, nodules and nodular opacities, overall decreased lung opacity, and overall increased lung opacity.

Figure 4.6.1 Lung Lobe Atelectasis (Feline)   CT

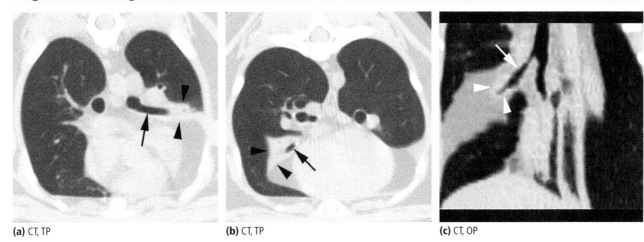

(a) CT, TP   **(b)** CT, TP   **(c)** CT, OP

4y MC Abyssinian cat with chronic respiratory disease. Images **a** and **b** are representative 1 mm collimated transverse images of the midthorax at the level of the left cranial (**a**) and right middle (**b**) lobar bronchi, respectively. Image **c** is an oblique long-axis reformatted image highlighting the right middle lung lobe. The left cranial lobar bronchus is aerated and in its normal position (**a**: arrow), but the lung lobe is volume depleted and of increased attenuation as a result of atelectasis (**a**: arrowheads). Similar findings are seen involving the right middle lobar bronchus (**b,c**: arrows) and lung (**b,c**: arrowheads). The oblique view clearly defines the path of the right middle lobe bronchus (**c**: arrow). The intermediate attenuation surrounding the atelectatic right middle lung lobe is pleural/pericardial fat. Multiple lobe atelectasis was secondary to chronic inflammatory pulmonary disease. Cultures from bronchial secretions documented a diagnosis of *Mycoplasma* pneumonia.

Figure 4.6.2 Emphysema (Feline)   CT

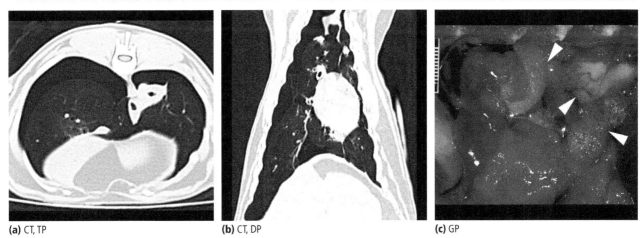

(a) CT, TP   **(b)** CT, DP   **(c)** GP

1.5y Domestic Shorthair with respiratory distress and radiographic evidence of pneumothorax. There is evidence of bilateral pneumothorax and multiple focal areas of atelectasis. Aerated lung appears somewhat more lucent than expected given the severity of the pneumothorax, and peripheral parenchyma attenuation averaged below −925 HU. Other specific morphologic features of emphysema were not seen on CT images, but the gross postmortem image of the lungs reveals pronounced emphysematous changes and bullae in multiple lung lobes (**c**: arrowheads). Microscopic features were consistent with congenital terminal bronchiolar dysplasia leading to emphysema and bulla formation.

Figure 4.6.3 Pulmonary Bullae (Canine) CT

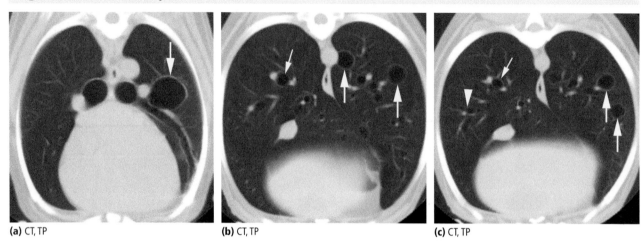

(a) CT, TP   **(b)** CT, TP   **(c)** CT, TP

13y M Fox Terrier with solitary pulmonary adenocarcinoma (not shown). Representative CT images of the middle and caudal thorax, ordered from cranial to caudal, reveal multiple thin-walled bullae of varying size. Bullae are documented to be spherical and distinguished from tubular airways by viewing multiple consecutive images. Bullae are also of larger diameter than expected for airways in the periphery of the lung (a–c: large arrows). Unlike bullae, airways also branch (c: arrowhead) and are flanked by pulmonary arteries and veins (b,c: small arrows). The multiple bullae were clinically silent and thought to be developmental in this dog. Gross and microscopic evaluation of representative bullae removed during lung lobectomy confirmed the imaging diagnosis.

Figure 4.6.4 Cardiogenic Pulmonary Edema (Feline)   CT

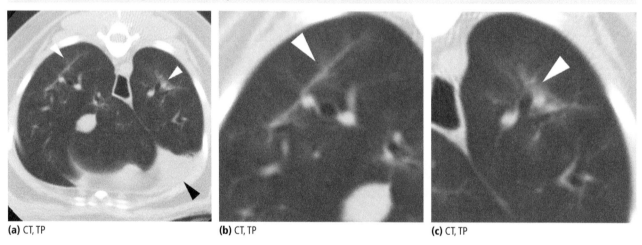

(a) CT, TP   **(b)** CT, TP   **(c)** CT, TP

4y FS Domestic Shorthair currently receiving dialysis for renal failure. The cat had echocardiographic signs of mild cardiomyopathy and was moderately fluid overloaded at the time of the CT examination. Image a is a representative image at the level of the caudal thorax, and images b and c are magnified views of image a. A small volume of dependent pleural fluid elevates aerated lung (a: black arrowhead). There is a mild, diffuse increase in pulmonary attenuation with additional multiple focal regions of ground-glass opacity. The latter infiltrates appear to be most pronounced surrounding the pulmonary vasculature (a–c: white arrowheads). Postmortem examination confirmed the infiltrates were due to pulmonary edema. In this cat, the edema was thought to be due to relative ventricular failure from the combination of cardiomyopathy and fluid overload.

Figure 4.6.5 Noncardiogenic Pulmonary Edema (Feline)   CT

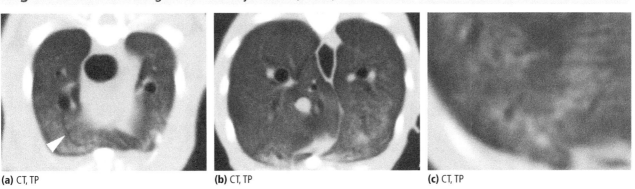

(a) CT, TP   (b) CT, TP   (c) CT, TP

11y MC Domestic Shorthair with chronic diarrhea and weight loss. Images **a** and **b** are representative of the cranial and caudal thorax, respectively. Image **c** is a magnified view of the caudoventral lung field. There is generalized, nonuniform increased pulmonary attenuation that is more pronounced in the dependent lung fields. Infiltrates have a diffuse ground-glass appearance with evidence of overtly alveolar infiltrates and air bronchogram formation in more affected regions (**a**: arrowhead). Postmortem examination revealed pronounced interstitial and alveolar pulmonary edema secondary to widespread arterial and venous pulmonary thrombosis. The underlying cause of pulmonary thromboembolism was not determined.

Figure 4.6.6 Pulmonary Contusion (Canine)   CT

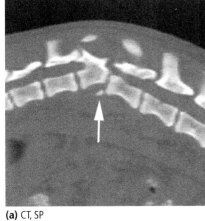

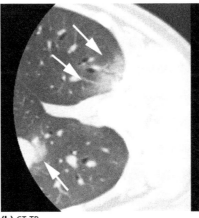

1y M Italian Greyhound hit by a car two times in one day. The CT examination was performed with the dog on a backboard in lateral recumbency. A spinal fracture/luxation is present at the level of L1–2 (**a**: arrow). Image **b** was acquired at the level of the caudal thoracic spine and is oriented with nondependent lung at the top. Focal mixed interstitial to alveolar infiltrates are evident in the dorsal peripheral region of the left caudal lung lobe and in the ventral peripheral region of the accessory lung lobe (**b**: arrows). CT features are consistent with pulmonary contusion and hemorrhage.

(a) CT, SP   (b) CT, TP

Figure 4.6.7 Right Middle Lung Lobe Torsion (Canine) CT

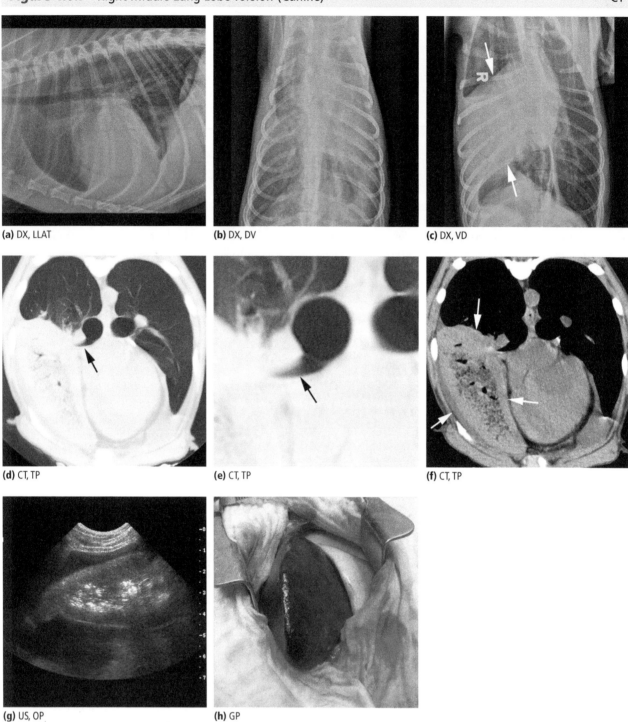

(a) DX, LLAT

(b) DX, DV

(c) DX, VD

(d) CT, TP

(e) CT, TP

(f) CT, TP

(g) US, OP

(h) GP

4y F Afghan Hound with chylous pleural effusion and increasing respiratory effort. Images **d** and **f** are lung and soft-tissue windowed images, respectively, acquired at the level of the right middle lung lobe bronchus. Image **e** is a magnified view of image **d**. There is moderate pleural effusion (**a–c**) and increased right lung lobe density and volume (**c**: arrows) on survey thoracic radiographs. The right middle lobar bronchus tapers abruptly near its origin (**d,e**: arrow), consistent with lung lobe torsion. Right middle lobe volume is increased because of congestion but is necrotic centrally with a characteristic emphysematous appearance (**f**: arrows). Although contrast medium was not administered, torsional vascular occlusion would most likely prevent contrast enhancement of the affected lung lobe. On ultrasound examination, the lung lobe is surrounded by hypoechoic fluid and is partially aerated centrally (**g**). At the time of surgery the devitalized lung lobe had a hepatized appearance (**h**). Right middle lung lobe torsion was confirmed and lobectomy was performed. Microscopic findings were consistent with widespread infarction due to vascular compromise.

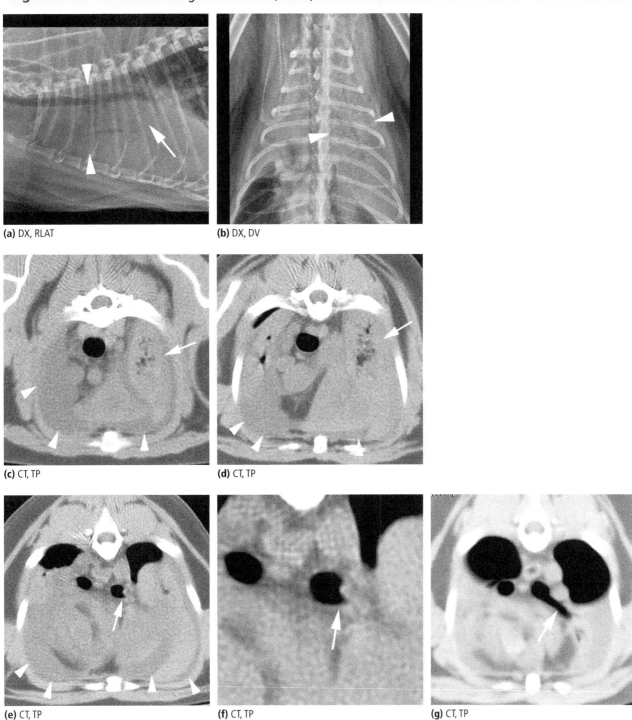

(a) DX, RLAT

(b) DX, DV

(c) CT, TP

(d) CT, TP

(e) CT, TP

(f) CT, TP

(g) CT, TP

13y MC Domestic Shorthair with 3-month history of idiopathic chylothorax. Radiographic and CT images were acquired at the time of most recent evaluation (a–f) and 2 months previously (g). Images c–e were acquired through the cranial thorax and ordered from cranial to caudal. Image **f** is a magnified view of image **e**. Image **g** was acquired at approximately the same level as image **e**. Radiographs revealed air bronchograms and alveolograms (a,b: arrowheads) and a possible truncated left cranial lobe bronchus (a: arrow) characteristic of lung lobe torsion. CT images reveal a characteristic heterogeneous air and soft-tissue lung pattern of pulmonary emphysema associated with lung lobe torsion (c,d: arrows). The origin of the left cranial lobar bronchus tapers and truncates abruptly (e,f: arrows). Although the images are windowed to best define the pulmonary parenchyma features and the lobar bronchus, pleural effusion can also be appreciated (c–e: arrowheads). On the CT image acquired 2 months previously (g), a moderate pleural effusion is present, causing collapse of the cranial and middle lung lobes. However, the left cranial lobe bronchus is clearly identified (g: arrow) and can be followed unimpeded peripherally on adjacent images, indicating the torsion was not present at that time. Microscopic examination of the left cranial lung following surgical excision revealed extensive coagulation necrosis and hemorrhage as a consequence of torsion.

Figure 4.6.9 Interstitial Pneumonia (Feline)   CT

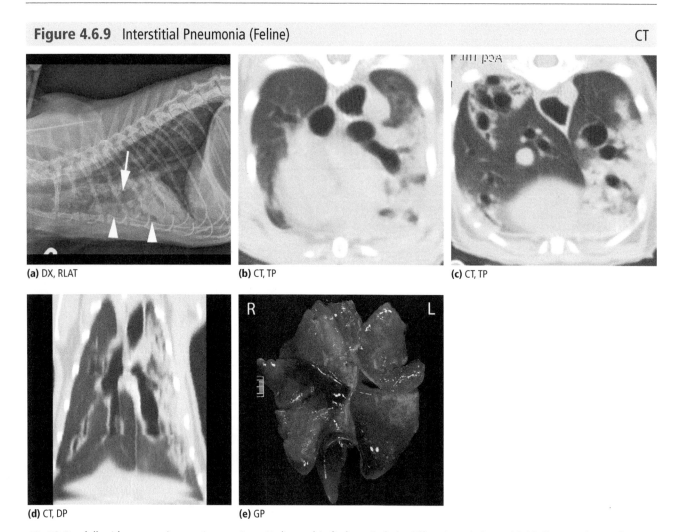

(a) DX, RLAT   **(b)** CT, TP   **(c)** CT, TP

(d) CT, DP   **(e)** GP

12y FS Ragdoll with progressive respiratory signs. Radiographic findings include diffuse bronchointerstitial infiltrates that coalesce to alveolar infiltrates ventrally (**a**: arrowheads) and marked bronchiectasis (**a**: arrow). CT images confirm the presence of generalized bronchiectasis and alveolar infiltrates involving the left cranial, right cranial, and left and right caudal lung lobes (**b–d**). Bronchoalveolar lavage revealed moderate suppurative inflammation without evidence of infectious agents. Postmortem examination documented bronchiectasis and severe, diffuse and acute interstitial pneumonia with fibrin exudation, alveolar histiocytosis, and septal fibrosis (**e**). Infectious agents were not detected on either routine or special stains.

Figure 4.6.10 Eosinophilic Bronchopneumopathy (Canine)   CT

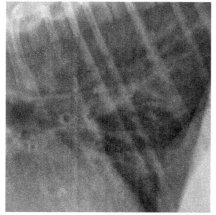

(a) DX, RLAT

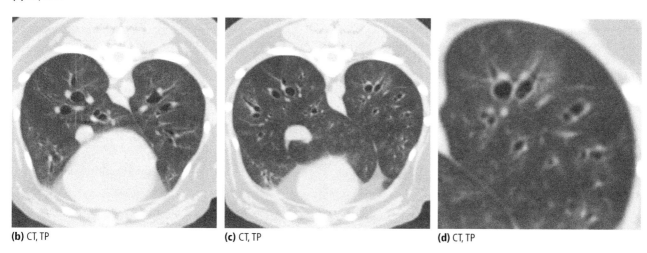

(b) CT, TP   **(c)** CT, TP   **(d)** CT, TP

6y MC Pomeranian with chronic cough. The dog also has a marked peripheral eosinophilia. Image **a** is a representative view of the caudo-dorsal lung field. Images **b** and **c** are representative 1 mm collimated CT images of the caudal thorax. Image **d** is a magnified view of image **c**. A diffuse airway oriented pattern is present radiographically and defined by bronchial wall thickening and mildly increased pulmonary opacity (**a**). Comparable features are present on CT images (**b–d**). Bronchoalveolar lavage cytology revealed moderate eosinophilic and mild suppurative inflammation with epithelial hyperplasia, consistent with the diagnosis of eosinophilic bronchopneumopathy. No microorganisms were detected, and microbial cultures were negative. The dog responded well following a course of steroid and cyclosporine therapy.

Figure 4.6.11 Eosinophilic Bronchopneumopathy (Canine)   CT

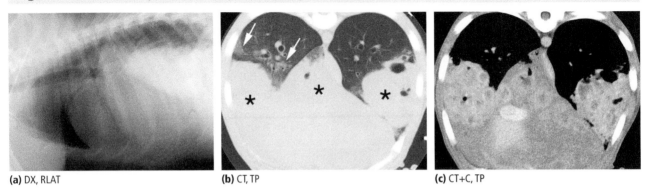

(a) DX, RLAT   **(b)** CT, TP   **(c)** CT+C, TP

4y MC Rottweiler with 3-month history of cough and recent progression to dyspnea and tachypnea, which has been unresponsive to cough suppressants and antibiotics. Radiographs revealed opacification of the accessory and dependent regions of the caudal lung lobes, consistent with consolidating alveolar infiltrates or pulmonary masses (a). Image **b** is representative of the caudal thorax in a lung window, and image **c** is a contrast-enhanced image at approximately the same level as image **b**. CT images reveal pulmonary masses in the accessory and dependent regions of the caudal lung lobes (**b**: asterisks). Ground-glass to alveolar infiltrates are also present in the nondependent regions of the caudal lung lobes (**b**: arrows). Patent airway lumina are evident within the masses in image **b**, and a complex grape cluster appearance in image C is indicative of additional thick-walled, fluid-filled airways incorporated within consolidated lung parenchyma. Lung biopsy revealed severe, diffuse, chronic eosinophilic bronchitis with eosinophilic granulomas. Microbial cultures were negative, and the dog responded to immunosuppressive doses of steroids but eventually developed severe bronchiectasis. (Same dog as in Figure 4.5.10 with end-stage bronchiectasis.)

Figure 4.6.12 Endogenous Lipid Pneumonia (Feline)   CT

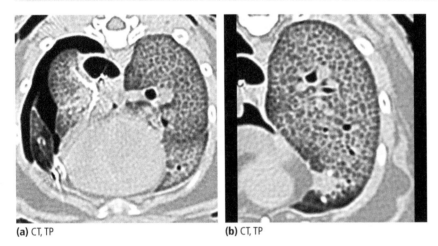

(a) CT, TP   **(b)** CT, TP

9y Domestic Shorthair with respiratory distress following thoracotomy and lung lobectomy for removal of a lung tumor. There is a diffuse reticulated interstitial to alveolar pattern throughout all lung fields (a, b). Average lung attenuation was approximately −250 HU. A right-sided pneumothorax is present as a sequela of right caudal lung lobectomy (a). Postmortem examination revealed severe diffuse lipid pneumonia characterized by flooding of alveoli by large numbers of macrophages containing lipid droplets, confirmed by Oil Red O staining. There was also extensive pleural and septal fibrosis. Review of lung tissue from the lung lobectomy performed 6 days prior to postmortem examination showed no evidence of alveolar histiocytes. In this patient, the endogenous lipid pneumonia was thought to be associated with acute respiratory distress syndrome following thoracotomy.

Figure 4.6.13 Bacterial Bronchopneumonia (Canine)   CT

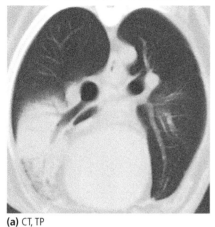

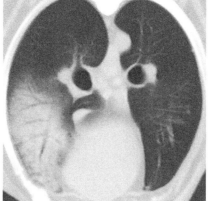

8y FS German Shepherd cross with a right axillary mass. Alveolar infiltrates were detected on thoracic radiographs. Images **a** and **b** are representative images acquired at the level of the right middle lung lobe. There are consolidating alveolar infiltrates of the right middle lung lobe with well-demarcated air bronchograms. The lobe retains normal volume, indicating the presence of infiltrates rather than atelectasis. Bronchoalveolar lavage revealed suppurative inflammation.

(a) CT, TP   **(b)** CT, TP

Figure 4.6.14 *Mycoplasma* Pneumonia (Feline)   CT

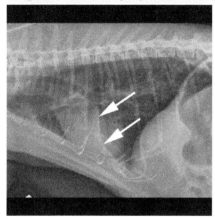

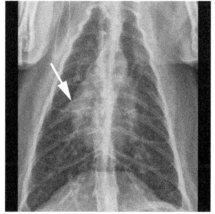

(a) DX, LLAT   **(b)** DX, DV

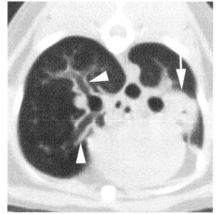

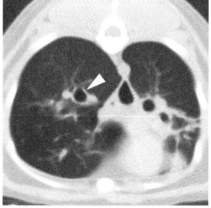

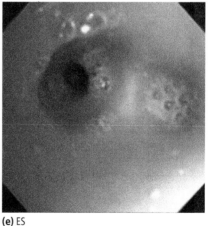

(c) CT, TP   **(d)** CT, TP   **(e)** ES

5y Domestic Shorthair with 5-month history of cough. Images **c** and **d** are representative images of the mid and caudal thorax and are ordered from cranial to caudal. There is a prominent diffuse bronchial pattern (**a,b**), pulmonary hyperinflation (**a,b**), and right middle lung lobe collapse (**a,b**: arrows) on the radiographic examination. On CT images, marked airway wall thickening is evident, and large bronchial lumina appear dilated (**c,d**: arrowheads). There are additional interstitial to consolidating alveolar pulmonary infiltrates peripherally. Both the right middle lung lobe (not shown) and the caudal component of the left cranial lung lobe (**c**: arrow) are collapsed. Copious mucoid exudate was encountered on bronchoscopic examination (**e**). Exudate cytology revealed marked suppurative inflammation and cultured positive for *Mycoplasma*.

Figure 4.6.15 Necrotizing Pleuropneumonia (Canine)   CT

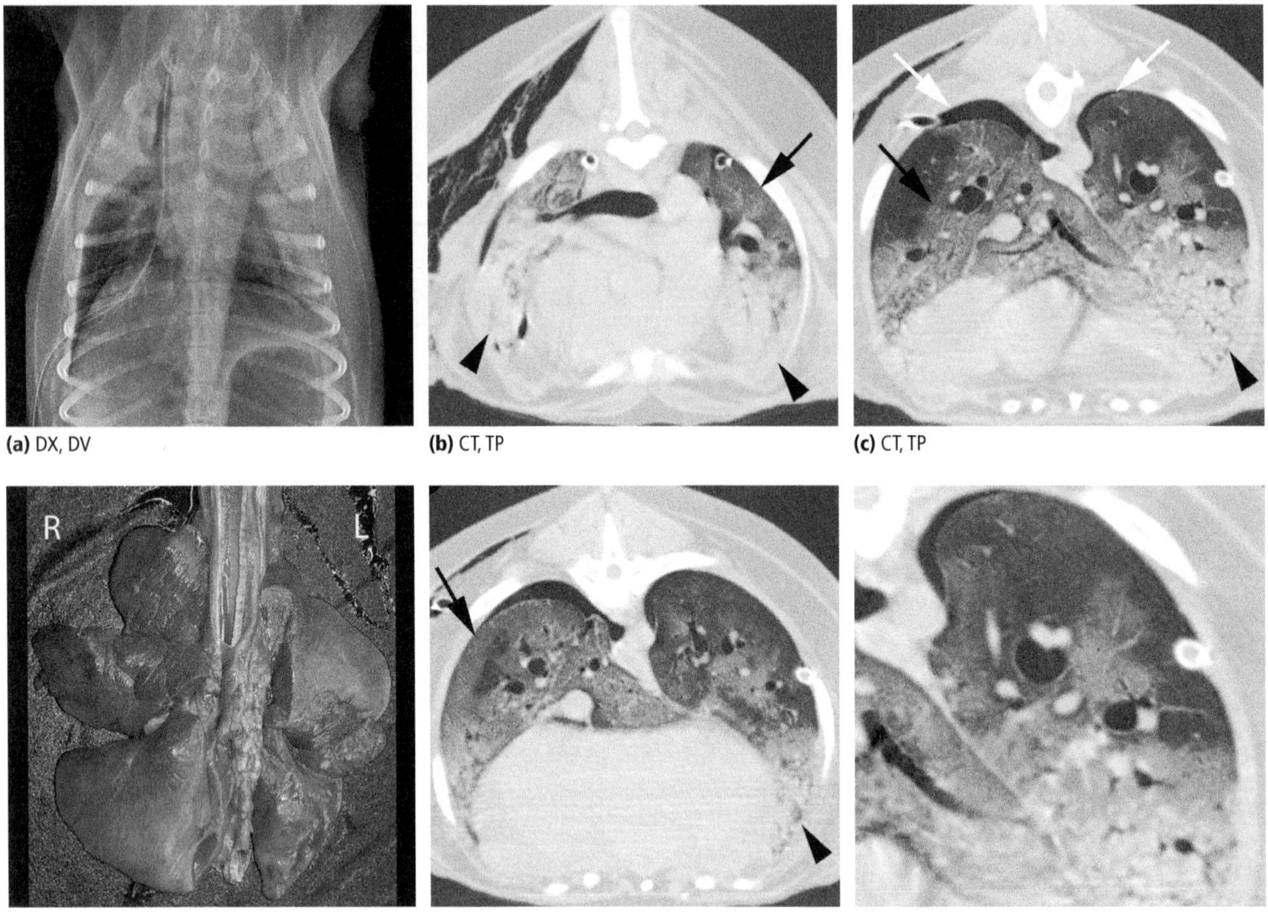

(a) DX, DV

(b) CT, TP

(c) CT, TP

(d) GP

(e) CT, TP

(f) CT, TP

12y FS Golden Retriever being treated for pneumonia and pneumothorax. Thoracostomy catheters were placed prior to acquiring the imaging studies. Radiographs revealed consolidating alveolar infiltrates in multiple lobes (**a**), which were more pronounced in the dependent regions of the lung (best seen on lateral radiographs, not included here) and consistent with bronchopneumonia. Representative CT images (**b,c,e**) are ordered from cranial to caudal. Image **f** represents a thinly collimated magnification of image **c**. There are generalized interstitial infiltrates with ground-glass appearance in all visible lung lobes (**b,c,e**: black arrow), which coalesce into alveolar infiltrates in dependent regions of the lungs (**b,c,e**: black arrowheads). Mild pneumothorax is present bilaterally (**c**: white arrows). The right thoracic wall emphysema is a sequela of thoracostomy catheterization. Pleural fluid cytology was interpreted as marked suppurative inflammation, and microbial culture yielded large numbers of hemolytic *E. coli*. Gross postmortem examination revealed lung discoloration and volume loss with palpable regions of consolidation (**d**).

Figure 4.6.16 Foreign Body Pneumonia (Canine)

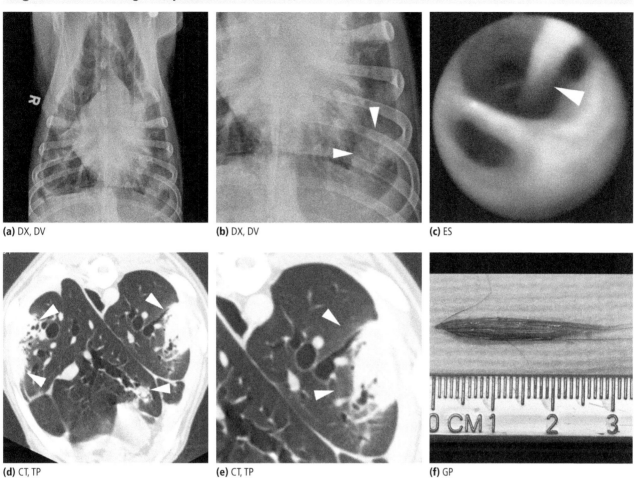

(a) DX, DV

(b) DX, DV

(c) ES

(d) CT, TP

(e) CT, TP

(f) GP

3y FS German Shorthair Pointer with chronic cough and more recent onset of weight loss and lethargy. Interstitial to alveolar infiltrates are present involving multiple lung lobes on thoracic radiographs (**a**), and there is an ill-defined mass in the periphery of the left caudal lung lobe (**b**: arrowheads). Peripheral consolidating alveolar infiltrates with air bronchograms are present in multiple lung lobes on CT images and appear to be centered on distal airways (**d**: arrowheads). Ground-glass opacity surrounds the larger lesions (**e**: arrowheads). The peripheral and multifocal distribution of alveolar infiltrates is characteristic of pneumonia induced by migrating plant awn foreign bodies lodged in distal airways. Multiple plant awns were detected (**c**: arrowhead). Representative image of a bronchoscopically retrieved plant awn (from a different patient) (**f**). Bronchoalveolar lavage revealed septic suppurative inflammation with intracytoplasmic organisms.

Figure 4.6.17 Pulmonary Abscess (Canine)

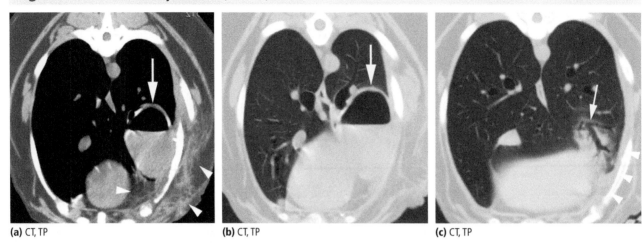

(a) CT, TP **(b)** CT, TP **(c)** CT, TP

8y MC Dalmatian with 2-month history of intermittent coughing. Images **a** and **b** are soft-tissue and lung windowed images at approximately the same level in the cranial thorax. Image **c** is caudal to image **b**. A large, partially fluid-filled, thick-walled oval cavitary mass is seen in the caudal part of the left cranial lung lobe (**a,b**: arrows). Diffuse mediastinal and subcutaneous edema is evident in close association with the mass (**a**: arrowheads). Regional alveolar infiltrates (**c**: small arrow) and focal pleural effusion (**c**: arrowheads) are also present caudal and adjacent to the mass. The cavitary lesion was found to be partially filled with hemorrhagic fluid at the time of lung lobectomy. Microscopic evaluation of the abscess capsule and adjacent lung revealed a marked inflammatory response. Ancillary CT findings were due to mediastinitis, pleuritis, and subcutaneous cellulitis.

Figure 4.6.18 Pyogranulomatous Pneumonia (Feline)

CT

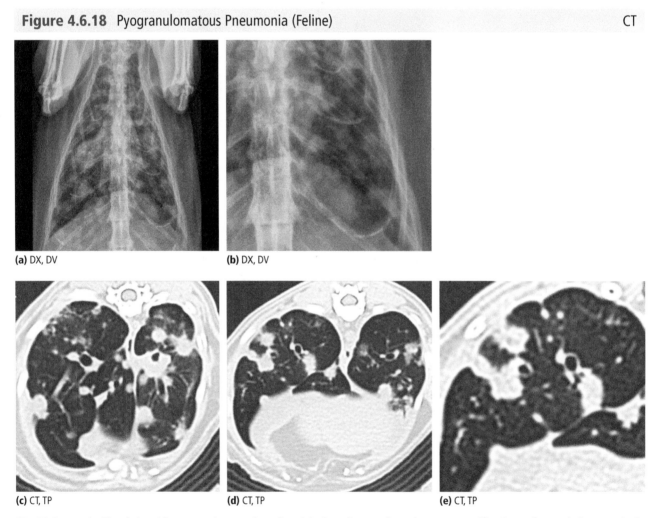

(a) DX, DV **(b)** DX, DV

(c) CT, TP **(d)** CT, TP **(e)** CT, TP

13y FS Domestic Shorthair with progressive cough and weight loss. Images **b** and **e** are magnifications of **a** and **d**, respectively. Radiographs reveal widespread, irregularly margined and coalescing nodules of varying size in all lung lobes (**a,b**). Similar findings are present on representative CT images (**c–e**). Bronchoalveolar lavage cytology was interpreted as pyogranulomatous inflammation. The underlying cause of the pyogranulomatous pneumonia was not determined but thought to be infectious. Tests for feline coronavirus, *Toxoplasma gondii*, *Dirofilaria immitis*, *Mycoplasma*, bacteria, and fungal organisms were all negative.

Figure 4.6.19 *Coccidioides immitis* Mycotic Pneumonia (Canine)   CT

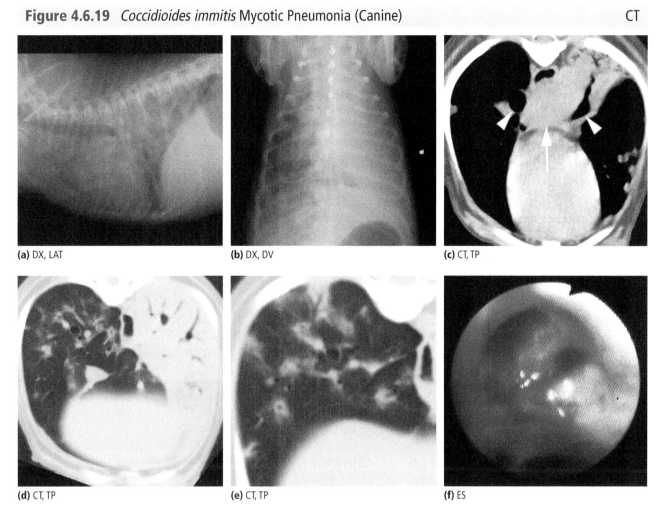

(a) DX, LAT   **(b)** DX, DV   **(c)** CT, TP

(d) CT, TP   **(e)** CT, TP   **(f)** ES

7y MC Dachsund with progressive increase in respiratory effort, weight loss, and diminished activity of 1-month duration. There is consolidation of the entire left lung and coalescing alveolar infiltrates in the right lung on thoracic radiographs (**a**,**b**). On CT images, the central tracheobronchial lymph node is markedly enlarged (**c**: arrow), causing compression and abaxial displacement of the mainstem bronchi (**c**: arrowheads). The left lung is consolidated with persisting air bronchograms (**d**). Multifocal, partially coalescing, and poorly margined alveolar infiltrates are present in the right lung lobes and appear to be centered on airways in many instances (**e**). On broncho-scopic examination, the carina has an abnormal blunted shape, and mucosa appears inflamed with regions of frank hemorrhage (**f**). Bronchoalveolar lavage cytology revealed pyogranulomatous inflammation, and a *Coccidioides immitis* titer was positive. Postmortem examination confirmed disseminated pyogranulomatous pneumonia with numerous intralesional fungal spherules.

Figure 4.6.20 *Pneumocystis carinii* Mycotic Pneumonia (Canine) CT

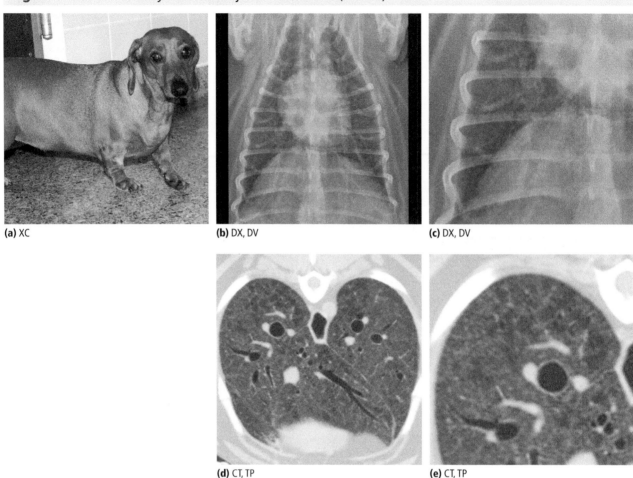

(a) XC

(b) DX, DV

(c) DX, DV

(d) CT, TP

(e) CT, TP

2y FS Dachshund with a 4-month history of exercise intolerance (**a**). There are moderate to marked diffuse interstitial infiltrates in the lung fields on the radiographic examination (**b,c**). A diffuse ground-glass pattern is seen on CT images (**d**), with an average attenuation of approximately −650 HU in the ventral lung fields. There is a more lucent reticulated pattern in the most dorsal regions of the lung (**e**). Bronchoalveolar lavage cytology was consistent with *Pneumocystis carinii* infection.

Figure 4.6.21 *Paragonimus* Parasitic Pneumonia (Canine) CT

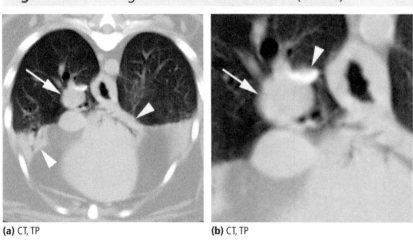

(a) CT, TP

(b) CT, TP

10y FS Kelpie with a mass involving the left optic nerve. Thoracic radiographs reveal a solitary pulmonary nodule in the right caudal lung lobe. Image **b** represents a magnification of image **a**. A well-demarcated soft-tissue attenuating mass is seen immediately dorsal to the caudal vena cava (**a,b**: arrow). Focal mineralization is present at the periphery of the mass (**b**: arrowhead). Increased attenuation and volume depletion in the accessory lobe and the dependent part of the right caudal lung lobe (**a**: arrowheads) are indicative of a combination of alveolar infiltrates and atelectasis. Microscopic evaluation of the pulmonary mass following lung lobectomy revealed a focal granulomatous pneumonia containing an aggregate of cysts filled with fluke eggs. The optic nerve mass proved to be a meningioma unrelated to the pulmonary lesion.

Figure 4.6.22 Bronchoalveolar Carcinoma (Canine)   CT

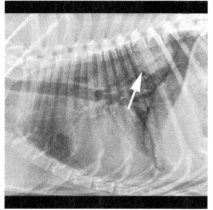

(a) DX, RLAT

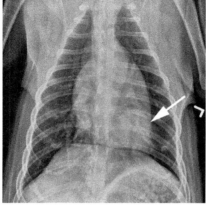

(b) DX, DV

11y M Australian Shepherd with no clinical signs referable to pulmonary disease. There is a large well-demarcated soft-tissue mass in the dorsal aspect of the left caudal lung lobe on survey radiographs (**a,b**: arrows). The soft-tissue attenuating mass is also seen on representative CT images (**c,d**: large arrows). Some airways are left relatively undisturbed (**c**: arrowhead), while others are compressed and displaced (**d**: arrowheads). Ground-glass opacities are present at the periphery of the mass (**c**: small arrow). Pathologic diagnosis following lung lobectomy was locally invasive well-differentiated bronchoalveolar carcinoma. The ground-glass infiltrates seen on CT images likely reflected the local tumor invasion.

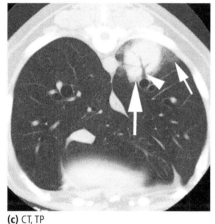

(c) CT, TP

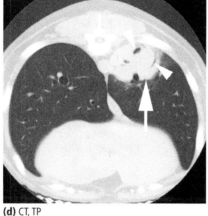

(d) CT, TP

Figure 4.6.23 Cavitary Bronchoalveolar Carcinoma (Canine)   CT

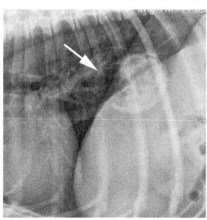

(a) DX, LLAT

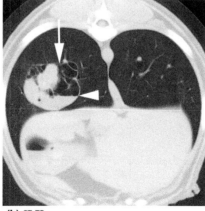

(b) CT, TP

11y FS Shepherd/Doberman Pinscher cross with no clinical signs referable to pulmonary disease. A well-demarcated cavitary mass is seen in the right caudal lung lobe on survey radiographs (**a**: arrow). The cavitary nature of the pulmonary mass is also evident on CT images (**b**: arrow), and the presence of a meniscus indicates that part of the soft-tissue attenuating component is fluid that has distributed in the dependent part of the mass (**b**: arrowhead). Pathologic diagnosis following lung lobectomy was bronchoalveolar carcinoma.

Figure 4.6.24   Regionally Invasive Pulmonary Adenocarcinoma (Canine)

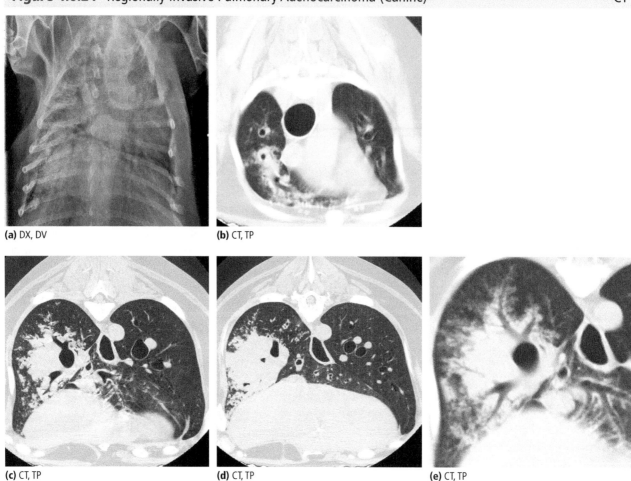

(a) DX, DV   **(b)** CT, TP

(c) CT, TP   **(d)** CT, TP   **(e)** CT, TP

13y MC Bassett Hound with progressively worsening cough of at least 6 months' duration. There is an ill-defined pulmonary mass in the right caudal thorax, which compresses the right mainstem bronchus and displaces the cardiac silhouette to the left (**a**). At the periphery of the mass, there is a mixed pulmonary pattern involving the entire right lung that includes bronchial, interstitial, and alveolar components. Images **b–d** are representative CT images ordered from cranial to caudal. Image **e** is a 7 mm collimated magnified view of the right caudal and accessory lobes. The presence of a right caudal lobe mass is confirmed on CT images (**b–e**). Large airways within the mass are preserved, although smaller airways are either compressed or displaced (**c,d**). There is extension of the mass into the right cranial, middle, and accessory lobes from peribronchial migration, best illustrated in image **e**. Fine-needle aspiration biopsy confirmed a diagnosis of pulmonary adenocarcinoma.

Figure 4.6.25 Histiocytic Sarcoma (Canine)   CT

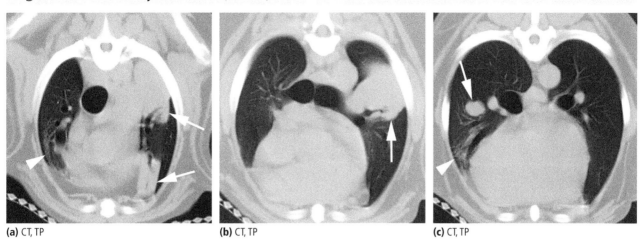

(a) CT, TP   **(b)** CT, TP   **(c)** CT, TP

10y M Labrador Retriever with increased respiratory effort and cough. Representative CT images are ordered from cranial to caudal. There are multiple well-demarcated bronchocentric soft-tissue attenuating pulmonary masses of variable size seen in the left cranial (**a**,**b**: arrows) and right middle (**c**: arrows) lung lobes. There is also partial atelectasis of the dependent part of the right cranial and middle lung lobes, likely associated with lateral recumbency during transport to the CT room while under anesthesia (**a**,**c**: arrowheads). Postmortem examination confirmed a diagnosis of histiocytic sarcoma.

Figure 4.6.26 Pulmonary Lymphoma (Canine)   CT

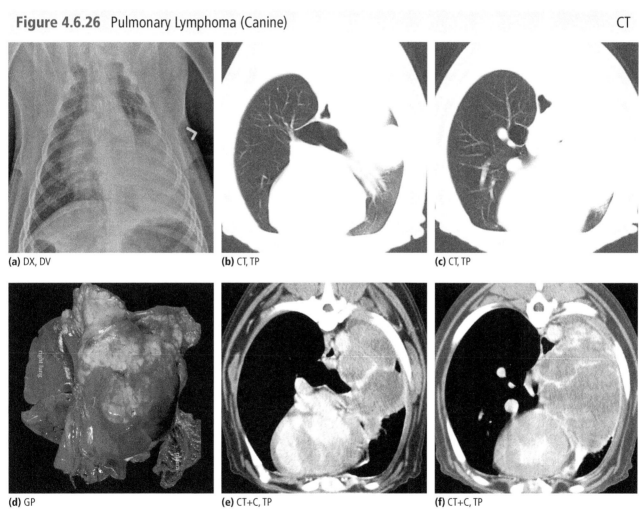

(a) DX, DV   **(b)** CT, TP   **(c)** CT, TP

(d) GP   **(e)** CT+C, TP   **(f)** CT+C, TP

9y MC Labrador Retriever with progressively worsening cough of 3 months' duration. Survey radiographs reveal a large soft-tissue mass in the left caudal lung lobe, which compresses and displaces the left mainstem and caudal lobar bronchi (**a**). CT images **b** and **c** are unenhanced and viewed with lung settings, and images **e** and **f** are comparable images acquired following contrast administration and viewed using soft-tissue settings. A soft-tissue attenuating lobular mass involves all of the left caudal and much of the left cranial lung lobes (**b**,**c**). The mass moderately and uniformly enhances centrally, with a thin rim of more intense enhancement peripherally (**e**,**f**). Postmortem examination confirmed a diagnosis of B-cell lymphoma that incorporated most of the left lung (**d**).

Figure 4.6.27 Pulmonary Metastasis (Canine)   CT

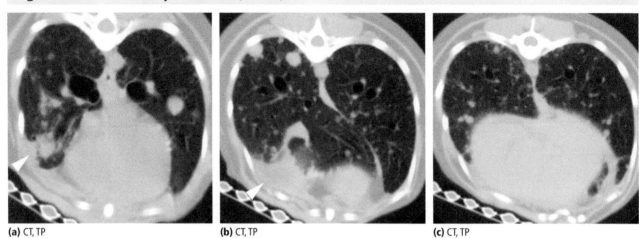

(a) CT, TP   **(b)** CT, TP   **(c)** CT, TP

13y FS Poodle cross with previous diagnosis of mammary carcinoma. Pulmonary nodules were detected during a recent thoracic radio-graphic examination. CT images are ordered from cranial to caudal. Multiple soft-tissue attenuating pulmonary nodules ranging from 1–6 mm in diameter are distributed throughout all lung lobes (**a–c**). There is a focal region in the ventral aspect of the right hemithorax, in which nodules appear to coalesce (**a,b**: arrowheads). Postmortem examination confirmed widespread pulmonary metastasis of mammary adenocarcinoma.

Figure 4.6.28   Progression of Pulmonary Metastasis (Canine)   CT

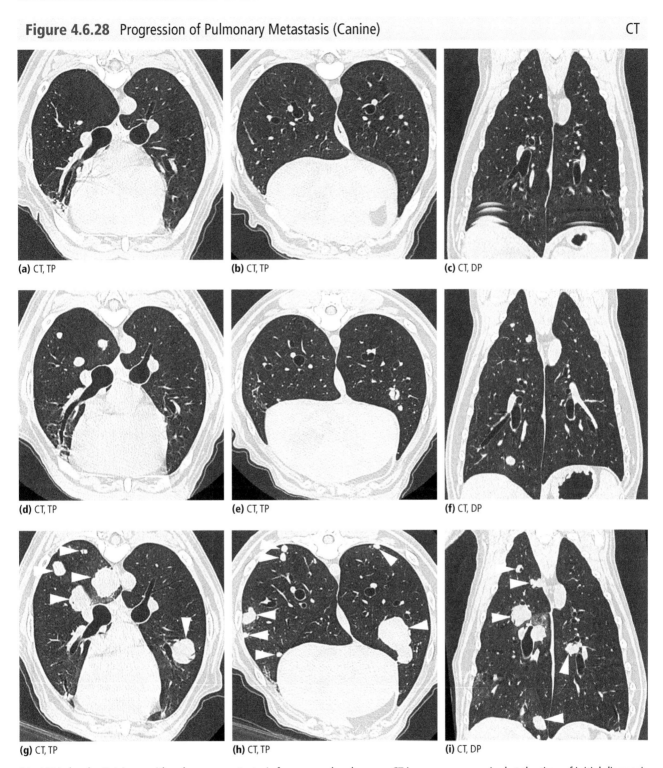

(a) CT, TP   (b) CT, TP   (c) CT, DP

(d) CT, TP   (e) CT, TP   (f) CT, DP

(g) CT, TP   (h) CT, TP   (i) CT, DP

11y MC Labrador Retriever with pulmonary metastasis from an oral melanoma. CT images were acquired at the time of initial diagnosis of primary disease (a–c) and at 73 days (d–f) and 157 days (g–i) following the initial scan. Multiple metastatic masses and nodules are easily detected on representative transverse and dorsal plane images acquired at day 157 (g–i: arrowheads). By viewing comparable images from the different dates in the vertical columns, one can appreciate the appearance and progression of metastasis over time. Postmortem examination confirmed the presence of widespread pulmonary metastasis. The curvilinear densities near the diaphragm in image c are due to diaphragmatic motion during image acquisition.

Figure 4.6.29 Well-demarcated Pulmonary Metastases (Canine)   CT

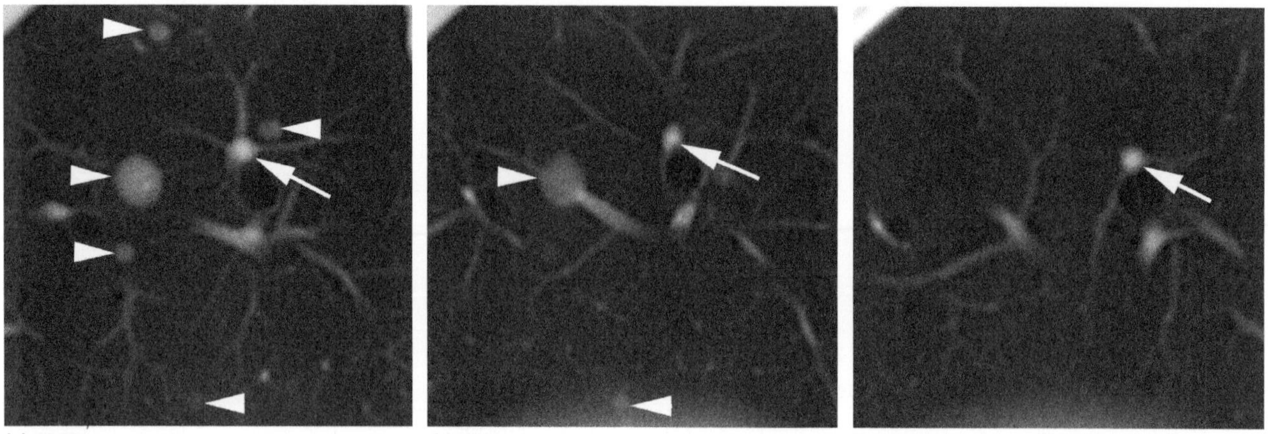

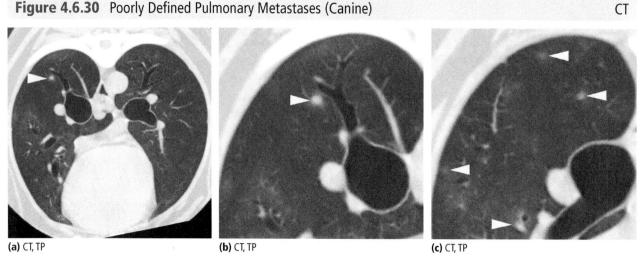

(a) CT, TP   **(b)** CT, TP   **(c)** CT, TP

7y FS Vizsla with metastatic hemangiosarcoma. Images **a–c** are consecutive 5 mm collimated images of the right caudal lung lobe. Multiple well-demarcated pulmonary nodules are seen (**a,b**: arrowheads). The nodules are of varying attenuation and appear translucent because of partial volume averaging effect with adjacent aerated lung (**a,b**). By comparison, end-on blood vessels of similar diameter are more attenuating (**a–c**: arrow).

Figure 4.6.30 Poorly Defined Pulmonary Metastases (Canine)   CT

(a) CT, TP   **(b)** CT, TP   **(c)** CT, TP

6y F Golden Retriever with metastatic hemangiosarcoma. Images **a–c** are 1 mm collimated images. Image **b** is a magnification of image **a**, and image **c** is a magnified image acquired cranial to image **b**. Multiple poorly defined soft-tissue attenuating nodules are seen (**a–c**: arrowheads). In addition, there is nonuniform ground-glass opacity around the periphery of the nodules and in other regions of the lung. Lack of definition of the nodules in this patient likely reflects inflammation or hemorrhage within or adjacent to the metastatic lesions.

Figure 4.6.31 Mucinous Adenocarcinoma with Osseous Metaplasia (Canine) CT

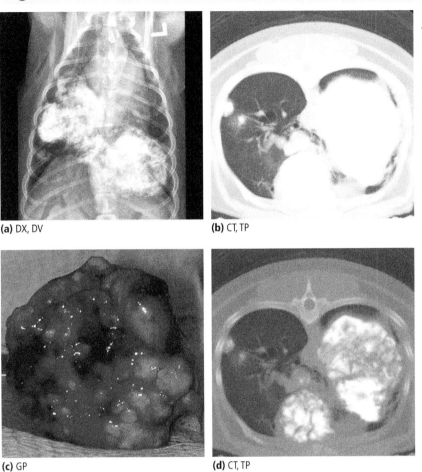

10y Jack Russell Terrier with progressively worsening nonproductive cough. There are multiple mineral-attenuating masses in the left caudal, right middle, and right caudal lung lobes on survey radiographs (a). Masses are highly yet incompletely mineralized on CT images, creating a complex multilobular appearance (b,d). Pathologic diagnosis following lung lobectomy was mucinous adenocarcinoma with extensive osseous metaplasia (c). The origin of the primary tumor was not determined.

(a) DX, DV

(b) CT, TP

(c) GP

(d) CT, TP

Figure 4.6.32 Maximum-Intensity Projection Imaging for Detection of Small Metastases (Canine) CT

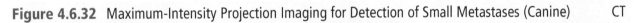

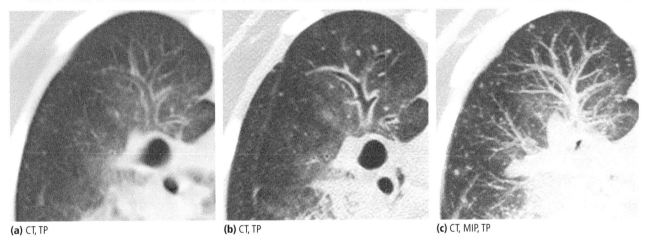

(a) CT, TP

(b) CT, TP

(c) CT, MIP, TP

11y FS Australian Cattle Dog with bronchoalveolar carcinoma with distant metastasis to other lung lobes. Representative CT images of the right caudal lung lobe were all acquired at the same level and include a 5 mm collimated image (a), a 1 mm collimated image (b), and a 15 mm thick maximum-intensity projection (MIP) image (c). Small peripheral miliary metastatic nodules are difficult to see on the 5 mm collimated image because of reduced contrast from partial volume averaging with aerated lung (a). A few nodules are seen on the 1 mm collimated image, but the number of images required to view the entire thorax makes thin collimation impractical for metastasis screening. Miliary nodules are clearly seen on the MIP image because of nearly complete elimination of partial volume averaging, and the number of images required to view the entire thorax is reduced. Postmortem examination confirmed the diagnosis of bronchoalveolar carcinoma arising from the left cranial lung lobe with bronchial migration and distant metastasis to other lobes.

Figure 4.6.33 Osseous Metaplasia (Canine)   CT

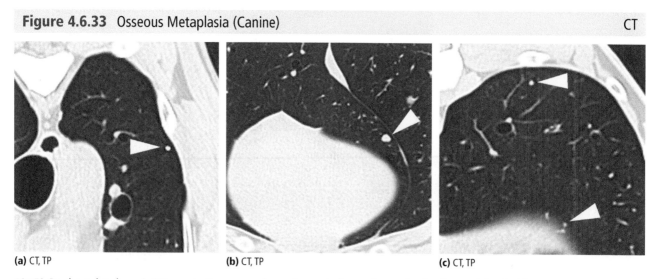

(a) CT, TP   **(b)** CT, TP   **(c)** CT, TP

12y FS Greyhound. A thoracic CT examination was performed as part of a staging evaluation for an abdominal hemangiosarcoma. Highly attenuating, well-demarcated miliary nodules are seen in the periphery of the pulmonary parenchyma in representative images (a–c: arrowheads). Given their small diameter, the level of attenuation exceeds what would be expected if nodules had soft-tissue density.

Figure 4.6.34 Pulmonary Fibrosis (Canine)   CT

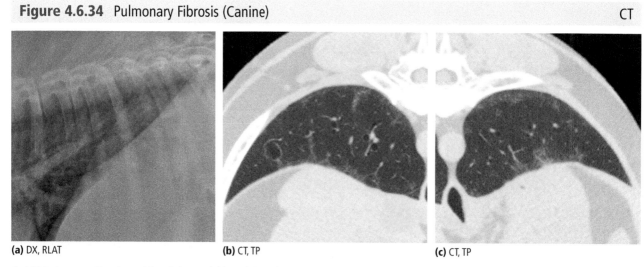

(a) DX, RLAT   **(b)** CT, TP   **(c)** CT, TP

9y MC Doberman Pinscher with a right caudal lung lobe adenoma. There is a moderate unstructured interstitial pattern in the caudodorsal lung field on thoracic radiographs (a). CT images of the caudal lung lobes reveal unstructured and linear regions of increased attenuation that are located primarily in the subpleural regions of the lung (b,c). A thin-walled bulla is also present in the right caudal lobe (b) and is considered an incidental finding. Right caudal lung lobectomy was performed to remove the pulmonary mass (not shown). Pathologic diagnosis of the unstructured and linear hyperattenuating lung lesions described above was marked multifocal to coalescing chronic interstitial fibrosis. The inciting cause for the fibrosis was not determined but was thought likely to be due to a previous inflammatory insult.

Figure 4.6.35 Pulmonary Fibrosis (Canine)   CT

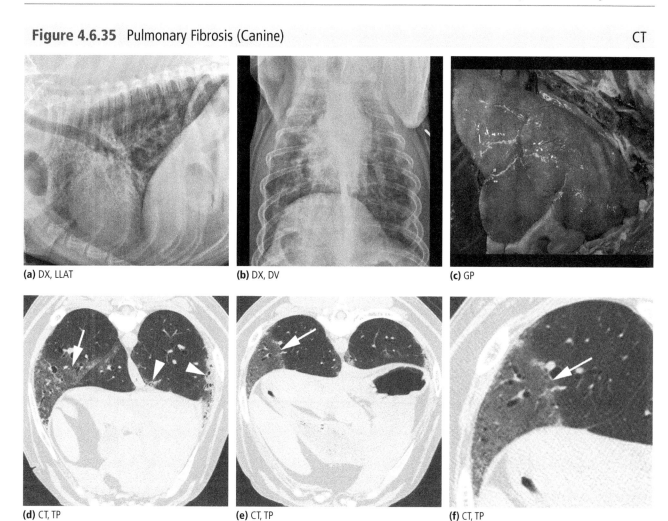

(a) DX, LLAT   (b) DX, DV   (c) GP

(d) CT, TP   (e) CT, TP   (f) CT, TP

4y MC Chesapeake Bay Retriever with 18-month history of interstitial pneumonia. Microbial cultures and serology were negative, and the dog has been partially responsive to steroid therapy until recently. There is a marked predominantly interstitial pattern in all lung fields, which is most pronounced on the right (**a**,**b**). CT images **d** and **e** are representative images of affected lung ordered from cranial to caudal, and image **f** is a magnification of image **e**. There is a uniform increase in attenuation of the lateroventral aspect of the right caudal lung lobe with retention of bronchovascular architecture (**d**–**f**: arrows). More focal regions of subpleural hyperattenuation are present in the left caudal lung lobe and appear to be associated with volume loss (**d**: arrowheads). Postmortem examination revealed severe chronic interstitial fibrosis with lung parenchyma diffusely affected (**c**). Pulmonary inflammation was minimal, consisting primarily of intra-alveolar macrophages. The initiating cause was not determined but was thought likely to be due to previously diagnosed interstitial pneumonia.

Figure 4.6.36 Pulmonary Fibrosis and Mineralization (Canine)   CT

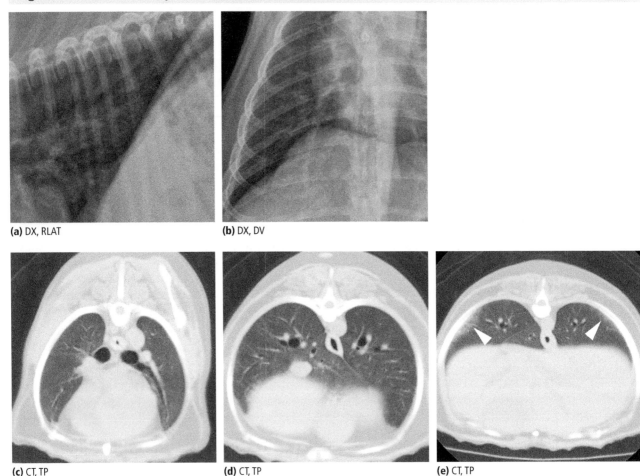

(a) DX, RLAT

(b) DX, DV

(c) CT, TP

(d) CT, TP

(e) CT, TP

12y FS Miniature Pinscher with chronic renal failure, probable hyperadrenocorticism, and recent onset of respiratory compromise. There is a generalized mild to moderate unstructured interstitial pattern on thoracic radiographs (**a,b**). There is diffuse and uniform increased pulmonary attenuation on CT images (**c–e**), with an average of approximately –635 HU. There are focal regions of more pronounced hyperattenuation in subpleural parenchyma of the caudal lung lobes (**e**: arrowheads). Pathologic diagnosis following postmortem examination was marked diffuse interstitial fibrosis and mineralization. Mineralization of the basement membrane in the lung was thought to contribute to acute tachypnea and dyspnea.

References

1. Scrivani PV, Thompson MS, Dykes NL, Holmes NL, Southard TL, Gerdin JA, et al. Relationships among subgross anatomy, computed tomography, and histologic findings in dogs with disease localized to the pulmonary acini. Vet Radiol Ultrasound. 2012;53:1–10.
2. Anderson WI, King JM, Flint TJ. Multifocal bullous emphysema with concurrent bronchial hypoplasia in two aged Afghan hounds. J Comp Pathol. 1989;100:469–473.
3. Gopalakrishnan G, Stevenson GW. Congenital lobar emphysema and tension pneumothorax in a dog. J Vet Diagn Invest. 2007;19:322–325.
4. Hoover JP, Henry GA, Panciera RJ. Bronchial cartilage dysplasia with multifocal lobar bullous emphysema and lung torsions in a pup. J Am Vet Med Assoc. 1992;201:599–602.
5. Ruth J, Rademacher N, Ogden D, Rodriguez D, Gaschen L. Imaging diagnosis – congenital lobar emphysema in a dog. Vet Radiol Ultrasound. 2011;52:79–81.
6. Au JJ, Weisman DL, Stefanacci JD, Palmisano MP. Use of computed tomography for evaluation of lung lesions associated with spontaneous pneumothorax in dogs: 12 cases (1999–2002). J Am Vet Med Assoc. 2006;228:733–737.
7. Lipscomb VJ, Hardie RJ, Dubielzig RR. Spontaneous pneumothorax caused by pulmonary blebs and bullae in 12 dogs. J Am Anim Hosp Assoc. 2003;39:435–445.
8. Reetz JA, Caceres AV, Suran JN, Oura TJ, Zwingenberger AL, Mai W. Sensitivity, positive predictive value, and interobserver variability of computed tomography in the diagnosis of bullae associated with spontaneous pneumothorax in dogs: 19 cases (2003–2012). J Am Vet Med Assoc. 2013;243:244–251.

9. Murphy KA, Brisson BA. Evaluation of lung lobe torsion in Pugs: 7 cases (1991–2004). J Am Vet Med Assoc. 2006;228:86–90.

10. Schultz RM, Peters J, Zwingenberger A. Radiography, computed tomography and virtual bronchoscopy in four dogs and two cats with lung lobe torsion. J Small Anim Pract. 2009;50: 360–363.

11. Seiler G, Schwarz T, Vignoli M, Rodriguez D. Computed tomographic features of lung lobe torsion. Vet Radiol Ultrasound. 2008;49:504–508.

12. Larsen BT, Colby TV. Update for pathologists on idiopathic interstitial pneumonias. Arch Pathol Lab Med. 2012;136:1234–1241.

13. Clercx C, Peeters D. Canine eosinophilic bronchopneumopathy. Vet Clin North Am Small Anim Pract. 2007;37:917–935.

14. Carminato A, Vascellari M, Zotti A, Fiorentin P, Monetti G, Mutinelli F. Imaging of exogenous lipoid pneumonia simulating lung malignancy in a dog. Can Vet J. 2011;52:310–312.

15. Himsworth CG, Malek S, Saville K, Allen AL. Endogenous lipid pneumonia and what lies beneath. Can Vet J. 2008;49:813–815.

16. Jerram RM, Guyer CL, Braniecki A, Read WK, Hobson HP. Endogenous lipid (cholesterol) pneumonia associated with bronchogenic carcinoma in a cat. J Am Anim Hosp Assoc. 1998;34:275–280.

17. Jones DJ, Norris CR, Samii VF, Griffey SM. Endogenous lipid pneumonia in cats: 24 cases (1985–1998). J Am Vet Med Assoc. 2000;216:1437–1440.

18. Raya AI, Fernandez-de Marco M, Nunez A, Afonso JC, Cortade LE, Carrasco L. Endogenous lipid pneumonia in a dog. J Comp Pathol. 2006;135:153–155.

19. Betancourt SL, Martinez-Jimenez S, Rossi SE, Truong MT, Carrillo J, Erasmus JJ. Lipoid pneumonia: spectrum of clinical and radiologic manifestations. AJR Am J Roentgenol. 2010;194:103–109.

20. Lee JS, Im JG, Song KS, Seo JB, Lim TH. Exogenous lipoid pneumonia: high-resolution CT findings. Eur Radiol. 1999;9:287–291.

21. Gurney JW. Diagnostic Imaging: Chest. Salt Lake City: Amirsys Inc., 2007.

22. Chandler JC, Lappin MR. Mycoplasmal respiratory infections in small animals: 17 cases (1988–1999). J Am Anim Hosp Assoc. 2002;38:111–119.

23. Foster SF, Barrs VR, Martin P, Malik R. Pneumonia associated with Mycoplasma spp in three cats. Aust Vet J. 1998;76:460–464.

24. Schultz RM, Zwingenberger A. Radiographic, computed tomographic, and ultrasonographic findings with migrating intrathoracic grass awns in dogs and cats. Vet Radiol Ultrasound. 2008;49:249–255.

25. Hagiwara Y, Fujiwara S, Takai H, Ohno K, Masuda K, Furuta T, et al. Pneumocystis carinii pneumonia in a Cavalier King Charles Spaniel. J Vet Med Sci. 2001;63:349–351.

26. Lopez A. Respiratory System. In: McGavin, MD, Zachary, JF (eds): Pathologic Basis of Veterinary Disease. St. Louis: Mosby Elsevier, 2007;463–558.

27. Marolf AJ, Gibbons DS, Podell BK, Park RD. Computed tomographic appearance of primary lung tumors in dogs. Vet Radiol Ultrasound. 2011;52:168–172.

28. Paoloni MC, Adams WM, Dubielzig RR, Kurzman I, Vail DM, Hardie RJ. Comparison of results of computed tomography and radiography with histopathologic findings in tracheobronchial lymph nodes in dogs with primary lung tumors: 14 cases (1999–2002). J Am Vet Med Assoc. 2006;228:1718–1722.

29. Tsai S, Sutherland-Smith J, Burgess K, Ruthazer R, Sato A. Imaging characteristics of intrathoracic histiocytic sarcoma in dogs. Vet Radiol Ultrasound. 2012;53:21–27.

30. Geyer NE, Reichle JK, Valdes-Martinez A, Williams J, Goggin JM, Leach L, et al. Radiographic appearance of confirmed pulmonary lymphoma in cats and dogs. Vet Radiol Ultrasound. 2010;51: 386–390.

31. Armbrust LJ, Biller DS, Bamford A, Chun R, Garrett LD, Sanderson MW. Comparison of three-view thoracic radiography and computed tomography for detection of pulmonary nodules in dogs with neoplasia. J Am Vet Med Assoc. 2012;240:1088–1094.

32. Nemanic S, London CA, Wisner ER. Comparison of thoracic radiographs and single breath-hold helical CT for detection of pulmonary nodules in dogs with metastatic neoplasia. J Vet Intern Med. 2006;20:508–515.

33. Syrja P, Heikkila HP, Lilja-Maula L, Krafft E, Clercx C, Day MJ, et al. The histopathology of idiopathic pulmonary fibrosis in West Highland White Terriers shares features of both non-specific interstitial pneumonia and usual interstitial pneumonia in man. J Comp Pathol. 2013;149:303–313.

34. Heikkila HP, Lappalainen AK, Day MJ, Clercx C, Rajamaki MM. Clinical, bronchoscopic, histopathologic, diagnostic imaging, and arterial oxygenation findings in West Highland White Terriers with idiopathic pulmonary fibrosis. J Vet Intern Med. 2011; 25:433–439.

Section 5

Abdomen

5.1

Body wall, retroperitoneum, and peritoneal cavity

Multislice CT can be used to rapidly acquire images with high contrast and high spatial resolution in anesthetized, sedated, or awake animals and is well suited for examination of the body wall, retroperitoneum, and peritoneal cavity.[1] MR is used less often in imaging these regions because of respiratory motion artifact during image acquisition.

The retroperitoneal space, which is often difficult to evaluate with other imaging modalities, is well visualized on cross-sectional and reformatted CT images. The abdominal aorta and caudal vena cava course through the fat contained in the retroperitoneal space. The major retroperitoneal organs include the kidneys and adrenal glands. Paraaortic lymph nodes are inconsistently seen unless enlarged. The larger medial iliac lymph nodes are located lateral to the iliac branches of the aorta, and the hypogastric lymph nodes can be detected between the iliac arteries.

The body wall consists of thin muscle layers interspersed with fat, which are readily evaluated on CT images. The peritoneal space is filled with fat that surrounds the serosal surface of the abdominal organs.

Trauma

Trauma to the spine can cause hemorrhage to extend into the spinal musculature and retroperitoneal space. On CT images, hemorrhage may be slightly hyperattenuating or isoattenuating and has ill-defined margins as it dissects through the retroperitoneal space (Figure 5.1.1). On MR images, edema and hemorrhage appear as T2 hyperintensity in the spinal musculature and retroperitoneal space.[2] Hemorrhage may also be seen in the pelvic retroperitoneal space (Figure 5.1.2).

Effusion

Perirenal fluid can accumulate in animals with acute renal failure due to infectious inflammatory disease, renal toxicity, or renal obstruction (Figure 5.1.3). Although this has not been described with CT or MR imaging, veterinary ultrasonographic studies have shown the association between unilateral or bilateral perirenal fluid accumulation and acute renal failure.[3]

Increased vascular pressure or permeability can lead to peritoneal effusion. This appears as dependent pockets of fluid attenuation conforming to the regional anatomy (Figures 5.1.4, 5.1.5).

Inflammatory disorders

Infectious inflammatory disease may be localized in the retroperitoneal space or body wall. Abscesses in certain geographic regions may be caused by penetration of migrating grass awns through the body wall, which may connect with external draining tracts or cause body wall masses. Alternatively, the foreign body may enter the retroperitoneal space via the pleural space secondary to inhalation. Pleural foreign bodies often migrate through the diaphragm into the lumbar musculature, causing cellulitis or abscess and clinical signs of acute abdominal or back pain. CT features of foreign bodies migrating from the pleural space include a round- or oval-walled tract with central fluid-attenuating material and gas, which extends from the diaphragm to the sublumbar musculature. On contrast-enhanced images, the wall of the tract is moderately contrast enhancing. The inflammation may

Atlas of Small Animal CT and MRI, First Edition. Erik R. Wisner and Allison L. Zwingenberger.
© 2015 John Wiley & Sons, Inc. Published 2015 by John Wiley & Sons, Inc.

extend into the retroperitoneal fat to cause increased attenuation and streaks of soft-tissue attenuation (Figure 5.1.6).

Foreign bodies that penetrate through the skin may cause multilobular, peripherally contrast-enhancing masses with fluid-attenuating centers in the subcutaneous tissues (Figure 5.1.7). They may also penetrate into the retroperitoneal space, causing an abscess in this region with a connecting draining tract to the skin (Figure 5.1.8). Other types of penetrating foreign bodies, such as projectiles, can introduce infection into the peritoneal or retroperitoneal space (Figure 5.1.9).

Abscesses due to fungal disease occasionally occur in the retroperitoneal space. On MR images, they appear as T2 hyperintense and T1 contrast-enhancing masses that may surround the vasculature or cause vascular thrombosis.[4]

Increased attenuation of peritoneal fat can be seen as "fat stranding" on CT images. The proposed mechanism of fat stranding is edema due to increased vascular permeability and engorgement of the lymphatics.[5] This can appear as a ground-glass (Figure 5.1.4) or linear, reticulated pattern and has been associated with inflammatory lesions, such as abscesses and gastrointestinal perforation, in dogs.[6] Localization of the fat stranding to a particular organ can help to pinpoint the source of the abnormality. CT is also capable of detecting free gas within the abdomen without the superimposition of organs encountered with ultrasonography.

Neoplasia

CT of the abdomen has become a mainstay in imaging lesions involving complex fascial planes of the abdomen, especially for surgical planning and surgical oncology.[7] Surgical margins surrounding inflammatory or neoplastic lesions can be assessed to determine the depth and width of resection, as well as removal of neighboring structures, such as ribs. Multiplanar reformatting is especially helpful in visualizing and measuring for surgical margins.

Lipomas are frequently encountered in the subcutaneous tissues and within the intermuscular fat depositions. These are rounded, fat-attenuating masses that may have soft-tissue septations present (Figure 5.1.10). Their often large size may displace neighboring organs or extend into the peritoneal or retroperitoneal space. Large lipomas may become hemorrhagic, with increased soft-tissue attenuation interspersed with fat on CT images (Figure 5.1.11). Infiltrative lipomas are characterized by dissection within surrounding musculature (Figure 5.1.10).[8] Lipomas may also infiltrate fat planes within the pelvis, causing additional mass effects (Figure 5.1.12).

Feline injection-site sarcomas occur in the abdominal wall or pelvic soft tissues because of extension of a distant tumor or misdirected injection meant for the distal extremity. Involvement of the musculature of the body wall appears as contrast enhancement of the tumor with extension to the musculature and surrounding tissues.[9] Differentiating postsurgical inflammation from tumor extension in animals scanned for radiation therapy can be challenging and is not always possible. Fibrosarcoma in dogs is an invasive neoplasm that may involve the peritoneal cavity or pelvic canal. Contrast-enhanced imaging of the lesions is necessary to accurately define the tumor margins and evaluate for local lymph node enlargement. Fibrosarcomas and other sarcomas are moderately to intensely contrast enhancing with poorly defined margins (Figures 5.1.13, 5.1.14, 5.1.15), and tendrils of neoplastic tissue may extend to regional tissues.

Hemangiosarcoma occasionally occurs as a mass in the pelvis or retroperitoneal space without apparent primary abdominal involvement. These masses are irregular and lobular in shape, with heterogeneous contents on both CT and MR images. Hemorrhagic components of the mass are hypoattenuating on CT (Figure 5.1.16) and T1 hypointense and T2 hyperintense on MR images (Figure 5.1.17). In both modalities, the masses tend to be peripherally contrast enhancing.

Various tumor types may occur on the abdominal wall and pelvis, causing mass effects and imaging characteristics ranging from solid to cystic (Figure 5.1.18). The medial iliac lymph nodes, internal iliac lymph nodes, and lumbar lymph nodes should be evaluated for enlargement and regions of poor contrast enhancement, indicative of metastatic disease from the body wall, peritoneum, pelvis, or pelvic limbs (Figures 5.1.18, 5.1.19).

Figure 5.1.1   Retroperitoneal Hemorrhage (Canine)   CT

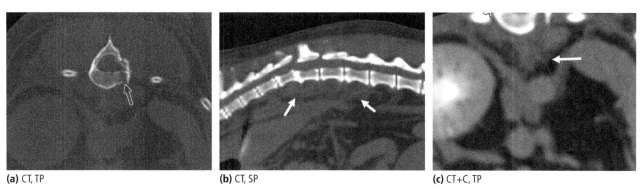

(a) CT, TP   **(b)** CT, SP   **(c)** CT+C, TP

11y MC Maltese with a T12–13 fracture/luxation sustained from an attack by a larger dog. A fracture of the left pedicle and body of T12 is shown on a transverse image (**a**: open arrow). There is ill-defined fluid attenuation within the retroperitoneal space due to hemorrhage dorsal to the descending aorta (**b**,**c**: arrows).

Figure 5.1.2   Spontaneous Pelvic Hematoma (Canine)   CT

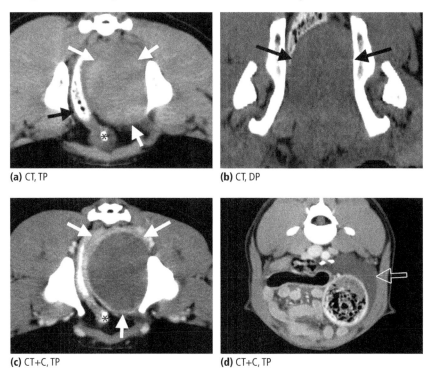

(a) CT, TP   **(b)** CT, DP

(c) CT+C, TP   **(d)** CT+C, TP

3y FS Boxer with history of straining to urinate and defecate. On unenhanced images, there is a heterogeneous soft-tissue attenuating (45 HU) mass in the left pelvic region (**a**: white arrows) causing rightward deviation of the colon (**a**: black arrow). The mass peripherally enhances following intravenous contrast administration (**c**: white arrows). A urinary catheter is seen within the bladder lumen (**a**,**c**: asterisk). The dorsal plane image shows the mass occupying the majority of the pelvic canal (**b**: arrows). More cranially, hemorrhage is present as hypoattenuating fluid in the left retroperitoneal space (**d**: open arrow). The mass was not neoplastic; however, it contained vascular structures that may have represented a preexisting vascular anomaly.

Figure 5.1.3 Retroperitoneal Fluid—Leptospirosis (Canine)   CT

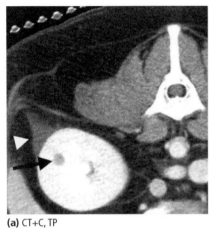 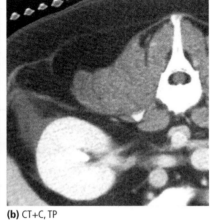

9y M mixed-breed dog with retroperitoneal fluid. Contrast CT was performed to rule out urine leakage into the retroperitoneal space. There is a triangular fluid accumulation lateral to the right kidney in the retroperitoneal space (a: arrowhead). There is an incidental renal cortical cyst (a: arrow). No contrast medium was observed to leak into the peritoneal space during the study. Definitive diagnosis was leptospirosis with acute renal failure.

(a) CT+C, TP   **(b)** CT+C, TP

Figure 5.1.4 Mesenteric Edema—Fluid Overload (Feline)   CT

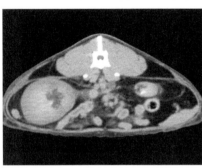 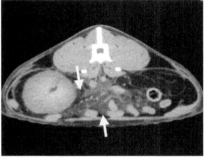

(a) CT+C, TP   **(b)** CT+C, TP

8y MC Bengal with ureteral obstruction. Aggressive intravenous fluid therapy had been initiated to treat acute chronic renal failure. The right kidney is enlarged with a dilated pelvis, and the left kidney is small. There is ground-glass fluid attenuation within the fat surrounding the small intestine, as well as more linear fat stranding surrounding the right kidney (b: arrows). Subcutaneous edema is also present. On these contrast-enhanced images, there is very little enhancement of the kidneys, indicating poor renal function.

Figure 5.1.5 Peritoneal Effusion (Canine)   CT

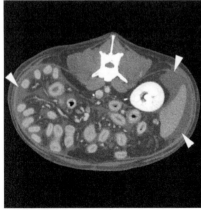 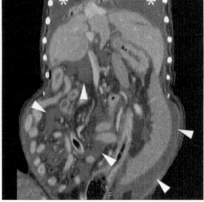

6y FS Pit Bull Terrier with bicavitary modified transudative effusion. Fluid is widely dispersed within the peritoneal cavity with prominent collections surrounding the small intestine and spleen (a,b: arrowheads). Pleural effusion is also evident in the caudal pleural space (b: asterisks). The effusion had both low cellularity and low protein and was thought to have resulted from abnormal hydrostatic or oncotic forces. A definitive diagnosis was not reached.

(a) CT+C, TP   **(b)** CT+C, DP

Figure 5.1.6 Migrating Foreign Body Abscess (Canine) CT

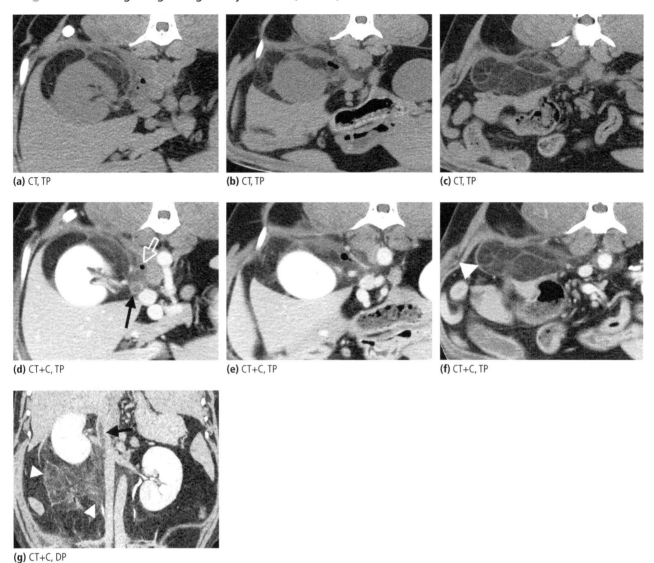

(a) CT, TP

(b) CT, TP

(c) CT, TP

(d) CT+C, TP

(e) CT+C, TP

(f) CT+C, TP

(g) CT+C, DP

12y FS Labrador Retriever with acute onset of abdominal pain, recent history of coughing, and fever. Unenhanced (**a–c**) and comparable contrast-enhanced (**d–f**) transverse images are ordered from cranial to caudal. There is a well-circumscribed tract and abscess in the right retroperitoneal space lateral to the diaphragmatic muscle (**d,g**: black arrow) with peripheral contrast enhancement. There is additional nonenhancing fluid dorsal to the inflammatory tract, which contains gas bubbles (**d**: open arrow). The retroperitoneal fat surrounding the kidney has fat stranding in a linear pattern with central regions of ground-glass opacity (**f,g**: arrowheads). A migrating grass awn was retrieved from the retroperitoneal space.

Figure 5.1.7 Abdominal Wall Abscess (Canine) CT

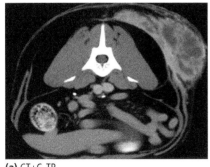

8y FS Border Collie with a recurrent abscess on the left flank. There is a multilobulated mass in the subcutaneous tissues of the left dorsolateral body wall. The mass does not enter the deeper layers of fat adjacent to the spine. There is peripheral contrast enhancement with nonenhancing central regions. Plant material from a migrating grass awn was discovered after surgical removal.

(a) CT+C, TP

Figure 5.1.8 Retroperitoneal Abscess and Superficial Draining Tract (Canine)   CT

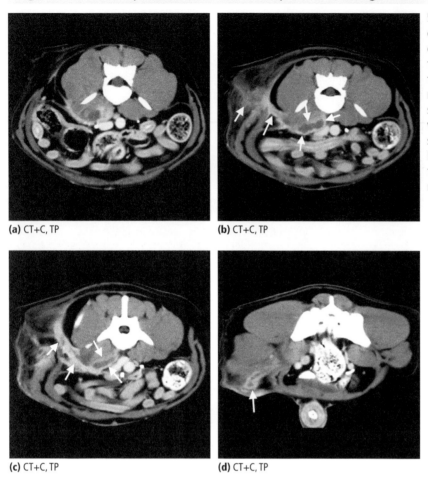

(a) CT+C, TP   (b) CT+C, TP

(c) CT+C, TP   (d) CT+C, TP

5y M German Shorthaired Pointer with a chronic draining tract in the inguinal region. On contrast-enhanced images ordered from cranial to caudal, there is a hyperattenuating tract in the sublumbar musculature. Additional abnormal enhancement is seen in the retroperitoneal space and subcutaneous tissues of the body wall (b,c: arrows). The tract exits the skin surface in the right inguinal region (d: arrow). Exploratory surgery was performed to resect the draining tracts; however, no foreign material was retrieved.

Figure 5.1.9 Retroperitoneal Perirenal Abscess—*Mycobacterium* (Feline)   CT

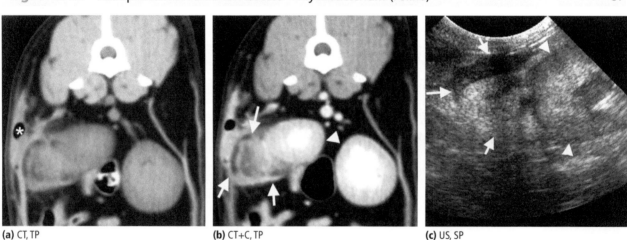

(a) CT, TP   (b) CT+C, TP   (c) US, SP

8y MC Domestic Longhair with draining tract present for 2½ years. A pellet was identified in the peritoneal cavity. There is gas in the subcutaneous tissues of the right abdominal wall (a: asterisk). On contrast-enhanced images, hyperattenuating tissue surrounds fluid-attenuating material (b: arrows) lateral to the cranial pole of the right kidney (b: arrowhead). This represents a chronic retroperitoneal abscess extending from the kidney to the body wall. The fluid and hyperechoic fat (c: arrows) surrounding the kidney (c: arrowhead) are also visible on ultrasonography. Mycobacterium was cultured from abscess fluid.

Figure 5.1.10   Abdominal Wall Infiltrative Lipoma (Canine)   CT

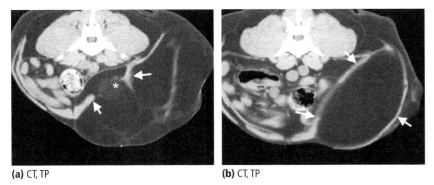

(a) CT, TP   **(b)** CT, TP

3y FS Vizsla with recurrent lipoma after surgery. Images are ordered from cranial to caudal. There is a large, lobular fat-attenuating mass in the left inguinal region. The mass separates and distorts the relationship of the internal and external oblique muscles and the rectus abdominis muscle (**a**: arrows). Widening and infiltration of the internal oblique muscle is visible in the center of the muscular discontinuity (**a**: asterisk). The more dorsal arrow denotes a region of muscular irregularity. The abdominal musculature is more regular in the caudal aspect of the mass (**b**: arrows).

Figure 5.1.11   Encapsulated Lipoma with Organizing Hematoma (Canine)   CT

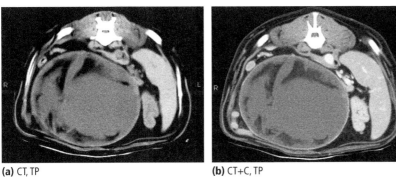

(a) CT, TP   **(b)** CT+C, TP

12y MC Labrador Retriever cross with a suspected splenic mass based on abdominal palpation. There is a large mass with a thick, regular capsule in the right cranial abdomen. The inner portion of the mass is heterogeneous soft-tissue attenuating material surrounded by fat. On contrast-enhanced images, the capsule of the mass is moderately enhancing. Histopathology showed a fibrous capsule with internal fat necrosis and hemorrhage.

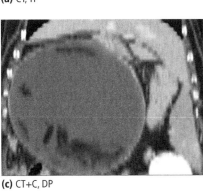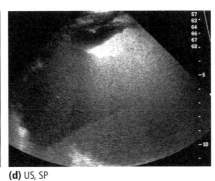

(c) CT+C, DP   **(d)** US, SP

Figure 5.1.12 Pelvic Lipoma (Canine)

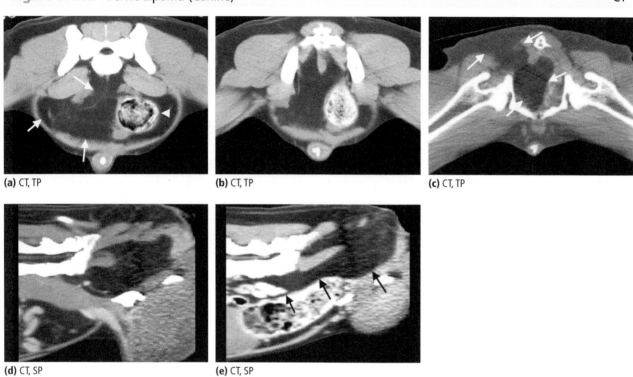

(a) CT, TP   **(b)** CT, TP   **(c)** CT, TP

(d) CT, SP   **(e)** CT, SP

7y MC Golden Retriever with a history of straining to defecate. Transverse images (**a–c**) are ordered from cranial to caudal. There is an ill-defined, fat-attenuating mass in the right caudal peritoneal cavity and pelvic canal (**a**: arrows). The mass displaces the colon to the left side of the abdomen (**a**: arrowhead). The fatty tissue occupies more than half of the pelvic canal caudally and separates the gluteal muscles to join with the subcutaneous fat over the right hip (**c**: arrows). On sagittal reformatted images, the continuity of the mass within the pelvis is appreciated (**e**: arrows).

Figure 5.1.13 Abdominal Wall Fibrosarcoma (Canine)

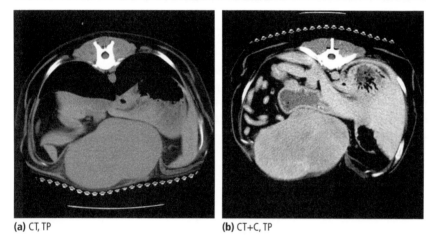

(a) CT, TP   **(b)** CT+C, TP

7y FS Golden Retriever with a previously diagnosed thoracic mass. On the unenhanced image, there is a large mass originating from the right ventral body wall and protruding both externally and internally in the cranial abdomen. The mass remains in a similar position in sternal (**a**) and dorsal (**b**) recumbency. The mass is soft-tissue attenuating and deviates the stomach dorsally within the abdomen. On the contrast-enhanced image, the mass is moderately and heterogeneously enhancing. Histopathology revealed a grade I fibrosarcoma.

Figure 5.1.14   Pelvic Fibrosarcoma (Feline)   CT

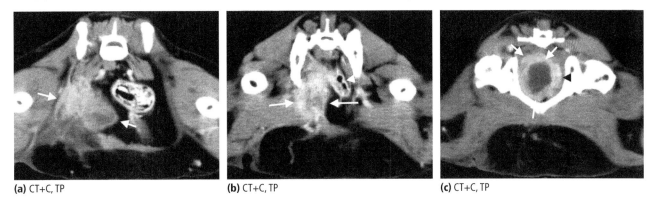

(a) CT+C, TP **(b)** CT+C, TP **(c)** CT+C, TP

15y Domestic Shorthair with a history of straining to defecate. Images are ordered from cranial to caudal. There is an ill-defined, contrast-enhancing mass in the right caudal abdomen (**a,b**: arrows) displacing the colon to the left (**b**: arrowhead). The mass infiltrates the muscles of the abdominal wall and lumbar spine, with fluid accumulation ventrally in the peritoneal space. Within the pelvic canal, the mass is peripherally contrast enhancing with a central, fluid-attenuating region (**c**: arrows). The colon is completely compressed by the mass at this level (**c**: arrowhead). Fine-needle aspiration cytology was consistent with a fibrosarcoma.

Figure 5.1.15   Spindle Cell Tumor (Canine)   CT

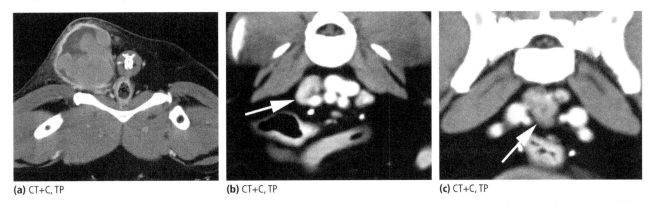

(a) CT+C, TP **(b)** CT+C, TP **(c)** CT+C, TP

15y FS Australian Shepherd cross presenting with an incompletely excised tail-base mass. There is a lobular soft-tissue and fluid-attenuating mass lateral to the tail base and dorsal to the pelvis (**a**). There is intense contrast enhancement of the periphery of the mass and moderate contrast enhancement of the lobular internal soft-tissue component. The fat peripheral to the mass contains soft-tissue nodules and fat stranding. The medial iliac and internal iliac lymph nodes are enlarged and heterogeneously contrast enhancing (**b,c**: arrows). Histopathology results were spindle cell sarcoma with cellulitis and metastatic lymphadenopathy.

Figure 5.1.16   Retroperitoneal Hemangiosarcoma (Canine)   CT

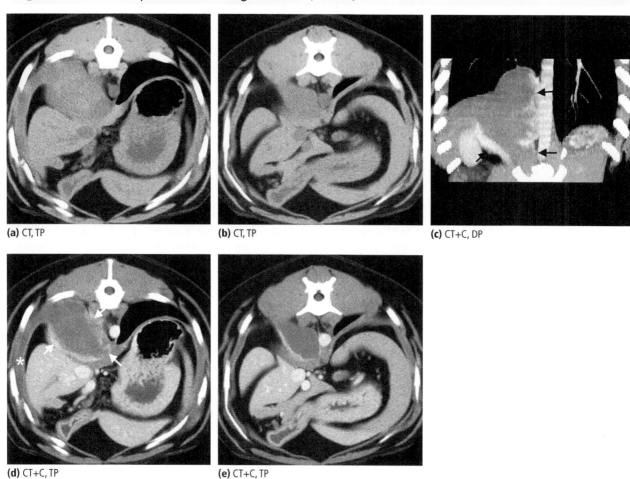

(a) CT, TP   **(b)** CT, TP   **(c)** CT+C, DP

(d) CT+C, TP   **(e)** CT+C, TP

3y MC Labrador Retriever with acute onset of lethargy. Transverse unenhanced (**a,b**) and comparable contrast-enhanced (**d,e**) images are ordered from cranial to caudal. There is a fluid-attenuating mass within the caudal mediastinum, which crosses the diaphragm and extends into the retroperitoneal space (**c,d**: arrows). The mass extends between the peritoneum and body wall on the right side (**d**: asterisk) and peripherally and intensely contrast enhances. Biopsy confirmed that the mass was a hemangiosarcoma.

Figure 5.1.17   Retroperitoneal Hemangiosarcoma (Canine)   MR

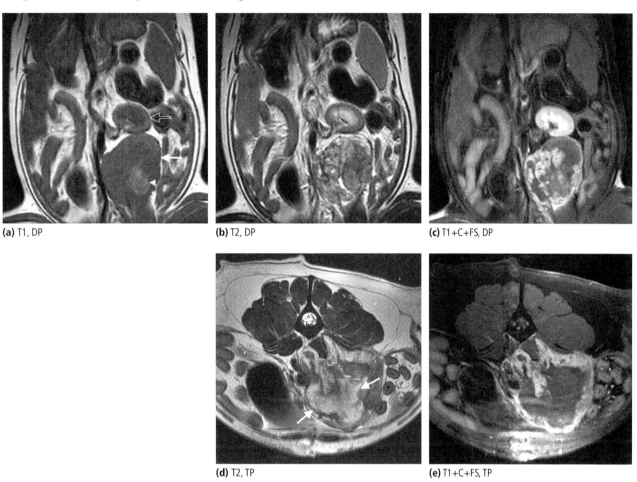

(a) T1, DP

(b) T2, DP

(c) T1+C+FS, DP

(d) T2, TP

(e) T1+C+FS, TP

6y FS Golden Retriever with acute onset of lethargy and anemia. There is a large mass in the left retroperitoneal space (**a,d**: arrows) displacing the left kidney cranially (**a**: open arrow). There is a focal, central T1 hyperintensity indicative of intratumoral hemorrhage (**a**: arrowhead). The internal portion of the mass is T1 hypointense (**a**) and heterogeneously T2 hyperintense (**b,d**). The mass is intensely and peripherally contrast enhancing (**c,e**).

Figure 5.1.18   Cystic Sublumbar Carcinoma (Canine)   CT

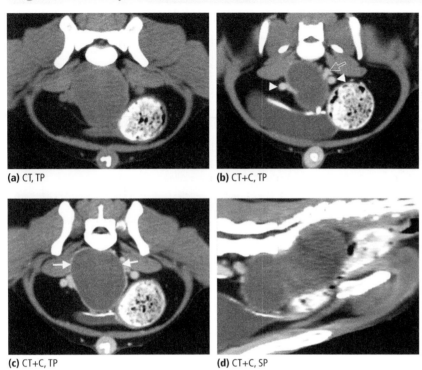

(a) CT, TP   (b) CT+C, TP

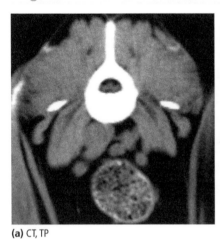

(c) CT+C, TP   (d) CT+C, SP

7y MC Golden Retriever cross with a history of straining to defecate. Images **a** and **c** are comparable unenhanced and contrast-enhanced images, and **b** is cranial to **c**. There is a large, central mass that is uniformly hypoattenuating on unenhanced images (**a**). There is rim enhancement of the mass following intravenous contrast administration (**c**: arrows), and the sublumbar vasculature deviates laterally as a result of the mass effect (**b**: arrowheads). Excisional biopsy confirmed regional metastatic carcinoma of probable anal gland origin. The normal left medial iliac lymph node is seen lateral to the vasculature (**b**: open arrow). The sagittal image shows the extent of the mass and colonic compression in the pelvic inlet (**d**).

Figure 5.1.19   Metastatic Mast Cell Tumor (Canine)   CT

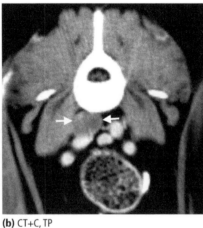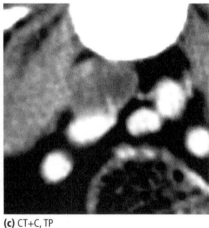

(a) CT, TP   (b) CT+C, TP   (c) CT+C, TP

7y MC Labrador Retriever with mast cell tumor on the right pelvic limb. Images **a** and **b** are comparable unenhanced and contrast-enhanced images, and **c** is a magnification of **b**. On a CT scan acquired for radiation therapy planning, the right medial iliac lymph node is enlarged and irregular, displacing the local vasculature ventrally. On the contrast-enhanced image, there is mild peripheral enhancement (**b**: arrows) and no enhancement centrally. Metastatic mast cell tumor was confirmed by fine-needle aspiration cytology.

References

1. Shanaman MM, Hartman SK, O'Brien RT. Feasibility for using dual-phase contrast-enhanced multi-detector helical computed tomography to evaluate awake and sedated dogs with acute abdominal signs. Vet Radiol Ultrasound. 2012;53:605–612.

2. Johnson P, Beltran E, Dennis R, Taeymans O. Magnetic resonance imaging characteristics of suspected vertebral instability associated with fracture or subluxation in eleven dogs. Vet Radiol Ultrasound. 2012;53:552–559.

3. Holloway A, O'Brien R. Perirenal effusion in dogs and cats with acute renal failure. Vet Radiol Ultrasound. 2007;48:574–579.

4. Clemans JM, Deitz KL, Riedesel EA, Yaeger MJ, Legendre AM. Retroperitoneal pyogranulomatous and fibrosing inflammation secondary to fungal infections in two dogs. J Am Vet Med Assoc. 2011;238:213–219.

5. Thornton E, Mendiratta-Lala M, Siewert B, Eisenberg RL. Patterns of fat stranding. American Journal of Roentgenology. 2011;197:W1–W14.

6. Shanaman MM, Schwarz T, Gal A, O'Brien RT. Comparison between survey radiography, B-mode ultrasonography, contrast-enhanced ultrasonography and contrast-enhanced multi-detector computed tomography findings in dogs with acute abdominal signs. Vet Radiol Ultrasound. 2013;54:591–604.

7. LeBlanc AK, Daniel GB. Advanced imaging for veterinary cancer patients. Vet Clin North Am Small Anim Pract. 2007;37:1059–1077.

8. McEntee MC, Thrall DE. Computed tomographic imaging of infiltrative lipoma in 22 dogs. Vet Radiol Ultrasound. 2001; 42:221–225.

9. Travetti O, Di GM, Stefanello D, et al. Computed tomography characteristics of fibrosarcoma – a histological subtype of feline injection-site sarcoma. J Feline Med Surg. 2013;15:488–493.

5.2

Hepatovascular disorders

Introduction

With the advent of multislice CT and advanced MR angiography protocols, cross-sectional imaging has become a gold standard diagnostic technique for hepatovascular anomalies. Congenital intrahepatic and extrahepatic portosystemic shunts are well seen, and their complex anatomy can be characterized using 3D renderings. This is advantageous for surgical planning and for detecting vasculature that courses through solid organs or crosses the diaphragm.

The normal hepatic arterial vasculature consists of three to five arterial branches that course ventral to the portal vein and parallel the portal branches within the hepatic parenchyma (Figure 5.2.1). The caudal vena cava receives short right veins from the right liver lobes, a large left vein from the left liver lobes, and a slightly smaller vein from the right medial and quadrate lobes (Figure 5.2.2). The phrenic vein courses parallel to the diaphragm and enters the left hepatic vein at its most cranial aspect. The portal tributaries include the jejunal veins collecting into the cranial mesenteric vein, the colic vein, the splenic vein from the left side, and the gastroduodenal vein from the right and ventral aspect. The portal vein diameter increases with the addition of each tributary. The portal vein then branches to the right lateral liver lobe, and two larger cranial branches supply the right medial lobe and left liver lobes (Figure 5.2.3). The left gastric vein joins the splenic vein from the cranial direction and is often involved in anomalous vessels.[1]

CT angiographic protocols can include single-phase or dual-phase imaging, depending on the anomaly and the capabilities of the scanner.[1] A simple extrahepatic shunt can be adequately imaged with a single portal phase angiogram with appropriate timing. Caveats include determining the correct scan initiation time delay relative to contrast administration and ensuring the image collimation is appropriate for the size of dog, with smaller 0.5–2 mm image collimation used for dogs weighing less than 10 kg. Multislice scanners are capable of acquiring arterial, portal, and delayed phase images in very thin collimation. Using a timing protocol calculated from a dynamic CT series with a small contrast dose results in the best arterial and portal phase timing. Automatic bolus detection may be used to initiate the arterial phase scan; however, timing of the portal phase scan is not possible with this technique. Suggested protocols are listed in Table 5.2.1.

Advanced CT tools, such as 3D imaging, maximum-intensity projection (MIP) of thick-slab images, and multiplanar reformatting, can all be used to show the relationship between the normal and abnormal vasculature, in addition to the native acquired images. Thin collimation (≤1.0 mm) on initial image acquisition provides the best spatial resolution in the resulting displays.

MR angiography has also been used for diagnosis of hepatovascular disorders because of its excellent depiction of the portal and abdominal vasculature. Images may be acquired with or without contrast medium; however, contrast-enhanced angiography with a 3D acquisition and fast spoiled gradient-echo pulse sequence (3D FSPGR) provide high-quality, high-contrast images. The 3D FSPGR series is acquired sequentially without timing of the bolus and has been successfully used to diagnose a variety of vascular anomalies.[2,3]

Atlas of Small Animal CT and MRI, First Edition. Erik R. Wisner and Allison L. Zwingenberger.
© 2015 John Wiley & Sons, Inc. Published 2015 by John Wiley & Sons, Inc.

Vascular disorders

Arterioportal fistula

Anomalous connections between the hepatic arterial and portal venous systems can occur congenitally. The presence of high-pressure flow in the portal vasculature causes portal hypertension, resulting in extreme dilation of portal branches, ascites, and multiple acquired extrahepatic shunts (Figure 5.2.4). With dual-phase CT angiography, one or more anastomoses of the arterial system with the portal system can often be identified as a plexus of small vessels. The presence of contrast in the portal vasculature during the arterial phase is diagnostic. The entire abdomen should be scanned to detect the multiple acquired shunts that are usually present between the abdominal portal vein and caudal vena cava.

Congenital intrahepatic shunts

Congenital intrahepatic shunts occur in large-breed dogs (Irish Wolfhounds, Golden Retrievers, Labrador Retrievers, Australian Cattle Dogs, Old English Sheepdogs) and rarely in cats, resulting in a large-diameter direct communication with the caudal vena cava. These vessels may be classified as left divisional (Figure 5.2.5, 5.2.6), as a remnant of the ductus venosus; central divisional (Figure 5.2.7), coursing relatively straight through the central liver; or right divisional (Figure 5.2.8), coursing through the right liver lobes.[4] The majority of intrahepatic shunts in cats are left divisional.[5]

CT or MR angiography demonstrates the anatomy of the abnormal vessel and helps with surgical planning for both open or minimally invasive procedures. Key findings include the anatomic path and termination of the shunt into the caudal vena cava and whether it intersects with large hepatic veins that might be occluded during surgery. The shape and size of the opening of the vessel into the caudal vena cava is also of importance when planning minimally invasive procedures. Caudal vena cava diameter is measured to determine the size of the stent required for shunt attenuation with coils.

Multiple intrahepatic shunts can also occur, either as a variant of the primary disorder or as an acquired consequence of attempted shunt attenuation.[6] These are small-diameter, irregular branches that connect to the hepatic veins and may mimic hepatic veins themselves (Figure 5.2.9).

Congenital extrahepatic shunts

Congenital extrahepatic shunts occur in smaller-breed dogs (Cairn Terriers, Yorkshire Terriers, Russell Terriers, Dachshunds, Miniature Schnauzers, Maltese) and cats. The majority of shunts are single; however, multiple congenital extrahepatic shunts are occasionally seen.[7] Extrahepatic shunts have been classified as splenocaval (Figure 5.2.10), splenophrenic (Figure 5.2.11), splenoazygos (Figure 5.2.12, 5.2.13), right gastric–caval (Figure 5.2.14, 5.2.15), and right gastric–caval or azygos with a caudal shunt loop.[8] Additional variations in shunt anatomy can be seen that do not conform to this general classification. A description of shunts involving the left gastric vein identified variants that entered the phrenic vein, the caudal vena cava, and the azygos vein.[9]

The diameter of the portal vein decreases after the exit of the shunt vessel, and the enlarged anomalous vessel should be followed to its termination. Multiplanar reformatting and 3D rendering can be helpful in defining the anatomy. The normal tributaries of the portal vein should also be identified and their junction with the portal vein or the shunt described. The entrance of tributaries to the shunt vessel (e.g. splenic vein, left gastric veins) may affect surgical placement of occlusion devices to avoid residual shunting.

Multiple acquired extrahepatic shunts

Multiple acquired extrahepatic portosystemic shunts form because of portal hypertension, often due to primary hepatic parenchymal disease. There are a variety of pathways arising from the portal vein and tributaries, including gastrophrenic, pancreaticoduodenal, splenorenal, mesenteric, and hemorrhoidal collateral vessels.[10] The anomalous vessels are often large when arising from the splenic vein and small when arising from other veins, describing a tortuous route between the portal and systemic circulation. They are best detected by scanning the entire abdomen and by using thin collimation for maximal spatial resolution. Small collateral vessels may appear as a "blush" rather than individual vessels because of limitations of spatial resolution (Figure 5.2.16).

Complex vascular anomalies

Interruption of the caudal vena cava occurs congenitally and is often without clinical signs, as blood flows through the azygos vein to return to the heart.[11] This may occur together with other anomalies, such as aplasia or interruption of the portal vein and situs inversus (Figure 5.2.17).[12] Complex anomalies, such as interrupted portal vein, result in a complete lack of intrahepatic portal vasculature, making these animals unsuitable for shunt attenuation. When CT angiography is performed in some dogs, the intrahepatic portal vein branches may not fill with contrast, as pressures are low. This should not be mistaken for portal interruption, as these dogs can experience normal postsurgical vascular development with shunt attenuation (Figure 5.2.18).

Table 5.2.1 Protocols for CT angiography. Choose whether to perform a single-phase or dual-phase protocol. The most thinly collimated images are appropriate for very small dogs (<10 kg) and multislice scanners. Timing is determined from the dynamic CT scan by creating a graph with regions of interest, or by counting the number of images (at 1 slice/second) until peak vessel enhancement. TA = time to peak contrast in aorta (s), TAPS = total time of arterial phase scan (s), Delay = time delay between arterial and portal phase scans. Pre-delay (TA) and interscan delay (Delay) are programmed into the dual-phase scan at setup. The portal phase scan should begin at plateau of portal enhancement, which can be estimated at 20–30 seconds depending on body weight, with moderate individual variability. Contrast medium used should be non-ionic and high concentration.

Series	Phase	Start	End	Direction	Collimation	Algorithm	Contrast medium	Delay
Survey abdomen	Precontrast	Diaphragm	Pelvic inlet	Cr–Cd	0.5–2.5 mm	Soft tissue	none	0
Dynamic	Timing	Porta hepatis	n/a	Stationary	2–5 mm	Soft tissue	0.25 ml/kg, 5 ml/s, 1 s rotation, 60 s duration	0 (start scan and injection simultaneously)
Dual-phase	Arterial	Porta hepatis	Diaphragm	Cd–Cr	0.5–2.5 mm	Soft tissue	2 ml/kg, 3–5 ml/s	(TA) Peak arrival in aorta (from dynamic)
	Portal	Diaphragm	Pelvic inlet	Cr–Cd	0.5–2.5 mm	Soft tissue		(TA + TAPS + Delay) Plateau of portal (from dynamic)
Multiphase	Delayed	Diaphragm	Pelvic inlet	Cr–Cd	0.5–2.5 mm	Soft tissue		60–180 s post injection
Single-phase	Portal	Diaphragm	Pelvic inlet	Cr–Cd	0.5–2.5 mm	Soft tissue	2 ml/kg, 3–5 ml/s	(TP) Plateau of portal (from dynamic). Estimate method 20–30 s post injection, increasing with body weight.

Legend for Figures 5.2.1–5.2.18

A	Aorta	LP	Left portal branch
AZ	Azygos vein	LG	Left gastric artery
C	Caudal vena cava	LGV	Left gastric vein
CD	Caudal mesenteric vein	P	Portal vein
CR	Cranial mesenteric vein	PH	Phrenic vein
GA	Gastroduodenal artery	RP	Right portal branch
GD	Gastroduodenal vein	RGA	Right gastric artery
H	Hepatic artery	RG	Right gastric vein
HB	Hepatic artery branch	RM	Right medial branch hepatic vein
J	Jejunal vein	RMP	Right medial portal branch
L	Left hepatic vein	S	Splenic vein

Figure 5.2.1 Hepatic Arteries (Canine)   CT

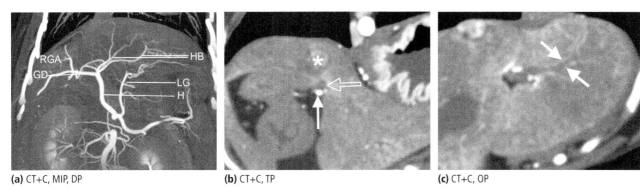

(a) CT+C, MIP, DP   **(b)** CT+C, TP   **(c)** CT+C, OP

The regional hepatic arteries branch from the hepatic artery and are between three and five in number (**a**). These branches supply the left, central, and right regions of the liver. The left gastric artery branches from the celiac artery more proximally and caudally, and travels cranially along the gastric wall. The gastroduodenal artery continues after the hepatic arteries branch toward the right and caudal abdomen. The right gastric artery arises cranially from the gastroduodenal artery on the right side. On transverse images, the hepatic artery and branches (**b**: arrow) are positioned ventral to the portal vein (**b**: open arrow) and caudal vena cava (**b**: asterisk). Within the hepatic parenchyma, the hepatic arteries follow the portal veins (**c**: arrows). See Legend for Figures 5.2.1–5.2.18.

Figure 5.2.2 Hepatic Veins (Canine)   CT

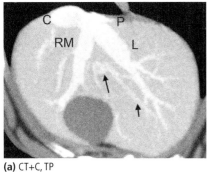 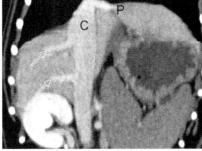

The largest vein draining the liver comes from the left liver lobes (**a**). The phrenic vein (**a,b**) is a small vein that enters the caudal vena cava parallel to the diaphragm. The right medial lobes are drained by a vein that spans the gallbladder (**a**). The portal vein branches (**a**: arrows) interdigitate with the hepatic veins. Small right veins enter the caudal vena cava from the dorsal right liver lobes (**b**: open arrows). See Legend for Figures 5.2.1–5.2.18.

(a) CT+C, TP   **(b)** CT+C, DP

Figure 5.2.3   Portal Vein (Canine)

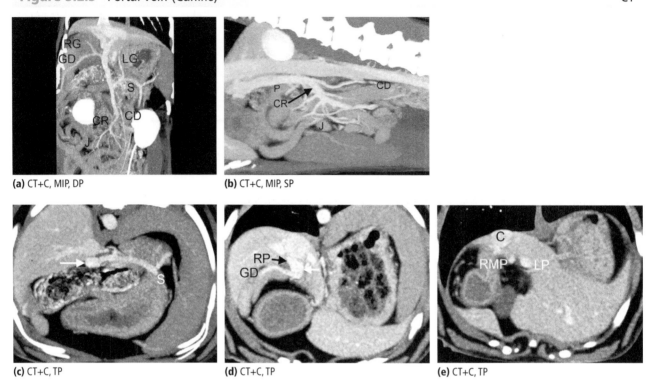

(a) CT+C, MIP, DP

(b) CT+C, MIP, SP

(c) CT+C, TP

(d) CT+C, TP

(e) CT+C, TP

The jejunal veins travel from the intestine to the cranial mesenteric vein (**a**). The caudal mesenteric vein joins the portal vein from the left dorsal abdomen. The next most cranial tributary of the portal vein (**b,c**: arrow) is the splenic vein (**c**) from the left side and then, slightly more cranial, the gastroduodenal vein (**d**) from the right lobe of the pancreas. The portal vein gives off a right branch to the right lateral lobe (**d**) and then branches to the right medial (often called central division) and left liver lobes. See page 507 for Legend for Figures 5.2.1–5.2.18.

Figure 5.2.4   Hepatic Arterioportal Fistula (Feline)   CT

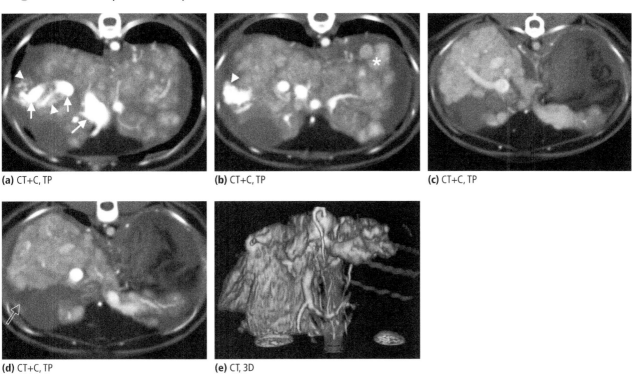

(a) CT+C, TP   **(b)** CT+C, TP   **(c)** CT+C, TP

(d) CT+C, TP   **(e)** CT, 3D

5mo MC Domestic Shorthair with ascites. Transverse images (**a–d**) are ordered from cranial to caudal. During the arterial phase scan, the liver is markedly and irregularly contrast enhancing (**b**: asterisk). The hepatic artery is enlarged, and high-attenuating blood is present in the dilated portal vasculature during this phase (**a**: arrows). There is a small plexus of vessels on the right lateral liver, representing a portion of the arterioportal anastomosis (**a,b**: arrowheads). Free fluid is present in the peritoneum (**d**: open arrow). A 3D image from the ventral perspective illustrates the multiple enlarged, intrahepatic vessels. See page 507 for Legend for Figures 5.2.1–5.2.18.

Figure 5.2.5   Congenital Intrahepatic Shunt—Left Divisional (Canine)   CT

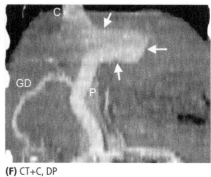

(a) CT+C, TP

(b) CT+C, TP

(c) CT+C, TP

(d) CT+C, TP

(e) CT+C, TP

(F) CT+C, DP

5mo FS Golden Retriever with poor growth. Transverse images (**a–e**) are ordered from caudal to cranial. There is a single intrahepatic shunt arising from the portal vein at the porta hepatis and traveling to the left side (**b–d**: arrows). The vessel forms a curve that returns to the caudal vena cava in the cranial liver near the diaphragm. The dorsal reformatted image demonstrates the typical shape of the patent ductus venosus (**f**: arrows). See page 507 for Legend for Figures 5.2.1–5.2.18.

Figure 5.2.6   Congenital Intrahepatic Shunt—Left Divisional (Canine)   CT

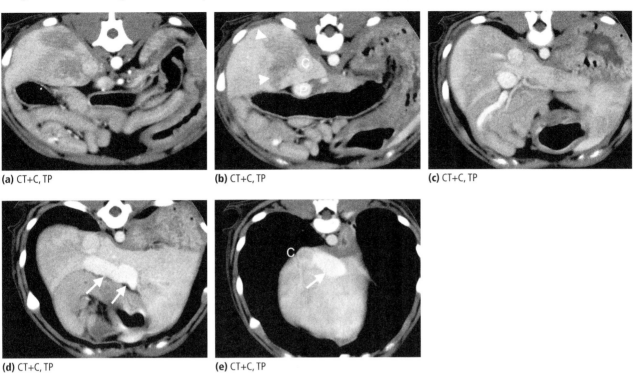

(a) CT+C, TP   **(b)** CT+C, TP   **(c)** CT+C, TP

(d) CT+C, TP   **(e)** CT+C, TP

3mo MC Rottweiler with stupor after meals. Images are ordered from caudal to cranial. An anomalous vessel arises from the left side of the portal vein within the liver (**d,e**: arrows), curving to join the caudal vena cava near the diaphragm. During the late arterial phase and early portal phase, there is mottled contrast enhancement of the liver (**b**: arrowheads), which is a common finding in dogs with shunts, and is presumed to be due to increased arterial blood supply. See page 507 for Legend for Figures 5.2.1–5.2.18.

Figure 5.2.7   Congenital Intrahepatic Shunt—Central Divisional (Canine)   CT

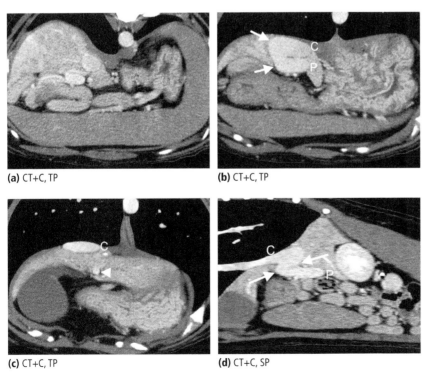

(a) CT+C, TP   **(b)** CT+C, TP

(c) CT+C, TP   **(d)** CT+C, SP

1y Labrador Retriever with aggression after meals and polydipsia. Transverse images (**a–c**) are ordered from caudal to cranial. There is a short anomalous vessel (**b,d**: arrows) arising from the right side of the portal vein and traveling dorsally to join with the caudal vena cava. Cranial to the shunt, there is a blind-ending portal branch that does not continue cranially (**c**: arrowhead). No other intrahepatic portal branches are present. The liver is small (**b,d**), and the parenchyma shows typical mottled enhancement in the early portal phase (**a**). See page 507 for Legend for Figures 5.2.1–5.2.18.

Figure 5.2.8   Congenital Intrahepatic Shunt—Right Divisional (Canine)   CT

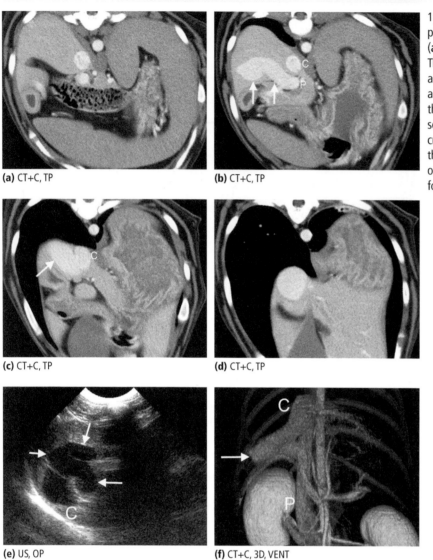

1y FS Doberman Pinscher with suspected portosystemic shunt. Transverse images (a–d) are ordered from caudal to cranial. There is a large, tortuous anomalous vessel arising from the right side of the portal vein and traveling through the right liver lobes to the caudal vena cava (b,c: arrows). The vessel was visible on ultrasound images in the cranial liver (e: arrows). A 3D rendering from the ventral aspect demonstrates the shape of the shunt vessel (f: arrow). See page 507 for Legend for Figures 5.2.1–5.2.18.

(a) CT+C, TP

(b) CT+C, TP

(c) CT+C, TP

(d) CT+C, TP

(e) US, OP

(f) CT+C, 3D, VENT

Figure 5.2.9   Multiple Intrahepatic Shunts (Canine)   CT

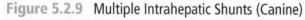
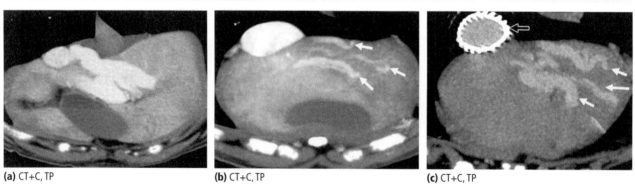

(a) CT+C, TP

(b) CT+C, TP

(c) CT+C, TP

6mo MC Labrador Retriever with failure to gain weight. Preoperatively, there are multiple small, tortuous vessels within the hepatic parenchyma (b: arrows), cranial to the main shunt vessel (a). After partial shunt occlusion with a stent (c: open arrow) and coil embolization, the multiple anomalous vessels have increased in diameter (c: arrows). See page 507 for Legend for Figures 5.2.1–5.2.18.

Figure 5.2.10 Congenital Extrahepatic Shunt—Splenocaval (Canine)

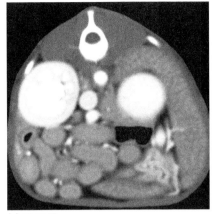

(a) CT+C, TP

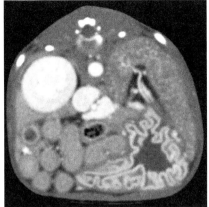

(b) CT+C, TP

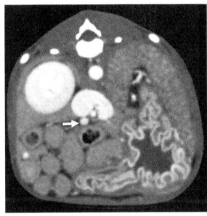

(c) CT+C, TP

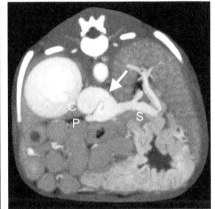

(d) CT+C, MIP, TP

2y MC Yorkshire Terrier with 2-year history of episodic ataxia and seizures. Images **a–c** are ordered from caudal to cranial. The short extrahepatic shunt vessel arises from the portal vein at the junction of the splenic vein and curves dorsally and to the left to join the caudal vena cava (**d**: arrow). The portal vein decreases in diameter cranial to the shunt exit (**c**: arrow). The MIP image shows the relationship between the splenic vein and the shunt (**d**). See page 507 for Legend for Figures 5.2.1–5.2.18.

Figure 5.2.11 Congenital Extrahepatic Shunt—Splenophrenic (Canine) CT

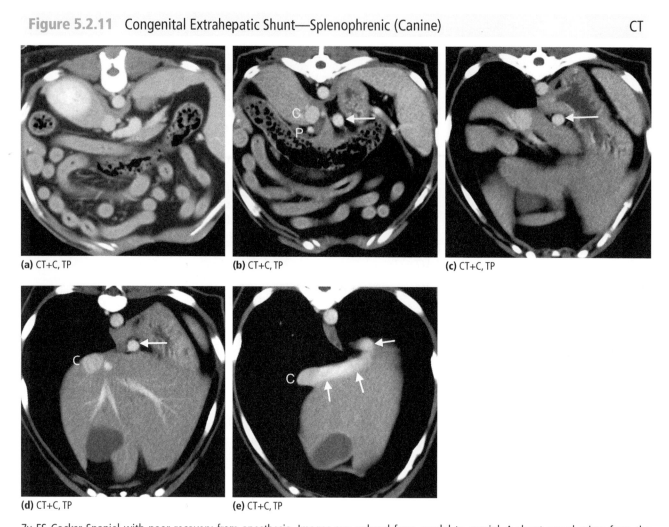

(a) CT+C, TP

(b) CT+C, TP

(c) CT+C, TP

(d) CT+C, TP

(e) CT+C, TP

7y FS Cocker Spaniel with poor recovery from anesthesia. Images are ordered from caudal to cranial. A shunt vessel arises from the splenic vein (**a**) and travels medial to the gastric fundus (**b–d**: arrow) toward the diaphragm. The vessel joins the phrenic vein and then travels to the caudal vena cava parallel to the diaphragm (**e**: arrows). See page 507 for Legend for Figures 5.2.1–5.2.18.

Figure 5.2.12   Congenital Extrahepatic Shunt—Splenoazygos (Canine)   CT

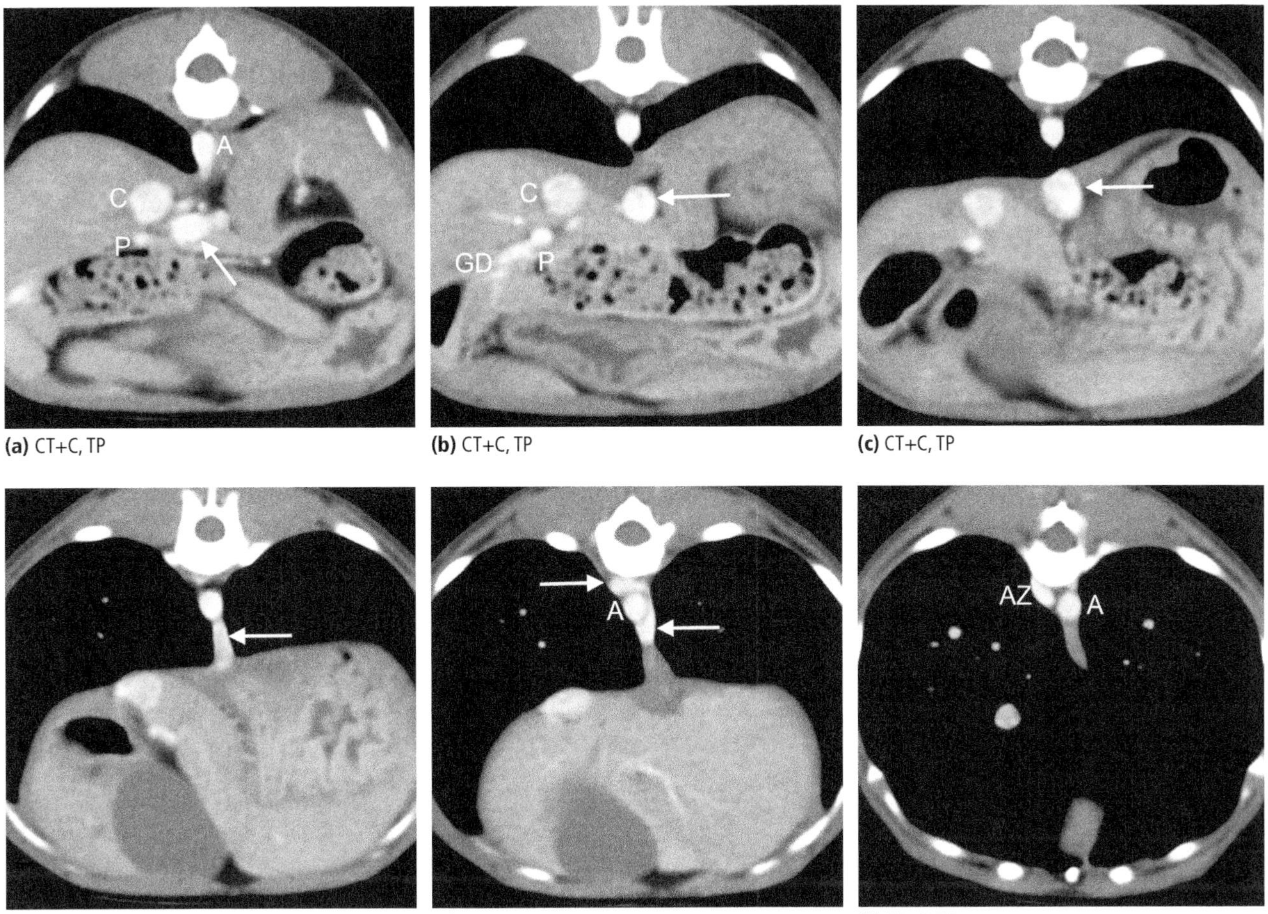

(a) CT+C, TP

(b) CT+C, TP

(c) CT+C, TP

(d) CT+C, TP

(e) CT+C, TP

(f) CT+C, TP

6mo F Yorkshire Terrier failing to gain weight. Images are ordered from caudal to cranial. On portal phase angiographic images, a shunt vessel (**a–e**: arrows) exits the portal vein through the splenic vein, traveling along midline dorsal to the liver and then rising dorsally at the diaphragm through the caudal vena cava to the azygos vein. See page 507 for Legend for Figures 5.2.1–5.2.18.

Figure 5.2.13   Congenital Extrahepatic Shunt—Splenoazygos (Canine)   MR

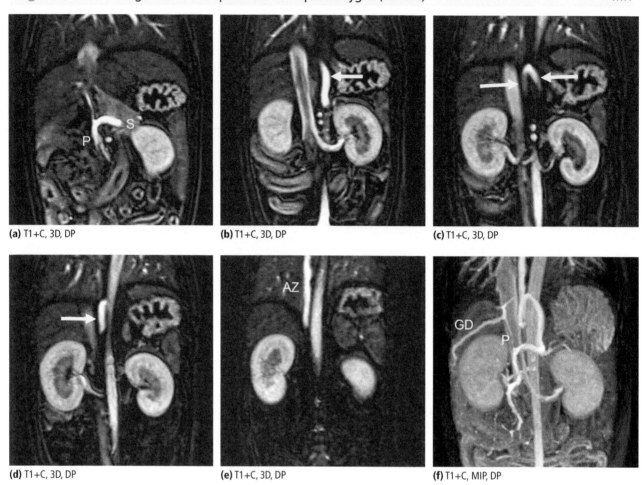

(a) T1+C, 3D, DP   **(b)** T1+C, 3D, DP   **(c)** T1+C, 3D, DP

(d) T1+C, 3D, DP   **(e)** T1+C, 3D, DP   **(f)** T1+C, MIP, DP

4y F Maltese Terrier with suspected portosystemic shunt. Images are ordered from ventral to dorsal (**a–e**) after subtraction. There is a congenital extrahepatic shunt vessel traveling from the portal vein (**a**: P), through the splenic vein (**a**: S), and then dorsally (**b–d**: arrows) to join the azygos vein (**e**: AZ). The MIP image shows the entire course of the shunt vessel (**f**). The gastroduodenal vein (**f**: GD) joins the portal vein cranial to the shunt origin. The portal vein decreases in diameter after the shunt exit (**f**: P). See page 507 for Legend for Figures 5.2.1–5.2.18. Clinic of Small Animal Surgery and Reproduction, Ludwig Maximillian Universität, Munich, Germany, 2014. Reproduced with permission from Ludwig Maximillian Universität.

Figure 5.2.14   Congenital Extrahepatic Shunt—Right Gastric–Caval (Canine)   CT

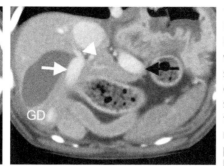

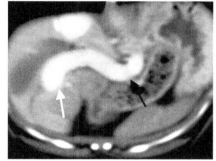

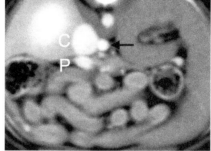

(a) CT+C, TP

(b) CT+C, TP

(c) CT+C, TP

(d) CT+C, TP

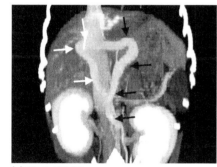

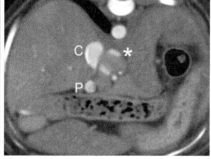

(e) CT+C, MIP, DP

(f) CT+C, TP

1y FS Terrier with failure to gain weight. Images **a–c** are ordered caudal to cranial, and images **d–f** are ordered cranial to caudal. The white arrows denote the cranial course of the shunt and the black arrows denote the caudal course to the shunt termination. The large shunt vessel (**a–c**: white arrow) arises from the gastroduodenal vein at the level of the right gastric vein and travels cranially to the porta hepatis, where it gives off a right intra-hepatic branch (**b**: arrowhead). It crosses to the left side (**a–c**: black arrow) and travels caudally to join the caudal vena cava near the right kidney (**d**: black arrow). The dorsal plane MIP image shows the right (**e**: white arrows) and left (**e**: black arrows) arms of the shunt vessel. A plastic ameroid constrictor was placed around the shunt vessel at its junction with the caudal vena cava (**f**: asterisk), occluding the blood flow. See page 507 for Legend for Figures 5.2.1–5.2.18.

Figure 5.2.15 Congenital Extrahepatic Right Gastric–Caval Shunt (Canine) MR

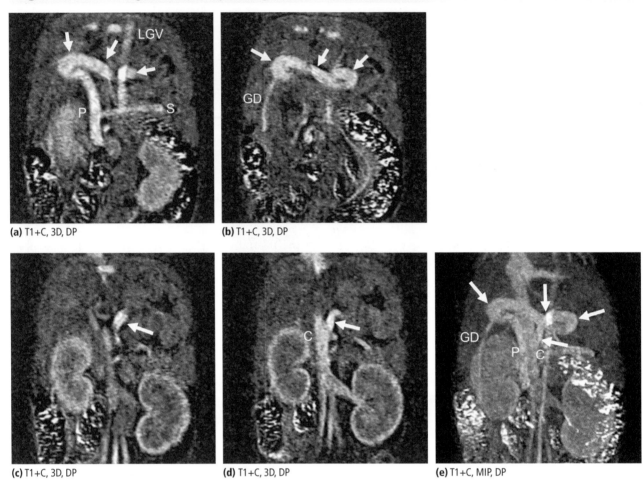

(a) T1+C, 3D, DP

(b) T1+C, 3D, DP

(c) T1+C, 3D, DP

(d) T1+C, 3D, DP

(e) T1+C, MIP, DP

4mo M Yorkshire Terrier with suspected portosystemic shunt. Images are ordered from ventral to dorsal (**a–d**) after subtraction. The shunt arises at the cranial aspect of the gastroduodenal vein (**b**: GD), travels from right to left in the cranial abdomen (**a–d**: arrows), and then terminates in the caudal vena cava (**d**: C). The shunt crosses the splenic and left gastric veins but does not anastamose with them (**a**: S,LGV). The MIP image shows the course of the shunt in its entirety (**e**: arrows). See page 507 for Legend for Figures 5.2.1–5.2.18. Clinic of Small Animal Surgery and Reproduction, Ludwig Maximillian Universität, Munich, Germany, 2014. Reproduced with permission from Ludwig Maximillian Universität.

Figure 5.2.16   Multiple Acquired Extrahepatic Shunts (Canine)   CT

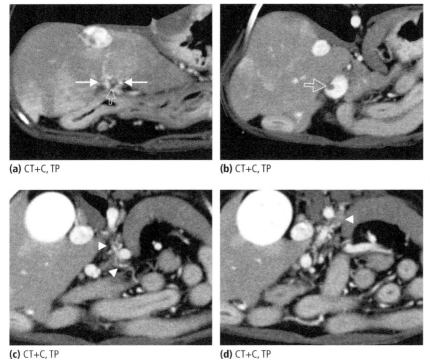

(a) CT+C, TP

(b) CT+C, TP

(c) CT+C, TP

(d) CT+C, TP

4y MC Pug with protein-losing enteropathy and seizures. Images are ordered from cranial to caudal. On portal-phase angiography, there is decreased size and a filling defect in the portal vein (**a**: open arrow), with hepatic arterial branches surrounding the vessel (**a**: arrows). A more discrete thrombus is visible in the distended portal vein, just caudal to the porta hepatis (**b**: open arrow). Near the right renal vein, there are multiple small, tortuous vessels surrounding the cranial mesenteric artery (**c,d**: arrowheads), which represent multiple extrahepatic shunts.

Figure 5.2.17   Complex Vascular Anomaly—Portal Aplasia (Canine)   CT

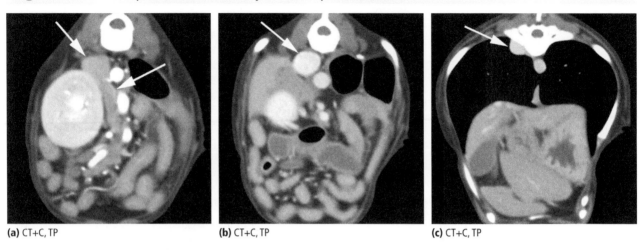

(a) CT+C, TP   **(b)** CT+C, TP   **(c)** CT+C, TP

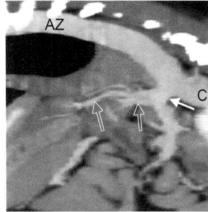

(d) CT+C, MIP, SP

1y M Dachshund with suspected portosystemic shunt. Transverse images (**a–c**) are ordered from caudal to cranial. The portal vein travels dorsally in the caudal abdomen (**a–c**: arrows) to join the caudal vena cava. The prehepatic caudal vena cava is absent cranial to the shunt, and the blood travels to the azygos vein (**d**). The sagittal image shows the portal tributaries traveling caudally (**d**: open arrows) toward the portal vein (**d**: arrow). There is no portal vein supplying the liver. See page 507 for Legend for Figures 5.2.1–5.2.18.

Figure 5.2.18   Postoperative Portal Development (Canine)   CT

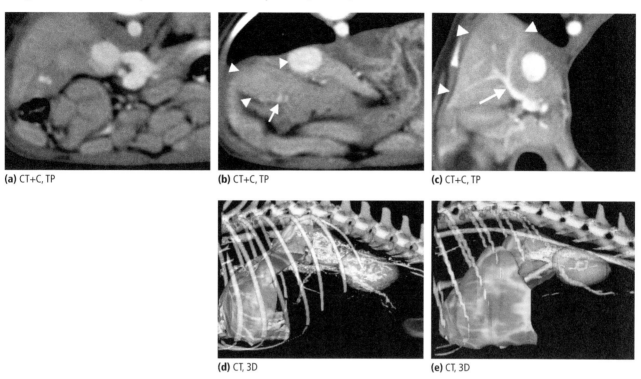

(a) CT+C, TP   **(b)** CT+C, TP   **(c)** CT+C, TP

(d) CT, 3D   **(e)** CT, 3D

3y M Yorkshire Terrier with obtundation and elevated bile acids. On preoperative CT angiography, a single extrahepatic shunt (**a**) was present, and cranially there was no evidence of portal vasculature. Hepatic arterial branches were visible (**b**: arrow), and the right liver was hypoplastic (**b**: arrowheads). Eight weeks after shunt attenuation, the right portal branch is normal in size (**c**: arrow), and the liver has increased in volume on transverse images (**c**: arrowheads) and comparative presurgical (**d**) and postsurgical (**e**) 3D volume renderings of the liver. See page 507 for Legend for Figures 5.2.1–5.2.18.

References

1. Zwingenberger AL, Schwarz T. Dual-phase CT angiography of the normal canine portal and hepatic vasculature. Vet Radiol Ultrasound. 2004;45:117–124.

2. Mai W, Weisse C. Contrast-enhanced portal magnetic resonance angiography in dogs with suspected congenital portal vascular anomalies. Vet Radiol Ultrasound. 2011;52:284–288.

3. Bruehschwein A, Foltin I, Flatz K, Zoellner M, Matis U. Contrast-enhanced magnetic resonance angiography for diagnosis of portosystemic shunts in 10 dogs. Vet Radiol Ultrasound. 2010;51:116–121.

4. Lamb CR, White RN. Morphology of congenital intrahepatic portacaval shunts in dogs and cats. Vet Rec. 1998;142:55–60.

5. Tivers M, Lipscomb V. Congenital portosystemic shunts in cats: investigation, diagnosis and stabilisation. J Feline Med Surg. 2011;13:173–184.

6. Mehl ML, Kyles AE, Case JB, Kass PH, Zwingenberger A, Gregory CR. Surgical management of left-divisional intrahepatic portosystemic shunts: outcome after partial ligation of, or ameroid ring constrictor placement on, the left hepatic vein in twenty-eight dogs (1995–2005). Vet Surg. 2007;36:21–30.

7. Leeman JJ, Kim SE, Reese DJ, Risselada M, Ellison GW. Multiple congenital PSS in a dog: case report and literature review. J Am Anim Hosp Assoc. 2013;49:281–285.

8. Nelson NC, Nelson LL. Anatomy of extrahepatic portosystemic shunts in dogs as determined by computed tomography angiography. Vet Radiol Ultrasound. 2011;52:498–506.

9. White RN, White RN, Parry AT, Parry AT. Morphology of congenital portosystemic shunts emanating from the left gastric vein in dogs and cats. J Small Anim Pract. 2013;54:459–467.

10. Bertolini G. Acquired portal collateral circulation in the dog and cat. Vet Radiol Ultrasound. 2010;51:25–33.

11. Fischetti AJ, Kovak J. Imaging diagnosis: Azygous continuation of the caudal vena cava with and without portocaval shunting. Vet Radiol Ultrasound. 2008;49:573–576.

12. Zwingenberger AL, Spriet M, Hunt GB. Imaging diagnosis – portal vein aplasia and interruption of the caudal vena cava in three dogs. Vet Rec. 2012;171:444–447.

5.3

Hepatobiliary disorders

Introduction

Disorders of the hepatic parenchyma and biliary tract are commonly seen in small animals. CT and MRI imaging are used to evaluate the size and extent of the lesions for diagnosis and surgical planning. The tissue characterization and perfusion imaging capabilities of MR and CT images allow investigation into the type of lesion present, increasing the probability of a specific imaging diagnosis. Multiphase imaging with contrast administration is recommended for CT and MR imaging of the liver to gain the most information, especially when evaluating nodules and masses.

Trauma

Liver lobe torsion occurs when a liver lobe, most frequently the left lateral or medial lobe, rotates on its axis and blood supply is occluded.[1,2] The resulting hypoperfusion of the lobe causes enlargement and rounding of the margins because of venous congestion. The lobe does not enhance after contrast administration if the arterial supply is occluded or necrosis is advanced (Figure 5.3.1).

In people, CT is used to assess the liver for blunt trauma. Lacerations appear as linear or branching hypoattenuating regions in the parenchyma on enhanced images. Acute parenchymal hematomas are hyperattenuating with a low-attenuating rim on unenhanced images. More chronic parenchymal hematomas are of low attenuation with irregular margins. Active bleeding can be seen as high-attenuating blood flow into a low-attenuating hematoma. Subcapsular hematomas appear as elliptical low-attenuating fluid between the liver capsule and parenchyma on enhanced images.[3]

Inflammatory disorders

Diffuse inflammatory disease of the liver may result in hepatic enlargement during the acute phase, with rounding of the liver margins. The affected region may contrast enhance on both CT and MRI images in hypervascular inflammation and may lack contrast enhancement if necrosis occurs (Figure 5.3.2). Focal lesions, such as hepatic abscesses, are peripherally, intensely contrast enhancing and will have a fluid-attenuating or T1 hypointense, T2 hyperintense center on CT and MR images, respectively. Cholecystitis results in strong contrast enhancement of the gall-bladder wall (see Degenerative disorders later in this chapter).[4] Emphysematous cystitis is recognized by gas accumulation within the wall of the gallbladder. The appearance of biliary mucoceles has not been reported on CT images, and ultrasound is currently the imaging modality of choice.

Parasitic masses secondary to *Echinococcus* sp. have been reported to result in multilobular, cystic, cavitary hepatic masses with regions of internal mineralization.[5]

Nodules and mass lesions

Many hepatic neoplasms derive their blood supply partly or entirely from the hepatic arterial system, whereas the normal hepatic parenchyma is supplied 75% from the portal system.[5] These characteristics allow

---

Atlas of Small Animal CT and MRI, First Edition. Erik R. Wisner and Allison L. Zwingenberger.
© 2015 John Wiley & Sons, Inc. Published 2015 by John Wiley & Sons, Inc.

differentiation to be made on multiphase CT and MR scans in people.[7,8]

Benign hepatic masses

The term nodular hyperplasia is often used to describe apparently spontaneous development of a somewhat unorganized mass consisting of relatively normal hepatic cellular elements. A regenerative nodule suggests a similar response to a known or suspected hepatic insult. Despite the nuanced differences, the terms are often used interchangeably. Nodular hyperplasia is nonencapsulated and may be either hypoattenuating during the arterial phase (Figure 5.3.3)[9] or diffusely hyperattenuating (Figure 5.3.4).[10] Nodular hyperplasia is often isointense to liver in the unenhanced, portal, and delayed phases, making detection difficult in protocols that do not include arterial phase imaging. Nodular hyperplasia lesions tend to be smaller than hepatocellular adenoma or carcinoma. On MR images, regenerative nodules are similar to hepatic parenchyma with T1, T2, and contrast imaging characteristics similar to normal liver.[11]

Hepatocellular adenomas are diffusely contrast enhancing in the arterial phase, similar to nodular hyperplasia. They may also be isoattenuating in the unenhanced and delayed phases, appearing similar to normal liver parenchyma (Figures 5.3.5, 5.3.6).

Myelolipomas are benign tumors composed of fat and myeloid elements, which occur in cats and wild felines.[12] On CT images, they are irregular, lobular masses with fat-attenuating characteristics (Figure 5.3.7).

Cholangiocellular adenoma (biliary cystadenoma) is a benign neoplasm occurring more frequently in cats. These masses are composed of multiple variably sized cystic regions with little or no peripheral contrast enhancement and central fluid attenuation on CT images (Figure 5.3.8).

Malignant hepatic masses

On arterial phase CT images in people, hepatocellular carcinoma has increased arterial enhancement compared to benign nodules and early washout in the portal phase.[12] This is beginning to be explored in veterinary medicine with CT and MRI although our experience suggests that variability in enhancement may limit diagnostic utility. Hepatocellular carcinoma is more cystic and has central hypoattenuating regions with peripheral arterial enhancement on CT images (Figure 5.3.9).[8,9] This may be partially due to the large size of typical hepatocellular carcinomas at time of diagnosis, with regions of poor perfusion and necrosis. On MR images, hepatocellular carcinoma is heterogeneous on T1 and T2 images (Figure 5.3.10) with increased signal intensity in the early contrast phase. Greater heterogeneity following contrast administration is associated with higher-grade lesions.[11] Liver-specific contrast medium has been investigated and is effective in differentiating benign from malignant lesions, with similar imaging characteristics compared to gadolinium-DTPA contrast medium.[13]

Cholangiocellular carcinomas (biliary adenocarcinomas) have been reported in cats and dogs.[8,9,11] They are poorly encapsulated with heterogeneous contrast enhancement and regions of absent contrast enhancement (Figure 5.3.11).

Metastatic lesions to the liver may be hypervascular or hypovascular, depending on their degree of arterial blood supply. Hypovascular lesions are more common in people, with hypoattenuation on the arterial phase (Figures 5.3.12, 5.3.13). A target lesion appearance in the delayed phase images has been identified as specific for hypervascular metastasis, such as those of neuroendocrine tumors (Figure 5.3.12).[14] Metastatic lesions tend to be hypointense on T1 and hyperintense on T2 images with contrast rim enhancement and multifocal distribution.[11]

Lymphoma often occurs as a diffuse hepatic abnormality, and is hypointense to skeletal muscle on T2-weighted MR images, compared to normal dogs that have hyperintense liver intensity.[15] Mass lesions may also occur, for example in the bile duct, causing partial obstruction (Figure 5.3.14). Hepatic lymphoma is hypoattenuating on CT and may have a central region of low intensity indicating necrosis. Enhancement may be absent, patchy, or peripheral.[16]

Hepatic sarcomas have a variable appearance in people depending on the specific cell type. Common features include hypoattenuation compared to normal liver on unenhanced images, an unorganized multicameral appearance when cysts are present, and variable but often inhomogeneous or peripheral contrast enhancement.[17] Primary sarcomas, such as hemangiosarcoma, spindle cell sarcoma, and histiocytic sarcoma, occur in the liver of dogs as large masses (Figure 5.3.15). On MR images, hemangiosarcoma is T1 hypointense and T2 hyperintense. On contrast-enhanced images, rim enhancement is seen in masses with internal hemorrhage and masses enhance progressively on delayed phase images.[11]

Neuroendocrine tumors, or carcinoids, arise from neuroendocrine cells present within the biliary tree, gallbladder, or hepatic progenitor cells. Hypervascularity is common on histopathology; however, imaging features have not been described.[12]

Degenerative and other disorders

Hepatic cysts develop for a variety reasons but can be associated with hepatic neoplasia, polycystic kidney disease, parasitic disease, and congenital hepatopathy.[18]

Cysts appear as single or multiple fluid-attenuating or T2 hyperintense lesions with a thin wall, central fluid accumulation and no enhancement (Figure 5.3.16). When large, cysts produce a mass effect.

Degenerative disease of the liver can result in vacuolar hepatopathy, fat accumulation, and cyst formation, changing the imaging characteristics of the parenchyma. Liver disease resulting in vacuolar hepatopathy may cause hepatic enlargement with rounded borders and focal regions of hypoattenuation (Figure 5.3.17). Steatosis of the liver results in more hypoattenuating parenchyma on CT images, although this may only be apparent on measurements with regions of interest. Hepatic lipidosis in cats also results in decreased hepatic attenuation on CT images.[19] Fat accumulation would be expected to be hyperintense on T1 and T2 MR images.

Degenerative or cirrhotic livers are variably sized, with chronic loss of normal parenchyma resulting in microhepatia. The combination of fibrosis and the lobular abnormal architecture created by septa is termed cirrhosis.[12]

Cholelithiasis and biliary obstruction

Cholelithiasis, mineralized sludge accumulation, or calculi in the biliary tree may be observed in asymptomatic animals (Figures 5.3.18, 5.3.19). When obstruction of the bile duct occurs, the gallbladder may be enlarged with surrounding inflammation, thickened wall, and peritoneal effusion (Figure 5.3.20). Neoplasia can also occur in the region of the bile duct, obstructing the flow of bile (Figure 5.3.14).

Figure 5.3.1 Liver Lobe Torsion (Canine)   CT

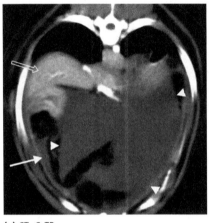 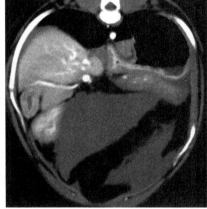 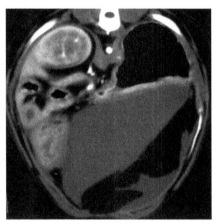

(a) CT+C, TP   (b) CT+C, TP   (c) CT+C, TP

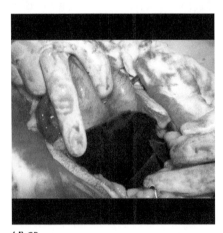

(d) GP

Unknown signalment and history. Images **a–c** are through the liver and ordered from cranial to caudal. The left liver lobes are enlarged, extending past the right kidney (**a–c**). The lobe is hypoattenuating on contrast-enhanced images (**a**: arrowheads). No vascularity is noted in the lobe, in contrast to the normal enhancement of the right liver lobes (**a**: open arrow). There is fluid-attenuating peritoneal effusion present (**a**: solid arrow). At surgery, the affected lobe was enlarged, engorged, and friable (**d**). Lee et al 2009.[19] Reproduced with permission from Wiley.

Figure 5.3.2 Hepatitis and Necrosis (Canine)

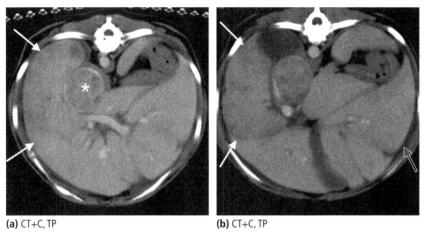

(a) CT+C, TP

(b) CT+C, TP

14y MC Welsh Terrier with pheochromocytoma and invasion of the caudal vena cava. The adrenal mass appears as heterogeneous tissue expanding the caudal vena cava (**a**: asterisk) and creating a filling defect. The liver lobes are enlarged and rounded. The right lateral lobe is heterogeneously contrast enhancing in the portal phase (**a,b**: arrows), which may be related to necrosis or differential perfusion due to the mass effect. Peritoneal effusion is present (**b**: open arrow). Postmortem examination confirmed extensive multifocal hepatocellular necrosis.

Figure 5.3.3 Nodular Hyperplasia (Canine)

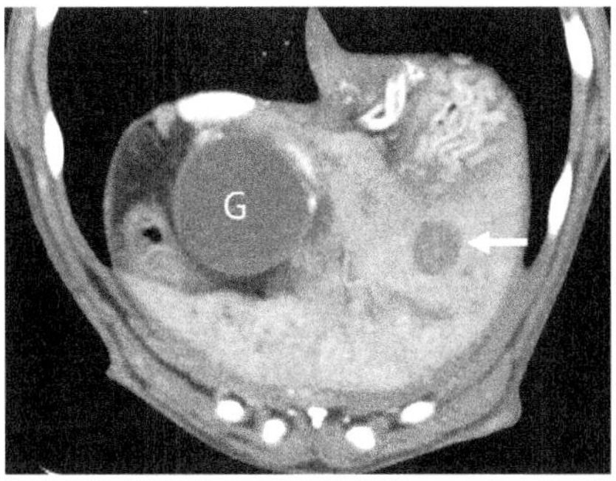

(a) CT+C, TP

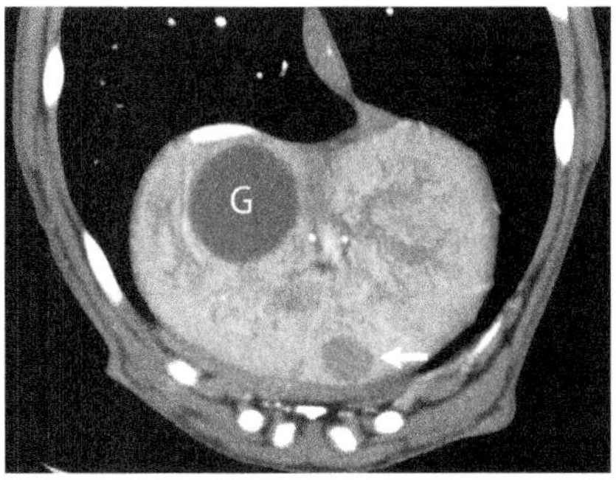

(b) CT+C, TP

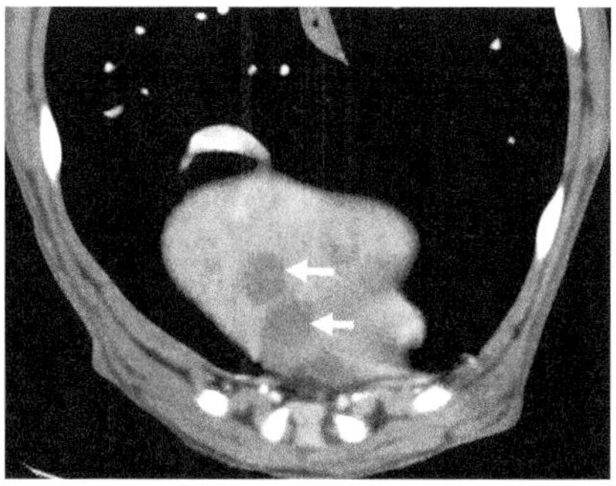

(c) CT+C, TP

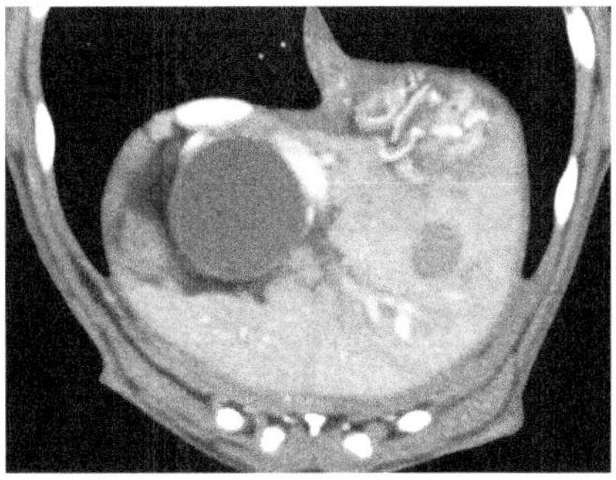

(d) CT+C, TP

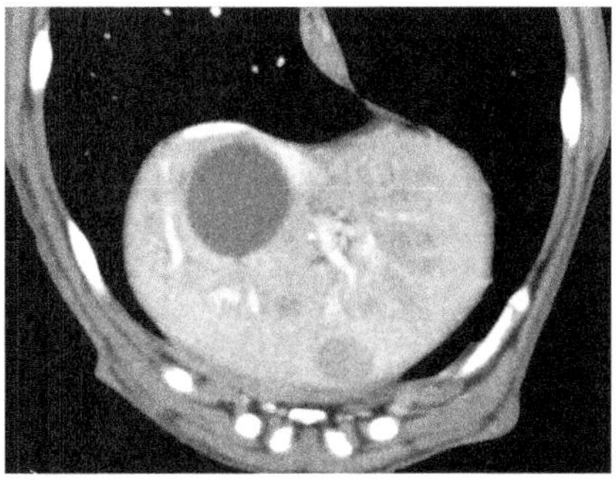

(e) CT+C, TP

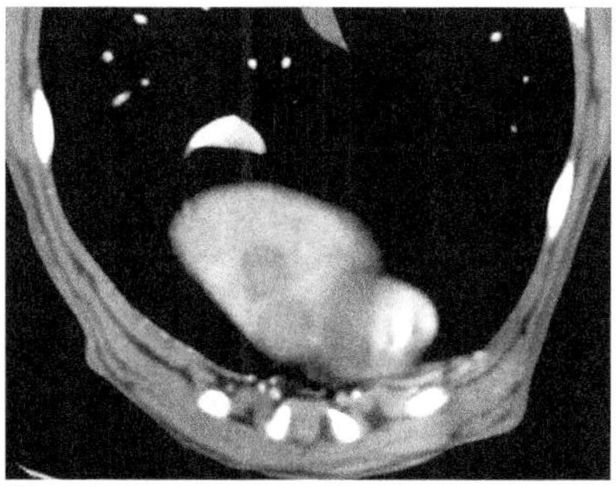

(f) CT+C, TP

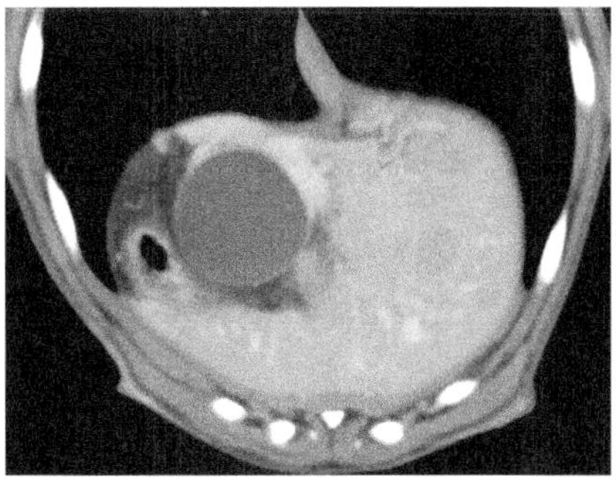

(g) CT+C, TP

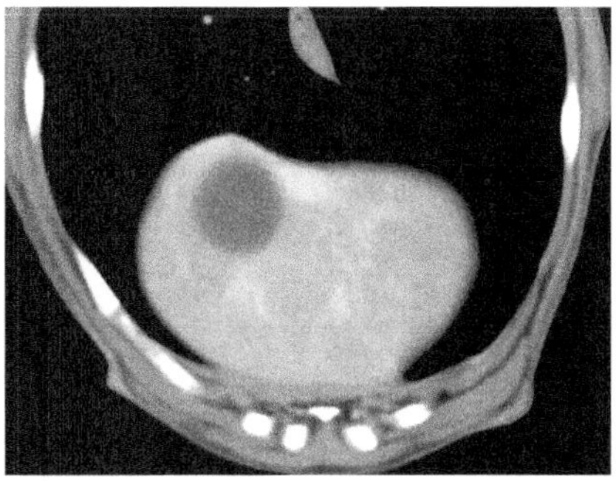

(h) CT+C, TP

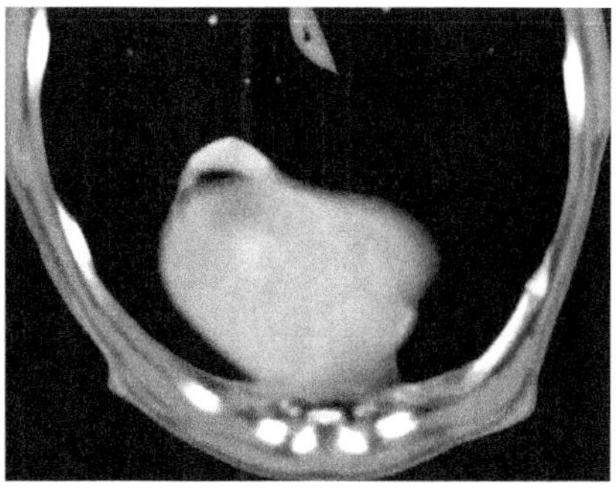

(i) CT+C, TP

3y F Pit Bull Terrier with elevated liver enzymes. Comparable arterial (**a–c**), portal (**d–f**), and delayed (**g–i**) phase images ordered caudal to cranial show multiple hypoattenuating, rounded liver nodules in the liver (**a–c**: arrows). The nodules become almost isoattenuating to liver in the delayed phase images, with mild rim enhancement. The gallbladder (**a,b**: G) is visible as a hypoattenuating structure in the right liver. Biopsy diagnosis of the nodules was nodular hyperplasia.

Figure 5.3.4 Nodular Hyperplasia (Canine)   CT

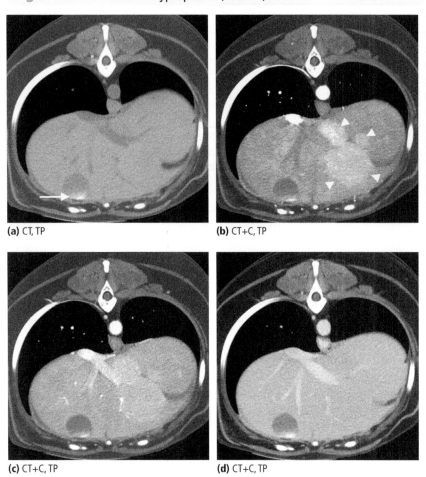

(a) CT, TP   (b) CT+C, TP

(c) CT+C, TP   (d) CT+C, TP

10y MC mixed-breed dog with liver mass. On the unenhanced image (**a**), the liver nodules are isoattenuating to the hepatic parenchyma, with a suggestion of mass effect on the left side. Multiple well-defined round masses are visible in the early arterial phase (**b**: arrowheads), with homogeneous contrast enhancement. The nodules become more isoattenuating in the portal phase (**c**) and are isoattenuating in the delayed phase (**d**). Hyperattenuating material is present in the dependent gallbladder (**a**: arrow). Biopsy diagnosis of the nodules was nodular hyperplasia.

Figure 5.3.5 Hepatic Adenoma (Canine)   CT

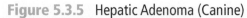
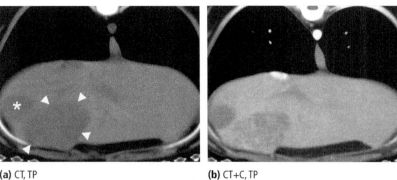

(a) CT, TP   (b) CT+C, TP

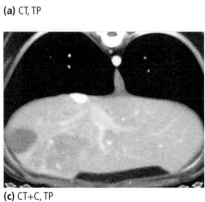
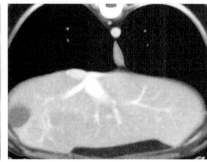

(c) CT+C, TP   (d) CT+C, TP

7y FS Maltese with elevated liver enzymes. There is a hypoattenuating mass with slightly irregular margins in the quadrate lobe (**a**: arrowheads), medial to the gallbladder (**a**: asterisk). On the arterial phase image (**b**), there is diffuse enhancement of the mass associated with an internal reticular pattern. During the portal (**c**) and delayed (**d**) phases, the mass becomes isoattenuating to normal liver. Surgical excisional biopsy confirmed hepatocellular adenoma.

Figure 5.3.6   Hepatic Adenoma (Canine)   CT

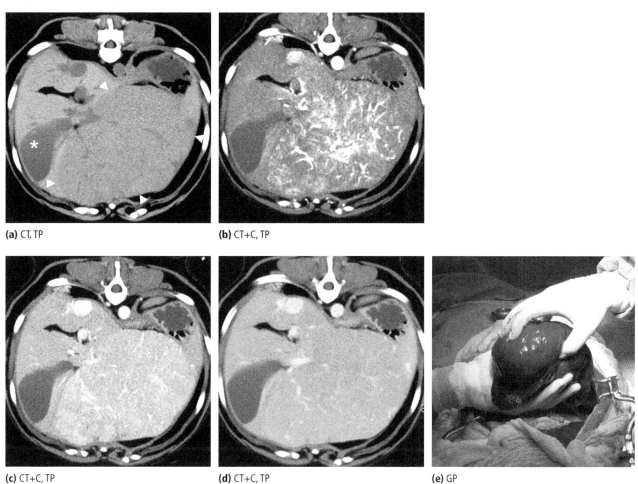

(a) CT, TP

(b) CT+C, TP

(c) CT+C, TP

(d) CT+C, TP

(e) GP

10y FS mixed-breed dog with elevated liver enzymes. The liver mass is located in the left lateral lobe and is hypoattenuating on the unenhanced image (**a**: arrowheads). The gallbladder (**a**: asterisk) is displaced by the mass effect. There is contrast enhancement of the entire mass during the arterial phase (**b**), mild hyperattenuation on the portal phase (**c**), and isoattenuation on the delayed phase image (**d**). Surgical excisional biopsy confirmed hepatocellular adenoma (**e**).

Figure 5.3.7 Myelolipoma (Feline)

CT

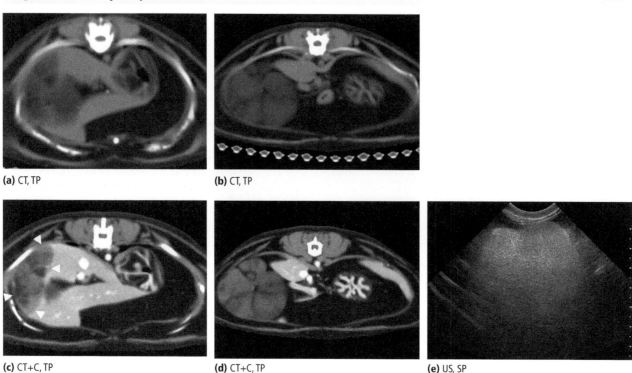

(a) CT, TP

(b) CT, TP

(c) CT+C, TP

(d) CT+C, TP

(e) US, SP

9y FS Domestic Shorthair with a palpable abdominal mass. Images **a–d** are comparable unenhanced (**a,b**) and contrast-enhanced (**c,d**) images of the liver ordered from cranial to caudal. A multilobular, fat-attenuating (−67 HU) mass is present in the right lateral lobe and extends caudally (**a,b**). The mass is poorly demarcated within the cranial liver (**c**: arrowheads) and is well encapsulated caudally. There is very mild contrast enhancement of the mass (**d**). On ultrasonography, the mass was hyperechoic, suggesting fat as the tissue of origin. Surgical excisional biopsy confirmed myelolipoma.

Figure 5.3.8 Cholangiocellular Adenoma (Feline)

CT

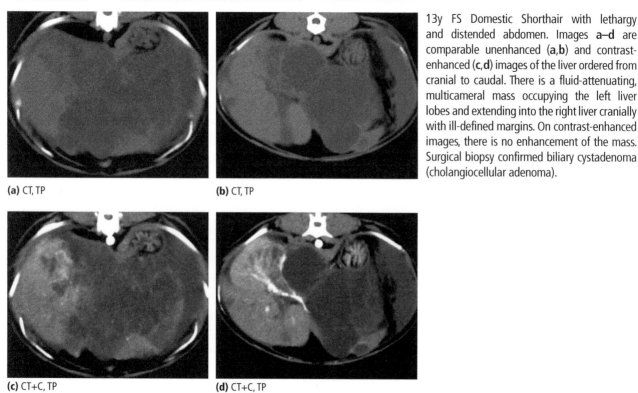

(a) CT, TP

(b) CT, TP

13y FS Domestic Shorthair with lethargy and distended abdomen. Images **a–d** are comparable unenhanced (**a,b**) and contrast-enhanced (**c,d**) images of the liver ordered from cranial to caudal. There is a fluid-attenuating, multicameral mass occupying the left liver lobes and extending into the right liver cranially with ill-defined margins. On contrast-enhanced images, there is no enhancement of the mass. Surgical biopsy confirmed biliary cystadenoma (cholangiocellular adenoma).

(c) CT+C, TP

(d) CT+C, TP

Figure 5.3.9   Hepatocellular Carcinoma (Canine)   CT

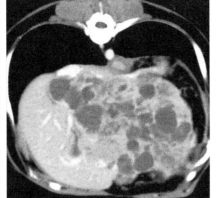

(a) CT, TP

(b) CT+C, TP

9y FS Dachshund with hemoabdomen. There is a large, multilobular and cystic mass in the left liver, extending across midline (**a**,**b**). The mass is poorly encapsulated cranially, with a more encapsulated portion in the caudate lobe (**c**: arrows). The borders of the mass are ill defined on enhanced images, with multiple unenhancing cystic structures and a more uniformly enhancing soft-tissue region. The mass was found to occupy the left medial and quadrate lobes during surgical exploration. Partial excisional biopsy confirmed hepatocellular carcinoma with capsular invasion (**d**).

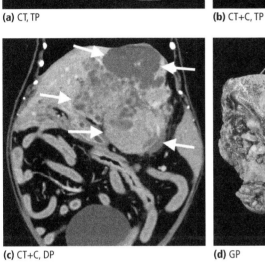

(c) CT+C, DP

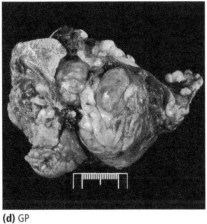

(d) GP

Figure 5.3.10 Carcinoma—Undetermined Origin (Canine)

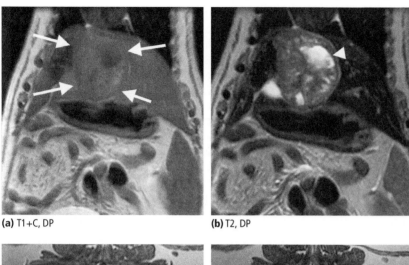

5y MC Norwegian Elkhound with episodes of collapse. On T1 contrast-enhanced images, there is a mildly enhancing mass (**a**, **c**: arrows) with a cystic, hypointense center. T2-weighted images confirm the cystic center because of hyperintensity within the cyst (**b**: arrowhead). A biopsy of the mass was consistent with carcinoma of undetermined origin.

(a) T1+C, DP

(b) T2, DP

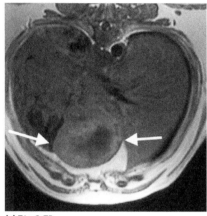

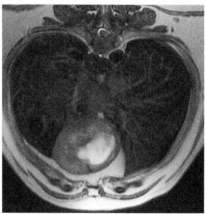

(c) T1+C, TP

(d) T2, TP

Figure 5.3.11 Feline Biliary Adenocarcinoma (Feline)

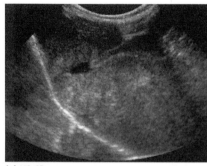

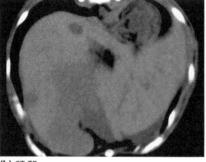

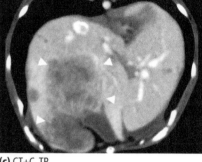

(a) US, SP

(b) CT, TP

(c) CT+C, TP

14y MC Domestic Shorthair with a hepatic mass discovered on ultrasound exam. On ultrasound imaging, the mass is distorting the right liver with mildly heterogeneous architecture (**a**). The mass is poorly encapsulated on CT images, with relative hypoattenuation on unenhanced (**b**) and contrast-enhanced (**c**) images. There is mild, heterogeneous contrast enhancement (**c**: arrowheads). Surgical excision and biopsy confirmed a diagnosis of biliary adenocarcinoma involving the right medial and lateral liver lobes.

Figure 5.3.12   Metastatic Hemangiosarcoma (Canine)   CT

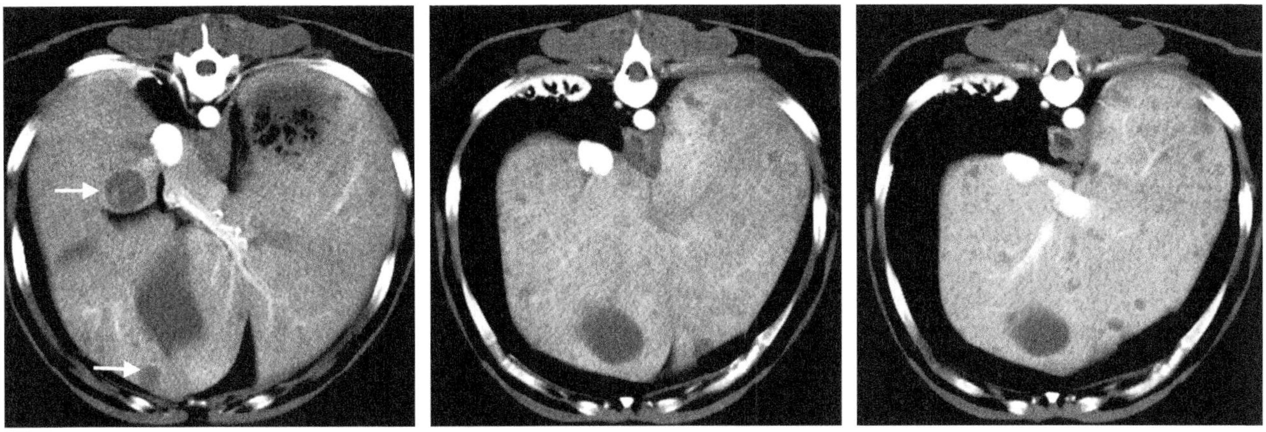

(a) CT+C, TP

(b) CT+C, TP

(c) CT+C, TP

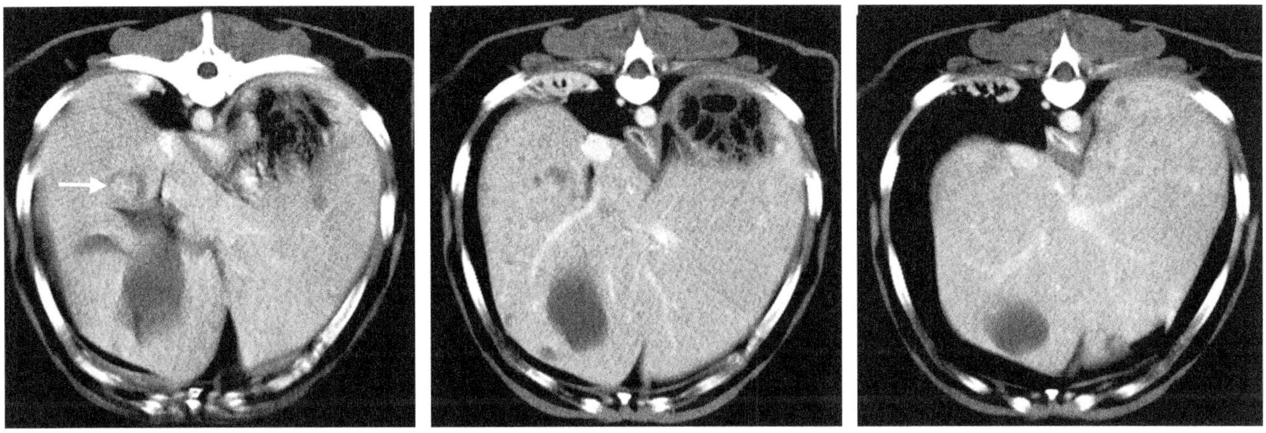

(d) CT+C, TP

(e) CT+C, TP

(f) CT+C, TP

8y M Labrador Retriever. Hemangiosarcoma of the neck treated previously with radiation therapy. Arterial phase (**a–c**) and comparable portal phase (**d–f**) images are ordered from caudal to cranial. There are multiple variably sized, hypoattenuating nodules throughout the liver parenchyma (**a**: arrows). The largest nodule has a central region of more hyperattenuating tissue that contrast enhances (**d**: arrow), producing a target-like lesion. The remainder of the nodules are hypoattenuating on late arterial phase images (**a–c**), and some become isoattenuating on portal phase images (**d–f**).

Figure 5.3.13   Benign Hepatocellular Adenoma and Metastatic Neuroendocrine Tumor (Canine)   CT

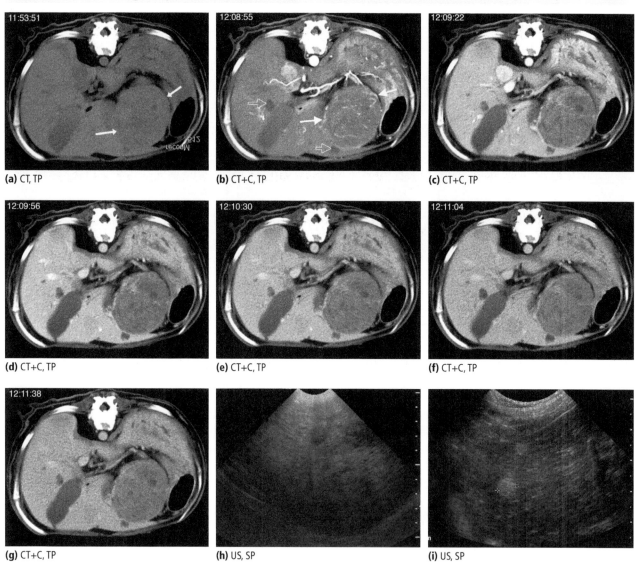

(a) CT, TP

(b) CT+C, TP

(c) CT+C, TP

(d) CT+C, TP

(e) CT+C, TP

(f) CT+C, TP

(g) CT+C, TP

(h) US, SP

(i) US, SP

12y MC Bulldog with liver mass discovered on screening ultrasound examination. Images **a–g** were acquired at the same location through the liver at varying time points following contrast administration. The time of scanning is annotated on each image. There is a large, encapsulated mass in the left lateral liver lobe, which is hypoattenuating on unenhanced images (**a**: arrows). On arterial phase images, the mass is diffusely, heterogeneously contrast enhancing (**b**: arrows). Additional hypoattenuating nodules become visible (**b**: open arrows) distant to the large mass. The mass remains hypoattenuating to normal liver, with heterogeneous enhancement throughout the portal and delayed phases (**c–g**). The large mass was confirmed to be a benign hepatocellular adenoma, and the smaller nodules were metastatic pancreatic beta cell tumor. The difference between the appearance of the large mass (**h**) and metastatic lesions (**i**) is apparent on ultrasound images.

Figure 5.3.14   Lymphoma with Bile Duct Obstruction (Feline)

CT

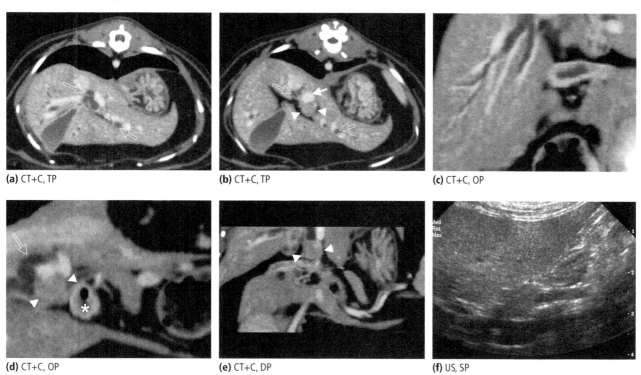

(a) CT+C, TP

(b) CT+C, TP

(c) CT+C, OP

(d) CT+C, OP

(e) CT+C, DP

(f) US, SP

12y MC Domestic Shorthair with hepatitis, anorexia, and vomiting. There is an irregular, isoattenuating mass (**b,d,e**: arrowheads) obstructing the common bile duct and causing intrahepatic biliary distension (**a,b,d**: open arrows). The mass is located ventral to the portal vein (**b**: arrow) and in close proximity to the duodenum (**d**: asterisk). The fluid-attenuating, branching bile ducts are visible parallel to the portal veins (**c**). The mass was also visible on ultrasound images near the duodenal papilla (**f**: calipers). Surgical biopsy confirmed lymphoma.

Figure 5.3.15 Spindle Cell Sarcoma (Canine)

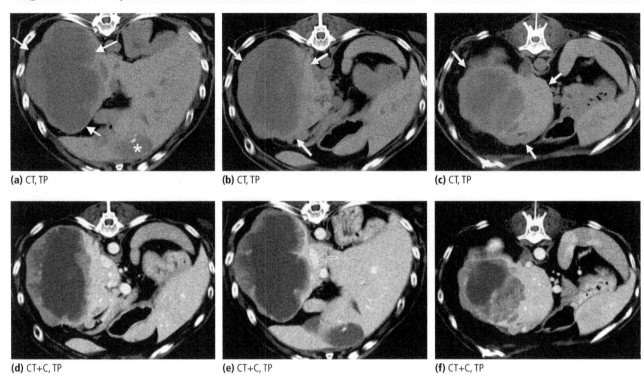

(a) CT, TP   **(b)** CT, TP   **(c)** CT, TP

(d) CT+C, TP   **(e)** CT+C, TP   **(f)** CT+C, TP

14y FS Labrador Retriever with liver mass discovered on screening ultrasound. Images are comparable unenhanced (**a–c**) and contrast-enhanced (**d–f**) images through the liver and ordered from cranial to caudal. There is a large, irregularly margined mass in the right lateral liver lobe with a fluid-attenuating center (**a–c**: arrows). The gallbladder is displaced to the left and contains mineral-attenuating material (**a**: asterisk). On contrast-enhanced images, the mass is peripherally enhancing and is poorly defined from the normal liver on the medial border. The mass effect is causing compression of the caudal vena cava (**e**: open arrow). Surgical biopsy confirmed spindle cell sarcoma.

Figure 5.3.16 Hepatic Cyst (Canine)

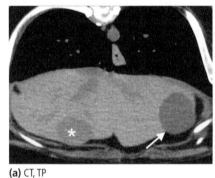 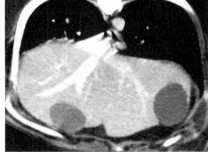

8y MC Pembroke Welsh Corgi with thymoma. A well-circumscribed, fluid-attenuating mass is present in the left lateral liver lobe (**a**: arrow) protruding from the capsular surface. The structure is opposite to the gallbladder (**a**: asterisk). On contrast-enhanced images, there is no enhancement of the structure (**b**). The hepatic cyst was incidental and was discovered during evaluation of the cranial mediastinal mass. Surgical excisional biopsy confirmed the diagnosis.

(a) CT, TP   **(b)** CT+C, TP

Figure 5.3.17   Vacuolar Hepatopathy (Canine)   CT

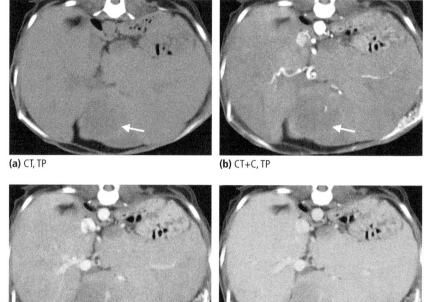

(a) CT, TP

(b) CT+C, TP

(c) CT+C, TP

(d) CT+C, TP

13y FS Brittany with a pulmonary mass. The liver was included in a thoracic CT scan. Images were acquired at the same location through the liver at varying time points following contrast administration. The hepatic borders are enlarged and rounded. There is a focal region of hypoattenuation in the left medial lobe on unenhanced, arterial, and portal phase images (**a–c**: arrows), which minimally contrast enhances on the delayed phase image (**d**). Fine needle aspiration biopsy revealed diffuse vacuolar hepatopathy.

Figure 5.3.18   Biliary Calculi (Canine)   CT

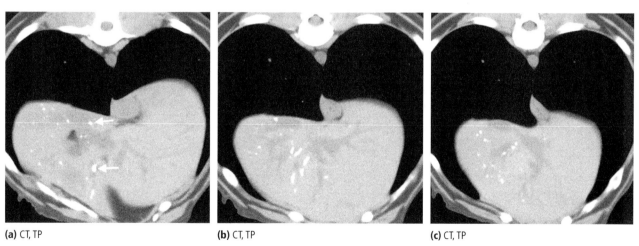

(a) CT, TP

(b) CT, TP

(c) CT, TP

4y MC Australian Cattle Dog imaged for a musculoskeletal sarcoma. Images are through the liver and ordered from caudal to cranial. There are multiple, small, rounded mineral opacities in the bile ducts throughout the liver (**a**: arrows). The calculi form linear opacities where they are clustered in close proximity. Biliary calculi were an incidental finding with no clinical signs.

Figure 5.3.19 Cholelithiasis (Canine) CT

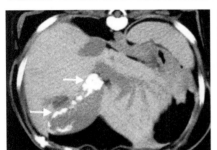

8y MC mixed breed with incidental choleliths and mineralized debris. The mineral opacities are rounded and clumped into larger collections (arrows). The CT scan was performed in dorsal recumbency, and the mineral debris is sedimenting to the dependent side of the gallbladder.

(a) CT, TP

Figure 5.3.20 Gallbladder Obstruction (Feline) CT

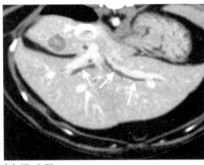 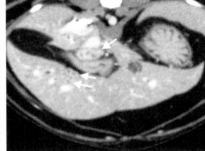

(a) CT+C, TP   **(b)** CT+C, TP

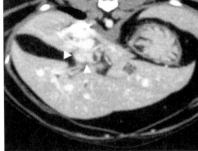 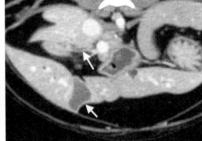

(c) CT+C, TP   **(d)** CT+C, TP

6y FS Domestic Shorthair with anorexia and lethargy. Images are ordered from cranial to caudal. There are multiple dilated bile ducts in the liver parallel to the portal branches (**a**: arrows). Additional cystic masses consistent with cholangiocellular adenoma are seen as multilobular, fluid-attenuating nodules in the parenchyma (**a**: open arrow). The walls of the bile ducts are contrast enhancing, as is the gallbladder wall, as a result of cholangitis and cholecystitis (**b,d**: arrows). There is contrast-enhancing soft tissue filling the lumen of the common bile duct at the junction of the cystic duct and hepatic ducts (**c**: arrowheads). The small gallbladder size in the face of obstruction is a result of chronic fibrosis observed intraoperatively. The position of the obstructive soft tissue precluded biopsy or surgical management, and differential diagnoses included inflammatory disease and neoplasia.

References

1. Schwartz SG, Mitchell SL, Keating JH, Chan DL. Liver lobe torsion in dogs: 13 cases (1995–2004). J Am Vet Med Assoc. 2006;228: 242–247.

2. Lee KJ, Yamada K, Hirokawa H, Shimizu J, Kishimoto M, Iwasaki T, et al. Liver lobe torsion in a Shih-tzu dog. The Journal of small animal practice. 2009;50:157.

3. Yoon W, Jeong YY, Kim JK, Seo JJ, Lim HS, Shin SS, et al. CT in blunt liver trauma. Radiographics. 2005;25:87–104.

4. Marolf AJ, Kraft SL, Dunphy TR, Twedt DC. Magnetic resonance (MR) imaging and MR cholangiopancreatography findings in cats with cholangitis and pancreatitis. J Feline Med Surg. 2013;15: 285–294.

5. Scharf G, Deplazes P, Kaser-Hotz B, Borer L, Hasler A, Haller M, et al. Radiographic, ultrasonographic, and computed tomographic appearance of alveolar echinococcosis in dogs. Vet Radiol Ultrasound. 2004;45:411–418.

6. El-Serag HB, Marrero JA, Rudolph L, Reddy KR. Diagnosis and Treatment of Hepatocellular Carcinoma. Gastroenterology. 2008;134:1752–1763.

7. Hussain SM, Zondervan PE, JN IJ, Schalm SW, de Man RA, Krestin GP. Benign versus malignant hepatic nodules: MR imaging findings with pathologic correlation. Radiographics. 2002;22:1023–1036– discussion 1037–1029.

8. Terayama N, Matsui O, Ueda K, Kobayashi S, Sanada J, Gabata T, et al. Peritumoral rim enhancement of liver metastasis: hemodynamics observed on single-level dynamic CT during hepatic

arteriography and histopathologic correlation. J Comput Assist Tomogr. 2002;26:975–980.

9. Taniura T, Marukawa K, Yamada K, Hikasa Y, Ito K. Differential diagnosis of hepatic tumor-like lesions in dog by using dynamic CT scanning. Hiroshima J Med Sci. 2009;58:17–24.

10. Fukushima K, Kanemoto H, Ohno K, Takahashi M, Nakashima K, Fujino Y, et al. CT characteristics of primary hepatic mass lesions in dogs. Vet Radiol Ultrasound. 2012;53:252–257.

11. Clifford CA, Pretorius ES, Weisse C, Sorenmo KU, Drobatz KJ, Siegelman ES, et al. Magnetic resonance imaging of focal splenic and hepatic lesions in the dog. J Vet Intern Med. 2004;18: 330–338.

12. Cullen JM. Summary of the World Small Animal Veterinary Association Standardization Committee Guide to Classification of Liver Disease in Dogs and Cats. Veterinary Clinics of NA: Small Animal Practice. 2009;39:395–418.

13. Yonetomi D, Kadosawa T, Miyoshi K, Nakao Y, Homma E, Hanazono K, et al. Contrast agent Gd-EOB-DTPA (EOB·Primovist®)

for low-field magnetic resonance imaging of canine focal liver lesions. Vet Radiol Ultrasound. 2012;53:371–380.

14. Kamaya A, Maturen KE, Tye GA, Liu YI, Parti NN, Desser TS. Hypervascular Liver Lesions. Seminars in Ultrasound, CT and MRI. 2009;30:387–407.

15. Feeney DA, Sharkey LC, Steward SM, Bahr KL, Henson MS, Ito D, et al. Parenchymal signal intensity in 3-T body MRI of dogs with hematopoietic neoplasia. Comp Med. 2013;63:174–182.

16. Noronha V, Shafi NQ, Obando JA, Kummar S. Primary non-Hodgkin's lymphoma of the liver. Crit Rev Oncol Hematol. 2005;53:199–207.

17. Levy AD. Malignant liver tumors. Clin Liver Dis. 2002;6:147–164.

18. Zatelli A, D'Ippolito P, Bonfanti U, Zini E. Ultrasound-assisted drainage and alcoholization of hepatic and renal cysts: 22 cases. J Am Anim Hosp Assoc. 2007;43:112–116.

19. Nakamura M, Chen H-M, Momoi Y, Iwasaki T. Clinical application of computed tomography for the diagnosis of feline hepatic lipidosis. J Vet Med Sci. 2005;67:1163–1165.

5.4

Gastrointestinal tract

Introduction

Contrast radiography and endoscopy continue to be the most common approaches for diagnosis of intraluminal disorders, mucosal/mural defects, and abnormal gastrointestinal position and motility disorders in human and veterinary medicine. Although diagnostic ultrasound is widely used for evaluation of mural masses and extramural diseases, such as regional metastasis, CT and, to a lesser extent, MR can sometimes be more specific and sensitive and are increasingly used for these purposes.[1–3] Cross-sectional imaging of the gastrointestinal tract is challenging because of variations in the volume of intraluminal gas, fluid, and solid contents that can markedly alter luminal diameter and shape, mural thickness, visibility of wall layers, and the appearance of the mucosal lining (Figure 5.4.1). In addition to routine scanning with or without intravenous contrast enhancement, virtual endoscopic examinations are currently performed in people following distension of the stomach or colon with gas or positive contrast medium.[4–12] Similar techniques have been reported in the veterinary literature but are not yet in widespread use.[13] Virtual gastroscopy and colonoscopy provide an excellent view of the gastrointestinal mucosal surface unencumbered by luminal collapse.

CT measurements of unenhanced and contrast-enhanced gastrointestinal wall thickness are in the range of those reported for abdominal ultrasonography. There is also a positive correlation between wall thickness and diameter with increasing body weight. The gastrointestinal wall may not be visible in segments that are collapsed.[14] Wall layers are visible in 22% of segments, most often in the stomach and jejunum.

Imaging of the stomach is traditionally performed using contrast gastrography, ultrasound, or endoscopy. However, prominent gastric rugal folds can sometimes mimic mural masses when viewed using these imaging modalities. In these instances, CT can be performed following distension of the stomach to rule out mural pathology. With the stomach distended, CT imaging enables noninvasive visualization of the entire gastric wall. The stomach can be distended with 30 ml/kg of water to reduce the gastric rugal folds normally present, and intravenous contrast medium can be used to define the soft-tissue layers of the gastric wall.[15] Gastric mucosa and submucosa intensely enhance immediately following intravenous contrast administration and remain enhanced during early delayed phase imaging.

Virtual endoscopy is an alternative approach to imaging the gastrointestinal tract. Following gas distension of the stomach or colon, a three-dimensional CT representation of the mucosal surface is computer generated from transverse images, with the resulting data set mimicking the anatomy viewed using traditional endoscopy techniques (Figure 5.4.2). Advantages are that all mucosal surfaces can be evaluated and, unlike conventional endoscopy, the technique is noninvasive. The two-dimensional CT images can also be used in combination with endoscopic images to evaluate mural and extramural pathology. A limitation of virtual endoscopy is that it is not possible to obtain functional real-time analysis of peristalsis or mural biopsies with this technique.

Atlas of Small Animal CT and MRI, First Edition. Erik R. Wisner and Allison L. Zwingenberger.
© 2015 John Wiley & Sons, Inc. Published 2015 by John Wiley & Sons, Inc.

Mechanical obstruction, trauma, and hemorrhage

In imaging the acute abdomen, mechanical obstruction of the gastrointestinal tract is often a primary differential diagnosis. Radiographs and ultrasonography are used most often to diagnose mechanical obstruction. However, large patient size, gas, and subtle abnormalities may hinder diagnosis. CT can be used to detect such imaging signs as intestinal dilation with gas and fluid, foreign bodies, and plication due to linear foreign body.[16] CT is less sensitive than ultrasonography for detection of secondary complications of gastrointestinal perforation, such as free air or small amounts of free fluid.[16] Foreign bodies may be identified within the lumen of the stomach (Figure 5.4.3). The inflammatory tracts associated with penetrating foreign bodies provide valuable diagnostic information regarding gastric or bowel wall perforation and extramural disease (Figure 5.4.4).[17,18] CT has been used in people to identify gastrointestinal mural pathology following blunt abdominal trauma, but some reports suggest it is not a sensitive test for lesion detection.[19-21]

CT angiography is sometimes used for diagnosis of acute gastrointestinal hemorrhage and mesenteric ischemia in people and is considered both sensitive and specific when performed on multidetector CT systems using rapid multiphase imaging protocols.[22] The technique has not been sufficiently explored to determine its diagnostic value in veterinary medicine.

Inflammatory and vascular disorders

Gastritis, enteritis, and colitis result in a diffuse thickening of the bowel wall, which may be visible on CT images (Figures 5.4.5). Diffuse, uniform to heterogeneous contrast enhancement results from the inflammatory process, and increased attenuation may be seen in surrounding fat (Figure 5.4.6). Ileus of the bowel causes marked dilation of the stomach and bowel segments with fluid (Figure 5.4.7). These conditions have not been well described in the veterinary literature to date, but the use of CT and MR has been extensively reported in people for evaluation of Crohn's disease and other inflammatory gastrointestinal disorders.[23-28]

Inflammatory polyps occur in the stomach and small intestine as mucosal masses that protrude into the lumen and may cause outflow obstruction (Figure 5.4.8). Their tendency to extend into the lumen of the stomach makes virtual endoscopy a viable method of visualization.[13]

Neoplasia

Leiomyoma and leiomyosarcoma

Leiomyoma and leiomyosarcoma are discrete masses of the gastric or bowel wall.[29,30] These may appear as a focal, eccentric mass with loss of layering and peripheral or heterogeneous contrast enhancement.[15] These tumors may be mineralized (Figure 5.4.9) and can cause partial bowel or gastric outflow obstruction (Figure 5.4.10).

Gastrointestinal stromal tumors

Gastrointestinal stromal tumors (GISTs) are rare in dogs and cats but have been reported in both species.[31-33] GISTs are neoplasms of mesenchymal origin arising in the colon (48%), small intestine (29%), stomach (19%), and mesentery (5%) according to one canine study.[31] CT imaging features described in people include well-defined masses with heterogeneous contrast enhancement sometimes with central fluid attenuation. Masses can become quite large before causing clinical signs because of their tendency to grow outward, which minimizes the likelihood of gastrointestinal obstruction (Figure 5.4.11).[34]

Lymphoma

Gastrointestinal lymphoma has been reported in both dogs and cats and is the most common tumor affecting the alimentary tract in cats.[35,36] Lymphoma causes moderate to severe mural thickening and may occur in any region of the stomach or intestine (Figure 5.4.12). It is often circumferential, with moderate heterogeneous contrast enhancement and hyperattenuating mucosa (Figure 5.4.13).[14,15] Increased, tortuous arteries may be seen supplying the affected portion of the stomach.[16] On MR images, lymphoma of the mesentery is isointense on T1 with moderate contrast enhancement and hyperintense on T2 images.[37]

Adenocarcinoma

Adenocarcinoma is the most common malignant gastric neoplasm in dogs, with Rough-Coated Collies, Staffordshire Terriers, Chow Chows, Hovawarts, and Belgian Shepherds predisposed.[33,35] Although rare, gastric adenocarcinoma is also occasionally seen in cats.[35] Adenocarcinoma of the stomach appears as a focal wall thickening without discrete wall layering. Contrast enhancement is heterogeneous with a hyperattenuating mucosa.[15] In the intestine, adenocarcinoma appears as circumferential wall thickening with heterogeneous contrast enhancement (Figures 5.4.14, 5.4.15).

Figure 5.4.1   Normal Gastrointestinal Tract (Canine) CT

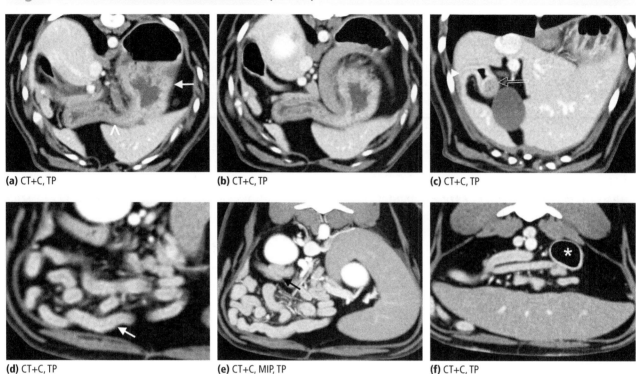

(a) CT+C, TP   **(b)** CT+C, TP   **(c)** CT+C, TP

(d) CT+C, TP   **(e)** CT+C, MIP, TP   **(f)** CT+C, TP

3y MC mixed-breed dog. The stomach is filled with a small amount of fluid and gas located in the fundus (**a**). The mucosa is intensely contrast enhancing, defining multiple rugal folds (**a**: arrow). The body of the stomach is smaller in size with a smoother wall (**a**: caret). The pylorus is thicker because of its musculature (**c**: open arrow) and joins with the duodenum (**c**: arrowhead) near the right body wall. The serosal layer of the small intestine is contrast enhancing (**d**: arrow). The ileocolic junction is located in the right abdomen (**e**: arrow). The ileum is medial, and the empty colon is lateral in these images. The colon contains a variable amount of gas, fluid, and feces, affecting the thickness of the wall (**f**: asterisk).

Figure 5.4.2   Virtual Colonoscopy (Canine) CT

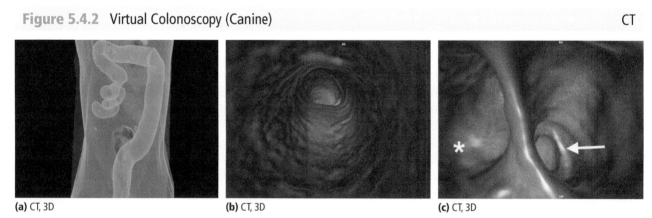

(a) CT, 3D   **(b)** CT, 3D   **(c)** CT, 3D

1y M mixed-breed dog. Pneumocolonography requires gas distension of the colonic wall, allowing the mucosal surface to be evaluated. A 3D rendering of the colon shows its size and course within the abdomen. The colon and cecum are distended (**a**). Internal renderings of the 3D image allow visualization of the mucosal surface (**b**). The ileocecocolic junction is visible as a small orifice (**c**: arrow) at the termination of the ascending colon (**c**: asterisk).

Figure 5.4.3   Gastric Foreign Body (Canine)   CT

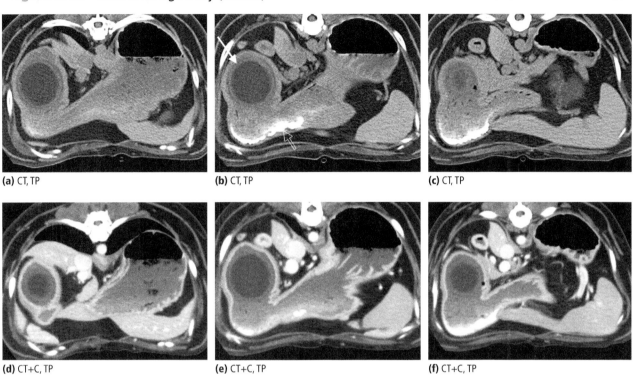

(a) CT, TP   **(b)** CT, TP   **(c)** CT, TP

(d) CT+C, TP   **(e)** CT+C, TP   **(f)** CT+C, TP

11y MC Golden Retriever presenting for radiation therapy of a soft-tissue sarcoma on the thoracic wall. Images **a–c** and comparable contrast enhanced images **d–f** are ordered from cranial to caudal. A large, round foreign body (**b**: arrow) is identified in the gastric pylorus as a clinically silent finding. The foreign body is located in a nondependent position, indicating that it is fixed. The stomach is moderately distended with fluid. There is particulate mineral-opacity material sedimenting ventrally, representing a gravel sign and partial outflow obstruction (**b**: open arrow). The gastric wall appears normal in thickness and enhances normally on contrast-enhanced images (**d–f**). A rubber ball was surgically removed from the stomach.

Figure 5.4.4 Penetrating Gastric Foreign Body (Canine)   CT

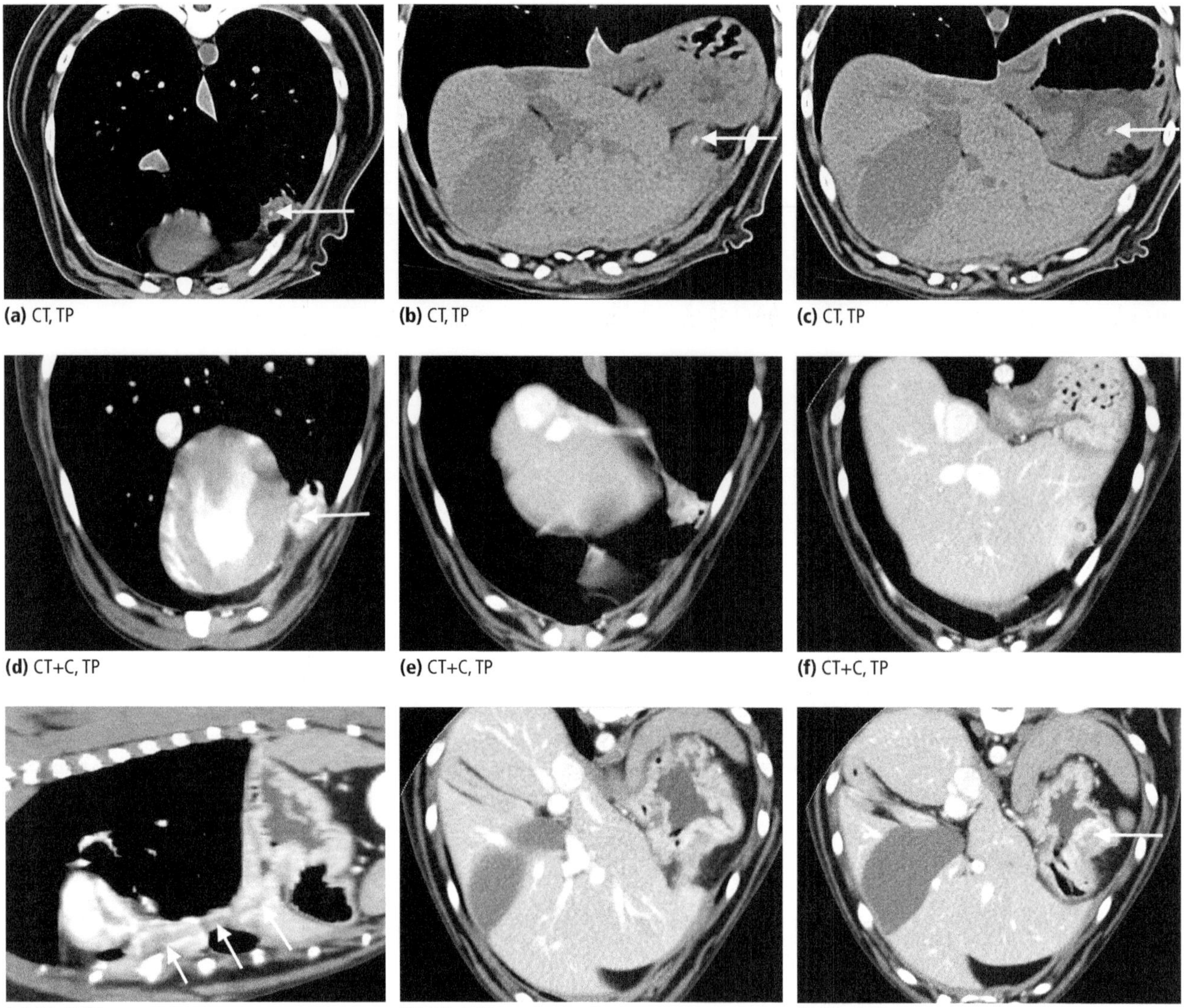

(a) CT, TP

(b) CT, TP

(c) CT, TP

(d) CT+C, TP

(e) CT+C, TP

(f) CT+C, TP

(g) CT+C, SP

(h) CT+C, TP

(i) CT+C, TP

5y MC Cocker Spaniel with persistent pulmonary infiltrates in the left caudal lung lobe. Unenhanced (**a–c**) and contrast-enhanced (**d–f,h,i**) transverse images are ordered from cranial to caudal. There is increased opacity in the left caudal lung lobe, with a central hyperattenuating linear structure that can be followed from the thorax to the ventral gastric wall (**a–c**: arrow). On contrast-enhanced images, the pulmonary infiltrates are intensely enhancing with a central lucent region of fluid attenuation (**d,i**: arrow). The hyperattenuating structure remains visible within the fluid tract and can be followed on the sagittal image through the diaphragm (**g**: arrows). The gastric wall has a focal thickening where the foreign body originates (**h,i**). A bamboo skewer was surgically removed.

Figure 5.4.5 Gastritis (Canine)

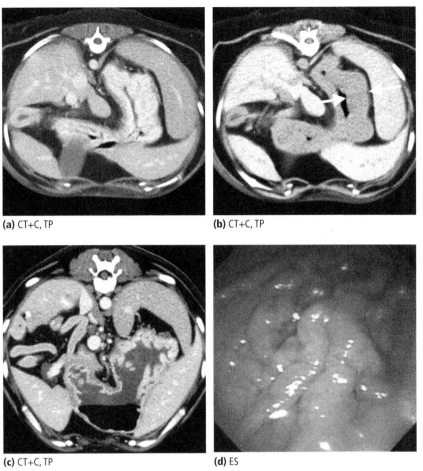

(a) CT+C, TP

(b) CT+C, TP

(c) CT+C, TP

(d) ES

6y MC Shetland Sheepdog with chronic bicavitary effusion. There is focal, marked thickening of the gastric wall in portal phase (**a**) and delayed phase (**b**: arrows) images. The rugal folds are thickened; however, wall layering is not disrupted. A normal stomach is included for comparison (**c**). Rugal thickening and nondistensibility of the stomach were found on endoscopy (**d**). The biopsy diagnosis was lymphoplasmacytic gastritis.

Figure 5.4.6 Colitis (Canine)

CT

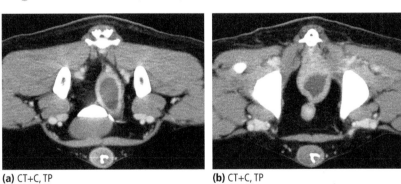

(a) CT+C, TP

(b) CT+C, TP

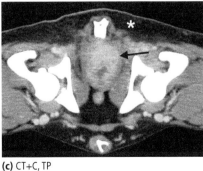

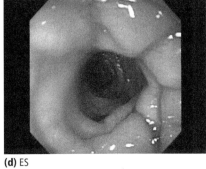

(c) CT+C, TP

(d) ES

7y MC Soft-Coated Wheaten Terrier with 2-month history of tenesmus and hematochezia. CT images are ordered from cranial to caudal. The terminal portion of the colon and rectum are fluid filled with a markedly thickened wall. The rectal wall is asymmetrically thickened near the anus (**c**: arrow), with partial obstruction of the lumen. Increased attenuation of adjacent fat is present in the subcutaneous tissue in this region, suggesting regional inflammation (**c**: asterisk). The affected colonic tissues are uniformly and intensely contrast enhancing. A colonoscopic image reveals irregular mucosal lining consistent with an annular mural lesion (**d**). Biopsy confirmed chronic, diffuse lymphoplasmacytic and eosinophilic colitis.

Figure 5.4.7 Enterocolitis and Ileus (Canine) CT

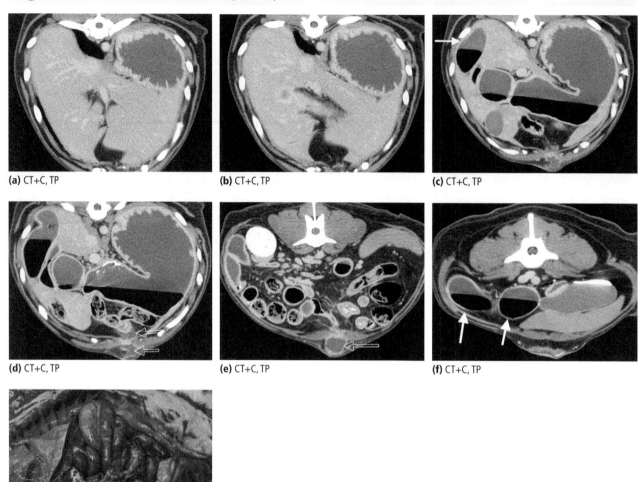

(a) CT+C, TP

(b) CT+C, TP

(c) CT+C, TP

(d) CT+C, TP

(e) CT+C, TP

(f) CT+C, TP

(g) GP, LAT

5y MC Labrador Retriever with a history of regurgitation and distended bowel for 1 week. Images were obtained in dorsal recumbency, and inverted fluid–gas interfaces are visible. CT images are ordered from cranial to caudal. The stomach is markedly distended with fluid (**c**: arrowhead), as is the duodenum (**c,f**: arrows). Other loops of small intestine are thickened with foamy gas and fluid contents. A fluid-attenuating seroma with peripheral contrast enhancement is visible on the ventral body wall secondary to a previous laparotomy (**d,e**: open arrows) that extends into the peritoneal cavity. Gross postmortem findings were consistent with enterocolitis and ileus, and the diagnosis was confirmed histologically as chronic lymphoplasmacytic gastroenterocolitis.

Figure 5.4.8 Adenomatous Polyp—Pylorus (Canine)

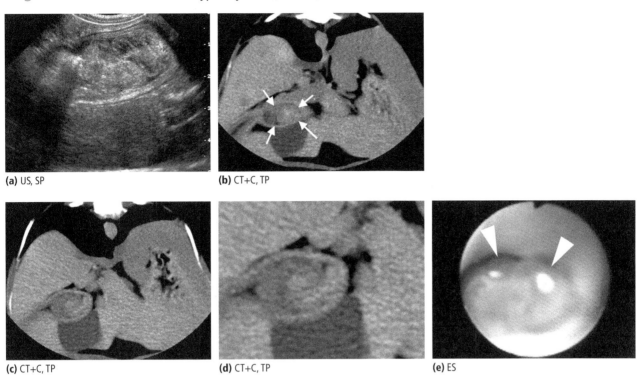

(a) US, SP

(b) CT+C, TP

(c) CT+C, TP

(d) CT+C, TP

(e) ES

14y MC Miniature Schnauzer with history of regurgitation. Ultrasonography was initially performed, which showed a hyperechoic mass occupying the lumen of the pylorus. Images **b** and **c** are ordered from caudal to cranial, and image **d** is a magnification of image **c**. Delayed-contrast CT images show a hypoattenuating to isoattenuating mass in the pyloric antrum (**b**: arrows). The mass is heterogeneous with a hyperattenuating center. The pyloric wall is not thickened in this region. An endoscopic examination revealed a mural mass protruding into the pyloric lumen (**e**: arrowheads). Excisional biopsy confirmed a diagnosis of adenomatous polyp.

Figure 5.4.9 Leiomyoma—Stomach (Canine)

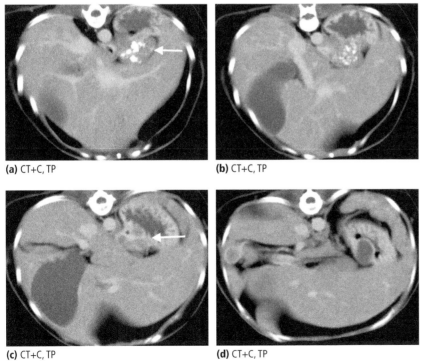

(a) CT+C, TP

(b) CT+C, TP

17y MC mixed-breed dog. Images are ordered from cranial to caudal. A gastric mass was identified on screening ultrasound. The well-defined mass on the medial wall of the fundus has multifocal mineralized regions (**a**: arrow). The gastric wall is focally thickened with hypoattenuating contents caudally and peripheral contrast enhancement (**c**: arrow). The most caudal aspect of the mass (**d**) remains centrally unenhanced. Surgical excisional biopsy confirmed a diagnosis of gastric leiomyoma.

(c) CT+C, TP

(d) CT+C, TP

Figure 5.4.10 Leiomyosarcoma—Colon (Feline)

CT

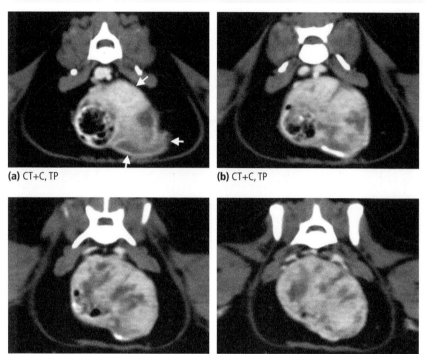

(a) CT+C, TP   (b) CT+C, TP

(c) CT+C, TP   (d) CT+C, TP

9y FS Domestic Mediumhair with hematochezia. Images are through the distal colon and are ordered from cranial to caudal. There is a large, eccentric, heterogeneously contrast-enhancing mass originating from the colonic wall (a: arrows). More caudally, the mass compresses the colonic lumen, which is identified by gas and mineral-opacity feces (b–d). Surgical excisional biopsy confirmed a diagnosis of colonic leiomyosarcoma.

Figure 5.4.11 Gastrointestinal Stromal Tumor—Cecum (Canine)

CT

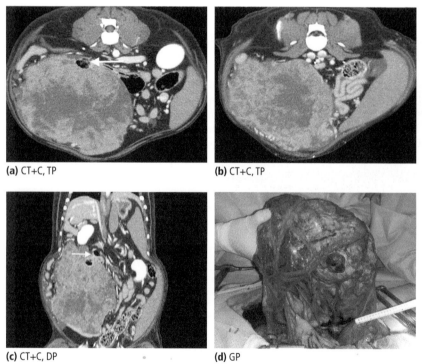

(a) CT+C, TP   (b) CT+C, TP

(c) CT+C, DP   (d) GP

7y FS Golden Retriever with progressive abdominal distension. There is an extremely large mass in the right abdomen, causing displacement of the remainder of the abdominal viscera to the left side. The mass is heterogeneously and peripherally contrast enhancing. A region of bowel containing gas, identified as the cecum, is visible in the dorsal and cranial aspect of the mass (a,c: arrow). The mass was surgically excised and histologically diagnosed as a gastrointestinal stromal tumor (d).

Figure 5.4.12   Lymphoma—Stomach (Canine)

MR

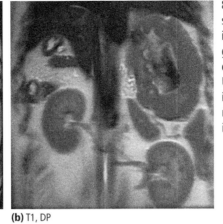

8y MC Rottweiler with multifocal neurologic signs. The gastric wall is markedly thickened in the region of the fundus (**c**: arrow). The gastric wall is homogeneously hypointense on T1 images and hyperintense on T2 images. Ultrasound images showed loss of wall layering in addition to thickening (**e**). The necropsy revealed disseminated T-cell lymphoma including the gastric wall (**f**).

(a) T1, TP

(b) T1, DP

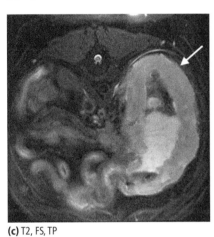

(c) T2, FS, TP

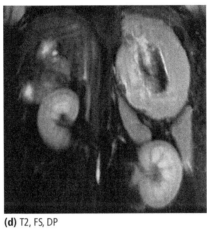

(d) T2, FS, DP

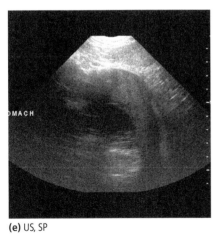

(e) US, SP

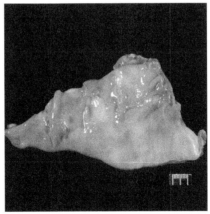

(f) GP

Figure 5.4.13 Lymphoma—Jejunum (Canine)

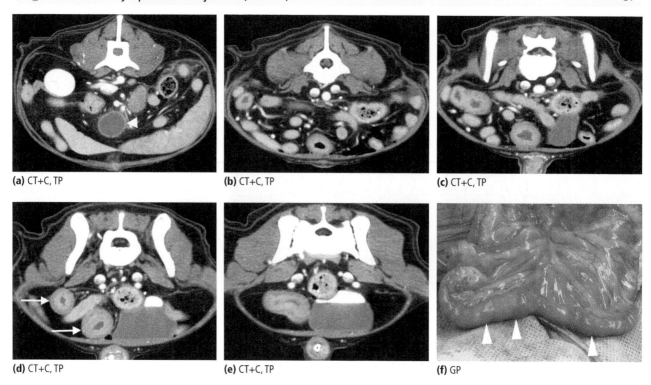

(a) CT+C, TP   **(b)** CT+C, TP   **(c)** CT+C, TP

(d) CT+C, TP   **(e)** CT+C, TP   **(f)** GP

10y MC Golden Retriever with vomiting with increasing frequency. CT images are ordered from cranial to caudal. The mesenteric lymph nodes are markedly enlarged and rounded with peripheral contrast enhancement (**a**: arrowhead). In the caudal abdomen, a segment of jejunum has thickened walls with a contrast-enhancing inner region and hypoattenuating outer region (**d**: arrows). Pneumoperitoneum is present secondary to previous surgery. T-cell lymphoma was present in the jejunum (**f**: arrowheads) and mesenteric lymph nodes.

Figure 5.4.14 Adenocarcinoma—Duodenum (Canine)

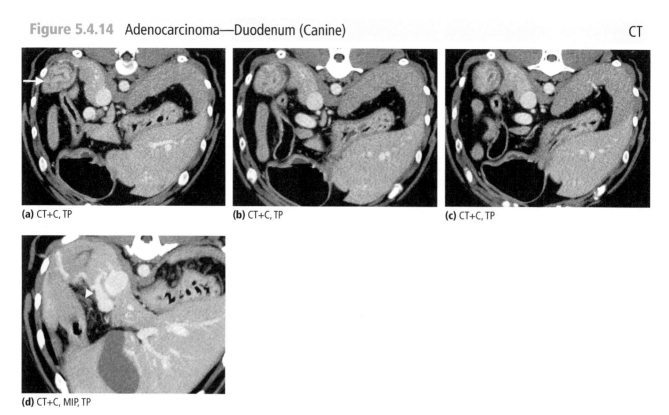

(a) CT+C, TP   **(b)** CT+C, TP   **(c)** CT+C, TP

(d) CT+C, MIP, TP

9y FS German Wirehaired Pointer with anorexia, vomiting, and weight loss for several months. Images **a–c** are ordered from cranial to caudal. The duodenum is markedly and eccentrically thickened. There is heterogeneous contrast enhancement (**a**: arrow), which is more prominent centrally in some regions. The bile duct enters the duodenum in a region of wall thickening; however, it does not appear to be obstructed (**d**: arrowhead). Excisional biopsy confirmed a diagnosis of adenocarcinoma.

Figure 5.4.15   Adenocarcinoma—Colon (Feline)

CT

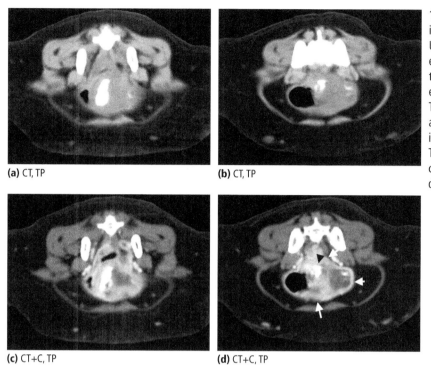

(a) CT, TP

(b) CT, TP

(c) CT+C, TP

(d) CT+C, TP

15y FS Siamese with a 2-week history of vomiting, hematochezia, and straining to defecate. Unenhanced (**a,b**) and comparable contrast-enhanced (**c,d**) images are ordered from caudal to cranial. On unenhanced images, there is an eccentric mass arising from the wall of the colon. The central region of the mass is mineralized (**d**: arrowhead). The colonic lumen is compressed, indicating partial obstruction by the mass. The mass is heterogeneously and peripherally contrast enhancing (**d**: arrows). The cytologic diagnosis was adenocarcinoma.

References

1. Federle MP. Gastroduodenal Anatomy and Imaging Issues. In: Federle MP (ed): Diagnostic Imaging: Abdomen. Salt Lake City: Amirsys, Inc., 2005;I:3–2–5.

2. Federle MP. Colon Anatomy and Imaging Issues. In: Federle MP (ed): Diagnostic Imaging: Abdomen. Salt Lake City: Salt Lake City, 2005;I:5–2–5.

3. Federle MP. Small Intestine Anatomy and Imaging Issues. In: Federle MP (ed): Diagnostic Imaging: Abdomen. Salt Lake City: Salt Lake City, 2005;I:4–2–5.

4. Boellaard TN, de Haan MC, Venema HW, Stoker J. Colon distension and scan protocol for CT-colonography: an overview. Eur J Radiol. 2013;82:1144–1158.

5. Boone D, Halligan S, Taylor SA. Evidence review and status update on computed tomography colonography. Curr Gastroenterol Rep. 2011;13:486–494.

6. Christensen KN, Fidler JL, Fletcher JG, Maccarty R, Johnson CD. Pictorial review of colonic polyp and mass distortion and recognition with the CT virtual dissection technique. Radiographics. 2010;30:e42; discussion e43.

7. Ghuman M, Bates N, Moore H. Computed tomographic colonography (CTC): a retrospective analysis of a single site experience and a review of the literature on the status of CTC. N Z Med J. 2012;125:60–67.

8. Rockey DC. Computed tomographic colonography: ready for prime time? Gastroenterol Clin North Am. 2010;39:901–909.

9. Rockey DC. Computed tomographic and magnetic resonance colonography: challenge for colonoscopy. Dig Dis. 2012;30 Suppl 2:60–67.

10. Rosenberg JA, Rubin DT. Performance of CT colonography in clinical trials. Gastrointest Endosc Clin N Am. 2010;20:193–207.

11. Shen Y, Kang HK, Jeong YY, Heo SH, Han SM, Chen K, et al. Evaluation of early gastric cancer at multidetector CT with multiplanar reformation and virtual endoscopy. Radiographics. 2011;31:189–199.

12. Yee J, Sadda S, Aslam R, Yeh B. Extracolonic findings at CT colonography. Gastrointest Endosc Clin N Am. 2010;20:305–322.

13. Yamada K, Morimoto M, Kishimoto M, Wisner ER. Virtual endoscopy of dogs using multi-detector row CT. Vet Radiol Ultrasound. 2007;48:318–322.

14. Hoey S, Drees R, Hetzel S. Evaluation of the gastrointestinal tract in dogs using computed tomography. Vet Radiol Ultrasound. 2013;54:25–30.

15. Terragni R, Vignoli M, Rossi F, Laganga P, Leone VF, Graham JP, et al. Stomach wall evaluation using helical hydro–computed tomography. Vet Radiol Ultrasound. 2012;53:402–405.

16. Shanaman MM, Schwarz T, Gal A, O'Brien RT. Comparison between survey radiography, B-mode ultrasonography, contrast-enhanced ultrasonography and contrast-enhanced multi-detector computed tomography findings in dogs with acute abdominal signs. Vet Radiol Ultrasound. 2013;54:591–604.

17. Furukawa A, Sakoda M, Yamasaki M, Kono N, Tanaka T, Nitta N, et al. Gastrointestinal tract perforation: CT diagnosis of presence, site, and cause. Abdom Imaging. 2005;30:524–534.

18. Ghahremani GG. Radiologic evaluation of suspected gastrointestinal perforations. Radiol Clin North Am. 1993;31:1219–1234.

19. Halvorsen RA, Jr., McKenney K. Blunt trauma to the gastrointestinal tract: CT findings with small bowel and colon injuries. Emerg Radiol. 2002;9:141–145.

20. Katz DS, Yam B, Hines JJ, Mazzie JP, Lane MJ, Abbas MA. Uncommon and unusual gastrointestinal causes of the acute abdomen: computed tomographic diagnosis. Semin Ultrasound CT MR. 2008;29:386–398.

21. Peters E, LoSasso B, Foley J, Rodarte A, Duthie S, Senac MO, Jr. Blunt bowel and mesenteric injuries in children: do nonspecific computed tomography findings reliably identify these injuries? Pediatr Crit Care Med. 2006;7:551–556.

22. Johnson JO. Diagnosis of acute gastrointestinal hemorrhage and acute mesenteric ischemia in the era of multi-detector row CT. Radiol Clin North Am. 2012;50:173–182.

23. Al-Hawary MM, Kaza RK, Platt JF. CT enterography: concepts and advances in Crohn's disease imaging. Radiol Clin North Am. 2013;51:1–16.

24. Amitai MM, Ben-Horin S, Eliakim R, Kopylov U. Magnetic resonance enterography in Crohn's disease: a guide to common imaging manifestations for the IBD physician. J Crohns Colitis. 2013;7:603–615.

25. Gee MS, Harisinghani MG. MRI in patients with inflammatory bowel disease. J Magn Reson Imaging. 2011;33:527–534.

26. Ilangovan R, Burling D, George A, Gupta A, Marshall M, Taylor SA. CT enterography: review of technique and practical tips. Br J Radiol. 2012;85:876–886.

27. Masselli G, Gualdi G. CT and MR enterography in evaluating small bowel diseases: when to use which modality? Abdom Imaging. 2013;38:249–259.

28. Pariente B, Peyrin-Biroulet L, Cohen L, Zagdanski AM, Colombel JF. Gastroenterology review and perspective: the role of cross-sectional imaging in evaluating bowel damage in Crohn disease. AJR Am J Roentgenol. 2011;197:42–49.

29. Kapatkin AS, Mullen HS, Matthiesen DT, Patnaik AK. Leiomyosarcoma in dogs: 44 cases (1983–1988). J Am Vet Med Assoc. 1992;201:1077–1079.

30. Swann HM, Holt DE. Canine gastric adenocarcinoma and leiomyosarcoma: a retrospective study of 21 cases (1986–1999) and literature review. J Am Anim Hosp Assoc. 2002;38:157–164.

31. Frost D, Lasota J, Miettinen M. Gastrointestinal stromal tumors and leiomyomas in the dog: a histopathologic, immunohisto-chemical, and molecular genetic study of 50 cases. Vet Pathol. 2003;40:42–54.

32. Morini M, Gentilini F, Pietra M, Spadari A, Turba ME, Mandrioli L, et al. Cytological, immunohistochemical and mutational analysis of a gastric gastrointestinal stromal tumour in a cat. J Comp Pathol. 2011;145:152–157.

33. von Babo V, Eberle N, Mischke R, Meyer-Lindenberg A, Hewicker-Trautwein M, Nolte I, et al. Canine non-hematopoietic gastric neoplasia. Epidemiologic and diagnostic characteristics in 38 dogs with post-surgical outcome of five cases. Tierarztl Prax Ausg K Kleintiere Heimtiere. 2012;40:243–249.

34. Burkill GJ, Badran M, Al-Muderis O, Meirion Thomas J, Judson IR, Fisher C, et al. Malignant gastrointestinal stromal tumor: distribution, imaging features, and pattern of metastatic spread. Radiology. 2003;226:527–532.

35. Gualtieri M, Monzeglio MG, Scanziani E. Gastric neoplasia. Vet Clin North Am Small Anim Pract. 1999;29:415–440.

36. Gustafson TL, Villamil A, Taylor BE, Flory A. A retrospective study of feline gastric lymphoma in 16 chemotherapy-treated cats. J Am Anim Hosp Assoc. 2014;50:46–52.

37. Yasuda D, Fujita M, Yasuda S, Taniguchi A, Miura H, Hasegawa D, et al. Usefulness of MRI compared with CT for diagnosis of mesenteric lymphoma in a dog. J Vet Med Sci. 2004;66:1447–1451.

5.5

Pancreas

The canine and feline pancreas is readily visible on unenhanced and contrast-enhanced CT images and on MR images. CT is preferred because of faster scanning times and the ability to eliminate motion artifact when viewing the thin tissue of the pancreas. However, MR has increased contrast resolution and provides excellent information in inflammatory diseases, such as chronic pancreatitis.[1]

The normal feline pancreatic thickness on T1 images is 9.5 ± 1.2 mm, and pancreatic duct size is 1.65 ± 0.05 mm.[2] The pancreas is T1 hyperintense and T2 hypointense compared to the liver, with a uniform architecture. The feline pancreatic duct is oriented in the long axis of each lobe and may be visualized as a hypoattenuating (CT), hypointense (T1), or hyperintense (T2, FSE) linear structure. The feline pancreas is hypoattenuating to liver on unenhanced CT images, with rapid contrast enhancement and gradual washout (Figure 5.5.1).[3] CT imaging features of the canine pancreas are similar (Figure 5.5.2).

Multiphase CT angiography allows the evaluation of pancreatic tissues in the native, arterial, portal, and delayed phases of contrast enhancement. The canine pancreas is isoattenuating to liver on unenhanced images, hyperattenuating on arterial phase images, and hypoattenuating on portal and delayed phase images. The attenuation differences are due to the purely arterial blood supply of the pancreas, which results in rapid enhancement following injection of contrast medium, compared to the predominantly portal enhancement of the liver. The pancreaticoduodenal artery is visible during the arterial phase, and the pancreaticoduodenal vein opacifies during the portal and delayed phases (Figure 5.5.3).[4]

Inflammatory disorders

Acute pancreatitis has been diagnosed using CT imaging in dogs and cats (Figures 5.5.4, 5.5.5). The pancreas is enlarged with irregular borders and is intensely contrast enhancing. Regions of hypoattenuation may be present in necrotic regions. The surrounding mesentery has fat stranding secondary to local inflammation.[5] Chronic pancreatitis resulting in fibrosis and fat replacement may be hypoattenuating and poorly contrast enhancing (Figures 5.5.6, 5.5.7).[6] Nodular regions and mild enlargement without surrounding mesenteric inflammation are characteristic of chronic pancreatitis.

Pancreatitis is a challenging disease to diagnose in cats using ultrasound and CT. MR imaging shows promise in detecting these changes with increased tissue contrast and 3D volume imaging. Pancreatitis appears as T1 hypointensity and T2 hyperintensity with pancreatic duct dilation. The signal intensity changes are likely caused by edema and fibrosis. Administration of secretin can be used to dilate the pancreatic duct. This improves visualization of the pancreatic duct in normal cats; however, in those with pancreatitis, it causes only minimal change to ducts that are already dilated.[1] Unenhanced and contrast-enhanced CT images cannot consistently differentiate normal cats from those with pancreatitis unless there is marked pancreatic enlargement.[7]

Complications of pancreatitis in both species include formation of pseudocysts, abscesses, and necrosis. Pancreatic cysts and pseudocysts can also occur as incidental findings (Figure 5.5.8). On CT images, pseudocysts and abscesses appear fluid

Atlas of Small Animal CT and MRI, First Edition. Erik R. Wisner and Allison L. Zwingenberger.
© 2015 John Wiley & Sons, Inc. Published 2015 by John Wiley & Sons, Inc.

attenuating with thin to irregularly thickened borders. Inflammatory lesions are often peripherally contrast enhancing. Regions of tissue necrosis may fail to enhance on contrast images. Inflammatory pancreatic cysts may occur, appearing as multilocular, fluid-filled masses on CT images.[8]

Neoplasia

Insulinomas of the pancreas cause hypoglycemia and can lead to seizures. These tumors are often of small size and are difficult to localize both on ultrasound and on CT images. The addition of dual-phase CT angiography in evaluating for insulinoma maximizes the chance that attenuation differences will be visible for a small mass. A report of three dogs with insulinoma found that masses were best seen during the arterial phase, where strong contrast enhancement was present (Figure 5.5.9).[9] Few cases have been reported, and alternate enhancement patterns are possible (Figure 5.5.10). An increase in the number of tortuous vessels may be visible in the arterial phase, with heterogeneous contrast enhancement in the delayed phase. If the mass is large enough, the contour of the pancreatic lobe may be focally altered. Angiography is also advantageous in evaluating for local vascular invasion.

Adenocarcinoma of the pancreas occurs in dogs and cats. Irregular masses that deform the pancreatic margins may be present with heterogeneous contrast enhancement and regions of necrosis (Figure 5.5.11). Local lymph nodes and liver should be evaluated for evidence of metastatic disease.

Figure 5.5.1   Normal Pancreas (Feline)

CT

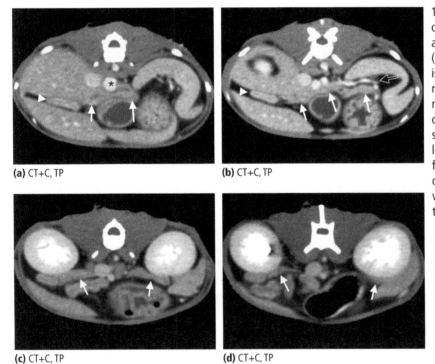

(a) CT+C, TP

(b) CT+C, TP

(c) CT+C, TP

(d) CT+C, TP

11y FS Rex. Images are ordered from cranial to caudal. The normal feline pancreas appears as an elongated structure in the cranial abdomen (a–d: white arrows). The body of the pancreas is ventral to the portal vein (a: asterisk). The right lobe is positioned medial to the duodenum (a,b: arrowheads), and the left lobe is cranial and dorsal to the colon, adjacent to the splenic vein (b: open arrow). The pancreatic lobes taper as they travel caudally (d). The feline left pancreatic lobe extends to the level of the left kidney (d). The pancreatic duct is visible as a hypoattenuating linear structure in the body of the pancreas (a).

Figure 5.5.2   Normal Pancreas (Canine)

CT

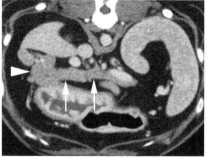

(a) CT+C, TP

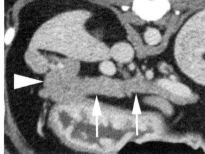

(b) CT+C, TP

10y MC Labrador Retriever. Images **a** and **c** are ordered cranial to caudal and **b** and **d** are magnifications of **a** and **c**, respectively. The body (**a**,**b**: arrowhead) and long axis of the left limb of the pancreas (**a**,**b**: arrows) are clearly seen on transverse images. The right limb of the pancreas often has a roughly triangular shape in cross-section (**c**,**d**: arrow) and is located medial to the descending duodenum (**c**,**d**: asterisk).

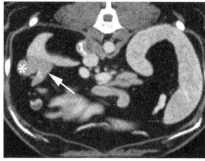

(c) CT+C, TP

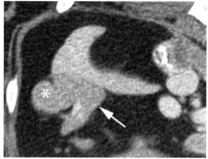

(d) CT+C, TP

Figure 5.5.3 Normal Pancreas—Four-Phase Angiographic Examination (Canine) CT

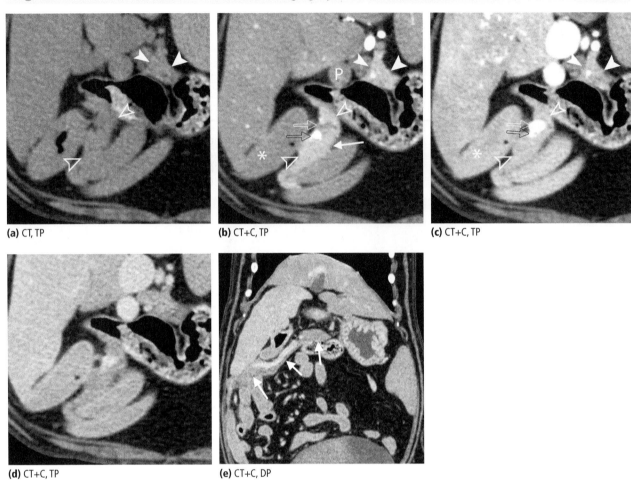

(a) CT, TP

(b) CT+C, TP

(c) CT+C, TP

(d) CT+C, TP

(e) CT+C, DP

2y M Border Collie presenting for portosystemic shunt. The four-phase angiographic images show the enhancement characteristics of a normal pancreas. The right pancreatic lobe (**a–c**: open arrowheads) is medial to the duodenum (**b,c**: asterisk), and the left pancreatic lobe (**a–c**: arrowheads) is medial to the portal vein (**b**: P). The pancreas is hyperattenuating to liver during the arterial phase (**b**: white arrow). The pancreaticoduodenal artery is contrast enhancing (**b**: black open arrow), while the pancreaticoduodenal vein is hypoattenuating (**b**: white open arrow). During the portal phase, the pancreas is isoattenuating to liver, and the pancreaticoduodenal vein contrast enhances (**c**: white open arrow) while the artery remains visible (**c**: black open arrow). The pancreas is hypoattenuating to liver during the delayed phase scan (**d**). The canine right pancreatic lobe is larger than the left (**e**: arrows).

Figure 5.5.4   Pancreatitis (Canine)   CT

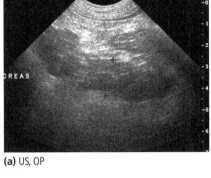

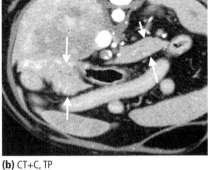

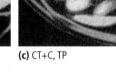

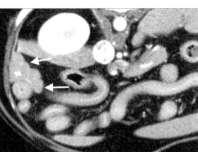

(a) US, OP   **(b)** CT+C, TP   **(c)** CT+C, TP

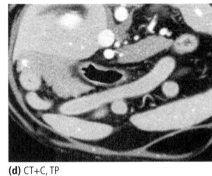

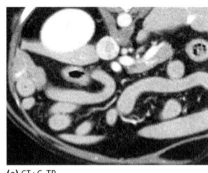

(d) CT+C, TP   **(e)** CT+C, TP

15y MC Cocker Spaniel with occasional decrease in appetite, invasive adrenal mass, and Spec cPL (canine pancreas-specific lipase) >1000 µg/L (normal range 0–200 µg/L). The pancreas is enlarged, hypoechoic, and surrounded by hyperechoic omentum on the ultrasound image (**a**: calipers). On arterial (**b,c**) and portal (**d,e**) phase CT images, there is enlargement of the pancreas with a lobular border (**b,c**: arrows). Contrast enhancement is uniform in both the arterial and portal phases. Mixed acute and chronic pancreatitis was found on histopathology.

Figure 5.5.5   Necrotizing Pancreatitis (Feline)   CT

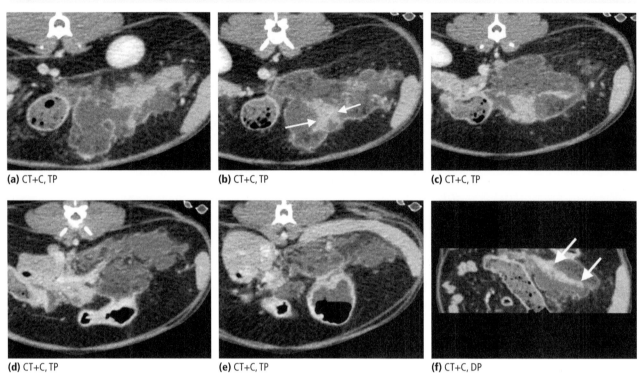

(a) CT+C, TP   **(b)** CT+C, TP   **(c)** CT+C, TP

(d) CT+C, TP   **(e)** CT+C, TP   **(f)** CT+C, DP

12y FS Domestic Shorthair with 1-week history of intermittent vomiting and anorexia. Images **a–e** are ordered from caudal to cranial. There is a large, irregular soft-tissue attenuating mass surrounding the left lobe of the pancreas. The pancreas is intensely contrast enhancing (**b,f**: arrows) and is enlarged. The central soft-tissue material is nonenhancing, consistent with fluid, with peripheral contrast enhancement. The fat surrounding this region is hyperattenuating, consistent with peritonitis and steatitis. Postmortem examination confirmed extensive suppurative and necrotizing pancreatitis with regional peritonitis, steatitis, and omental adhesions.

Figure 5.5.6   Chronic Pancreatitis (Canine)   CT

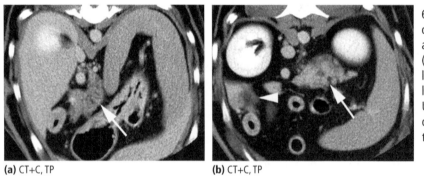

(a) CT+C, TP   **(b)** CT+C, TP

6y MC Rottweiler with a mast cell tumor. The owners report occasional vomiting. Images are ordered from cranial to caudal. The body (**a**: arrow), right limb (**b**: arrowhead), and left limb (**b**: arrow) of the pancreas are enlarged, lobular, and heterogeneously attenuating. Ultrasound-guided fine-needle aspiration cytology revealed moderate suppurative inflammation consistent with chronic pancreatitis.

Figure 5.5.7   Chronic Pancreatitis (Feline)   CT

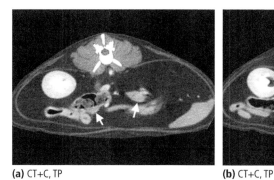
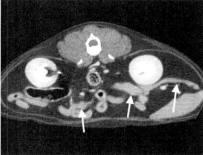

11y MC Domestic Shorthair with chronic vomiting. Images are ordered from cranial to caudal. The pancreas is moderately enlarged on both the left and right sides (**a,b**: arrows). The left lobe is clearly visible ventral and lateral to the left kidney (**b**). As is true for other modalities, CT imaging features of chronic pancreatitis in the cat can be subtle. The diagnosis was confirmed by an elevated spec fPL result.

(a) CT+C, TP   **(b)** CT+C, TP

Figure 5.5.8   Pancreatic Pseudocyst (Canine)   CT

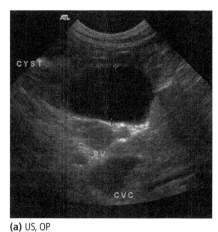
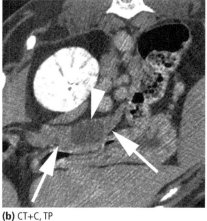

10y FS Labrador Retriever cross with a nasal squamous cell carcinoma. The CT examination was performed for staging purposes after a fluid-filled mass of uncertain origin was identified on a routine ultrasound examination (**a**: calipers). There is a well-demarcated, thin-walled fluid-attenuating mass (**b–d**: arrowhead) within the left limb of the pancreas (**b–d**: arrows). The pancreas is otherwise unremarkable, as is the surrounding mesenteric fat. The dog had no clinical signs associated with pancreatic disease, and the pseudocyst was considered an incidental finding.

(a) US, OP   **(b)** CT+C, TP

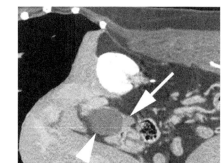
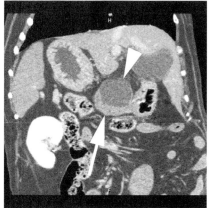

(c) CT+C, SP   **(d)** CT+C, DP

Figure 5.5.9   Pancreatic Insulinoma (Canine)   CT

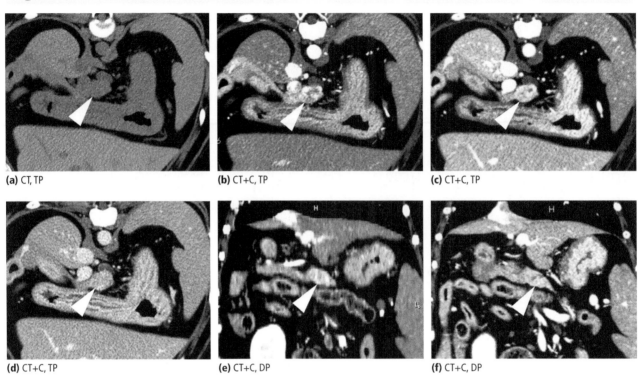

(a) CT, TP   (b) CT+C, TP   (c) CT+C, TP

(d) CT+C, TP   (e) CT+C, DP   (f) CT+C, DP

8y M Golden Retriever with hypoglycemic seizures. Images **a–d** are transverse images acquired at the level of the left limb of the pancreas and represent unenhanced, arterial, mixed arteriovenous and delayed phases of a four-phase pancreatic CT angiogram, respectively. Images **e** and **f** are dorsal plane images acquired during the arterial and mixed arteriovenous phase, respectively. The left pancreatic limb is enlarged, rounded, and isoattenuating to liver on the unenhanced image (**a**: arrowhead); markedly hyperatenuating during the early vascular phases (**b,c,e,f**: arrowhead); and moderately attenuating as a result of slow washout in the delayed phase (**d**: arrowhead). Surgical excisional biopsy confirmed a diagnosis of malignant insulinoma.

Figure 5.5.10   Pancreatic Insulinoma (Canine)

CT

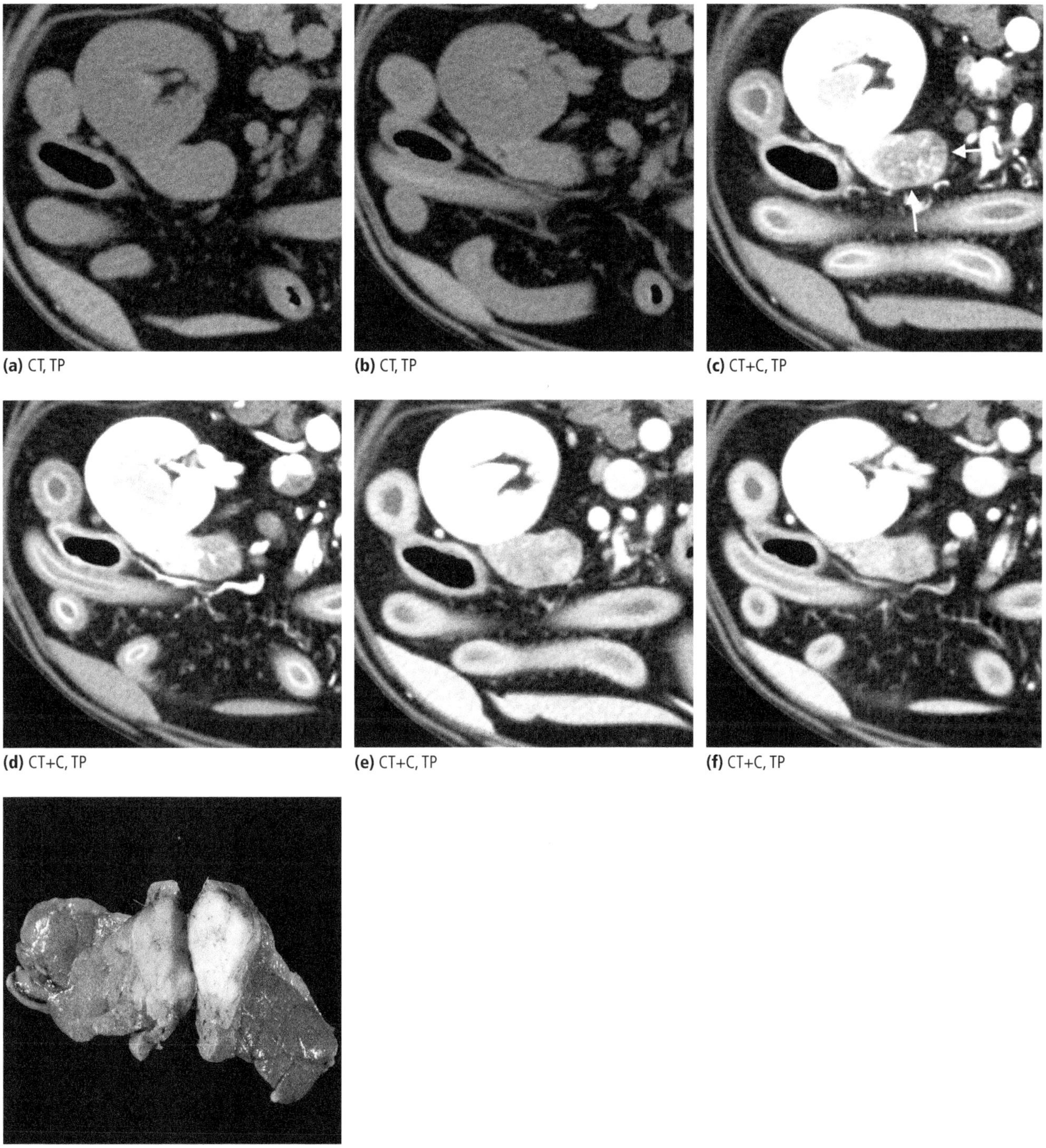

(a) CT, TP

(b) CT, TP

(c) CT+C, TP

(d) CT+C, TP

(e) CT+C, TP

(f) CT+C, TP

(g) GP

10y MC Terrier mix with seizures and persistent hypoglycemia. There is a focal enlargement and rounding of the right pancreatic lobe on unenhanced images (a,b). During the arterial phase (c,d), the pancreatic mass is hypoattenuating medially (c: arrows). The delayed phase images (e,f) show delayed washout compared to the lateral pancreas. Liver is not present in the same image for comparison. Surgical excisional biopsy confirmed a diagnosis of pancreatic islet cell carcinoma (g).

Figure 5.5.11   Pancreatic Adenocarcinoma (Feline)   CT

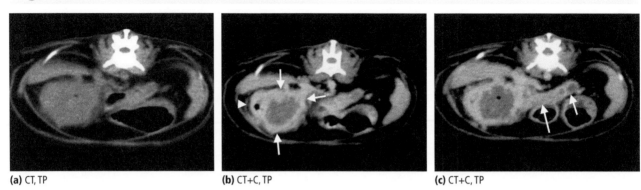

(a) CT, TP   **(b)** CT+C, TP   **(c)** CT+C, TP

14y MC Domestic Longhair with weight loss and lethargy. There is a soft-tissue attenuating mass in the region of the right pancreatic lobe. The duodenum is not clearly visible on the unenhanced images. On contrast-enhanced images, there is peripheral contrast enhancement of a large pancreatic mass with a central fluid-attenuating region (**b**: arrows). The mass compresses the lumen of the duodenum (**b**: arrowhead); however, it appears separate. The mass is contiguous with the left pancreatic lobe (**c**: arrows). Surgical biopsy revealed a diagnosis of exocrine pancreatic adenocarcinoma.

References

1. Marolf AJ, Kraft SL, Dunphy TR, Twedt DC. Magnetic resonance (MR) imaging and MR cholangiopancreatography findings in cats with cholangitis and pancreatitis. J Feline Med Surg. 2013;15: 285–294.
2. Marolf AJ, Stewart JA, Dunphy TR, Kraft SL. Hepatic and pancreaticobiliary MRI and MR cholangiopancreatography with and without secretin stimulation in normal cats. Vet Radiol Ultrasound. 2011;52:415–421.
3. Head LL, Daniel GB, Tobias K, Morandi F, DeNovo RC, Donnell R. Evaluation of the feline pancreas using computed tomography and radiolabeled leukocytes. Vet Radiol Ultrasound. 2003;44:420–428.
4. Cáceres AV, Zwingenberger AL, Hardam E, Lucena JM, Schwarz T. Helical computed tomographic angiography of the normal canine pancreas. Vet Radiol Ultrasound. 2006 ed. 2006;47:270–278.
5. Shanaman MM, Schwarz T, Gal A, O'Brien RT. Comparison between survey radiography, B-mode ultrasonography, contrast-enhanced ultrasonography and contrast-enhanced multi-detector computed tomography findings in dogs with acute abdominal signs. Vet Radiol Ultrasound [Internet]. 2013;54:591–604.
6. Hylands R. Veterinary diagnostic imaging. Chronic pancreatitis resulting in marked infiltrative fibrosis and necrosis. Can Vet J. 2006;47:1214–1217.
7. Forman MA, Marks SL, De Cock HEV, et al. Evaluation of serum feline pancreatic lipase immunoreactivity and helical computed tomography versus conventional testing for the diagnosis of feline pancreatitis. J Vet Intern Med. 2004;18:807–815.
8. Branter EM, Viviano KR. Multiple recurrent pancreatic cysts with associated pancreatic inflammation and atrophy in a cat. J Feline Med Surg. 2010;12:822–827.
9. Mai W, Cáceres AV. Dual-phase computed tomographic angiography in three dogs with pancreatic insulinoma. Vet Radiol Ultrasound. 2008;49:141–148.

5.6

Adrenal gland

The adrenal glands of dogs are bilobed and located cranial and medial to the left and right kidneys. The right adrenal gland is normally in contact with the caudal vena cava on its dorsolateral aspect. The adrenal glands are located in variable positions close to the celiac and cranial mesenteric arteries.[1] On CT images, the adrenal glands are soft-tissue attenuating on unenhanced images and isoattenuating to liver on contrast-enhanced images (Figure 5.6.1). The volume of the left adrenal gland is larger than the right in normal dogs. There is significant individual animal variation in size of the adrenal glands and no significant correlation with weight.[2] On MR images, the glands are T1 isointense to surrounding organs. On T2 images, the adrenal glands are isointense to the renal cortex and hyperintense to liver and musculature. The medulla is sometimes visible as a hyperintense region compared to the cortex on fast spin-echo T1, T2, or T1 contrast-enhanced images (Figure 5.6.2).[1] Adrenal glands are intensely contrast enhancing on both CT and MR images.

The feline adrenal glands are more oval in shape compared to those of the dog. They are similarly positioned medial and lateral to the caudal vena cava and cranial to the left and right kidneys. In CT dual-phase imaging of both species, arterial enhancement is intense in the cortex, and the gland is more uniformly enhancing in the venous phase (Figure 5.6.3). Feline adrenal glands are also visible on MR images, with imaging characteristics similar to those of the dog (Figure 5.6.4).

The common trunk of the caudal phrenic vein and cranial abdominal vein (previously termed the phrenicoabdominal vein) passes lateral and ventral to each adrenal gland to drain into the caudal vena cava. The common trunk receives the adrenal veins, which are short and not visible on imaging exams. However, they do form a point of entry to the vascular system in the case of invasive adrenal neoplasia.

Vascular disorders

Adrenal masses can invade local vasculature, as described above. In addition, they may rupture and cause intra-abdominal or retroperitoneal hemorrhage. The hemorrhage may be contained within the adrenal gland capsule or free in the peritoneal or retroperitoneal space. Hemorrhage appears as fluid-attenuating, nonenhancing tissue within the retroperitoneal or peritoneal cavity (Figure 5.6.5). Hemorrhage can occur in both vascularly invasive and noninvasive masses and may be life-threatening.[3]

Neoplasia

Pituitary adenomas are responsible for pituitary-dependent hyperadrenocorticism (PDHAC), which is the most commonly diagnosed cause of Cushing's syndrome in dogs and cats. Imaging features include bilaterally and generally symmetrically enlarged adrenal glands without evidence of a mass (Figure 5.6.6, 5.6.7). In adrenal-dependent hyperadrenocorticism (ADHAC), there is a primary adrenal mass (adenoma or carcinoma) that is responsible for the clinical signs (Figure 5.6.8). CT imaging can be used to evaluate both the brain and the adrenal glands to differentiate these two diseases.

Pituitary macroadenomas are intensely contrast enhancing and are discussed further in Chapter 2.9. However, pituitary glands affected by functional

Atlas of Small Animal CT and MRI, First Edition. Erik R. Wisner and Allison L. Zwingenberger.
© 2015 John Wiley & Sons, Inc. Published 2015 by John Wiley & Sons, Inc.

microadenomas appear normal in size and account for approximately 39–56% of patients with PDHAC.[4,5] Dogs with pituitary macroadenomas have greater enlargement of the adrenal glands compared to those with microadenomas, and the adrenal glands are of similar soft-tissue opacity.[6]

The maximum diameter of glands affected by PDHAC can exceed 20 mm, making it difficult to differentiate between PDHAC and ADHAC based on the diameter of the adrenal gland alone. By using the ratio of the maximum diameter of the larger adrenal gland to the maximum diameter of the smaller gland, the discrepancy between the gland with a functional mass and the normal gland can be quantified and used to differentiate PDHAC from ADHAC. When measuring the maximum diameter of each gland, reformatting thinly collimated images to obtain true diameters results in less overlap between PDHAC and ADHAC animals. Dogs with an adrenal gland ratio greater than 2.08 using reformatted images can be classified as ADHAC with 100% sensitivity and 98% specificity.[4]

Primary adrenal neoplasia in cats may be unilateral or bilateral adrenal adenomas or carcinomas, causing signs of hyperadrenocorticism or hyperaldosteronism. Hypoaldosteronism causes hypokalemia and muscle weakness in affected cats (Figure 5.6.9). One CT imaging report documents vascular invasion of an adenoma in a cat.[7]

Primary neoplasia of the canine adrenal gland may be caused by adrenal gland adenoma, carcinoma, or pheochromocytoma and may be unilateral or bilateral. Both carcinomas and adenomas can mineralize and contain cystic regions (Figure 5.6.10). The proximity of the adrenal gland to the caudal vena cava predisposes to vascular invasion and the formation of tumor thrombus within the common trunk of the cranial abdominal and caudal phrenic vein and into the caudal vena cava (Figures 5.6.11, 5.6.12). If large enough, the tumor thrombus may occlude the caudal vena cava and cause development of collateral circulation and ascites (Figure 5.6.13). The tumor may also invade the caudal phrenic vein to the level of the epaxial musculature or the renal vein.[8] These findings are significant for surgical planning since evidence of muscular or renal vein invasion carries a poorer prognosis. Metastatic disease may affect the adrenal gland as a solitary nodule, most often as a component of widespread metastasis (Figure 5.6.14).

Degenerative disorders

Nodular hyperplasia may cause mass lesions in the adrenal glands and results from degenerative change. These nodules have not been well described in the literature; however, they would be expected to be smaller than neoplastic nodules and to be without vascular invasion. Adrenal mineralization is a relatively common degenerative change that can be seen as an incidental finding. Older cats appear to be predisposed.

Figure 5.6.1   Normal Adrenal Glands (Canine)

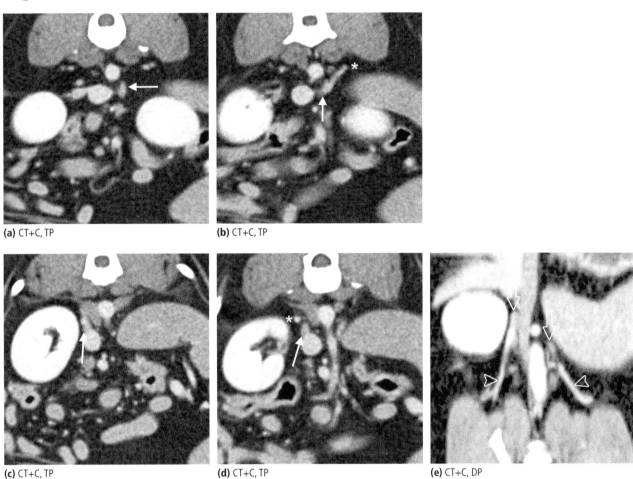

(a) CT+C, TP

(b) CT+C, TP

(c) CT+C, TP

(d) CT+C, TP

(e) CT+C, DP

3y FS mixed-breed dog. The left (**a**,**b**: arrow) and right (**c**,**d**: arrow) adrenal glands are slender, soft-tissue attenuating structures craniomedial to the left and right kidneys, respectively. The right adrenal gland is normally in contact with the caudal vena cava (**c**,**d**). The common trunk of the cranial abdominal and caudal phrenic veins passes lateral and ventral to the adrenal glands (**b**,**d**: asterisk). The large cranial abdominal veins (**e**: open arrowheads) can be seen caudal and lateral to the adrenal glands (**e**: arrows).

Figure 5.6.2 Normal Adrenal Glands (Canine)

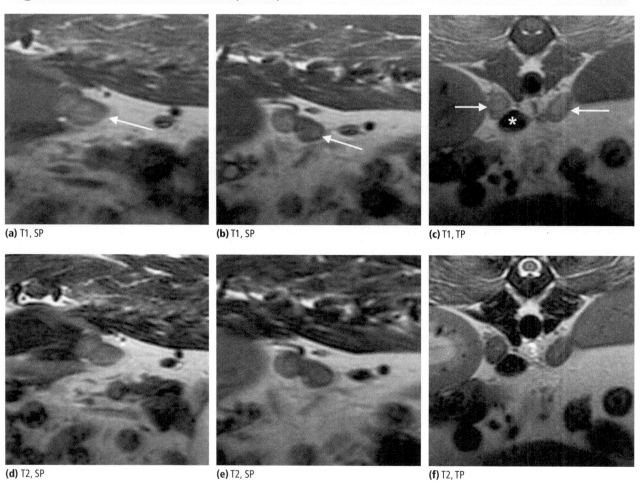

(a) T1, SP   **(b)** T1, SP   **(c)** T1, TP

(d) T2, SP   **(e)** T2, SP   **(f)** T2, TP

8y MC Dachshund. The left (**a,c,d**) and right (**b,c,e**) adrenal glands are small lobular structures located lateral to the caudal vena cava (**c:** asterisk). The outer cortex is slightly hypointense to the medulla on T1 images (**a–c**). On T2 images, the cortex is hyperintense compared to liver, and the medulla is slightly hyperintense to the cortex (**d–f**).

Figure 5.6.3 Normal Adrenal Glands (Feline)

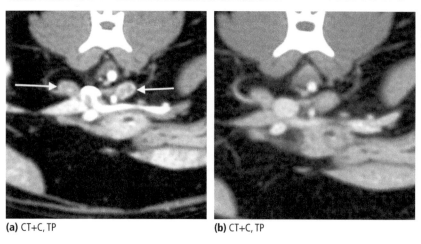

6y FS Domestic Shorthair. The normal, oval-shaped feline adrenal glands are situated lateral to the caudal vena cava. The cortex enhances strongly in the arterial phase (**a:** arrows) and is more uniform in the venous phase image (**b**).

(a) CT+C, TP   **(b)** CT+C, TP

Figure 5.6.4 Normal Adrenal Glands (Feline)

MR

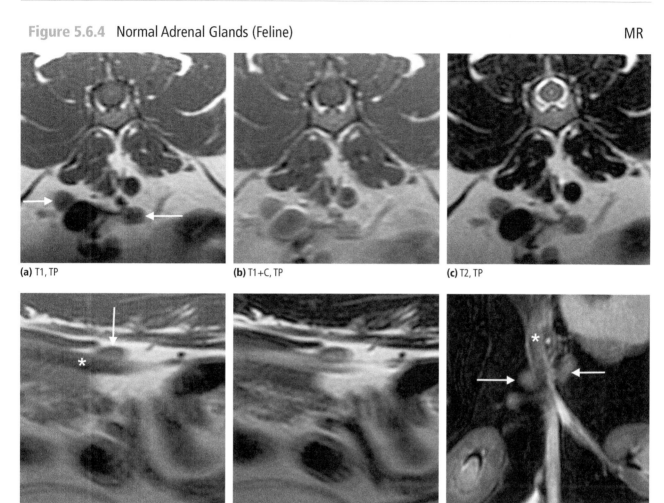

(a) T1, TP

(b) T1+C, TP

(c) T2, TP

(d) T1, SP

(e) T2, SP

(f) T2+FS DP

4y FS Domestic Shorthair. The adrenal glands are isointense to muscle on T1 images (**a**: arrows) with intense contrast enhancement (**b**). They are slightly hyperintense to muscle on T2 images (**c**). These oval glands (**d**,**f**: arrows) are located dorsal and lateral to the caudal vena cava (**d**,**f**: asterisk).

Figure 5.6.5   Adrenal Carcinoma with Hemorrhage (Canine) CT

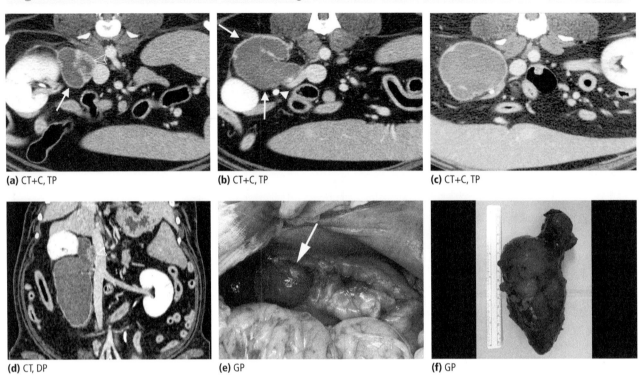

(a) CT+C, TP   **(b)** CT+C, TP   **(c)** CT+C, TP

(d) CT, DP   **(e)** GP   **(f)** GP

7y M Rottweiler with known adrenal mass and recent onset of abdominal discomfort. Image **a–c** are ordered from cranial to caudal. The right adrenal gland is enlarged (**a,d**: open arrowhead) with an eccentric, caudal cystic component of fluid attenuation (**a,b**: arrows). The remaining tissue of the mass and the adrenal capsule are peripherally contrast enhancing. The cystic component of the mass was hemorrhage, which extended caudally through the retroperitoneal space (**d**). The ureter is visible ventral to the hemorrhage (**b**: arrowhead). The gross and histological diagnosis was confirmed by excisional biopsy (**e**: arrow). Compare the appearance of the mass on the CT image (**d**) to the gross excisional specimen (**f**).

Figure 5.6.6   Pituitary-dependent Hyperadrenocorticism (Canine) CT

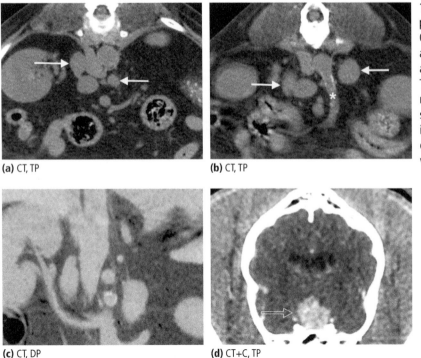

(a) CT, TP

(b) CT, TP

(c) CT, DP

(d) CT+C, TP

12y MC Boston Terrier with suspected pituitary-dependent hyperadrenocorticism. On unenhanced images, the right and left adrenal glands (**a,b**: arrows) are enlarged and rounded with uniform soft-tissue opacity. There is mineralization of the wall of the cranial mesenteric artery, secondary to Cushing's syndrome (**b**: asterisk). A contrast-enhanced image of the brain shows a large, intensely enhancing pituitary mass (**d**: open arrow), which was presumed to be functional.

Figure 5.6.7 Adrenal Cortical Adenoma (Feline) CT

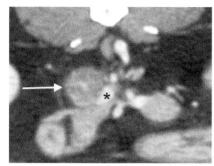

11y MC Domestic Shorthair with suspected hyperadrenocorticism. A right adrenal mass is present with irregular borders (arrow). The mass is peripherally contrast enhancing and is compressing but not invading the caudal vena cava (asterisk). The adrenal mass was excised and diagnosed as a cortical adenoma with capsular invasion.

(a) CT+C, TP

Figure 5.6.8 Adrenal Cortical Adenoma (Canine) CT

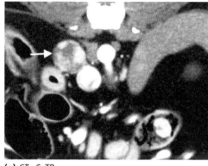 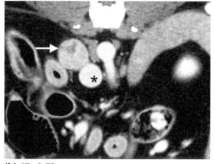 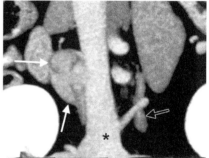

(a) CT+C, TP   (b) CT+C, TP   (c) CT+C, MIP, DP

10y FS Samoyed with an incidentally discovered adrenal mass and hypertension. The large right adrenal gland mass (a,b: arrow) does not appear to invade the local vasculature but slightly compresses the caudal vena cava (b: asterisk). An arterial phase image (a) shows patchy regions of contrast enhancement with subsequent infilling in the venous phase (b). The dorsal reformatted image shows the right adrenal mass (c: arrows) compressing the caudal vena cava slightly (c: asterisk) and the normal left adrenal gland (c: open arrow). Biopsy revealed an adrenal cortical adenoma that was nonfunctional, rather than a pheochromocytoma causing systemic hypertension as was clinically suspected.

Figure 5.6.9 Adrenal Cortical Adenoma (Feline)

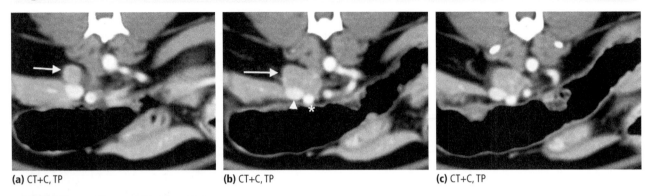

(a) CT+C, TP   **(b)** CT+C, TP   **(c)** CT+C, TP

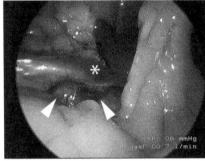

(d) GP, VENT

8y FS Domestic Longhair with hypokalemia. CT images are ordered from cranial to caudal. There is a large, irregular, heterogeneously enhancing right adrenal gland mass (**a**,**b**: arrow). The mass is compressing the caudal vena cava (**b**: arrowhead) and contacts the portal vein (**b**: asterisk) but does not appear to invade the vasculature. The mass was diagnosed as an adenoma causing clinical signs of hyperaldosteronism. A laparoscopic image shows the adrenal mass (**d**: arrowheads) located dorsal to the caudal vena cava (**d**: asterisk). The mass was histologically confirmed to be an adrenal adenoma.

Figure 5.6.10 Adrenal Cortical Adenoma (Canine)

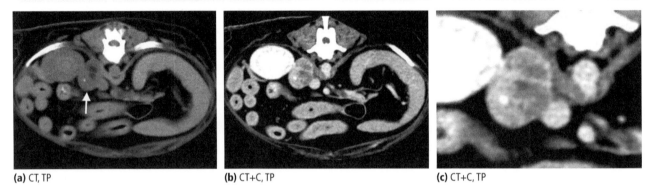

(a) CT, TP   **(b)** CT+C, TP   **(c)** CT+C, TP

16y FS Pekingese with multiple system failure. Image **c** represents a magnification of image **b**. The right adrenal gland is enlarged (**a**: arrow), with two fluid-attenuating cystic structures as well as a small, focal region of mineralization. There is heterogeneous tissue enhancement on the contrast-enhanced images (**b**,**c**). Postmortem examination confirmed the presence of multiple adenomas involving both adrenal glands.

Figure 5.6.11   Adrenal Carcinoma (Canine)   MR

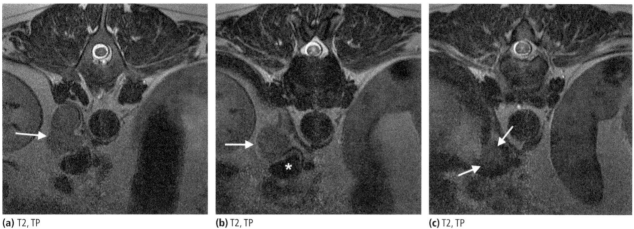

(a) T2, TP   **(b)** T2, TP   **(c)** T2, TP

14y FS Labrador Retriever with a spinal nerve sheath tumor. Images are ordered from cranial to caudal. There is a right-sided lobular adrenal mass, which is hyperintense on T2 images (**a,b**: arrows) and is in contact with the caudal vena cava (**b**: asterisk). The mass is invading the caudal vena cava, causing a tumor thrombus with incomplete venous obstruction (**c**: arrows). The mass was incidental to the primary nerve sheath tumor. The hypointense splenic nodules were diagnosed as nodular hyperplasia (**b,c**). Right adrenal cortical carcinoma with invasion into the vena cava lumen was confirmed on postmortem examination.

Figure 5.6.12   Pheochromocytoma (Canine)   CT

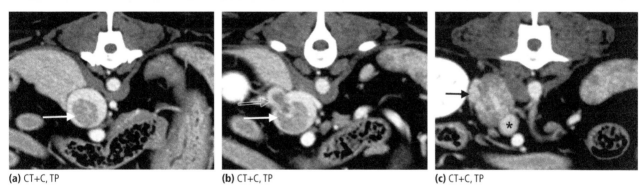

(a) CT+C, TP   **(b)** CT+C, TP   **(c)** CT+C, TP

13y MC Shih Tzu with episodes of collapse and vomiting. Images are ordered from cranial to caudal. Cranial to the right adrenal gland, there is a tumor thrombus causing a contrast filling defect in the caudal vena cava lumen (**a**: arrow). The adrenal mass has invaded the common trunk of the cranial abdominal and caudal phrenic vein (**b**: open arrow) and extends into the caudal vena cava (**b**: arrow), causing partial obstruction. The enlarged, irregular, heterogeneous adrenal gland mass is visible (**c**: arrow) in contact with the caudal vena cava more caudally (**c**: asterisk). Surgical excision, which included caval venotomy, confirmed the mass to be malignant pheochromocytoma. Schultz et al 2009.[8] Reproduced with permission from Wiley.

Figure 5.6.13   Pheochromocytoma (Canine)   CT

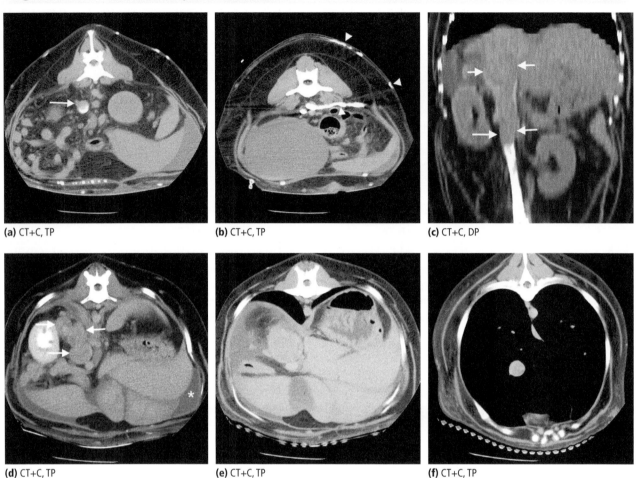

(a) CT+C, TP   **(b)** CT+C, TP   **(c)** CT+C, DP

(d) CT+C, TP   **(e)** CT+C, TP   **(f)** CT+C, TP

7y MC mixed-breed dog with ascites. Transverse images **a**, **d**, **e**, and **f** are ordered from caudal to cranial. Image **b** is caudal to image **a**. A contrast injection into the saphenous vein documents complete occlusion of the caudal vena cava by a tumor thrombus (**a,c**: arrows). Caudal to the obstruction, there is collateral circulation coursing laterally to the body wall and subcutaneous tissues (**b**: arrowheads). The tumor thrombus extends from caudal to the adrenal gland to the thoracic caudal vena cava (**c,f**). The mass arose from the right adrenal gland (**d**: arrows), causing caudal vena cava obstruction, enlargement (**e**), and ascites (**d**: asterisk). Postmortem examination confirmed a diagnosis of locally invasive pheochromocytoma.

Figure 5.6.14   Metastatic Hemangiosarcoma (Canine)   CT

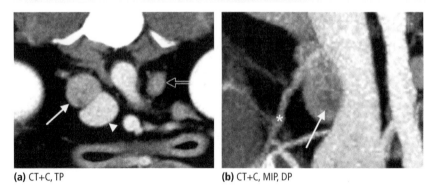

(a) CT+C, TP   **(b)** CT+C, MIP, DP

12y FS Alaskan Malamute with a splenic mass. The right adrenal gland (**a,b**: arrow) is enlarged with a slightly hypointense caudal pole. The phrenicoabdominal vein courses over the adrenal gland (**b**: asterisk) and is not invaded by the mass. The caudal vena cava is compressed by the mass but contains no tumor (**a**: arrowhead). The left adrenal gland is normal in size (**a**: open arrow). The primary splenic hemangiosarcoma was metastatic to multiple sites, including the adrenal gland. Schultz et al 2009.[8] Reproduced with permission from Wiley.

References

1. Llabres-Diaz FJ, Dennis R. Magnetic resonance imaging of the presumed normal canine adrenal glands. Vet Radiol Ultrasound. 2003;44:5–19.

2. Bertolini G, Furlanello T, De Lorenzi D, Caldin M. Computed tomographic quantification of canine adrenal gland volume and attenuation. Vet Radiol Ultrasound. 2006;47:444–448.

3. Whittemore JC, Preston CA, Kyles AE, Hardie EM, Feldman EC. Nontraumatic rupture of an adrenal gland tumor causing intra-abdominal or retroperitoneal hemorrhage in four dogs. J Am Vet Med Assoc. 2001;219:329–324.

4. Rodriguez Pineiro MI, de Fornel-Thibaud P, Benchekroun G, et al. Use of computed tomography adrenal gland measurement for differentiating ACTH dependence from ACTH independence in 64 dogs with hyperadenocorticism. J Vet Intern Med. 2011;25:1066–1074.

5. Kooistra HS, Voorhout G, Mol JA, Rijnberk A. Correlation between impairment of glucocorticoid feedback and the size of the pituitary gland in dogs with pituitary-dependent hyperadrenocorticism. J Endocrinol. 1997;152:387–394.

6. Bertolini G, Furlanello T, Drigo M, Caldin M. Computed tomographic adrenal gland quantification in canine adrenocorticotroph hormone-dependent hyperadrenocorticism. Vet Radiol Ultrasound. 2008;49:449–453.

7. Rose SA, Kyles AE, Labelle P, et al. Adrenalectomy and caval thrombectomy in a cat with primary hyperaldosteronism. J Am Anim Hosp Assoc. 2007;43:209–214.

8. Schultz RM, Wisner ER, Johnson EG, MacLeod JS. Contrast-enhanced computed tomography as a preoperative indicator of vascular invasion from adrenal masses in dogs. Vet Radiol Ultrasound. 2009;50:625–629.

5.7

Spleen

Introduction

CT and MR imaging have not been widely used for evaluation of patients with splenic disease because conventional radiography and ultrasonography are both excellent alternative imaging approaches. Many splenic lesions are identified on thoracic or abdominal studies acquired for other purposes. Some of these lesions may be incidental findings, while others may represent a key component of the animal's primary disorder. Abdominal CT to evaluate the spleen may be appropriate for accurate cancer staging and in animals with acute abdominal disease in which traumatic, vascular, or inflammatory disease of the spleen is suspected. CT for characterization and diagnosis of diffuse splenic disease is less compelling since CT features can be nonspecific, and diagnosis can usually be made using ultrasound and guided fine-needle or tissue core biopsy.

On unenhanced CT images, the spleen has a uniform density of approximately 50 HU. The splenic parenchyma consists predominantly of reticular connective tissue and blood vessels (red pulp) and lymphoreticular nodules (white pulp). The open circulatory (venous sinus) architecture of the red pulp causes a nonuniform distribution of contrast medium in early arterial phase contrast-enhanced imaging of the spleen. The mottled appearance of the parenchyma becomes increasingly uniform as contrast concentration equilibrates within the venous sinuses during portal and delayed phases (Figure 5.7.1).

The feline spleen is hypointense to liver on T1 images and hyperintense to liver on T2 images (Figure 5.7.2).[1] The canine spleen has similar MR imaging characteristics (Figure 5.7.3).

Trauma

CT has not been widely used for evaluation of the traumatic acute abdomen in veterinary medicine, largely because ultrasonography has historically been a more accessible alternative imaging modality. In people, CT is often used in trauma patients to identify fractures of the spleen and liver, which can lead to surgical hemoabdomen. Although CT has not been widely used for this purpose in veterinary medicine, CT should be considered as a presurgical diagnostic step in trauma patients with uncontrolled hemoabdomen when parenchymal organ fracture is suspected but cannot be verified using other imaging approaches. Experimental splenic trauma results in a discontinuous splenic capsule and local peritoneal effusion, with a nonenhancing focal splenic lesion (Figure 5.7.4). Intraparenchymal contrast collections and extraparenchymal contrast leakage may also be seen.[2] CT performed under sedation can provide rapid assessment of traumatic injuries.[3]

Splenic hematomas are periodically identified as complex, heterogeneously contrast-enhancing masses that distort the splenic capsule. These can occur as the result of known trauma or can be apparently spontaneous. Splenic hematomas may be difficult or impossible to distinguish from splenic neoplasia since the constellation of imaging findings overlaps. Unfortunately, fine-needle aspiration biopsy and tissue core biopsy may be misleading because of the presence of concurrent hemorrhage in association with splenic neoplasia.

Ectopic splenic tissue may be present as a result of congenital causes, trauma, or splenectomy. This tissue has the same imaging characteristics as normal spleen

Atlas of Small Animal CT and MRI, First Edition. Erik R. Wisner and Allison L. Zwingenberger.
© 2015 John Wiley & Sons, Inc. Published 2015 by John Wiley & Sons, Inc.

and may develop regenerative nodules, hematomas, or inflammation (Figures 5.7.5, 5.7.6).

Vascular disorders

Splenomegaly due to anesthetic drugs is likely caused by a combination of splenic smooth muscle relaxation and systemic hypotension causing sequestration of red blood cells in the spleen. Increased splenic volume results from administration of propofol, acepromazine, and thiopental.[4] The spleen appears uniform in attenuation with slightly rounded margins.

CT imaging characteristics of splenic torsion include the presence of abdominal effusion, generalized splenic enlargement, absence of contrast enhancement, and a dorsal midabdominal mass.[5] Vascular occlusion, particularly on the venous return side, results in splenic congestion and a resultant transcapsular effusion. Compromised arterial flow results in lack of contrast enhancement (Figure 5.7.7).

Splenic infarction may occur in isolation or as a component of a systemic disorder. Infarcted spleen may appear iso- or mildly hypoattenuating compared to perfused spleen on unenhanced images. Following contrast administration, infarcts appear nonenhancing or nonuniformly enhancing. The appearance of the infarct may vary depending on size and chronicity (Figure 5.7.8). Splenic venous thrombosis can occur concurrently with splenic infarction (Figure 5.7.9).

Some severe vascular and developmental anomalies, such as portal aplasia and situs ambiguus, have been associated with a lobular spleen that is partially divided into segments. This is somewhat difficult to appreciate on CT images because of splenic folding, but the incomplete divisions cause a lobular shape. This finding is benign; however, it may alert the clinician to the potential for vascular anomalies.[6]

Inflammatory disorders

CT is not commonly employed to evaluate diffuse inflammatory disease of the spleen. Splenitis, regardless of cause, will produce splenic enlargement and may result in heterogeneous contrast enhancement even on delayed portal phase contrast images. The splenic capsule may become thickened and contrast enhance if capsulitis is a significant component of the inflammatory disease (Figure 5.7.6).

Neoplasia

Benign masses of the spleen include leiomyoma, fibroma, and myelolipoma. With the exception of myelolipomas, which have a complex, mixed fat and soft-tissue attenuation pattern (Figure 5.7.10), benign splenic masses are likely to be more uniformly enhancing and more similar in inherent attenuation and contrast enhancement to normal splenic parenchyma than malignant neoplasms.

CT has not been used extensively in veterinary medicine for evaluation of infiltrative splenic neoplasms.

In people, splenic lymphoma results in splenic enlargement that may be generalized or regional and is present in conjunction with regions of low attenuation. The spectrum of CT appearances of lymphoma in people include homogeneous splenic enlargement, solitary mass, multifocal lesions, and diffuse involvement. CT or MRI are unlikely to provide a definitive diagnosis of lymphoma in veterinary patients (Figure 5.7.11).[7] However, positron emission tomography (PET)/CT shows promise in detecting metabolically active lesions secondary to round cell neoplasia in the spleen.[8] This may be of particular benefit when monitoring response to therapy.

The most common malignant splenic masses include hemangiosarcoma and fibrosarcoma. Generally, splenic hemangiosarcomas are large, complex, and hypoattenuating on unenhanced images (Figures 5.7.12, 5.7.13). Malignant splenic masses tend to contrast enhance to a lesser degree than benign masses, with 55 HU being a reasonable discriminating threshold.[9] Diagnosis of malignant splenic masses is often complicated by concurrent hematoma formation from a bleeding tumor.

The spleen is a frequent site of metastatic disease.[10] Metastases often appear as hypoattenuating nodules or masses distributed throughout the splenic parenchyma or in a subcapsular location. Following contrast administration, conspicuity of the nodules is accentuated because of relatively greater contrast enhancement of the surrounding normal splenic parenchyma (Figures 5.7.14, 5.7.15). Mild peripheral or nonuniform contrast enhancement is sometimes seen. On MR images, metastatic lesions are T1 hypointense, T2 hyperintense, and hyperintense on contrast-enhanced images.[11] These characteristics allow differentiation of malignant from benign disease.[12]

Degenerative disorders

Extramedullary hematopoiesis originates in the splenic red pulp, and lymphoid hyperplasia originates in the white pulp. Both forms of hyperplastic tissue have diffuse and nodular forms; however, on imaging examinations, generally only the nodular forms are evident as focal lesions.

Foci of extramedullary hematopoiesis may not be evident on unenhanced CT images since most are the same attenuation as normal splenic parenchyma and may not be large enough to distort the splenic capsule. Small foci are typically uniformly and moderately contrast enhancing and have variable margin definition (Figure 5.7.16). Nodules are generally less than 1–2 cm in diameter, and multiple nodules may be distributed throughout the splenic parenchyma. Larger masses may also occur in some cases (Figure 5.7.17).

Lymphoid hyperplasia arises from the splenic white pulp and may be up to 5–6 cm in diameter. Larger, mass-like nodules can distort the splenic capsule and may have a nonuniform, stellate contrast-enhancement pattern (Figures 5.7.18, 5.7.19). Contrast-enhanced HU

values of greater than 55 are more likely with benign nodules.

On MR images, benign splenic nodules, including lymphoid hyperplasia and extramedullary hematopoiesis, are hypointense on T1 and T2 images, with decreased enhancement relative to normal splenic parenchyma.[11]

Mineralization of the spleen may occur in small foci or in a lacy pattern secondary to hyperadrenocorticism or chronic steroid administration (Figure 5.7.20). This is a benign finding.

Figure 5.7.1 Normal Spleen (Canine)   CT

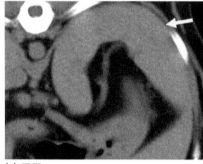 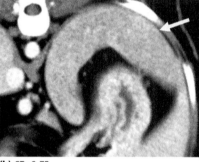 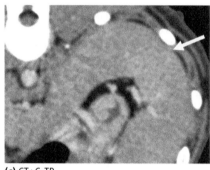

(a) CT, TP   **(b)** CT+C, TP   **(c)** CT+C, TP

10y FS Australian Shepherd. The spleen is uniform in attenuation on unenhanced images (**a**: arrow). During the arterial phase of contrast enhancement, the spleen has a high-attenuation, mottled enhancement pattern (**b**: arrow). Later in the venous phase, the enhancement is more uniform (**c**: arrow).

Figure 5.7.2 Normal Spleen (Feline)   MR

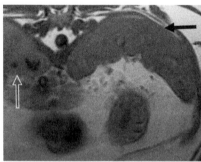 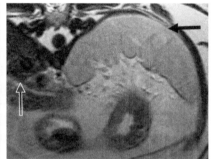

(a) T1, TP   **(b)** T2, TP

12y MC Domestic Shorthair. The spleen is moderately enlarged due to anesthesia. Compared to liver (**a,b**: open arrow), the spleen (**a,b**: arrow) is isointense on T1 images (**a**) and hyperintense on T2 images (**b**).

Figure 5.7.3   Normal Spleen (Canine)

MR

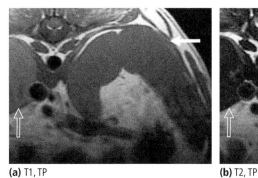
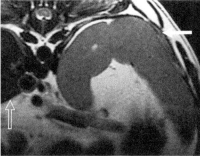

8y MC Dachshund. Compared to liver (**a**,**b**: open arrow), the normal canine spleen (**a**,**b**: arrow) is isointense to hypointense to liver on T1 images (**a**) and hyperintense on T2 images (**b**).

(**a**) T1, TP

(**b**) T2, TP

Figure 5.7.4   Splenic Rupture (Canine)

CT

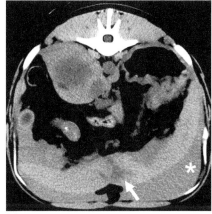
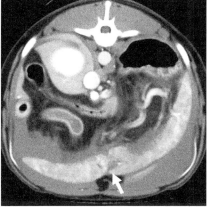
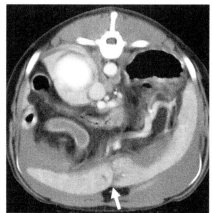

(**a**) CT, TP

(**b**) CT+C, TP

(**c**) CT+C, TP

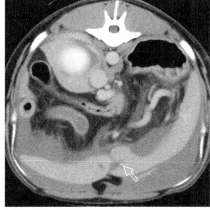
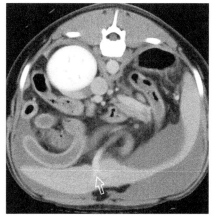

(**d**) CT+C, TP

(**e**) CT+C, TP

1.5y MC Labrador Retriever mix found recumbent with pale mucous membranes. On unenhanced images, there is a moderate amount of effusion in the dependent portion of the abdomen (**a**: asterisk). A hypoattenuating, irregular, linear separation of the splenic capsule and parenchyma is visible (**a**: arrow). On arterial phase (**b**: arrow) and venous phase (**c**: arrow) images, the region is nonenhancing. The splenic vein to this region is smaller (**d**: open arrow) than a neighboring intraparenchymal vessel (**e**: open arrow) on late-phase venous images. Reproduced with permission from S Specchi and K Alexander, University of Montreal, Montreal, Canada, 2014.

Figure 5.7.5   Ectopic Splenic Tissue—Hematoma (Canine)   CT

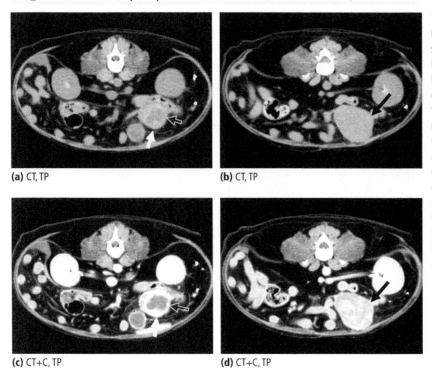

(a) CT, TP

(b) CT, TP

(c) CT+C, TP

(d) CT+C, TP

12y FS Pembroke Welsh Corgi with immune-mediated thrombocytopenia and previous splenectomy. Images **a** and **b** are cranial to images **c** and **d**. Several round, slightly irregularly margined masses are present in the left cranial abdomen. A normal spleen is not identified, and metallic staples are visible in this region. One mass is centrally hypoattenuating (**a,b**: open arrow) with peripheral hyperattenuating tissue (**a**: white arrow) and contrast enhancement (**b**: white arrow), suggesting central fluid or hemorrhage. The second mass is more homogeneously soft-tissue attenuating (**c**: black arrow) with more uniform enhancement (**d**: black arrow). Surgical excisional biopsy revealed extramedullary hematopoiesis and hematoma formation.

Figure 5.7.6   Ectopic Splenic Tissue—Splenitis and Capsulitis (Feline)   CT

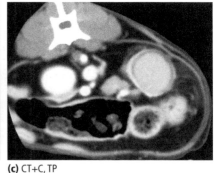

(a) CT, TP

(b) CT+C, TP

(c) CT+C, TP

12y MC Domestic Shorthair with weight loss and anemia. Images **b** and **c** are ordered from cranial to caudal. There is a round, soft-tissue attenuating mass in the left dorsal abdomen (**a**: white arrow). The margin is indistinct on unenhanced images, and there is fat stranding in the surrounding mesentery (**a**: open arrows). On contrast-enhanced images, there is intense, peripheral enhancement of the mass (**b**: black arrow) and uniform, moderate enhancement of the central region. A normal spleen was not identified. Excisional biopsy was performed, and splenitis and capsulitis of the ectopic spleen were associated with acute pancreatitis.

Figure 5.7.7   Splenic Torsion (Canine)   CT

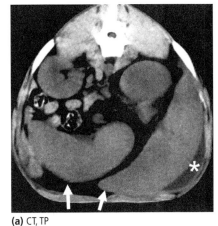
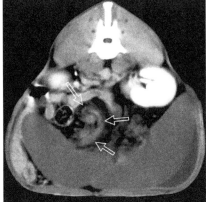

(a) CT, TP   **(b)** CT+C, TP

3y F German Shepherd Dog with hematuria and mild anorexia. The spleen is markedly enlarged and hypoattenuating (**a**: arrows) with associated free peritoneal fluid (**a**: asterisk). The rotated splenic pedicle appears as a mass effect with a spiral shape (**b**: open arrows). On the contrast-enhanced image (**b**), the spleen is nonenhancing. Patsikas et al. 2005.[5] Reproduced with permission from Wiley.

Figure 5.7.8   Acute Splenic Infarction (Canine)   CT

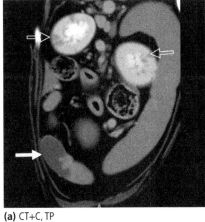
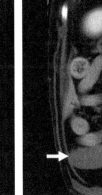

(a) CT+C, TP   **(b)** CT+C, TP

7y FS Labrador Retriever with left flank cellulitis. Images **a** and **b** are ordered from cranial to caudal. On contrast-enhanced images, the spleen is moderately enlarged with a nonenhancing region in the distal extremity (**a**,**b**: white arrow) and a more ill-defined region in the body of the spleen (**b**: arrowhead). The capsule of the spleen enhances in this region, and there is geographic demarcation with normal splenic parenchyma. Wedge-shaped, nonenhancing infarcts are also visible in both kidneys (**a**: open arrows).

Figure 5.7.9   Venous Thrombosis and Infarction (Canine)   CT

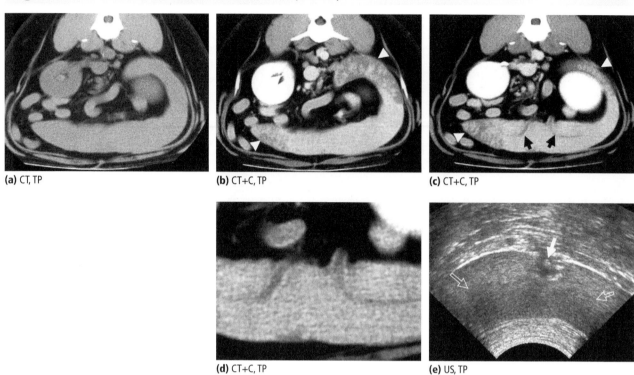

(a) CT, TP   **(b)** CT+C, TP   **(c)** CT+C, TP

(d) CT+C, TP   **(e)** US, TP

2y MC Labrador Retriever with coagulopathy. Images **b** and **c** are ordered from cranial to caudal and image **d** is a magnified view of image **c**. The spleen is moderately enlarged on the unenhanced image (**a**). Following intravenous contrast administration, there is heterogeneous enhancement of the parenchyma in several regions (**b,c**: arrowheads). There are soft-tissue attenuating filling defects in the splenic veins (**c**: black arrows), representing thrombosis. The thrombus was visualized as a hyperechoic filling defect on ultrasound (**e**: white arrow), as well as the hypoechoic infarcted regions of the parenchyma (**e**: open arrows).

Figure 5.7.10   Myelolipoma (Canine)   CT

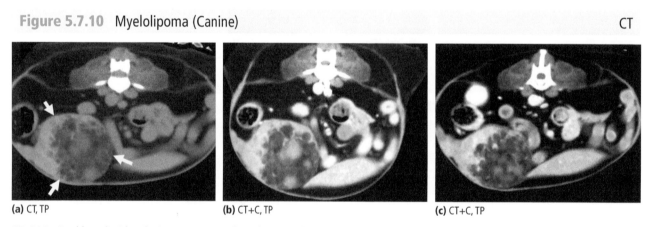

(a) CT, TP   **(b)** CT+C, TP   **(c)** CT+C, TP

17y MC mixed breed with splenic mass. Images **b** and **c** are ordered from cranial to caudal. There is a complex, round mass arising from the midbody of the spleen (**a**: arrows). The mass is heterogeneous with a soft-tissue attenuating rim and lobular regions of mixed attenuation approaching fat in the central region. On contrast-enhanced images (**b,c**), the soft-tissue regions are enhancing. Surgical excisional biopsy confirmed the diagnosis of myelolipoma.

Figure 5.7.11   Lymphoma with Hematoma (Canine)   CT

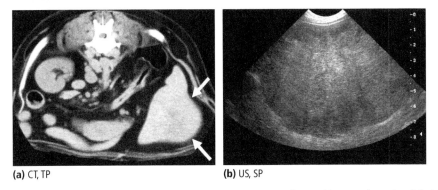

(a) CT, TP   (b) US, SP

12y FS Labrador Retriever with a splenic mass. On an unenhanced image, there is a lobular mass deforming the capsule of the spleen (a: arrows). Centrally, the mass is decreased in attenuation. The mass is ill defined and heterogeneous in appearance on an ultrasound examination (b). The spleen was excised, and marginal zone lymphoma was identified on histopathology with a large hematoma. Hematomas are often associated with marginal zone lymphomas.

Figure 5.7.12   Hemangiosarcoma (Canine)   CT

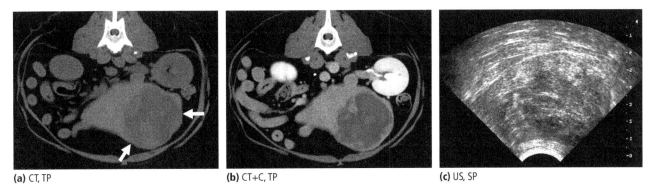

(a) CT, TP   (b) CT+C, TP   (c) US, SP

13y MC Dalmatian with a splenic mass. There is a large, heterogeneous, hypoattenuating mass deforming the splenic capsule (a: arrows). On the contrast-enhanced image, the mass is nonenhancing (b). The mass is heterogeneous in appearance on an ultrasound examination (c). Splenectomy was performed, and the mass was diagnosed as a hemangiosarcoma. Pulmonary nodules were discovered on thoracic CT and were presumed to be metastatic disease.

Figure 5.7.13 Hemangiosarcoma (Canine)   CT

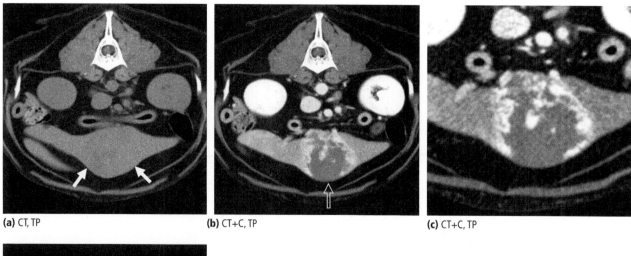

(a) CT, TP   **(b)** CT+C, TP   **(c)** CT+C, TP

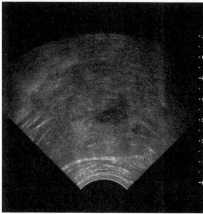

(d) US, TP

12y FS Alaskan Malamute with a splenic mass. Image **c** is a magnified view of image **b**. The heterogeneous, hypoattenuating mass is deforming the splenic contour in the midabdomen (**a**: arrows). Following intravenous contrast administration, the mass is centrally nonenhancing (**b**: open arrow) and peripherally, intensely enhancing. The mass is ill defined, heterogeneous and has a hypoechoic core on an ultrasound examination (**d**). The spleen was surgically removed and hemangiosarcoma was diagnosed on histopathology.

Figure 5.7.14 Splenic Metastasis (Canine)   CT

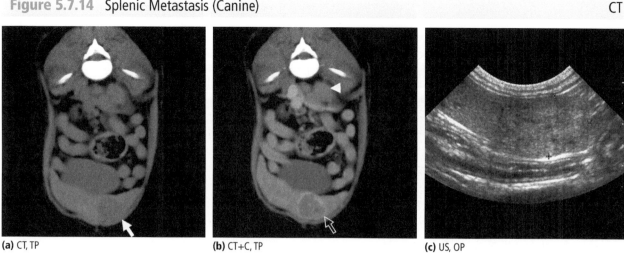

(a) CT, TP   **(b)** CT+C, TP   **(c)** US, OP

15y FS Dachshund with anal sac adenocarcinoma. There is a splenic mass in the distal extremity that is hypoattenuating on the unenhanced image (**a**: arrow). On the contrast-enhanced image, there is no central enhancement but moderate peripheral enhancement (**b**: open arrow). Enlarged lymph nodes are visible lateral to the aorta, resulting from regional metastasis of the anal sac adenocarcinoma (**b**: arrowhead). The mass is heterogeneous in appearance on an ultrasound examination (**c**). Splenic metastasis was diagnosed by ultrasound-guided fine-needle aspirate.

Figure 5.7.15   Splenic Metastasis (Canine)

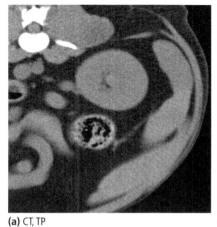 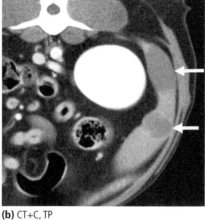

9y MC Labrador Retriever with cutaneous hemangiosarcoma. There are ill-defined, mildly hypoattenuating masses in the proximal extremity of the spleen, which are nonenhancing centrally with mild peripheral enhancement (**b**: arrows). Histology was performed after splenectomy, and a diagnosis of metastatic hemangiosarcoma was made.

(a) CT, TP   **(b)** CT+C, TP

Figure 5.7.16   Extramedullary Hematopoiesis (Canine)

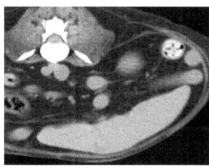 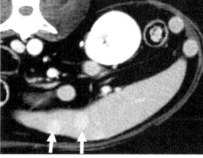 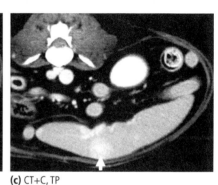

(a) CT, TP   **(b)** CT+C, TP   **(c)** CT+C, TP

12y FS Labrador Retriever with splenic nodules. Images **b** and **c** are ordered from cranial to caudal. There are moderately contrast-enhancing, well-defined nodules within the splenic parenchyma (**b,c**: arrows). The nodules are not well visualized on the unenhanced image (**a**). The nodules were diagnosed as extramedullary hematopoiesis on histopathology.

Figure 5.7.17   Extramedullary Hematopoiesis (Canine)

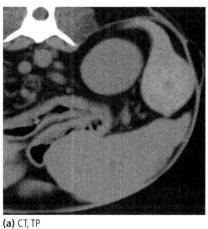 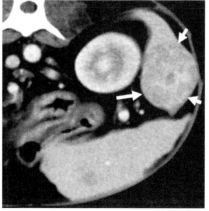

13y FS Brittany Spaniel with a splenic mass. There is a heterogeneous mass in the proximal extremity of the spleen, deforming the capsule. On the contrast-enhanced image, the mass is moderately, heterogeneously enhancing (**b**: arrows). Extramedullary hematopoiesis was diagnosed by fine-needle aspiration cytology.

(a) CT, TP   **(b)** CT+C, TP

Figure 5.7.18 Nodular lymphoid hyperplasia (Canine)   CT

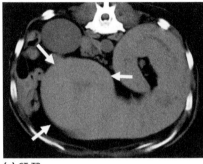 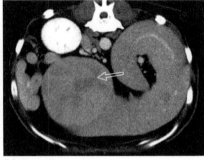

13y MC Giant Schnauzer with a splenic mass. There is a large mass within the distal extremity of the spleen (**a**: arrows), with a relatively hypoattenuating, stellate center on the contrast-enhanced image (**b**: open arrow). The mass is otherwise isoattenuating to normal spleen on the enhanced image.

(a) CT, TP   **(b)** CT+C, TP

Figure 5.7.19 Nodular Lymphoid Hyperplasia (Canine)   MR

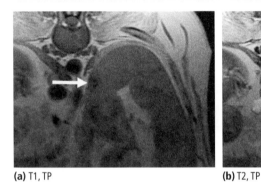 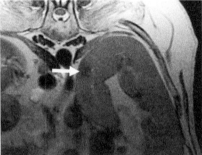

13y FS Basset Hound with intervertebral disc disease. Splenic nodules were seen incidentally, which are hypointense on T1 and T2 images (**a,b**: arrow). The nodules were diagnosed as nodular lymphoid hyperplasia at the time of postmortem examination.

(a) T1, TP   **(b)** T2, TP

Figure 5.7.20 Splenic Mineralization (Canine)   CT

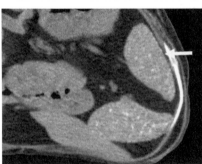

12y MC Boston Terrier with pituitary-dependent hyperadrenocorticism. There is lacy mineralization within the splenic parenchyma (arrow). A pituitary mass was diagnosed causing hyperadrenocorticism.

(a) CT, TP

References

1. Newell SM, Graham JP, Roberts GD, et al. Quantitative magnetic resonance imaging of the normal feline cranial abdomen. Vet Radiol Ultrasound. 2000;41:27–34.

2. Tang J, Li W, Lv F, et al. Comparison of gray-scale contrast-enhanced ultrasonography with contrast-enhanced computed tomography in different grading of blunt hepatic and splenic trauma: an animal experiment. Ultrasound Med Biol. 2009; 35:566–575.

3. Shanaman MM, Hartman SK, O'Brien RT. Feasibility for using dual-phase contrast-enhanced multi-detector helical computed tomography to evaluate awake and sedated dogs with acute abdominal signs. Vet Radiol Ultrasound. 2012;53:605–612.

4. Baldo CF, Garcia-Pereira FL, Nelson NC, Hauptman JG, Shih AC. Effects of anesthetic drugs on canine splenic volume determined via computed tomography. Am J Vet Res. 2012;73: 1715–1719.

5. Patsikas MN, Rallis T, Kladakis SE, Dessiris AK. Computed tomography diagnosis of isolated splenic torsion in a dog. Vet Radiol Ultrasound. 2005;42:235–237.

6. Zwingenberger AL, Spriet M, Hunt GB. Imaging diagnosis – portal vein aplasia and interruption of the caudal vena cava in three dogs. Vet Radiol Ultrasound. 2011;52:444–447.

7. Feeney DA, Sharkey LC, Steward SM, et al. Parenchymal signal intensity in 3-T body MRI of dogs with hematopoietic neoplasia. Comp Med. 2013;63:174–182.

8. Ballegeer EA, Hollinger C, Kunst CM. Imaging diagnosis – multicentric lymphoma of granular lymphocytes imaged with FDG PET/CT in a dog. Vet Radiol Ultrasound. 2013;54:75–80.

9. Fife WD, Samii VF, Drost WT, Mattoon JS, Hoshaw-Woodard S. Comparison between malignant and nonmalignant splenic masses in dogs using contrast-enhanced computed tomography. Vet Radiol Ultrasound. 2004;45:289–297.

10. Rossi F, Aresu L, Vignoli M, et al. Metastatic cancer of unknown primary in 21 dogs. Vet Comp Oncol. doi: 10.1111/vco.12011; 2013.

11. Clifford CA, Pretorius ES, Weisse C, et al. Magnetic resonance imaging of focal splenic and hepatic lesions in the dog. J Vet Intern Med. 2004;18:330–338.

12. Elsayes KM, Narra VR, Mukundan G, Lewis JS, Menias CO, Heiken JP. MR imaging of the spleen: spectrum of abnormalities. Radiographics. 2005;25:967–982.

5.8

Urinary tract

Introduction

The urinary tract is frequently evaluated with CT because of its excellent spatial resolution for examining small structures, such as ureters or small calculi. The function of each kidney can also be subjectively evaluated by evaluation of the renal and urine enhancement with contrast medium. Quantitative functional analysis has also been investigated using dynamic CT and perfusion techniques.[1,2]

The kidneys, ureters, bladder, and urethra can be imaged with CT and MR (Figures 5.8.1, 5.8.2). Renal contrast enhancement is multiphasic as contrast medium is filtered by the urinary system (Figure 5.8.3). The cortex enhances to a greater degree than the medulla on the initial corticomedullary phase. The nephrogram phase shows uniform renal enhancement prior to urine collecting in the renal pelvis. The renal pelvis and medulla are enhanced during the excretory phase. The ureters fill segmentally with contrast medium as a result of peristaltic contractions during the excretory phase. The ureters enter the dorsal bladder wall near the trigone. The urethra is less commonly evaluated with cross-sectional imaging but is easily included by scanning through the pelvis, and CT urethrography can be performed to better delineate the urethral lumen.

CT angiography is used to evaluate the anatomy of the renal vasculature, which is advantageous for surgical planning.[3,4] There is normally one artery and one vein supplying each kidney; however, anatomic variants of additional arteries and veins occur frequently in cats.[4] MR angiography of the canine renal vasculature has also been described.[5] CT software applications can be used to quantify renal volume with good accuracy.[6] Contrast-enhanced MR urography gives excellent information on renal anatomy and function, but it is less commonly used.

Contrast-induced nephropathy (CIN) has been described in people, which results in acute kidney injury, causing an increase of creatinine of more than 0.5 mg/dl or 25% over baseline within 48 hours of contrast administration.[7] This has not been fully characterized in dogs and cats; however, similar risk factors and prevention measures can be extrapolated. Hypovolemia, existing renal dysfunction, nephrotoxic drugs, hypotension, heart failure, and diabetes are risk factors for CIN. The use of iso- and low-osmolar contrast medium decreases risk of CIN, as does pre- and postcontrast hydration with intravenous saline.[7]

Developmental disorders

Renal cysts

Autosomal dominant polycystic kidney disease results in progressive development and enlargement of low-attenuation cysts in the renal cortex in cats. The disease has also been reported in dogs. In adult animals, the origin of cysts, whether congenital or degenerative, may be undetermined. Cysts may deform the capsule and distort the renal pelvis and are best seen on contrast-enhanced images (Figure 5.8.4).[8] Solid tumors and/or replacement of renal tissue with cystic structures occurs in hereditary multifocal renal cystadenocarcinomas in German Shepherd Dogs, along with nodular dermatofibrosis and uterine neoplasia.[9] These cysts often have attenuation greater than 5 HU, presumably as

Atlas of Small Animal CT and MRI, First Edition. Erik R. Wisner and Allison L. Zwingenberger.
© 2015 John Wiley & Sons, Inc. Published 2015 by John Wiley & Sons, Inc.

a result of necrotic tissue, tumor tissue, and hemorrhage. Renal dysplasia may also result in cyst formation, and affected kidneys are usually small, differentiating them from polycystic kidney disease.[10]

Ectopic ureters

Abnormal termination of one or both ureters distal to the trigone of the bladder results in urinary incontinence and hydroureter in female dogs.[11] Ectopic ureters are uncommon in male dogs and in cats. Multiple modalities are used to diagnose ectopic ureters, including CT, cystoscopy, ultrasonography, excretory urography, and vaginourethrography. CT is among the most sensitive methods to detect ectopic ureters and has the advantage of evaluating the kidneys, ureters, and urethral termination, without interference from the pelvis, and providing functional information (Figure 5.8.5).[12] The ureters fill with contrast approximately 2 minutes following intravenous contrast administration and are normally segmentally opacified as a result of peristalsis.[13] Furosemide injection can improve the number of ureteral segments visualized and the diameter of the segments during the pyelogram phase.[14]

The stream of contrast entering the bladder trigone is hyperattenuating to urine and can demarcate the vesiculoureteral junction. Ureters terminating in the caudal trigone or urethra travel close to midline and intramurally or occasionally extramurally. Ureteroceles can occur as dilations of the terminal ureter in dogs with ureteral ectopia, causing a thin-walled structure partially obstructing the ureter at the junction with the trigone (Figure 5.8.6). Secondary abnormalities include ipsilateral hydroureter and hydronephrosis resulting from chronic obstruction or pyelonephritis. In hydronephrotic kidneys, decreased renal function can be inferred from delayed pelvic and ureteral opacification although dilution of contrast may occur from urine stasis.

Retrocaval ureter

Retrocaval ureter, also termed circumcaval ureter, results from a developmental anomaly of the caudal vena cava and ureter. The prevalence in cats is approximately 35% and is normally right sided, although left or bilateral circumcaval ureter may be present. The anomaly is sometimes associated with double caudal vena cava.[15] Fewer reports are available in dogs, with left retrocaval ureter and transposition of the caudal vena cava reported (Figure 5.8.7). Contrast-enhanced MR urography was deemed a good diagnostic technique.[16] Ureters may circumnavigate the caudal vena cava and have been associated with strictures in cats.[17]

Trauma

Abdominal trauma can result in injury to renal parenchyma or vasculature. Although reports in the literature are lacking, expected abnormalities could include renal or perirenal hematoma, renal capsule tear, and renal vasculature avulsion (Figure 5.8.8). CT is the imaging modality of choice in people although MR is used when iodinated contrast medium is contraindicated or CT is unavailable.

Traumatic imaging characteristics can be extrapolated from findings in people. Intrarenal hematomas result in hypoattenuating foci in the renal cortex on contrast-enhanced images. Subcapsular hematoma appears as a hypoattenuating collection conforming to the outer renal capsule, highlighted by the contrast-enhanced renal parenchyma. When laceration of the kidney also occurs, hemorrhage can extend to the retroperitoneal space. Deep lacerations or avulsion can result in disruption or disconnection of the collecting system and renal vasculature. Contrast may extravasate, and renal parenchymal enhancement is poor.[18]

Lower urinary tract disruption results in leakage of urine into the retroperitoneal and/or peritoneal space. Expected imaging signs include extravasation of contrast medium from the ureter or bladder, similar to excretory urography or cystography. CT can eliminate superimposition of structures and is expected to have greater sensitivity to small volumes of contrast leakage compared to radiographs. In our experience, images acquired with the patient in both dorsal and ventral recumbency are sometimes required to detect the region of bladder rupture.

Vascular disorders

Renal infarcts are recognized as wedge-shaped areas of decreased attenuation in the renal cortex.[19] Acute infarcts may be subtle regions of hypoattenuation, progressing to larger regions as time progresses (Figure 5.8.9). The renal vasculature has three to four large interlobar arteries centrally and smaller interlobular arteries peripherally, obstruction of which may cause segmental or smaller peripheral infarcts, respectively (Figure 5.8.10). In chronic infarcts, the renal contour may be depressed because of tissue atrophy and fibrous replacement. These are frequently seen in animals with and without clinical signs of renal dysfunction. On MR images, acute infarcts are expected to be T1 and T2 hypointense, changing to T1 and T2 hyperintense from 1 day to 1 week post infarction, and T1 and T2 hypointense after 2 weeks as fibrosis replaces normal tissue.[20]

Inflammatory disorders

Inflammatory disorders of the urinary tract have not been well characterized in small animals, and expected imaging findings are extrapolated from people. Pyelonephritis results from ascending infections of the urinary tract and is most commonly encountered in animals with ectopic ureters or ureteral obstruction. In acute pyelonephritis, the kidney may be acutely enlarged with mild pelvic dilation and perirenal fat stranding on CT images. The affected renal parenchyma appears similar to infarction, with wedge-shaped hypoattenuating regions on contrast-enhanced images, which may enhance several hours after contrast administration.[21] Chronic pyelonephritis results in dilation of the collecting system and contrast enhancement of the wall of the renal pelvis. This may extend into the ureter as ureteritis. Chronic disease may result in renal abscessation, with a rounded, peripherally enhancing thick-walled fluid collection that may be contained within the renal capsule or extend into the retroperitoneal space. MR imaging is used in patients in which radiation or contrast medium is contraindicated. Expected imaging features include hyperintensity on T2 images and isointensity on T1 images, with decreased early and increased delayed contrast enhancement.[22]

Cross-sectional imaging is not routinely employed to image lower urinary tract infections. Image findings are expected to be similar to ultrasonographic findings, such as thickened bladder wall, presence of irregular mucosa, or mural polyps extending into the bladder lumen (Figure 5.8.11). Emphysematous cystitis would be characterized by intramural gas collections. Contrast medium normally forms a dependent layer in the bladder because of increased density; however, inverted layering of indeterminate cause has been described.[23]

Neoplasia

Primary and metastatic neoplasia may affect the upper and lower urinary tract and are characterized by disruption of normal renal architecture and the presence of disorganized nonfunctional tissue on contrast-enhanced images. CT and MR imaging can be used to detect and characterize the lesions and for surgical planning. Tumor types include renal cell carcinoma, sarcoma, adenoma, nephroblastoma, transitional cell carcinoma, and lymphoma. Smaller, benign masses, such as hemangioma, are more rarely encountered (Figure 5.8.12).

Primary renal cell carcinoma can be histologically divided into subtypes of clear cell, chromophobe, papillary, and multilocular cystic renal call carcinomas.[24] In human medicine, these subtypes have different enhancement patterns when viewed with multiphase CT, including unenhanced, corticomedullary, nephrographic, and excretory phases. Clear cell carcinomas are less frequent in dogs than in people; however, enhancement (125 HU) is expected to be higher in the corticomedullary phase than that of other tumors. The other tumor types are less intensely contrast enhancing during all phases (<106 HU).[25] Renal masses do not contain functional renal tissue, and enhancement is due to neovascularization (Figure 5.8.13). The masses tend to enhance during the vascular phase and then become hypoattenuating to normal renal tissue during the nephrographic and excretory phases.[26]

Nephroblastoma occurs most commonly in young dogs from 3 months to 4 years of age.[27,28] These tumors are derived from embryonic metanephric blastema and occur more commonly in the spine; however, concurrent renal and spinal nephroblastoma has been reported.[29] These large masses contain disorganized, immature renal tissue and may be partially functional (Figure 5.8.14). Ectopic nephroblastoma of the spine is described in Chapter 3.4, Figure 3.4.13.

Transitional cell carcinoma occurs more commonly in the urinary bladder and urethra but can affect the kidney through ureteral obstruction or invasion of the mass into the renal parenchyma. Transitional cell carcinoma has been reported as a heterogeneously enhancing, cystic renal mass with associated hydronephrosis and thickened ureteral wall.[30] Hydronephrosis secondary to ureteral obstruction results in a thin rim of enhancing tissue surrounding a dilated, fluid-attenuating renal pelvis. Hydroureter may be seen proximal to the site of the ureteral mass (Figure 5.8.15). The degree of contrast-enhanced urine in the pelvis gives an indication of renal function.

Transitional cell carcinoma of the bladder is characterized by a raised mass or flattened thickening of the bladder wall on MR and CT images. On CT images in people, the mass enhances to a greater degree than the bladder wall and can be seen as an enhancing mass or plaque-like filling defect surrounded by low-attenuation urine in the early contrast phase, although enhancement may be masked by surrounding high-attenuation urine (Figure 5.8.16). More invasive tumors may cause irregularity of the serosal surface and extend into local fat or musculature. Metastasis to local lymph nodes in people is characterized by enlargement greater than 10 mm in the short axis with rounding of the lymph node margins. False negatives are possible in normal-sized lymph nodes. Metastasis to bone, liver, skeletal muscle, spinal cord, and lungs has been reported.[31] Distension of the bladder with carbon dioxide has been recommended to increase the conspicuity of tumor margins from urine;[32] however, these masses are often intensely contrast enhancing and easily visualized. Urethral involvement causes thickening of the urethral wall and contrast enhancement of the tissues.[33]

There is little reported on MR imaging of bladder transitional cell carcinoma in dogs, but this modality is frequently employed in people. Tumors are isointense to muscle on T1 images and hyperintense to muscle and the bladder muscularis on T2 images. Tumors are intensely contrast enhancing on MR images and, similar to CT, show greatest enhancement within 90 seconds of contrast injection prior to contrast enhancement of the urine. In people, lymph nodes are considered metastatic when either oval and greater than 10 mm in diameter or round and greater than 8 mm in diameter. Distant metastases to liver, lymph node, and bone may also be contrast enhancing.[33]

Transitional cell carcinoma may originate from or extend to the urethra and may involve the prostate gland or vestibule (Figure 5.8.17). Other tumors occurring in the soft tissues surrounding the urethra include leiomyosarcoma or undifferentiated sarcoma. Imaging features include thickening, irregularity, or discrete masses with contrast enhancement on CT or MR images.

Lymphoma occurs unilaterally or bilaterally in kidneys of dogs and cats. CT and MR reports are lacking; however, similarities with lymphoma in people are expected. CT imaging is the modality of choice, with lymphoma appearing hypoattenuating compared to normal parenchyma in contrast-enhanced images. Single or multiple masses can be encountered. In people, lymphoma can extend to the retroperitoneal space with an amorphous mass that extends beyond the renal border and envelops the vasculature. Lymphoma may also surround the kidney without disrupting the underlying parenchyma, or diffusely infiltrate the kidney causing primarily renal enlargement with patchy contrast enhancement. [34]

Degenerative disorders

Chronic renal changes are common primary and incidental findings on CT and MR images. Various diseases of the upper urinary tract result in renal atrophy and fibrosis, altering the normal renal parenchyma. The kidneys may have unilateral or bilateral decreased size with irregularity of the cortical margin (Figure 5.8.18). Mineralization of the renal parenchyma and cystic changes may also be present. End-stage kidneys have minimal or absent urine contrast-enhancement, which is an indication of decreased functional tissue.

Urinary tract obstruction

CT is used most commonly in assessing cats, and less frequently dogs, for ureteral obstruction. Calculi are generally the cause of ureteral obstruction, with strictures or blood clots occurring less frequently. The obstruction may be unilateral or bilateral, with varying degrees of hydronephrosis depending on the completeness and duration of urethral obstruction. The size and number of calculi, as well as precise measurement of the distance from the kidney, are parameters that aid in surgical planning for ureterotomy.[35] Contrast enhancement of the obstructed kidney may be diminished because of chronic decreased function (Figure 5.8.19). Poor enhancement and the potential for renal toxicity may be contraindications for contrast administration. Contrast does not add information to the precontrast estimate of number and location of calculi.[36]

Urethral stricture may also result in obstruction of the urinary tract. Although often imaged using conventional radiographic contrast studies, urethrography is possible with CT imaging using the same technique. Multiplanar reformatting of thinly collimated images is advantageous for displaying the entire urethra with fine spatial resolution, allowing evaluation of the extent and degree of stricture (Figure 5.8.20). Extramural obstruction of the urethra may also be caused by malposition of the bladder or pelvic masses (Figure 5.8.21).

Figure 5.8.1 Normal Urinary Tract (Canine)   CT

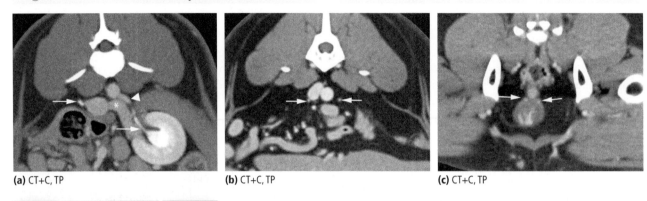

(a) CT+C, TP   **(b)** CT+C, TP   **(c)** CT+C, TP

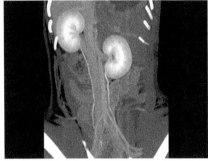

(d) CT+C, MIP, DP

1y FS Hound cross. Images **a–c** are ordered from cranial to caudal. The renal artery is smaller than the vein and arises from the lateral aspect of the aorta (**a**: arrowhead). The renal vein is larger, arising from the caudal vena cava (**a**: asterisk). The ureters can be seen exiting the renal pelvis (**a**: arrows) and coursing ventrolateral to the aorta and caudal vena cava (**b**: arrows) in the pyelogram phase. The ureters terminate near the bladder trigone (**c**: arrows) and cascades of contrast-enhanced urine stream to the dependent bladder (**c**). The course of the ureters can be seen through the retroperitoneal space on a ventrodorsal MIP projection (**d**).

Figure 5.8.2 Normal Urinary Tract (Canine)   MR

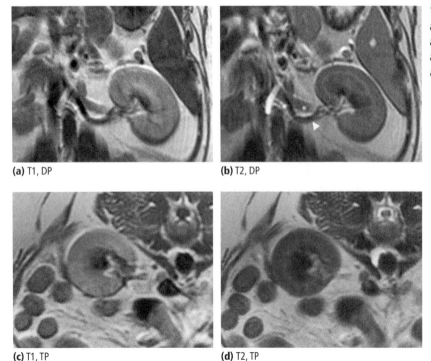

(a) T1, DP   **(b)** T2, DP

14y MC Norwegian Elkhound. The kidneys are hyperintense to spleen on T1 images and isointense on T2 images. The renal artery (**b**: arrowhead) and vein (**b**: asterisk) are best seen on the dorsal plane images.

(c) T1, TP   **(d)** T2, TP

Figure 5.8.3   Normal Renal Contrast Enhancement (Canine)   CT

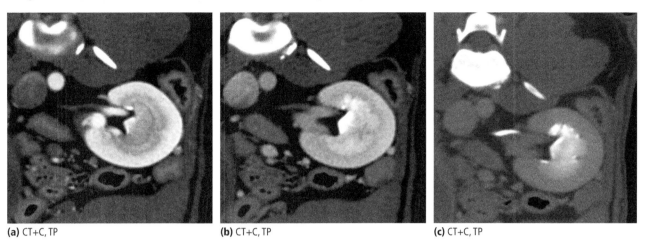

(a) CT+C, TP   **(b)** CT+C, TP   **(c)** CT+C, TP

7y FS German Shepherd Dog imaged for a right adrenal mass (not shown). Dual-phase CT angiography was performed with arterial, venous, and late-phase series, as seen by the enhancement of the aorta and caudal vena cava (**a–c**). The arterial phase image (**a**) shows intense cortical enhancement, indicating the renal corticomedullary phase. The venous phase image has relatively isoattenuating cortex and medulla, indicating the nephrogram phase, with early renal pelvic enhancement. The late venous excretory phase image has mainly pelvic, ureteral, and medullary enhancement.

Figure 5.8.4   Renal Cortical Cysts (Canine)   CT

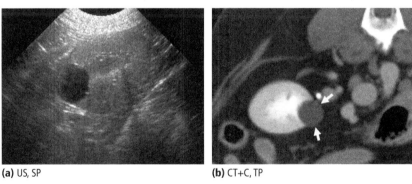

(a) US, SP   **(b)** CT+C, TP

5y MC Alaskan Malamute. Anechoic cysts are present in the right kidney on an ultrasound examination (**a**). On CT images, the cysts are fluid attenuating and distributed throughout the cortex (**b–d**), with one cyst deforming the renal capsule (**b**: arrows). The cysts are nonenhancing, as opposed to the marked enhancement of the renal cortex.

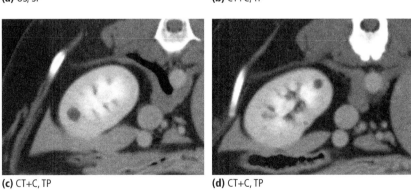

(c) CT+C, TP   **(d)** CT+C, TP

Figure 5.8.5   Bilateral Ureteral Ectopia (Canine)   CT

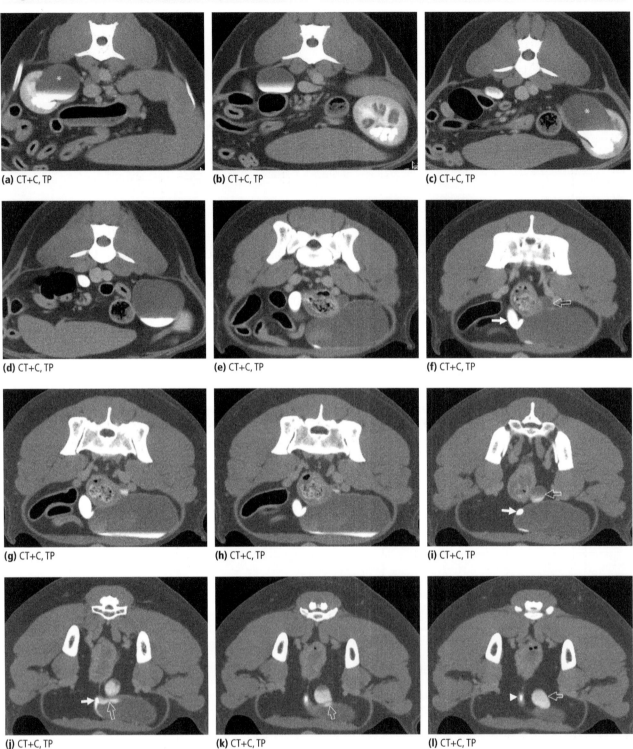

(a) CT+C, TP   **(b)** CT+C, TP   **(c)** CT+C, TP

(d) CT+C, TP   **(e)** CT+C, TP   **(f)** CT+C, TP

(g) CT+C, TP   **(h)** CT+C, TP   **(i)** CT+C, TP

(j) CT+C, TP   **(k)** CT+C, TP   **(l)** CT+C, TP

6.5y MC Labrador Retriever with incidentally discovered bilateral hydronephrosis and isosthenuria. Contrast-enhanced CT images are ordered from cranial to caudal from the kidneys to the urinary bladder. Both renal pelves are severely dilated, with layering of nonenhancing and contrast-enhancing urine (**a,c**: asterisk). The right ureter contains more uniform contrast as it travels distally toward the bladder (**f**: arrow). The left ureter is nonenhancing proximally and fills with lower attenuating contrast distally (**f**: open arrow). The right ureter enters the bladder at the trigone, and urine cascades into the dependent bladder (**i,j**: arrow). The left ureter has a caudal blind-ending dilation (**l**: open arrow); however, it enters the bladder wall and tunnels to the urethra without apparent connection to the bladder lumen (**i–k**: open arrow). The high-attenuation urine in the urethra (**l**: arrowhead) is likely due to both ureters continuing to tunnel in the urethral wall, as no backflow of urine appears in the bladder. The gender of the dog may have prevented typical incontinence symptoms.

Figure 5.8.6   Ectopic Ureters, Ureterocele (Canine)   CT

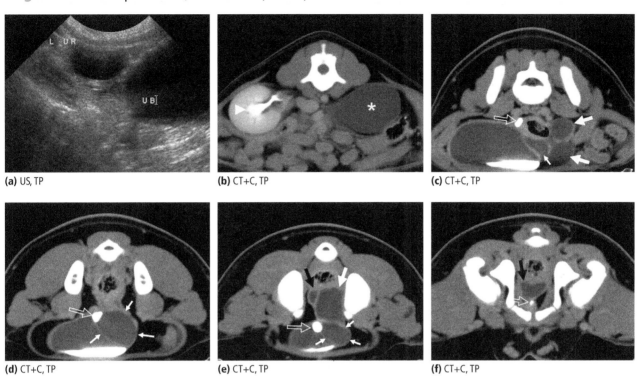

(a) US, TP

(b) CT+C, TP

(c) CT+C, TP

(d) CT+C, TP

(e) CT+C, TP

(f) CT+C, TP

2mo F Labrador Retriever with urinary incontinence. Images **b–f** are ordered from cranial to caudal. The left ureter was severely dilated on ultrasound examination (**a**: L UR). The left renal pelvis is hydronephrotic without contrast enhancement (**b**: asterisk), and residual left renal parenchyma is minimal. The right renal pelvis is also moderately dilated (**b**: arrowhead). The dilated left ureter is tortuous and dilated and extends beyond the bladder trigone into the pelvis as a blind-ending sac (**c,e**: white arrows). The right ureter is dilated, tunneling through the bladder wall and emptying contrast-enhancing urine into the bladder, before continuing into the urethra (**c–f**: open arrows). The ureterocele is seen as a thin-walled compartment (**d,e**: small arrows) in the left caudal bladder with connection to the ureter (**c**: small arrow). The vagina is filled with unenhanced urine dorsal to the urethra (**e,f**: black arrow).

Figure 5.8.7   Retrocaval Ureter (Canine)   CT

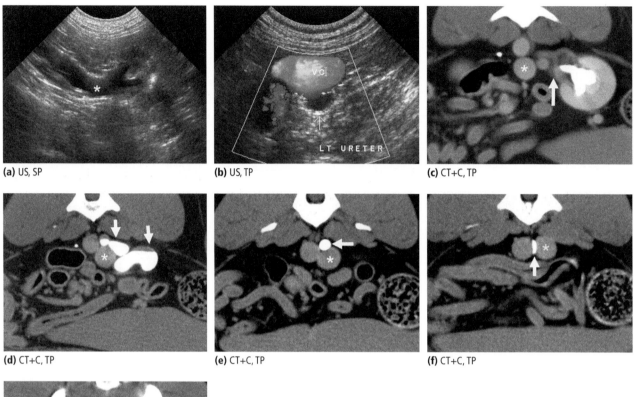

(a) US, SP   (b) US, TP   (c) CT+C, TP

(d) CT+C, TP   (e) CT+C, TP   (f) CT+C, TP

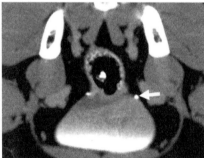

(g) CT+C, TP

3y FS Bernese Mountain Dog with incidentally discovered hydroureter. Images **c–g** are ordered from cranial to caudal. The dilated ureter was visible on ultrasound examination ventral to the caudal vena cava (**b**: arrow). On both ultrasonographic and CT images, the caudal vena cava was located on the left side, forming a curved lateral deviation caudal to the kidneys (**a,c–f**: asterisk). The left renal pelvis and ureter are dilated (**c–e**: arrows), and the ureter takes a dorsal course relative to the caudal vena cava. The ureter is compressed between the caudal vena cava and aorta more caudally (**f**: arrow) before entering the bladder normally at the trigone (**g**: arrow).

Figure 5.8.8   Traumatic Renal Capsule Tear (Feline)   CT

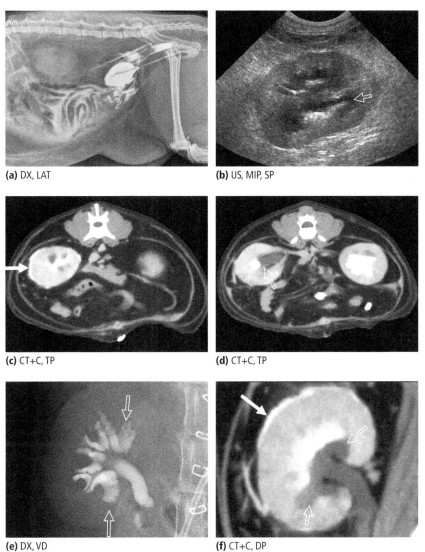

(a) DX, LAT

(b) US, MIP, SP

(c) CT+C, TP

(d) CT+C, TP

(e) DX, VD

(f) CT+C, DP

2y FS Domestic Shorthair with uroabdomen. A cystogram (**a**) revealed a ruptured bladder, which was repaired surgically. The uroabdomen continued following surgical repair, and the right renal pelvis was dilated on ultrasound examination (**b**: open arrow), CT (**d,f**: open arrows), and nephropyelography (**e**: open arrows), indicating ureteral obstruction. On contrast-enhanced CT images, there was subcapsular leakage of contrast from the kidney (**c,f**: white arrow), revealing that the source of the uroabdomen was a renal capsular tear. Ureteral necrosis, subcapsular hemorrhage, and inflammation were found on histopathology after nephrectomy, with trauma and ureteral obstruction as the differential diagnoses for renal capsular rupture.

Figure 5.8.9 Acute Renal Infarcts (Canine)

CT

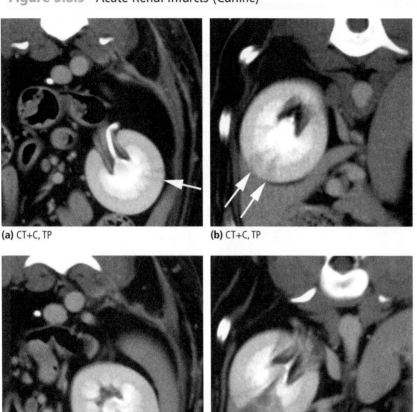

6y FS Labrador Retriever with cutaneous pyo-granulomatous inflammation and fever. The top and bottom rows of images were taken 1 week apart. In the acute phase of infarction, there are faint, triangular or wedge-shaped hypoattenuating regions in the right (**a**: arrow) and left (**b**: arrows) renal cortex and medulla. After 1 week, these progress to larger, markedly hypoattenuating triangular regions affecting the cortex and medulla (**c,d**: arrow).

(**a**) CT+C, TP   (**b**) CT+C, TP

(**c**) CT+C, TP   (**d**) CT+C, TP

Figure 5.8.10 Renal Infarcts (Canine)

CT

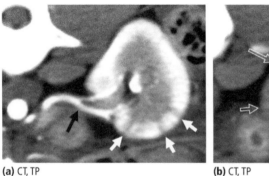 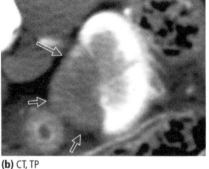 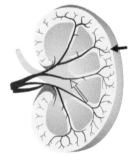

(**a**) CT, TP   (**b**) CT, TP   (**c**) IL

5mo F German Shepherd Dog with multiple congenital cardiac anomalies including cor triatriatum dexter. Images were acquired during the arterial phase of contrast administration. The bifurcating left renal artery is evident (**a**: black arrow). Multiple focal regions of cortical hypoperfusion are seen near the hilus (**a**: arrows), likely representing infarcts in the peripheral interlobular arteries (**c**: black arrow). A regional infarct involving the caudal pole of the kidney is present (**b**: open arrows), most likely representing infarction of one or more interlobar arteries (**c**: open arrow). The impaired cardiac circulation and/or previous cardiac surgery may be related to the infarcts.

Figure 5.8.11   Polypoid Cystitis (Canine)

CT

(a) CT, TP

(b) CT, TP

(c) CT, TP

(d) CT+C, TP

(e) CT+C, TP

(f) CT+C, TP

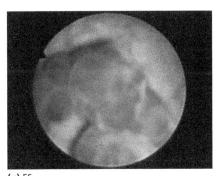

(g) ES

9y MC German Shepherd Dog with hematuria for several years. Unenhanced (**a–c**) and corresponding contrast-enhanced (**d–f**) images of the urinary bladder are ordered from cranial to caudal. On unenhanced images, there is a hypoattenuating, rounded structure in the bladder lumen (**a–c**: arrow), which is surrounded by more hyperattenuating urine. On contrast-enhanced images, the bladder wall is moderately thickened and enhancing (**d**: open arrow). There is a mass arising from the ventral bladder wall with a stalk and polypoid expansion. The mass has peripheral and heterogeneous contrast enhancement (**d–f**: arrow). Contrast-enhanced urine is located in the dorsal aspect of the bladder as the dog was imaged in dorsal recumbency. Polypoid cystitis was seen endoscopically (**g**).

Figure 5.8.12 Hemangioma (Canine)

CT

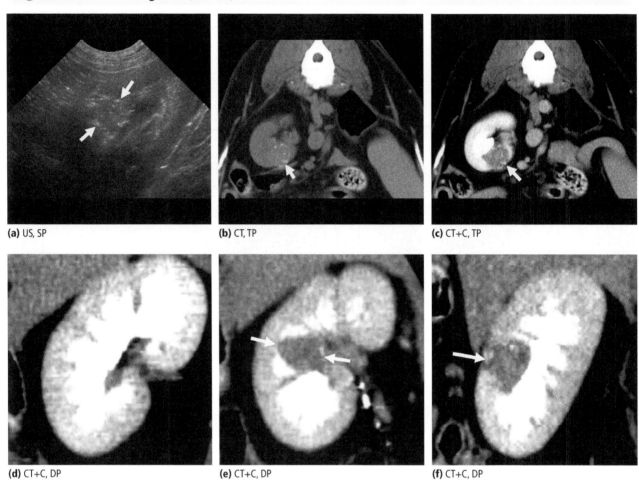

(a) US, SP

(b) CT, TP

(c) CT+C, TP

(d) CT+C, DP

(e) CT+C, DP

(f) CT+C, DP

9y FS German Shepherd Dog with a 5-month history of hematuria. A renal cortical mass with fine multifocal mineralization was seen in the cortex of the right kidney on ultrasound examination (**a**: arrows) and unenhanced CT (**b**: arrow). The mass was nonenhancing and is seen on transverse (**c**: arrow) and dorsal reformatted images (**e,f**: arrows) ventral to the renal pelvis (**d**). A nephrectomy was performed, and the mass was diagnosed as a hemangioma.

Figure 5.8.13   Renal Carcinoma (Canine)

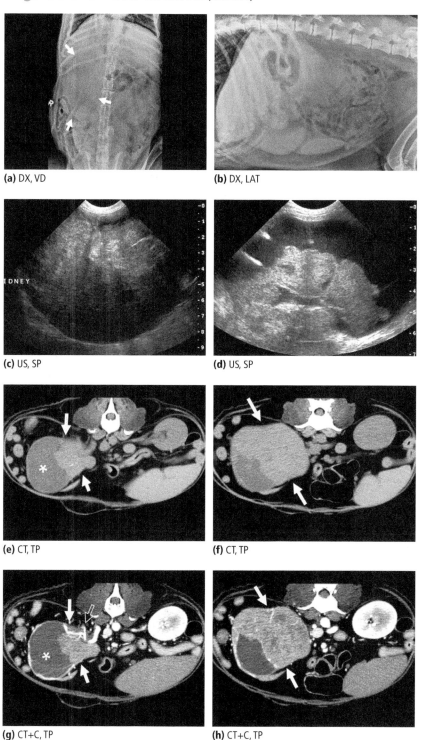

(a) DX, VD

(b) DX, LAT

(c) US, SP

(d) US, SP

(e) CT, TP

(f) CT, TP

(g) CT+C, TP

(h) CT+C, TP

8y MC mixed-breed dog with weight loss, inappetence, and elevated creatinine and blood urea nitrogen (BUN). Radiographs (**a**,**b**) revealed a mass effect arising from the right kidney (**a**: arrows). Ultrasonography confirmed the presence of a mass and greatly expanded right renal capsule (**c**,**d**). CT images show an enlarged, irregular right renal mass (**e**,**f**: arrows) with disorganized, heterogeneously enhancing tissue (**g**,**h**: arrows) near the pelvis and a peripheral fluid collection (**e**,**g**: asterisk). There is abundant arterial supply to the periphery of the mass (**g**: open arrow). On scintigraphic examination, the left kidney was normal (**i**: arrowhead—next page), and the right kidney had little radiopharmaceutical uptake in the cranial pole (**i**: open arrowhead) and an area of photopenia corresponding to the mass in the caudal pole (**i**: arrow). A nephrectomy was performed, and the mass was diagnosed as a renal carcinoma effacing the kidney (**j**). (Figure continues on next page.)

Figure 5.8.13 (*Continued*)

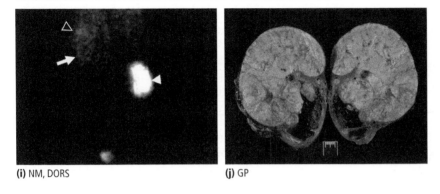

(i) NM, DORS   **(j)** GP

Figure 5.8.14 Nephroblastoma (Canine)

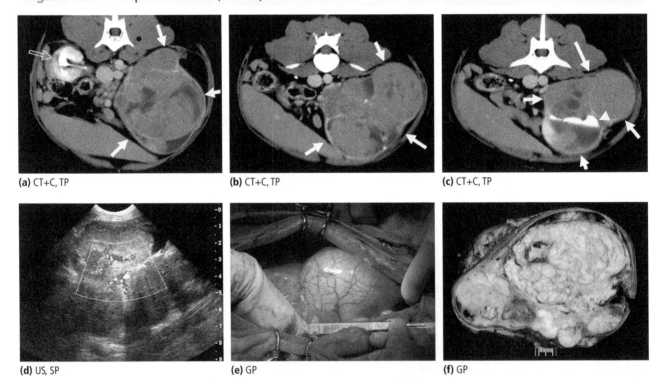

(a) CT+C, TP   **(b)** CT+C, TP   **(c)** CT+C, TP

(d) US, SP   **(e)** GP   **(f)** GP

2y MC Doberman Pinscher with hematuria. Images **a–c** are ordered from cranial to caudal. There is a large, heterogeneous, cavitary mass replacing the left kidney (**a–c:** arrows). The mass is heterogeneously contrast enhancing, and urine production is present in the most caudal cavitary region (**c:** arrowhead). The CT scan was performed in dorsal recumbency, hence the inverted fluid-contrast interface. The left ureter is not identified. The right kidney has mild pelvic dilation with a thin lateral cortex (**a:** open arrow) and cortical infarct (not shown). The mass is vascular on Doppler ultrasound (**d**). A nephrectomy was performed and nephroblastoma with disorganized renal tissue was diagnosed (**e,f**).

Figure 5.8.15 Ureteral Transitional Cell Carcinoma (Canine)   CT

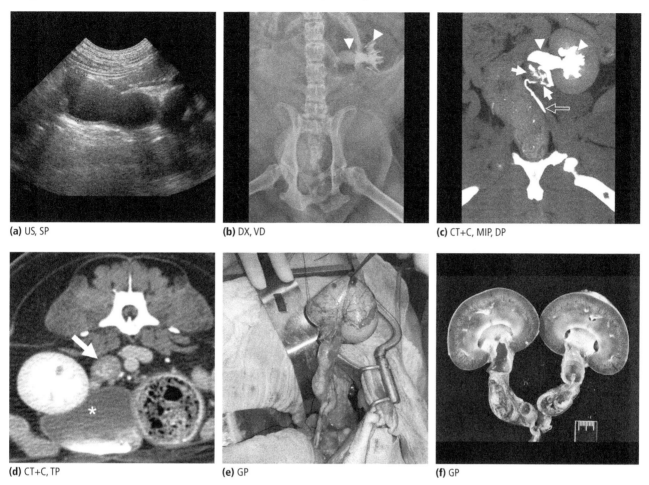

(a) US, SP

(b) DX, VD

(c) CT+C, MIP, DP

(d) CT+C, TP

(e) GP

(f) GP

8y MC English Bulldog with respiratory distress and incidentally discovered left ureteral obstruction on ultrasound examination (**a**). A nephropyelogram was performed, demonstrating the dilated left renal pelvis and proximal ureter (**b**: arrowheads) without visualization of the distal ureter. Urine enters the bladder, suggesting a partial obstruction. On CT images, the dilated left renal pelvis and proximal ureter are again seen (**c**: arrowheads). There is a soft-tissue mass enlarging the left ureter distal to the ureteral dilation (**c,d**: arrows), and the contrast-enhanced urine traces a complex, tortuous path through this region. The distal ureter is a more normal diameter (**c**: open arrow). The bladder is visible (**d**: asterisk) ventral to the ureteral mass (**d**: arrow) on transverse images. A nephrectomy was performed, and transitional carcinoma of the ureter was diagnosed.

Figure 5.8.16 Bladder Transitional Cell Carcinoma (Canine)   CT

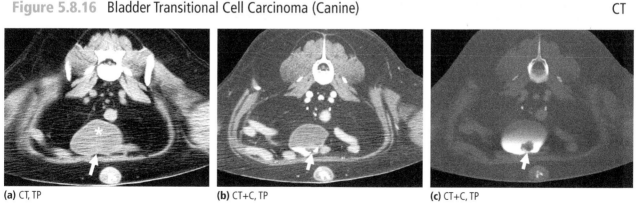

(a) CT, TP

(b) CT+C, TP

(c) CT+C, TP

10y MC German Shepherd Dog mix with lumbosacral intervertebral disc herniation and incidental bladder mass. The mass (**a**: arrow) is slightly hyperattenuating to urine (**a**: asterisk) on the unenhanced images, with small regions of mineralization. The mass becomes apparent as a filling defect (**b,c**: arrow) within the contrast-enhanced urine during the venous and late phase images. The mass was surgically excised and diagnosed as a focal papillary transitional cell carcinoma.

Figure 5.8.17 Urethral Transitional Cell Carcinoma (Canine)   CT

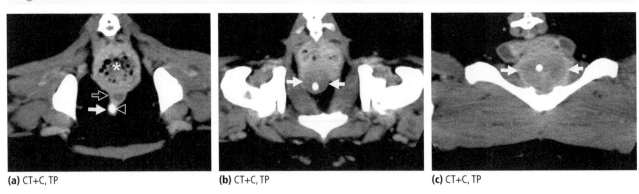

(a) CT+C, TP   **(b)** CT+C, TP   **(c)** CT+C, TP

10y FS German Shepherd Dog mix with pollakiuria. Images are ordered from cranial to caudal. The high-density structure centrally represents a catheter within the urethral lumen (**a**: open arrowhead). The walls of the urethra are of normal thickness in the most cranial image (**a**: white arrow). More caudally, the urethral wall is markedly thickened with moderate, heterogeneous contrast enhancement (**b**,**c**: arrows). The vagina (**a**: open arrow) and colon (**a**: asterisk) become displaced dorsally by the enlarged urethra, which extends caudally into the vestibule (**c**).

Figure 5.8.18 Multiple Urinary Tract Calculi (Feline)   CT

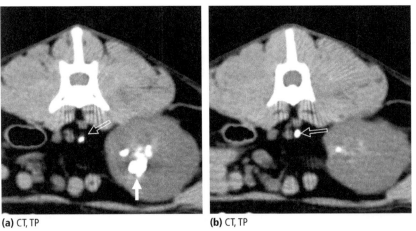

8y MC Japanese Bobtail with azotemia. Images are ordered from cranial to caudal. On unenhanced images, the left kidney is enlarged with an irregular contour (**a**,**b**), and multiple mineral-attenuating calculi are present in the renal pelvis (**a**: arrow). There are calculi within the left ureter (**a**,**b**: open arrow) causing ureteral obstruction. Small calculi are also present in the right ureter (**c**,**d**: open arrow). The right kidney was atrophied (not shown) as a result of previous obstruction. There are multiple small calculi in the urinary bladder (**d**: arrowhead).

(a) CT, TP   **(b)** CT, TP

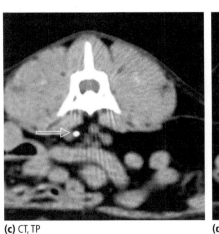
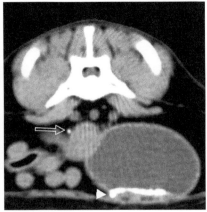

(c) CT, TP   **(d)** CT, TP

Figure 5.8.19   Ureteral Obstruction (Feline)

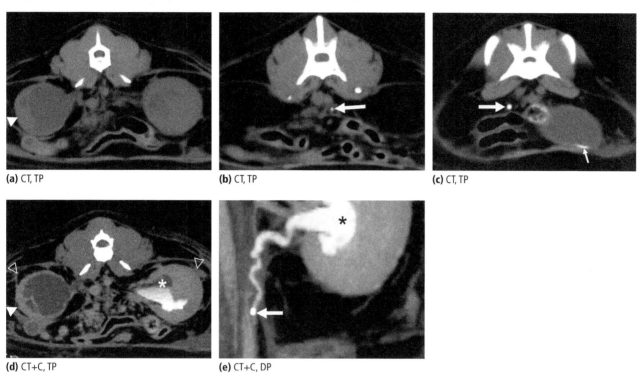

(a) CT, TP

(b) CT, TP

(c) CT, TP

(d) CT+C, TP

(e) CT+C, DP

11y MC Domestic Shorthair with renal failure and ureteral obstruction. Images **a–c** are ordered from cranial to caudal. The kidneys are enlarged and hydronephrotic on comparable unenhanced (**a**) and contrast-enhanced (**d**) images. There are ureteral calculi present in the left (**b**: arrow) and right (**c**: large arrow) ureters, causing bilateral ureteral obstruction. Calculi are also present in the urinary bladder (**c**: small arrow). On contrast-enhanced images, the right renal cortex enhances mildly (**d**: arrowhead) compared to unenhanced images (**a**: arrowhead); however, there is no enhancement in the renal pelvis, indicating minimal filtration function. The left kidney is functional with contrast-enhanced urine present in the dilated pelvis (**d,e**: asterisk). There is retroperitoneal effusion surrounding both kidneys (**d**: open arrowheads). The left proximal ureter is dilated and tortuous proximal to the ureteral calculus obstruction (**e**: arrow).

Figure 5.8.20   Urethral Stricture (Feline)   CT

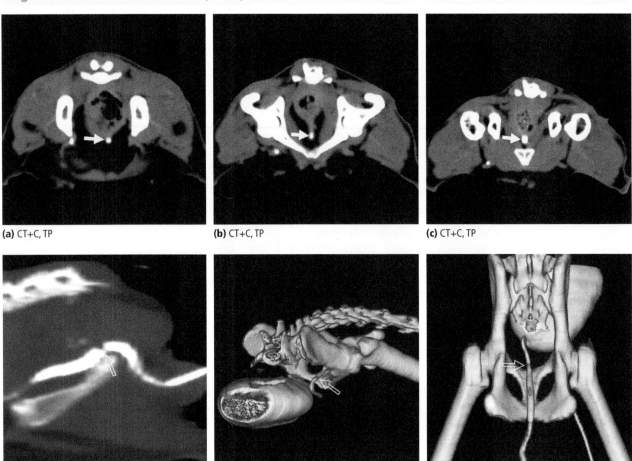

(a) CT+C, TP   (b) CT+C, TP   (c) CT+C, TP

(d) CT+C, SP   (e) CT+C, 3D, OBL   (f) CT+C, 3D, VENT

11y MC Domestic Longhair with stranguria. Images **a–c** are ordered from cranial to caudal. A urethrogram was performed to outline the lumen of the urethra. Cranial and caudal to the pubis, the urethra is normal in diameter (**a,c**: arrow). The urethral lumen narrows in a medial to lateral direction at the level of the pubis (**b**: arrow). The stricture is also seen on a sagittal reformatted image (**d**: open arrow) and on 3D reformatted images (**e,f**: open arrow).

Figure 5.8.21   Pelvic Bladder (Canine)   CT

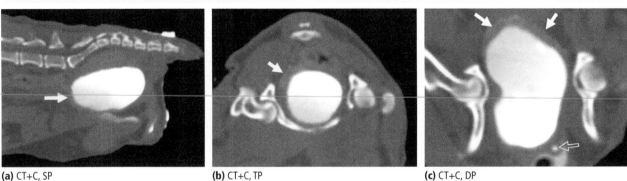

(a) CT+C, SP   (b) CT+C, TP   (c) CT+C, DP

14y FS Chihuahua with stranguria and pollakiuria. A cystourethrogram was performed under fluoroscopy prior to CT. Images are displayed in a wide window to counteract artifact from high-attenuation contrast medium in the bladder. The bladder is located entirely within the pelvis (**a–c**: arrows). The wall is thickened, most particularly in the cranioventral aspect. The caudal position of the bladder has caused lateral displacement of the urethra (**c**: open arrow), with partial outflow obstruction. A cystopexy was performed that relieved the clinical signs of stranguria, and no bacteria were cultured from the urine.

References

1. Alexander K, Ybarra N, del Castillo JR, Morin V, Gauvin D, Bichot S, et al. Determination of glomerular filtration rate in anesthetized pigs by use of three-phase whole-kidney computed tomography and Patlak plot analysis. Am J Vet Res. 2008;69: 1455–1462.

2. Schmidt DM, Scrivani PV, Dykes NL, Goldstein RM, Erb HN, Reeves AP. Comparison of glomerular filtration rate determined by use of single-slice dynamic computed tomography and scintigraphy in cats. Am J Vet Res. 2012;73:463–469.

3. Bouma JL, Aronson LR, Keith DG, Saunders HM. Use of computed tomography renal angiography for screening feline renal transplant donors. Vet Radiol Ultrasound. 2003;44:636–641.

4. Cáceres AV, Zwingenberger AL, Aronson LR, Mai W. Characterization of normal feline renal vascular anatomy with dual-phase CT angiography. Vet Radiol Ultrasound. 2008;49:350–356.

5. Cavrenne R, Mai W. Time-resolved renal contrast-enhanced MRA in normal dogs. Vet Radiol Ultrasound. 2009;50:58–64.

6. Tyson R, Logsdon SA, Werre SR, Daniel GB. Estimation of feline renal volume using computed tomography and ultrasound. Vet Radiol Ultrasound. 2013;54:127–132.

7. Cronin RE. Contrast-induced nephropathy: pathogenesis and prevention. Pediatr Nephrol. 2010;25:191–204.

8. Reichle JK, DiBartola SP, Léveillé R. Renal ultrasonographic and computed tomographic appearance, volume, and function of cats with autosomal dominant polycystic kidney disease. Vet Radiol Ultrasound. 2002;43:368–373.

9. Moe L, Lium B. Computed tomography of hereditary multifocal renal cystadenocarcinomas in German shepherd dogs. Vet Radiol Ultrasound. 1997;38:335–343.

10. Kim J, Choi H, Lee Y, Jung J, Yeon S, Lee H, et al. Multicystic dysplastic kidney disease in a dog. Can Vet J. 2011;52:645–649.

11. Davidson AP, Westropp JL. Diagnosis and management of urinary ectopia. Vet Clin North Am Small Anim Pract. 2014;44: 343–353.

12. Samii VF, McLoughlin MA, Mattoon JS, Drost WT, Chew DJ, DiBartola SP, et al. Digital fluoroscopic excretory urography, digital fluoroscopic urethrography, helical computed tomography, and cystoscopy in 24 dogs with suspected ureteral ectopia. J Vet Intern Med. 2004;18:271–281.

13. Rozear L, Tidwell AS. Evaluation of the ureter and ureterovesicular junction using helical computed tomographic excretory urography in healthy dogs. Vet Radiol Ultrasound. 2003;44:155–164.

14. Secrest S, Essman S, Nagy J, Schultz L. Effects of furosemide on ureteral diameter and attenuation using computed tomographic excretory urography in normal dogs. Vet Radiol Ultrasound. 2013;54:17–24.

15. Bélanger R, Shmon CL, Gilbert PJ, Linn KA. Prevalence of circumcaval ureters and double caudal vena cava in cats. Am J Vet Res. 2014;75:91–95.

16. Duconseille AC, Louvet A, Lazard P, Valentin S, Molho M. Imaging diagnosis–left retrocaval ureter and transposition of the caudal vena cava in a dog. Vet Radiol Ultrasound. 2010;51:52–56.

17. Zaid MS, Berent AC, Weisse C, Caceres A. Feline Ureteral Strictures: 10 Cases (2007–2009). J Vet Intern Med. 2011;25: 222–229.

18. Szmigielski W, Kumar R, Al Hilli S, Ismail M. Renal trauma imaging: Diagnosis and management. A pictorial review. Pol J Radiol. 2013;78:27–35.

19. Antopolsky M, Simanovsky N, Stalnikowicz R, Salameh S, Hiller N. Renal infarction in the ED: 10-year experience and review of the literature. Am J Emerg Med. 2012;30:1055–1060.

20. Choo SW, Kim SH, Jeong YG, Shin YM, Kim JS, Han MC. MR imaging of segmental renal infarction: an experimental study. Clin Radiol. 1997;52:65–68.

21. Ifergan J, Pommier R, Brion M-C, Glas L, Rocher L, Bellin MF. Imaging in upper urinary tract infections. Diagn Interv Imaging. 2012;93:509–519.

22. Runge VM, Timoney JF, Williams NM. Magnetic resonance imaging of experimental pyelonephritis in rabbits. Invest Radiol. 1997;32:696–704.

23. Samii VF. Inverted contrast medium-urine layering in the canine urinary bladder on computed tomography. Vet Radiol Ultrasound. 2005;46:502–505.

24. Edmondson EF, Hess AM, Powers BE. Prognostic Significance of Histologic Features in Canine Renal Cell Carcinomas: 70 Nephrectomies. Vet Pathol. 2014.

25. Young JR, Margolis D, Sauk S, Pantuck AJ, Sayre J, Raman SS. Clear cell renal cell carcinoma: discrimination from other renal cell carcinoma subtypes and oncocytoma at multiphasic multidetector CT. Radiology. 2013;267:444–453.

26. Yuh BI, Cohan RH. Different phases of renal enhancement: role in detecting and characterizing renal masses during helical CT. AJR Am J Roentgenol. 1999;173:747–755.

27. Michael HT, Sharkey LC, Kovi RC, Hart TM, Wünschmann A, Manivel JC. Pathology in practice. Renal nephroblastoma in a young dog. J Am Vet Med Assoc. 2013;242:471–473.

28. Pancotto TE, Rossmeisl JH, Zimmerman K, Robertson JL, Werre SR. Intramedullary spinal cord neoplasia in 53 dogs (1990–2010): distribution, clinicopathologic characteristics, and clinical behavior. J Vet Intern Med. 2013;27:1500–1508.

29. Gasser AM, Bush WW, Smith S, Walton R. Extradural spinal, bone marrow, and renal nephroblastoma. J Am Anim Hosp Assoc. 2003;39:80–85.

30. Zotti A, Corsi F, Ratto A, Petterino C. What is your diagnosis? Transitional cell carcinoma. J Am Vet Med Assoc. 2010;237: 777–778.

31. Vignoli M, Terragni R, Rossi F, Frühauf L, Bacci B, Ressel L, et al. Whole body computed tomographic characteristics of skeletal and cardiac muscular metastatic neoplasia in dogs and cats. Vet Radiol Ultrasound. 2013;54:223–230.

32. Naughton JF, Widmer WR, Constable PD, Knapp DW. Accuracy of three-dimensional and two-dimensional ultrasonography for measurement of tumor volume in dogs with transitional cell carcinoma of the urinary bladder. Am J Vet Res. 2012;73:1919–1924.

33. Setty BN, Holalkere N-S, Sahani DV, Uppot RN, Harisinghani M, Blake MA. State-of-the-art cross-sectional imaging in bladder cancer. Curr Probl Diagn Radiol. 2007;36:83–96.

34. Urban BA, Fishman EK. Renal lymphoma: CT patterns with emphasis on helical CT. Radiographics. 2000;20:197–212.

35. Berent AC. Ureteral obstructions in dogs and cats: a review of traditional and new interventional diagnostic and therapeutic options. J Vet Emerg Crit Car. 2011;21:86–103.

36. Carr AH, Wisner ER, Westropp JL, Mayhew PD. Feline obstructive ureterolithiasis: utility of computed tomography and ultrasound in clinical decision making. Vet Radiol Ultrasound. 2012;53:680.

5.9

Reproductive tract

Introduction

Cross-sectional imaging of the reproductive tract is often complementary to other modalities, including ultrasonography. The ovaries are located lateral and caudal to the kidneys in the dorsal peritoneal space. In anestrus, the ovary is a small triangular soft-tissue attenuating structure that often has no visible follicles. Follicles are smooth, round, fluid-attenuating structures that may protrude from the edge of the ovarian tissue. The uterine horns are smaller than small intestinal loops and can be followed caudally and medially in the lateral abdomen to join the uterine body between the bladder and colon. The cervix forms an enlargement at the junction of the uterine body and vagina. The vagina is located within the pelvic canal dorsal to the urethra (Figure 5.9.1).

The testes migrate from the region of the kidneys to the inguinal canal and scrotum during development. Normal testes are uniform in attenuation and intensity on CT and MR images. The prostate gland surrounds the urethra caudal to the trigone of the bladder. It is small and uniform in attenuation and intensity in neutered dogs. Intact animals have larger glands because of hyperplasia, and parenchymal cysts may also develop. The central region near the urethra is hyperintense on contrast-enhanced images, and radiating striations can be seen in the parenchyma (Figures 5.9.2, 5.9.3).

Female reproductive tract

The female reproductive tract has not been studied using CT or MR imaging; however, findings during the different phases of the reproductive cycle can be extrapolated from studies performed using ultrasound imaging.[1] Developmental anomalies of the reproductive tract can result in clinical signs related to incontinence. Fluid pooling in the vagina may be due to anatomical malposition, malformation of the urethra and/or vagina, and hermaphroditism (Figure 5.9.4).

Inflammation of the uterus may occur postpartum or after estrus and results in thickening of the uterine wall, with possible folding of the mucosa and fluid-attenuating contents with uterine enlargement. The wall of the uterus is enhancing in the inflammatory or hypertrophic state (Figure 5.9.5).

Masses arising from the ovary may be due to cysts or neoplastic lesions, such as carcinoma, adenocarcinoma, teratoma, granular cell tumor, or rhabdomyosarcoma.[2–4] Characteristics of aggressive adnexal masses on ultrasound imaging in people include an irregular solid tumor, presence of ascites, more than four papillary structures, irregular multilocular tumor larger than 10 cm, and very strong blood flow. Benign mass characteristics include a unilocular tumor, mass with solid components of less than 7 mm, presence of acoustic shadows, smooth multilocular mass <10 cm, and no blood flow.[5] On MR images, benign masses are purely cystic, endometrial, or fatty with an absence of wall enhancement with a low T2 signal in the solid component of the mass. Malignant mass characteristics include a mass >4 cm, bilateral masses, necrosis in a solid lesion, and cystic lesion with wall or septal thickness >3 mm or papillary projections, and ascites.[6] Other studies have shown intermediate T2 signal intensity and high b = 1,000 signal intensity on diffusion-weighted imaging to be predictors of malignancy.[7]

Atlas of Small Animal CT and MRI, First Edition. Erik R. Wisner and Allison L. Zwingenberger.
© 2015 John Wiley & Sons, Inc. Published 2015 by John Wiley & Sons, Inc.

Male reproductive tract

The most common developmental anomaly of the male reproductive tract is retained testicle. These can be occasionally challenging to locate using ultrasound, and CT imaging can be considered for surgical planning. Intra-abdominal testicles may be located near the inguinal ring lateral to the bladder or along the lateral body wall from the inguinal ring to the kidney. Retained testicles may be atrophied and therefore smaller than the descended testicle. Inguinal testicles lie between the inguinal ring and the scrotum in the subcutaneous tissues. These tend to be slightly larger than intra-abdominal testicles, with moderate contrast enhancement (Figure 5.9.6). Neoplasia is common in undescended testicles, including seminomas, mixed germ cell stromal cell tumors, and Sertoli cell tumors, which can predispose to testicular torsion.[8,9] Descended testicles are additionally affected by interstitial cell tumors.

Degenerative and inflammatory diseases include prostatitis and paraprostatic cysts. These large, fluid-filled cavitary lesions arise from the prostate gland and cause a mass effect in the region of the bladder. Prostatitis alone or concurrent with a paraprostatic cyst causes enlargement of the prostate gland with cavitary lesions that may connect with the urethra and shows strong enhancement. Paraprostatic cysts have thickened enhancing walls, nonenhancing fluid-filled centers, and occasionally mineralization. They may displace the bladder cranially and predispose to cystitis and urethritis (Figure 5.9.7). A urethrogram or intravenous contrast administration may demonstrate communication from the urethra to the paraprostatic cyst.

Trauma to the vascular portion of the penis may cause disruption of the urethra and hematoma formation along the perineal fascial planes. Hematomas are characterized by thin enhancing walls and a central non-enhancing fluid-attenuating center (Figure 5.9.8).

Prostatic carcinoma is most commonly caused by transitional cell carcinoma. These tumors may be solid or cavitary with cystic lesions and regions of mineralization. The solid neoplastic tissue is heterogeneous on CT and MR imaging, with variable intense contrast enhancement. The urethra may be invaded by the mass, causing communications to the cystic cavities and irregular enhancing mucosa on enhanced and urethrogram studies (Figure 5.9.9). Secondary effects include urethral obstruction leading to hydroureter and hydronephrosis (Figure 5.9.10).

Figure 5.9.1 Normal Female Reproductive Tract (Canine)   CT

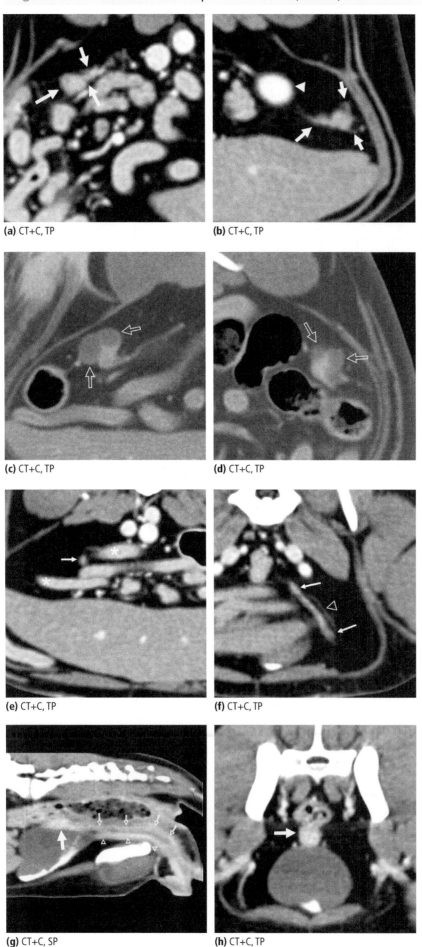

(a) CT+C, TP

(b) CT+C, TP

(c) CT+C, TP

(d) CT+C, TP

(e) CT+C, TP

(f) CT+C, TP

(g) CT+C, SP

(h) CT+C, TP

Mature mixed-breed female dogs. In anestrus, the ovary is a triangular soft-tissue attenuating structure (**a,b**: arrows) in the dorsal abdomen, caudal and lateral to the kidneys (**b**: arrowhead). Follicles appear as round fluid-attenuating structures protruding from the ovarian tissue (**c,d**: open arrows). The uterine horns (**e,f**: small arrows) are smaller than small intestinal loops (**e**: asterisks). The uterine vein can be seen parallel to the right uterine horn (**f**: open arrowhead). The cervix is a thickened structure between the bladder and colon (**g,h**: arrow). The vagina (**g**: small open arrows) exits the pelvis dorsal to the urethra (**g**: small open arrowheads). There is mild contrast enhancement of the normal tissues.

Figure 5.9.2   Normal Prostate Gland (Canine)   CT

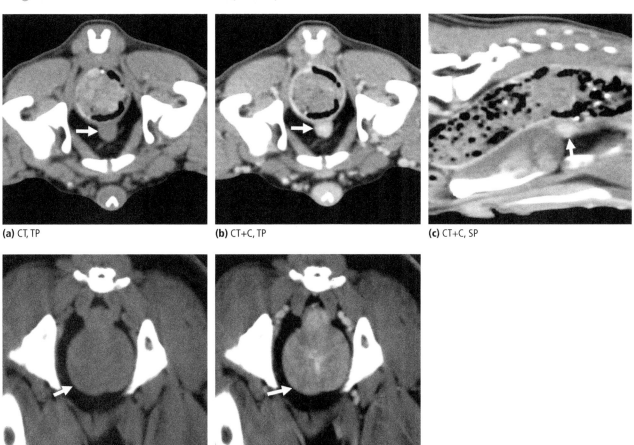

(a) CT, TP   **(b)** CT+C, TP   **(c)** CT+C, SP

(d) CT, TP   **(e)** CT+C, TP

Normal adult neutered and intact male dogs. The neutered dog's prostate gland is small and homogeneous with uniform contrast enhancement (**a–c**: arrow). Intact dogs undergo benign hyperplasia, causing enlargement of the prostate gland to a slightly bilobed structure with central and radiating striations of contrast enhancement (**d,e**: arrow).

Figure 5.9.3 Normal Prostate Gland (Canine)

MR

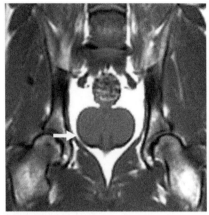

(a) T1, DP

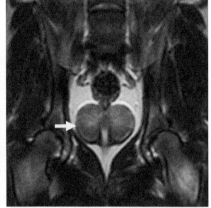

(b) T2, DP

10y M Belgian Malinois. There is prostatic enlargement due to benign hyperplasia. The prostate gland is isointense to muscle on T1 images (**a**: arrow) and hyperintense on T2 and STIR images (**b**,**c**: arrows). Contrast enhancement is present more centrally with a radiating pattern (**d**: arrow).

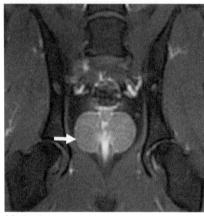

(c) ST, DP

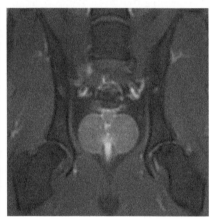

(d) T1+C+FS, DP

Figure 5.9.4   Pseudohermaphrodite (Canine)

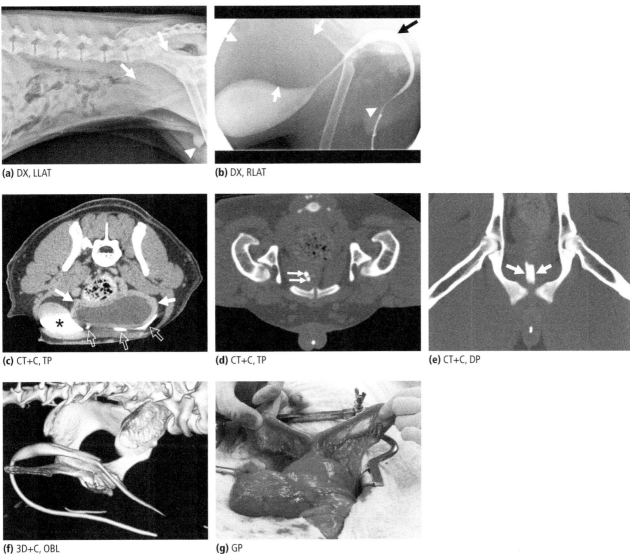

(a) DX, LLAT

(b) DX, RLAT

(c) CT+C, TP

(d) CT+C, TP

(e) CT+C, DP

(f) 3D+C, OBL

(g) GP

9mo F Viszla with urinary incontinence. A vestigial penis was present on radiographs (**a**: arrowhead). A large soft-tissue opacity mass is present between the bladder and the colon (**a**: arrows). The urethra is slightly widened in the pelvic region on the urethrogram (**b**: black arrow). A vestigial os penis is present (**b**: arrowhead). On contrast-enhanced CT images, the ovaries and uterine horns are normal (not shown). The uterine body or vagina is markedly enlarged and fluid filled with thickened, contrast-enhancing walls (**c**: arrows). The bladder (**c**: asterisk) and ureters (**c**: open arrows) are displaced by the enlarged structure. A urethrogram was performed, and within the pelvic canal there are two distinct lumens, one connecting with the urethra (**d,e**: arrows), cranial to the dilated segment of urethra (**f**). A small amount of contrast was present within the enlarged uterine structure, indicating probable communication (not shown). An ovariohysterectomy was performed, and inflammation of the uterine structures was found on histopathology (**g**). The urinary incontinence was presumed to be fluid leaking from the enlarged uterus or vagina with poor drainage secondary to developmental anomaly.

Figure 5.9.5   Endometrial Hyperplasia (Feline)   CT

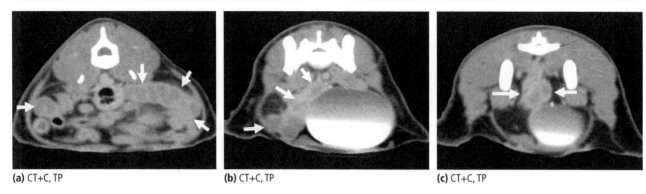

(a) CT+C, TP   **(b)** CT+C, TP   **(c)** CT+C, TP

5y F Persian imaged for ureteral obstruction. Images are ordered from cranial to caudal. The uterus is markedly enlarged and fluid filled with enhancing walls (**a–c**: arrows). Folds are visible in the wall of the uterus, causing an undulating pattern. The ovaries were unremarkable (not shown). An ovariohysterectomy was performed, and marked endometrial hyperplasia and endometritis were found on histopathology, possibly related to recent pregnancy.

Figure 5.9.6   Retained Testicles (Canine)   CT

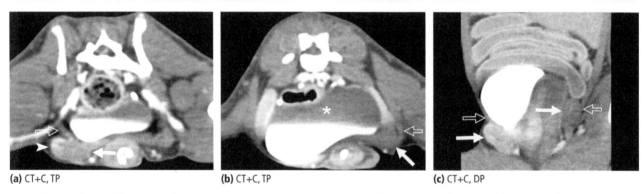

(a) CT+C, TP   **(b)** CT+C, TP   **(c)** CT+C, DP

1y M Shih Tzu imaged for an extrahepatic portosystemic shunt. Images **a** and **b** are ordered from caudal to cranial. The right testicle is mildly atrophied (**a**: solid arrow) and is located in the inguinal region external to the body wall (**a**: open arrow). The epididymis is visible laterally as a more strongly enhancing curvilinear structure (**a**: arrowhead). The left testicle (**b**: solid arrow) is located internal to the abdominal wall (**b**: open arrow) and lateral to the bladder (**b**: asterisk). There is minimal contrast enhancement, and the epididymis is not visualized. On the dorsal plane image, the testicles (**c**: arrows) are internal to (left) and external to (right) the musculature of the body wall (**c**: open arrows).

Figure 5.9.7 Paraprostatic Cyst (Canine)   CT

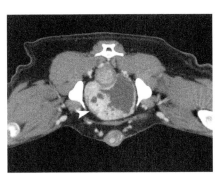

(a) CT+C, TP

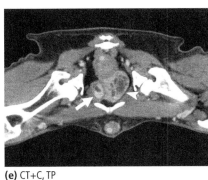

(b) CT+C, TP

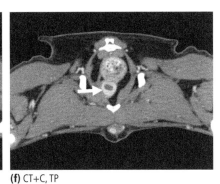

(c) CT+C, TP

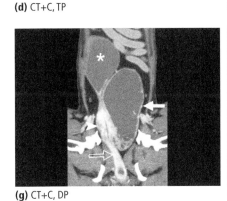

(d) CT+C, TP

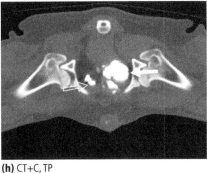

(e) CT+C, TP

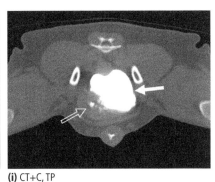

(f) CT+C, TP

(g) CT+C, DP   **(h)** CT+C, TP   **(i)** CT+C, TP

2y MC Dachshund with urinary incontinence. Images **a–f** are ordered from cranial to caudal. There is a large fluid-filled structure with a thickened contrast-enhancing wall on the left side of the caudal abdomen (**a–c,g**: solid arrow). The urinary bladder (**a,g**: asterisk) and urethra (**b,c,g**: open arrow) also have thickened walls and are displaced to the right. The cyst is continuous, with irregular enhancing prostatic tissue that contains multiple smaller cysts (**c–e,g**: arrowhead). The thickened urethra continues through the right side of the prostate gland and caudal to it (**e,f**: arrow). The relative positions of the structures are shown on the dorsal reformatted image (**g**). A urethrogram was performed, and the paraprostatic cyst filled with contrast medium (**h,i**: solid arrow). The lumen of the urethra is moderately irregular indicating urethritis (**h,i**: open arrows). The cyst was surgically resected with the remnant omentalized. Cystitis and cyst sepsis were present on microbial culture.

Figure 5.9.8 Penile Hemorrhage (Canine)

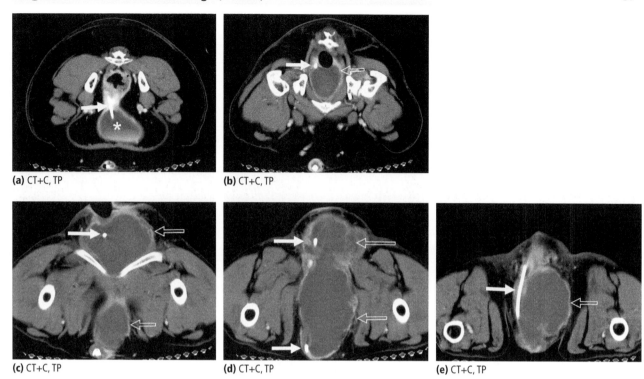

(a) CT+C, TP

(b) CT+C, TP

(c) CT+C, TP

(d) CT+C, TP

(e) CT+C, TP

4y MC Doberman Pinscher with a mass extending from rectum to penis. Images are ordered from cranial to caudal. A catheter is present in the urethra (**a–e**: solid arrows), extending to the urinary bladder (**a**: asterisk). There is a large tubular soft-tissue and fluid attenuating mass parallel to the urethra that extends from the pelvic canal to the penis (**b–e**: open arrows). The mass does not contrast enhance centrally and has a rim of peripheral enhancement. Fine-needle aspirates revealed blood and fat cells, and the mass was presumed to be a hematoma. Coagulopathy was not identified; however, there was a history of trauma, and the mass began to reduce in size after 48 hours.

Figure 5.9.9 Prostatic Carcinoma (Canine)

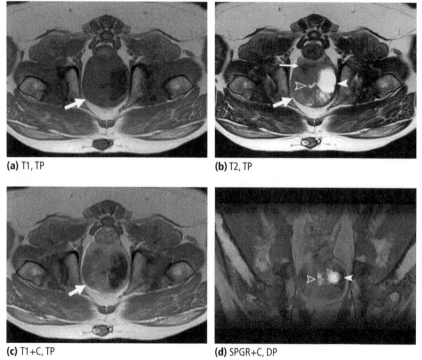

(a) T1, TP

(b) T2, TP

(c) T1+C, TP

(d) SPGR+C, DP

13y MC Leonberger with stranguria and pollakiuria. The prostate gland is enlarged (**a–c**: arrows) with a large cavitary region in the left lobe (**b**: solid arrowhead) that is hyperintense on T2 images and hypointense on T1 images. The urethra (**b**: open arrowhead) appears to communicate with this cavity on unenhanced images and has an irregularly shaped lumen (**a–c**). There is mineralization of the dorsal parenchyma (**b**: small arrow). The prostatic mass shows heterogeneous contrast enhancement (**c**: arrow). Contrast-enhanced urine fills the urethra (**d**: open arrowhead) and the cavity (**d**: solid arrowhead), confirming the urethral communication. The mass was diagnosed as a transitional cell carcinoma.

Figure 5.9.10 Prostatic Carcinoma (Canine)　　　　　　　　　　　　　　　　　　　CT

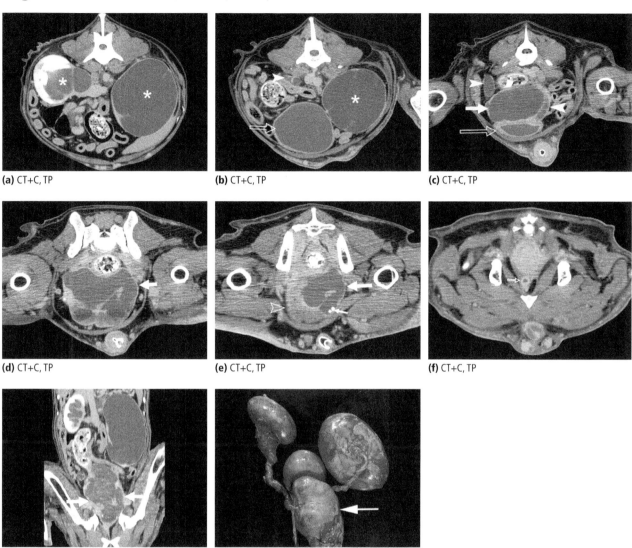

(a) CT+C, TP　　　　　**(b)** CT+C, TP　　　　　**(c)** CT+C, TP

(d) CT+C, TP　　　　　**(e)** CT+C, TP　　　　　**(f)** CT+C, TP

(g) CT+C, DP　　　　　**(h)** GP

4y M German Shepherd Dog with difficulty urinating. Images **a–f** are ordered from cranial to caudal. There is hydronephrosis of both kidneys, which is more pronounced on the left (**a,b**: asterisks). The right kidney is enhancing with a small amount of urine production, and the left appears nonfunctional. There is hydroureter on both the left and right sides (**b,c**: arrowheads), secondary to obstruction by the prostatic mass. A large cystic structure arising from the prostate gland (**c**: solid arrow) is present dorsal to the urinary bladder (**b,c**: open arrow). The cystic mass extends to the pelvic canal (**d,e**: arrows) and is continuous with enhancing prostatic parenchyma (**e**: open arrowhead). The urethra appears normal caudal to the prostate (**f**: small open arrow). The dorsal reformatted image shows the cystic mass extending from the pelvis into the abdomen (**g**: arrows). The mass was diagnosed as transitional cell carcinoma on necropsy, with metastasis to the kidneys and ureters (**h**). The gross pathology specimen is oriented the same as in the dorsal plane CT image (**g**), highlighting the appearance of the prostatic mass (**h**: arrow) in relation to the ureters, kidneys, and urinary bladder.

References

1. England GC, Yeager AE. Ultrasonographic appearance of the ovary and uterus of the bitch during oestrus, ovulation and early pregnancy. J Reprod Fertil. 1993;47:107–117.

2. Banco B, Antuofermo E, Borzacchiello G, Cossu-Rocca P, Grieco V. Canine ovarian tumors: an immunohistochemical study with HBME-1 antibody. J Vet Diagn Invest. 2011;23:977–981.

3. Coggeshall JD, Franks JN, Wilson DU, Wiley JL. Primary ovarian teratoma and GCT with intra-abdominal metastasis in a dog. J Am Anim Hosp Assoc. 2012;48:424–428.

4. Boeloni JN, Reis AMS, Nascimento EF, Silva JF, Serakides R, Ocarino NM. Primary ovarian rhabdomyosarcoma in a dog. J Comp Pathol. 2012;147:455–459.

5. Kaijser J, Vandecaveye V, Deroose CM, et al. Imaging techniques for the pre-surgical diagnosis of adnexal tumours. Best Pract Res Clin Obstet Gynaecol. 2014;28:683–695.

6. Hricak H, Chen M, Coakley FV, et al. Complex adnexal masses: detection and characterization with MR imaging – multivariate analysis. Radiology. 2000;214:39–46.

7. Thomassin-Naggara I, Daraï E, Cuenod CA, et al. Contribution of diffusion-weighted MR imaging for predicting benignity of complex adnexal masses. Eur Radiol. 2009;19:1544–1552.

8. Quartuccio M, Marino G, Garufi G, Cristarella S, Zanghì A. Sertoli cell tumors associated with feminizing syndrome and spermatic cord torsion in two cryptorchid dogs. J Vet Sci. 2012;13:207–209.

9. Foster RA. Common lesions in the male reproductive tract of cats and dogs. Vet Clin N Am Sm Anim Pract. 2012;42:527–545.

Section 6

Musculoskeletal System

6.1

Developmental and metabolic disorders

Developmental disorders

Developmental disorders of the skeletal system represent a wide array of etiologies and clinical manifestations of disease. Conventional radiographic examinations are often satisfactory for diagnosis of bone and joint lesions, but cross-sectional imaging is sometimes necessary for diagnosis or accurate characterization, particularly when the lesion is small or obscured because of complex skeletal anatomy. The predominant or significant imaging features of developmental disorders are often those of secondary degenerative disease.

Disorders primarily affecting joints

Osteochondrosis
Osteochondrosis is a disruption of endochondral ossification involving articular cartilage and underlying subchondral bone. Disturbances in cartilage growth result in necrosis, separation of cartilage from underlying subchondral bone, and subchondral bone defects. The disorder occurs most commonly in large- to giant-breed dogs during periods of rapid growth, and male dogs are overrepresented. The caudal humeral head, medial humeral condyle, lateral and medial femoral condyles, and lateral and medial trochlear ridges of the talus are the most commonly involved regions in the appendicular skeleton.[1]

Radiographic examination is usually adequate for detecting lesions that have subchondral bone manifestations, and radiographic features have been widely reported. Computed tomography and MRI can be useful when lesions are obscured by complex skeletal anatomy

(elbow and tarsus) or when articular cartilage or other soft tissues are affected.[2–4]

Typical CT features include focal subchondral bone surface defects with surrounding sclerosis (Figures 6.1.1, 6.1.2, 6.1.3, 6.1.4).[2,3] Hyperattenuating intraarticular osteochondral bodies are sometimes present.

Similar features are reported in osteochondrosis MR examinations in people, including subchondral bone defects and T1 and T2 subchondral hypoattenuation resulting from sclerosis. The intensity of subchondral bone can vary depending on the stage of disease and the relative effects of new subchondral bone formation, bone edema, and marrow replacement (Figure 6.1.5).[5] Imaging features of joint effusion and secondary degenerative disease can be seen with both modalities.

Elbow dysplasia
The term elbow dysplasia encompasses a number of pathologic entities of the developing elbow. The most common disorders include ununited anconeal process, medial coronoid disease, and osteochondrosis of the humeral condyle. Underlying causes for elbow dysplasia are not well understood, but the usual suspects—genetics, nutrition, growth disturbances, and trauma—have been proposed. Rapidly growing large- to giant-breed dogs are highly overrepresented although there does not appear to be a gender predilection other than for ununited anconeal process, which affects primarily males.[1] Elbow dysplasia is often bilateral, and concurrent developmental orthopedic disease of other joints is common. Although we describe the specific disorders

---

Atlas of Small Animal CT and MRI, First Edition. Erik R. Wisner and Allison L. Zwingenberger.

separately, they likely represent secondary manifestations of underlying growth disturbances and can occur separately or in combination. Further, many of the imaging features represent secondary degenerative changes rather than primary lesions.

Normal elbow

Because of the complexity of the elbow, CT provides improved diagnostic accuracy compared to conventional radiography, which is limited by anatomic superimposition.[6,7] Anatomic studies in clinically normal dogs have shown that CT is excellent for evaluation of bone and that muscles, large blood vessels, and nerves can also be evaluated when multiple imaging planes are used.[8] MRI is used extensively in people, but there are few reports in the veterinary literature other than descriptions of the normal canine joint, incomplete humeral condyle ossification, and flexor enthesiopathy.[9–13] In one cadaveric study of the canine normal elbow joint, the authors concluded all musculoskeletal structures could be visualized using a combination of all three major imaging planes and that T1 images provided the best anatomic detail, while T2 images were best for characterizing synovial cavities.[9]

CT images should be acquired with the limb moderately extended, and the limb should be positioned in relation to the body to minimize streak artifacts due to motion and beam-attenuation of other body parts outside the field-of-view. This is most easily accomplished with the patient in dorsal recumbency. A small field-of-view maximizes anatomic resolution, and thin collimation is necessary for multiplanar reformatting. In addition to native transverse images, the elbow should be viewed using sagittal and dorsal plane reformatted images. Oblique long axis plane reformatted images through the long dimension of the medial coronoid process and perpendicular to the radioulnar articular margin provide for a more complete assessment of the coronoid process and the congruity of the elbow joint (Figure 6.1.6).

Ununited anconeal process

The anconeal process is sometimes a separate center of ossification in large-breed dogs. This should fuse with the olecranon within a few months of age. When fusion fails, the anconeal process remains attached by a fibrous union, which results in joint instability. Ununited anconeal process is easily detected by radiographic examination, so CT is unnecessary for diagnosis. It is most often encountered on CT as a known abnormality when examining the elbow for other features of developmental elbow disease.

The fibrous region is soft-tissue attenuating, and the anconeal process and adjacent olecranon process are often misshapen because of remodeling. Affected elbows almost always have signs of degenerative joint disease, including periarticular remodeling and subchondral bone sclerosis (Figure 6.1.7).[14]

Medial coronoid disease

Although remodeling or fragmentation of the medial coronoid process is considered a manifestation of elbow dysplasia, it is generally assumed to be a secondary effect of underlying abnormal elbow development. Alterations to the medial coronoid process can include abnormal shape, reduced density associated with osteomalacia, fissures, and overt fragmentation. This is often accompanied by radioulnar incongruity with a shorter than expected radius leading to a "stair-step" involving the proximal articular surfaces of the two bones. Other features include irregularity of the radial incisura of the ulna, periarticular remodeling, and subchondral bone sclerosis associated with secondary degenerative joint disease. Articular cartilage erosions have also been positively correlated with radioulnar incongruency (Figures 6.1.8, 6.1.9, 6.1.10).[6,15–19]

Osteochondrosis of the medial humeral condyle

Imaging features of osteochondrosis involving the medial aspect of the humeral condyle are the same as those described for other anatomic sites and are described in an earlier section of this chapter (Figure 6.1.4).

Hip dysplasia

Hip dysplasia is a developmental disorder that has a genetic component and that affects primarily large-breed dogs. Hip joint laxity, incongruence, and subluxation cause pelvic limb lameness and chronic instability, eventually resulting in secondary degenerative joint disease. Radiographic examination, though imperfect, is the most widely used imaging modality for both screening and diagnosis, and limb-extended ventrodorsal views and distraction techniques are most commonly employed.

Weightbearing and nonweightbearing pelvic CT has been used to measure parameters such as dorsolateral subluxation, dorsal acetabular rim angle, femoral head and acetabular cup diameter, femoral neck anteversion angle, and distraction distance, as well as to subjectively evaluate hip conformation (Figures 6.1.11, 6.1.12).[20–25] MRI has also been used to estimate a synovial fluid index reflecting passive joint laxity.[23] Although quantitative data have been generated from these studies, it is unclear whether these techniques have significant clinical utility beyond that of currently used radiographic approaches.

Aseptic necrosis of the femoral head (Legg–Calve–Perthes disease)

Legg–Calve–Perthes Disease is a disorder thought to be the result of regional vascular obstruction to the femoral head due to infarction or extramural compression from coxafemoral joint effusion. Impaired blood flow results in subchondral bone necrosis and subsequent articular cartilage injury.[26,27] Femoral head and neck remodeling and degenerative joint disease are long-term sequelae.[28] Immature small- and toy-breed dogs are predisposed, but Australian Shepherds are also highly overrepresented.[29] Although radiographic features vary depending on the stage of the disease, common findings include flattening or irregularity of the femoral head subchondral bone margin, heterogeneous opacity of the epiphyseal and metaphyseal bone, shortening and thickening of the femoral neck, and increased apparent joint space width.[30]

CT features of an induced model of canine aseptic femoral head necrosis parallel those seen radiographically.[31]

MR findings associated with aseptic necrosis include inhomogeneous low to intermediate T1 intensity and inhomogeneous T2 intensity of the femoral head and neck compared to muscle. These regions inhomogeneously enhance following intravenous contrast administration.[32]

Disorders primarily affecting bone

Agenesis or malformation

Genetic mutations and in utero and postpartum errors in development can lead to agenesis, hypoplasia, or malformation of bone elements.[33–38] Gross abnormalities are easily recognized clinically and radiographically, so cross-sectional imaging is rarely employed for diagnosis. However, CT is used for surgical planning for correction of angular, torsional, or other limb deformities (Figure 6.1.13).[39–41] Three-dimensional computer simulations or printed replicas can be used to precisely contour bone plates and other orthopedic appliances.

Idiopathic disorders

Panosteitis

Panosteitis is a self-limiting idiopathic bone disorder that occurs predominantly in large-breed dogs 5–18 months of age, with German Shepherd Dogs highly overrepresented.[1] Clinical manifestations include shifting limb lameness with pain on palpation of affected limbs. Radiographic features include ill-defined regions of increased medullary opacity, which often originate near a long bone nutrient canal. A periosteal productive response is also occasionally present. Underlying pathologic features include proliferation of well-differentiated medullary woven bone and fibrous tissue.[28]

Survey radiographs are usually satisfactory for diagnosis, and the disorder is therefore often noted as a secondary finding on CT appendicular examinations performed for other reasons. Computed tomography features are similar to those described for conventional radiography (Figure 6.1.14). MR features have not been reported.

Hypertrophic osteodystrophy (metaphyseal osteodystrophy)

Hypertrophic osteodystrophy is a systemic disorder occurring primarily in immature dogs (2–9 months), with Great Danes, Weimaraners, Boxers, and Irish Setters overrepresented.[29] The underlying cause is unknown, but clinical signs include fever, lethargy, lameness, and appendicular pain on palpation during early stages of the disease. Early radiographic manifestations include linear lysis of metaphyseal bone, which parallels the physes and is most evident in the distal radius and ulna.[42,43] Osteolysis results from suppurative and fibrinous inflammation within metaphyseal bone. In later stages, adjacent periosteal inflammation leads to a reactive productive response involving the metaphyses.[28] CT and MR features of hypertrophic osteodystrophy have not been reported although CT features would likely parallel radiographic findings.

Epiphyseal and metaphyseal dysplasias
Incomplete ossification of the humeral condyle

This disorder is the result of incomplete ossification of the medial and lateral humeral condylar ossification centers, with the two centers separated by a thin fibrous band. Spaniels are highly overrepresented although the disorder has been reported in a variety of breeds.[44] The degree of incomplete ossification is variable, and the majority of dogs are bilaterally affected though often asymmetrically.[44–46] Survey radiographic studies in a large population of Springer Spaniels has also revealed small interosseous fissures in 14% of elbows in dogs with no clinical signs of lameness.[46] Structural compromise from incomplete fusion can lead to instability, with resulting lameness referable to the elbow. Catastrophic condylar or intercondylar Y or T fracture of the distal humerus during normal activity is often a sequela to the disorder.[45]

CT features of incomplete humeral condyle ossification include a complete to incomplete, saw-tooth to linear, hypoattenuating region between the medial and lateral condyles surrounded by hyperattenuating sclerotic bone. Affected joints may also have evidence of medial coronoid disease and articular incongruity (Figure 6.1.15).[47] We have also recognized intercondylar sclerosis without fissures in limbs contralateral to an affected elbow (Figure 6.1.15).

MR features include intercondylar STIR and T1 heterogeneity corresponding to the hypoattenuating linear regions seen on CT. Central T1 hyperintensity is surrounded by signal void due to adjacent sclerosis. Normal condyles are described as having uniform intercondylar STIR and T1 intensity.[48]

CT appears to be more sensitive than radiography for detection of incomplete humeral condylar ossification, particularly when fissures are incomplete. Numbers reported for MR diagnosis are not yet sufficient to determine the merit of this modality.

Disruptions of endochondral ossification

Disorders of enchondral ossification, such as multiple cartilaginous exostoses and retained ulnar cartilage core, are due to interruption or alteration of normal endochondral ossification. These disorders are readily recognized on survey radiographic examinations and are therefore most likely to be seen as secondary findings on CT or MR examinations.

Metabolic disorders

Hypertrophic osteopathy

Hypertrophic osteopathy most often results from neoplastic or inflammatory masses in the thoracic, abdominal, or pelvic cavities or from direct alterations in vascular perfusion.[49-52] The disorder manifests radiographically as dense, but often irregularly margined, periosteal new bone formation of the diaphysis and metaphysis of long bones, which seems to preferentially involve the distal extremities although all long bones are sometimes affected. New bone is often, but not always, symmetrically distributed, and thoracic and pelvic limbs may be affected to different degrees. Computed tomographic features of hypertrophic osteopathy have not been previously reported but generally parallel survey radiographic findings (Figure 6.1.16).

Secondary hyperparathyroidism

The two most common causes of secondary hyperparathyroidism are chronic hyperphosphatemic renal disease and diets deficient in calcium or with low calcium to phosphorus ratio. Low serum calcium levels cause an increase in parathyroid hormone production. This in turn leads to bone calcium mobilization that results in fibrous osteodystrophy. Affected animals have clinical signs of systemic disease, but the imaging manifestations are reduced bone density and pathologic fractures.

The skeletal manifestations of renal secondary hyperparathyroidism are not uniform, with bones of the skull being more affected early in the course of the disease. Nutritional secondary hyperparathyroidism, particularly in skeletally immature animals, appears to affect the bones more uniformly because of the overall higher bone metabolic activity in young animals.

CT features include reduced bone density and cortical thinning, which can be striking in some patients (Figure 6.1.17). Pathologic fractures are a common sequela in both the appendicular and axial skeleton.[53]

Soft-tissue mineralization due to hyperadrenocorticism

Elevated cortisol levels are thought to a have catabolic effect on collagen, elastin, and other proteins, resulting in increased calcium binding. Calcinosis cutis, mineralization within the skin, occurs in about 30% of dogs with hyperadrenocorticism, but other soft tissues, such as skeletal muscle, lung, and stomach, can also mineralize.[54]

CT features include plaque-like hyperattenuation in the skin (Figure 6.1.18). Similar changes also seem to occur frequently in muscle and along fascial planes.

Other metabolic disorders

Although there is a plethora of metabolic disorders that affect the skeletal system, they are uncommon, and there are few reports of the use of CT or MR for diagnosis.

Figure 6.1.1 Osteochondrosis of the Lateral Trochlear Ridge of the Talus (Canine)   CT

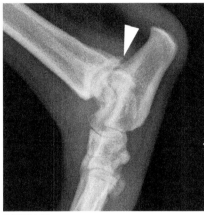

(a) DX, LAT

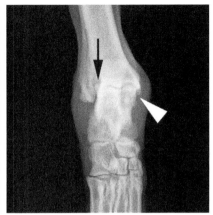

(b) DX, DP

5y MC Rottweiler with recent-onset right pelvic limb lameness. There is periarticular remodeling of the tarsocrural joint, indicative of degenerative joint disease (**a**,**b**: arrowhead). The dorsal margin of the lateral trochlear ridge of the talus appears mildly flattened and irregular (**b**: arrow). A transverse CT image through the dorsal trochlear ridge reveals multiple subchondral bone fragments in the lateral articular space (**c**: arrowhead). Flattening of the lateral trochlear ridge is also seen in the 3D rendering (**d**: arrow). Multiple subchondral bone fragments were removed by lateral arthrotomy.

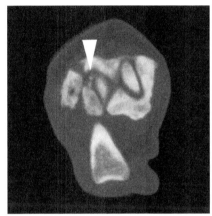

(c) CT, TP

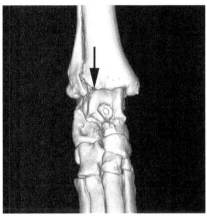

(d) CT, 3D, DORS

Figure 6.1.2 Osteochondrosis of the Medial Trochlear Ridge of the Talus (Canine)   CT

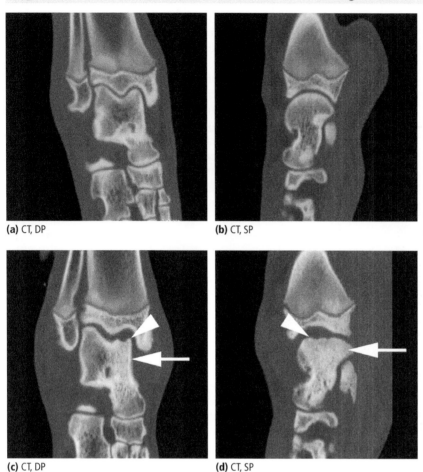

(a) CT, DP

(b) CT, SP

(c) CT, DP

(d) CT, SP

6mo MC Mastiff with right pelvic limb lameness. Images **a** and **b** are dorsal and sagittal plane images, respectively, of the normal left tarsocrural joint. The sagittal image is through the medial trochlear ridge of the talus. Images **c** and **d** are of the abnormal right tarsocrural joint and are oriented similar to images **a** and **b**. There is a large subchondral bone defect of the dorsal aspect of the right medial trochlear ridge (**c,d**: arrowhead), which is associated with joint space widening and marked subchondral bone sclerosis (**c,d**: arrow). Periarticular new bone formation involving the right tarsocrural joint is indicative of secondary degenerative disease.

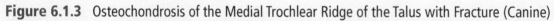

Figure 6.1.3 Osteochondrosis of the Medial Trochlear Ridge of the Talus with Fracture (Canine)   CT

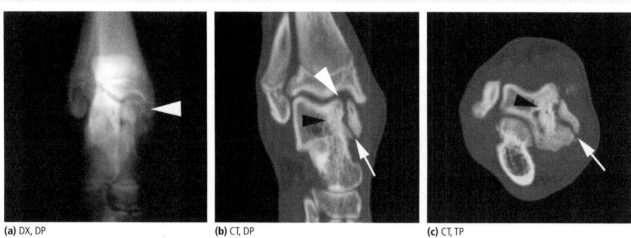

(a) DX, DP

(b) CT, DP

(c) CT, TP

6mo F Labrador Retriever with right pelvic limb lameness of 3 months' duration. The medial trochlear ridge subchondral bone contour is irregular, and the tarsocrural joint space is widened on the radiographic image (**a**: arrowhead). There is a subchondral defect of the dorsal margin of the medial trochlear ridge of the talus (**b**: white arrowhead), associated with surrounding subchondral bone sclerosis (**b,c**: black arrowhead) and a sagittally oriented fracture (**b,c**: arrow).

Figure 6.1.4 Osteochondrosis of the Medial Humeral Condyle (Canine)   CT

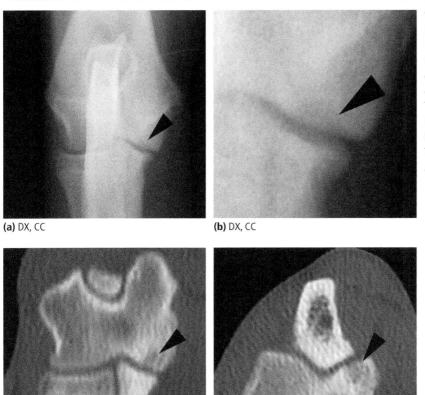

9mo MC Labrador Retriever with a 6-week history of left thoracic limb lameness. Image **b** is a magnification of image **a**. There is a subtle lucency of the subchondral bone of the medial aspect of the humeral condyle on the radiographic image (**a**,**b**: arrowhead). The subchondral defect is clearly seen on CT images (**c**,**d**: arrowhead) and is surrounded by a wide rim of sclerotic subchondral bone. The osteochondral defect was confirmed arthroscopically.

(a) DX, CC   **(b)** DX, CC

(c) CT, DP   **(d)** CT, TP

Figure 6.1.5 Osteochondrosis of the Lateral Femoral Condyle (Canine)   MR

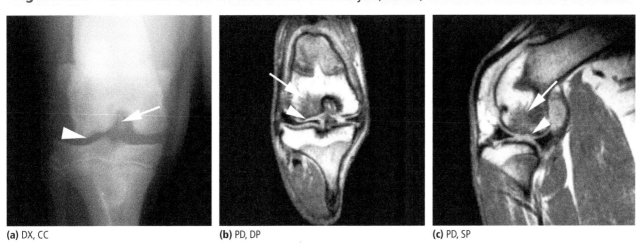

(a) DX, CC   **(b)** PD, DP   **(c)** PD, SP

1y FS Mastiff with left pelvic limb lameness. The sagittal MR image (**c**) is centered on the lateral femoral condyle. There is a lateral condylar subchondral defect with surrounding sclerosis on the radiographic image (**a**: arrowhead). A separate intraarticular osseous body is seen in the intercondyloid fossa (**a**: arrow). MR images reveal flattening and irregularity of the lateral condylar subchondral bone margin (**b**,**c**: arrowhead) and PD hypointensity of adjacent subchondral bone (**b**,**c**: arrow) consistent with sclerosis and marrow replacement. The osteochondral defect was confirmed arthroscopically.

Figure 6.1.6 Normal Elbow (Canine)   CT

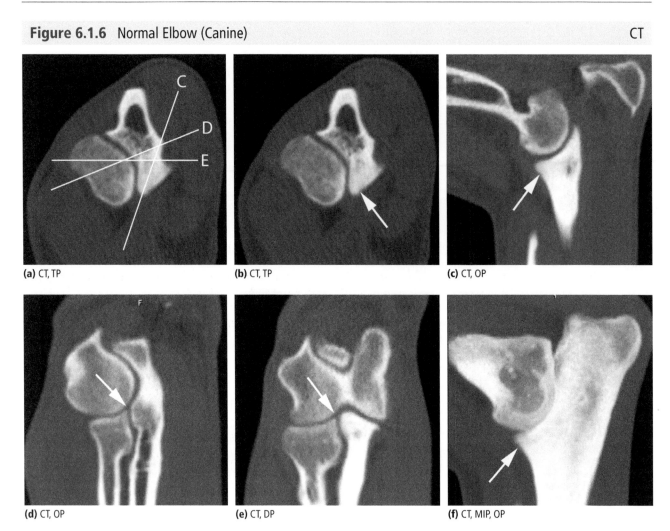

(a) CT, TP   **(b)** CT, TP   **(c)** CT, OP

(d) CT, OP   **(e)** CT, DP   **(f)** CT, MIP, OP

4y FS Golden Retriever with polyarthritis of unknown cause. Image **a** is a transverse image through the elbow at the level of the medial coronoid process. The labeled lines (**a**: C–E) correspond with the reformatted viewing plane of their respective images **c–e**. Image **f** is a maximum-intensity projection of the medial coronoid process in the same plane as image **c**. The medial coronoid process is smoothly margined and uniformly attenuating (**b,c,f**: arrow). The articular surfaces of the proximal radius and ulna are congruent, forming an uninterrupted surface (**d,e**: arrow).

Figure 6.1.7 Ununited Anconeal Process (Canine)

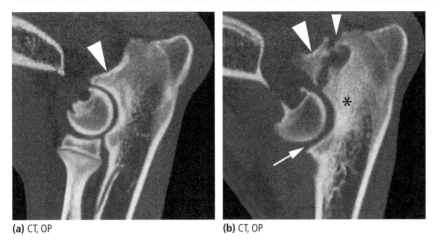

(a) CT, OP **(b)** CT, OP

10mo MC German Shepherd Dog/Mastiff cross with a 4-month history of left thoracic limb lameness. The clinically unaffected right elbow is shown in image **a**, and the abnormal left elbow is shown in image **b**. Images are in the plane of the long axis of the anconeal process. The right elbow had evidence of mild joint incongruity and medial coronoid process remodeling (not shown), but the anconeal process is intact (**a**: arrowhead). The left anconeal process is ununited (**b**: large arrowhead). The soft-tissue attenuating irregular linear area between the anconeal process and underlying parent bone (**b**: small arrowhead) represents a fibrous union that makes the joint inherently unstable. The anconeal process is misshapen and poorly mineralized, the humeroulnar joint is incongruent (**b**: arrow), and the subchondral bone of the trochlear notch is sclerotic (**b**: asterisk).

Figure 6.1.8 Fragmented Medial Coronoid Process (Canine) CT

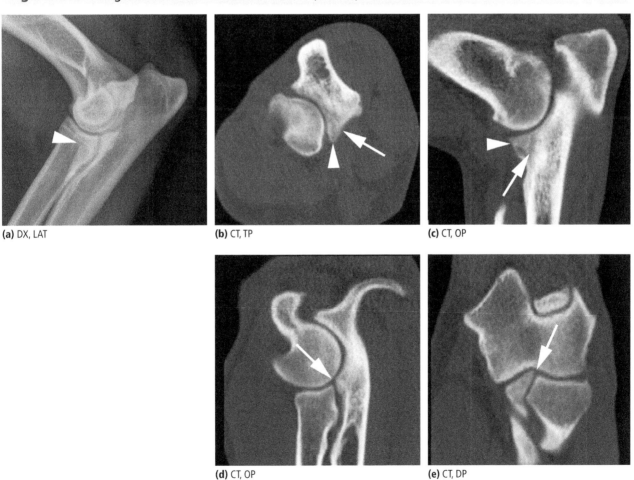

(a) DX, LAT **(b)** CT, TP **(c)** CT, OP

(d) CT, OP **(e)** CT, DP

6y MC Labrador Retriever with left thoracic limb lameness of 1-month duration. The margin of the medial coronoid process is poorly delineated on a lateral radiographic image (**a**: arrowhead). There is heterogeneous diminished attenuation of the medial coronoid process (**b,c**: arrowhead) and a thin lucent curvilinear fissure within the basilar part of the process (**b,c**: arrow) on CT images. Dorsal and long-axis oblique plane images show no significant radioulnar incongruity (**d,e**: arrow). An arthroscopic subcoronoidectomy was performed. The bone of the coronoid process showed malacia with overlying articular cartilage erosion.

Figure 6.1.9 Fragmented Medial Coronoid Process (Canine)

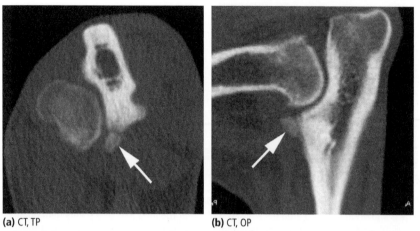

1y FS Golden Retriever with left thoracic limb lameness of 6 months' duration. The medial coronoid process is small and misshapen, has reduced density, and is clearly separate from adjacent bone (**a**,**b**: arrow). Dorsal and long-axis oblique plane images show radioulnar incongruity with nonuniform joint space width (**c**,**d**: arrow). The shorter length of the radius relative to the ulna causes disproportionate contact between the humeral condyle and proximal ulnar articular surface, leading to subchondral bone sclerosis in the medial aspect of the condyle (**d**: arrowhead).

(a) CT, TP

(b) CT, OP

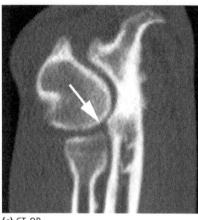

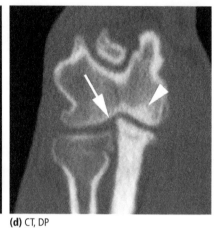

(c) CT, OP

(d) CT, DP

Figure 6.1.10 Fragmented Medial Coronoid Process (Canine)   CT

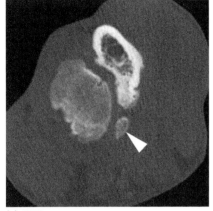

(a) CT, TP

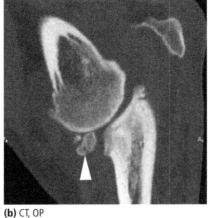

(b) CT, OP

1y MC Bernese Mountain Dog with bilateral thoracic limb lameness that is more pronounced on the right. The medial coronoid process is fragmented and grossly misshapen (**a,b**: arrowhead). There is marked incongruity of the humeroradioulnar articulation (**a–c**) with a pronounced "stair-step" between the radius and ulna (**d**: arrow). Periarticular remodeling and subchondral bone sclerosis are secondary degenerative changes (**a–d**).

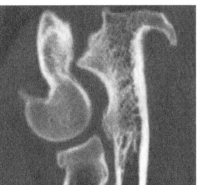

(c) CT, OP

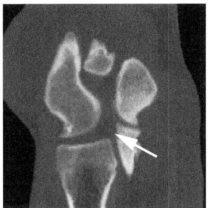

(d) CT, DP

Figure 6.1.11 Hip Dysplasia (Canine)   CT

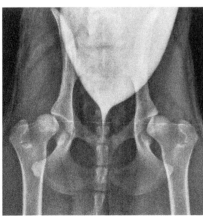

(a) DX, VD

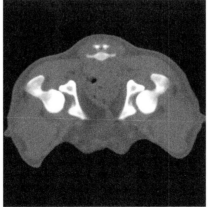

(b) CT, TP

9mo FS Portuguese Water Spaniel with chronic pelvic limb lameness. The CT examination was acquired to evaluate a medical problem unrelated to the coxofemoral joints. There is bilateral incongruity and subluxation of the coxofemoral joints, which is more pronounced on the right (**a**). These findings are also present on a CT image (**b**). Although it is unlikely that CT provides significantly more diagnostic information than conventional radiography, hip dysplasia is often encountered on CT examinations acquired for other purposes.

Figure 6.1.12 Hip Dysplasia (Canine)

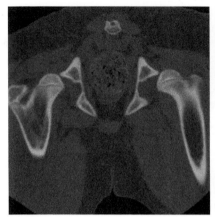

(a) CT, TP

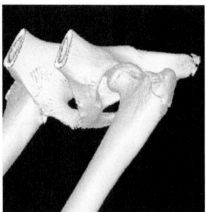

(b) CT, 3D, OBL

9mo FS Labrador Retriever with bilateral elbow and hip dysplasia. The pelvis was included in a CT examination performed primarily to preoperatively evaluate the elbows. Bilateral, marked coxofemoral subluxation is evident on the transverse image (**a**). A 3D rendering shows the degree of dorsal subluxation of the left femoral head (**b**).

Figure 6.1.13 Complex Developmental Abnormality with Patellar Hypoplasia (Canine)   CT

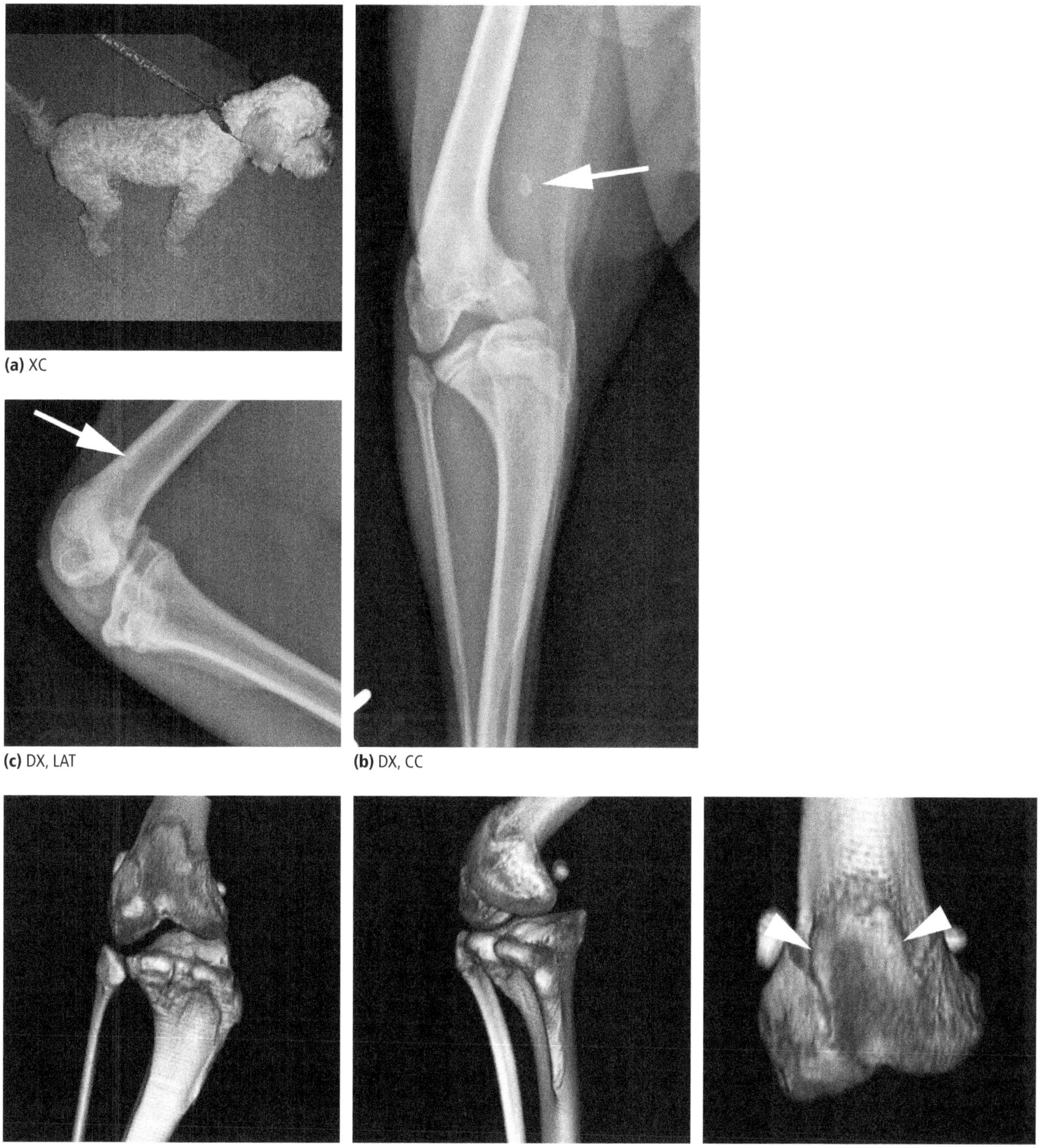

(a) XC

(c) DX, LAT

(b) DX, CC

(d) CT, 3D, CRAN

(e) CT, 3D, LAT

(f) CT, 3D, CRAN

10mo MC Labrador cross with bilateral pelvic limb deformities and abnormal gait (a). Radiographs reveal a complex angular and rotational deformity of the right pelvic limb centered on the stifle joint. A small osseous body dorsal and medial to the distal femur represents the hypoplastic patella (b,c: arrow). Images d and e show the angular and rotational deformities in three dimensions. Image f shows the distal femur in isolation and highlights the misshapen and hypoplastic trochlear ridges (f: arrowheads). The patella is not included in the 3D renderings.

Figure 6.1.14 Panosteitis (Canine) CT

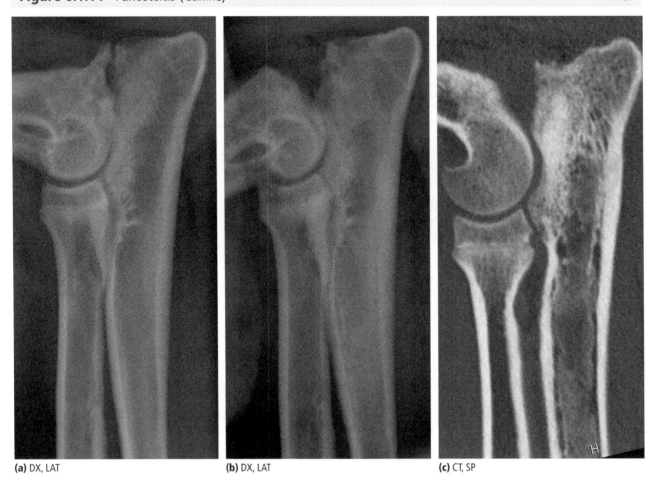

(a) DX, LAT **(b)** DX, LAT **(c)** CT, SP

14mo MC Mastiff with previously diagnosed ununited anconeal processes. All images are of the right elbow and proximal antebrachium. Image **a** was acquired at the time of initial presentation, and images **b** and **c** are postoperative examinations acquired 6 weeks later. There is ill-defined increased medullary opacity within the proximal metaphysis of the ulna on the initial radiographic examination (**a**). This finding is more pronounced 6 weeks later, and there is now an associated loss of endosteal margin definition (**b**). CT findings are similar to those seen on the radiographic examination (**c**).

Figure 6.1.15 Incomplete Humeral Condylar Ossification (Canine) CT

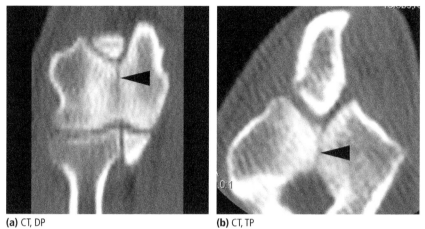

(a) CT, DP

3y MC Cocker Spaniel with chronic right thoracic limb lameness. Images **a** and **b** are of the right elbow, and images **c** and **d** are of the left elbow. Images have all been oriented with the lateral aspect of the limb to the left for easier comparison. An ill-defined fissure is seen in the right humeral condyle (**a**,**b**: arrowhead), surrounded by marked sclerosis. The central region of the left humeral condyle is also sclerotic, but a comparable fissure is not identified (**c**,**d**).

(b) CT, TP

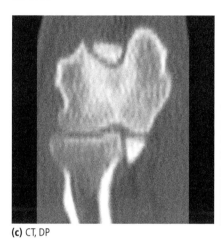

(c) CT, DP

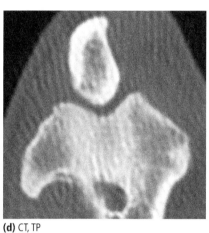

(d) CT, TP

Figure 6.1.16 Hypertrophic Osteopathy (Canine) CT

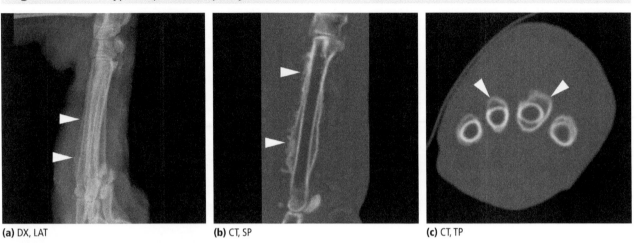

(a) DX, LAT   (b) CT, SP   (c) CT, TP

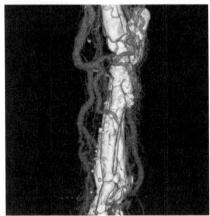

(d) CT+C, 3D, OBL

11y MC Mastiff with an acquired arteriovenous malformation of the right tarsus. Image **a** shows dense periosteal productive new bone involving the diaphyseal and metaphyseal regions of the metatarsal bones (**a**: arrowheads). The character and distribution of the productive response is more clearly seen on sagittal and transverse CT images through the metatarsus (**b**,**c**: arrowheads). A 3D rendering of a CT angiogram (**d**) shows the abnormal vascular network leading to regional hyperperfusion.

Figure 6.1.17 Renal Secondary Hyperparathyroidism (Canine)   CT

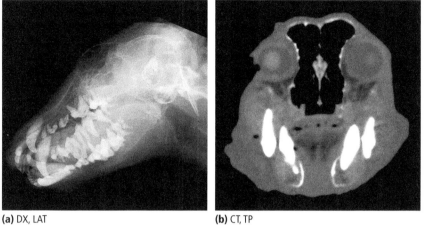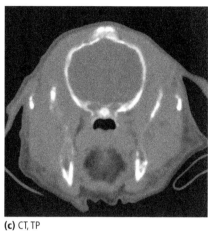

(a) DX, LAT   **(b)** CT, TP   **(c)** CT, TP

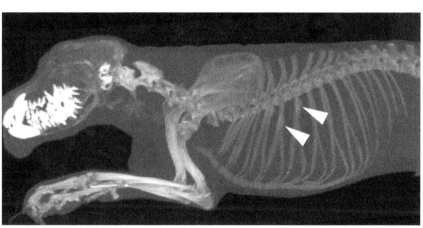

(d) CT, MIP, LAT

9y MC Cocker Spaniel with facial swelling and hemoptysis of 3-week duration. Clinical chemistry profile was indicative of severe chronic renal insufficiency. Images **b** and **c** are ordered rostral to caudal. A lateral skull radiograph reveals diffuse markedly decreased bone opacity (**a**). CT images show similar findings although the severity of bone loss, though diffuse, is nonuniform. An MIP image reveals skeletal demineralization to be most pronounced in the skull (**d**). Pathologic fractures of the ribs are also seen (**d**: arrowheads). Reproduced with permission from Dr. Shimizu Junichiro, Uni Animal Hospital, Hokkaido, Japan, 2014.

Figure 6.1.18 Soft-tissue Mineralization from Hyperadrenocorticism (Canine)   CT

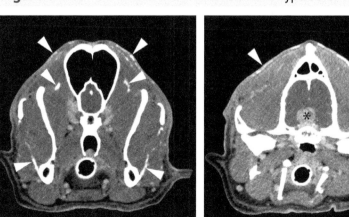

8y MC Newfoundland with pituitary-dependent hyperadrenocorticism. CT images of the skull reveal plaque-like mineralization in the skin (calcinosis cutis) and intermuscular fascia (**a,b**: arrowheads). A large contrast-enhancing pituitary mass is also seen (**b**: asterisk). Postmortem examination confirmed a pituitary adenoma.

(a) CT+C, TP   **(b)** CT+C, TP

References

1. Demko J, McLaughlin R. Developmental orthopedic disease. Vet Clin North Am Small Anim Pract. 2005;35:1111–1135.

2. Dingemanse WB, Van Bree HJ, Duchateau L, Gielen IM. Comparison of clinical and computed tomographic features between medial and lateral trochlear ridge talar osteochondrosis in dogs. Vet Surg. 2013;42:340–345.

3. Gielen I, van Bree H, Van Ryssen B, De Clercq T, De Rooster H. Radiographic, computed tomographic and arthroscopic findings in 23 dogs with osteochondrosis of the tarsocrural joint. Vet Rec. 2002;150:442–447.

4. Kippenes H, Johnston G. Diagnostic imaging of osteochondrosis. Vet Clin North Am Small Anim Pract. 1998;28:137–160.

5. Moktassi A, Popkin CA, White LM, Murnaghan ML. Imaging of osteochondritis dissecans. Orthop Clin North Am. 2012;43:201–211.

6. Kunst CM, Pease AP, Nelson NC, Habing G, Ballegeer EA. Computed tomographic identification of dysplasia and progression of osteoarthritis in dog elbows previously assigned OFA grades 0 and 1. Vet Radiol Ultrasound. 2014;55:511–520.

7. Lappalainen AK, Molsa S, Liman A, Laitinen-Vapaavuori O, Snellman M. Radiographic and computed tomography findings in Belgian shepherd dogs with mild elbow dysplasia. Vet Radiol Ultrasound. 2009;50:364–369.

8. De Rycke LM, Gielen IM, van Bree H, Simoens PJ. Computed tomography of the elbow joint in clinically normal dogs. Am J Vet Res. 2002;63:1400–1407.

9. Baeumlin Y, De Rycke L, Van Caelenberg A, Van Bree H, Gielen I. Magnetic resonance imaging of the canine elbow: an anatomic study. Vet Surg. 2010;39:566–573.

10. de Bakker E, Gielen I, Kromhout K, van Bree H, Van Ryssen B. Magnetic resonance imaging of primary and concomitant flexor enthesopathy in the canine elbow. Vet Radiol Ultrasound. 2013;55:56–62.

11. Janach KJ, Breit SM, Kunzel WW. Assessment of the geometry of the cubital (elbow) joint of dogs by use of magnetic resonance imaging. Am J Vet Res. 2006;67:211–218.

12. Probst A, Modler F, Kunzel W, Mlynarik V, Trattnig S. Demonstration of the articular cartilage of the canine ulnar trochlear notch using high-field magnetic resonance imaging. Vet J. 2008;177:63–70.

13. Snaps FR, Saunders JH, Park RD, Daenen B, Balligand MH, Dondelinger RF. Comparison of spin echo, gradient echo and fat saturation magnetic resonance imaging sequences for imaging the canine elbow. Vet Radiol Ultrasound. 1998;39:518–523.

14. Gasch EG, Labruyere JJ, Bardet JF. Computed tomography of ununited anconeal process in the dog. Vet Comp Orthop Traumatol. 2012;25:498–505.

15. Eljack H, Bottcher P. Relationship between axial radioulnar incongruence with cartilage damage in dogs with medial coronoid disease. Vet Surg. 2014 doi: 10.1111/j.1532-950X

16. Gemmill TJ, Mellor DJ, Clements DN, Clarke SP, Farrell M, Bennett D, et al. Evaluation of elbow incongruency using reconstructed CT in dogs suffering fragmented coronoid process. J Small Anim Pract. 2005;46:327–333.

17. House MR, Marino DJ, Lesser ML. Effect of limb position on elbow congruity with CT evaluation. Vet Surg. 2009;38:154–160.

18. Samoy Y, Gielen I, Van Caelenberg A, van Bree H, Duchateau L, Van Ryssen B. Computed tomography findings in 32 joints affected with severe elbow incongruity and fragmented medial coronoid process. Vet Surg. 2012;41:486–494.

19. Vermote KA, Bergenhuyzen AL, Gielen I, van Bree H, Duchateau L, Van Ryssen B. Elbow lameness in dogs of six years and older: arthroscopic and imaging findings of medial coronoid disease in 51 dogs. Vet Comp Orthop Traumatol. 2010;23:43–50.

20. Farese JP, Todhunter RJ, Lust G, Williams AJ, Dykes NL. Dorsolateral subluxation of hip joints in dogs measured in a weight-bearing position with radiography and computed tomography. Vet Surg. 1998;27:393–405.

21. Fujiki M, Kurima Y, Yamanokuchi K, Misumi K, Sakamoto H. Computed tomographic evaluation of growth-related changes in the hip joints of young dogs. Am J Vet Res. 2007;68:730–734.

22. Fujiki M, Misumi K, Sakamoto H. Laxity of canine hip joint in two positions with computed tomography. J Vet Med Sci. 2004;66:1003–1006.

23. Ginja MM, Ferreira AJ, Jesus SS, Melo-Pinto P, Bulas-Cruz J, Orden MA, et al. Comparison of clinical, radiographic, computed tomographic, and magnetic resonance imaging methods for early prediction of canine hip laxity and dysplasia. Vet Radiol Ultrasound. 2009;50:135–143.

24. Ginja MM, Gonzalo-Orden JM, Jesus SS, Silvestre AM, Llorens-Pena MP, Ferreira AJ. Measurement of the femoral neck anteversion angle in the dog using computed tomography. Vet J. 2007;174:378–383.

25. Kishimoto M, Yamada K, Pae SH, Muroya N, Watarai H, Anzai H, et al. Quantitative evaluation of hip joint laxity in 22 Border Collies using computed tomography. J Vet Med Sci. 2009;71:247–250.

26. Alpaslan AM, Aksoy MC, Yazici M. Interruption of the blood supply of femoral head: an experimental study on the pathogenesis of Legg-Calve-Perthes Disease. Arch Orthop Trauma Surg. 2007;127:485–491.

27. Kemp HB. Perthes' disease: the influence of intracapsular tamponade on the circulation in the hip joint of the dog. Clin Orthop Relat Res. 1981;105–114.

28. Weisbrode SE. Bone and Joints. In: McGavin MD, Zachary JF (eds): Pathologic Basis of Veterinary Disease. St. Louis: Mosby Elsevier, 2007;1041–1105.

29. LaFond E, Breur GJ, Austin CC. Breed susceptibility for developmental orthopedic diseases in dogs. J Am Anim Hosp Assoc. 2002;38:467–477.

30. Lee R. A study of the radiographic and histological changes occurring in Legg-Calve-Perthes disease (LCP) in the dog. J Small Anim Pract. 1970;11:621–638.

31. Wang C, Wang J, Zhang Y, Yuan C, Liu D, Pei Y, et al. A canine model of femoral head osteonecrosis induced by an ethanol injection navigated by a novel template. Int J Med Sci. 2013;10:1451–1458.

32. Bowlus RA, Armbrust LJ, Biller DS, Hoskinson JJ, Kuroki K, Mosier DA. Magnetic resonance imaging of the femoral head of normal dogs and dogs with avascular necrosis. Vet Radiol Ultrasound. 2008;49:7–12.

33. Balfour RJ, Boudrieau RJ, Gores BR. T-plate fixation of distal radial closing wedge osteotomies for treatment of angular limb deformities in 18 dogs. Vet Surg. 2000;29:207–217.

34. Deruddere K, Snelling S. A retrospective review of antebrachial angular and rotational limb deformity correction in dogs using intraoperative alignment and type 1b external fixation. N Z Vet J. 2014;62:290–296.

35. Hildreth BE 3rd, Johnson KA. Ulnocarpal arthrodesis for the treatment of radial agenesis in a dog. Vet Comp Orthop Traumatol. 2007;20:231–235.

36. Kim J, Blevins WE, Breur GJ. Morphological and functional evaluation of a dog with dimelia. Vet Comp Orthop Traumatol. 2006;19:255–258.

37. Sereda CW, Lewis DD, Radasch RM, Bruce CW, Kirkby KA. Descriptive report of antebrachial growth deformity correction in 17 dogs from 1999 to 2007, using hybrid linear-circular external fixator constructs. Can Vet J. 2009;50:723–732.

38. Weh JL, Kowaleski MP, Boudrieau RJ. Combination tibial plateau leveling osteotomy and transverse corrective osteotomy of the proximal tibia for the treatment of complex tibial deformities in 12 dogs. Vet Surg. 2011;40:670–686.

39. Coutin JV, Lewis DD, Kim SE, Reese DJ. Bifocal femoral deformity correction and lengthening using a circular fixator construct in a dog. J Am Anim Hosp Assoc. 2013;49:216–223.

40. Crosse KR, Worth AJ. Computer-assisted surgical correction of an antebrachial deformity in a dog. Vet Comp Orthop Traumatol. 2010;23:354–361.

41. Meola SD, Wheeler JL, Rist CL. Validation of a technique to assess radial torsion in the presence of procurvatum and valgus deformity using computed tomography: a cadaveric study. Vet Surg. 2008;37:525–529.

42. Grondalen J. Metaphyseal osteopathy (hypertrophic osteodystrophy) in growing dogs. A clinical study. J Small Anim Pract. 1976; 17:721–735.

43. Safra N, Johnson EG, Lit L, Foreman O, Wolf ZT, Aguilar M, et al. Clinical manifestations, response to treatment, and clinical outcome for Weimaraners with hypertrophic osteodystrophy: 53 cases (2009–2011). J Am Vet Med Assoc. 2013;242:1260–1266.

44. Marcellin-Little DJ, DeYoung DJ, Ferris KK, Berry CM. Incomplete ossification of the humeral condyle in spaniels. Vet Surg. 1994;23:475–487.

45. Martin RB, Crews L, Saveraid T, Conzemius MG. Prevalence of incomplete ossification of the humeral condyle in the limb opposite humeral condylar fracture: 14 dogs. Vet Comp Orthop Traumatol. 2010;23:168–172.

46. Moores AP, Agthe P, Schaafsma IA. Prevalence of incomplete ossification of the humeral condyle and other abnormalities of the elbow in English Springer Spaniels. Vet Comp Orthop Traumatol. 2012;25:211–216.

47. Carrera I, Hammond GJ, Sullivan M. Computed tomographic features of incomplete ossification of the canine humeral condyle. Vet Surg. 2008;37:226–231.

48. Piola V, Posch B, Radke H, Telintelo G, Herrtage ME. Magnetic resonance imaging features of canine incomplete humeral condyle ossification. Vet Radiol Ultrasound. 2012;53:560–565.

49. Brodey RS. Hypertrophic osteoarthropathy in the dog: a clinico-pathologic survey of 60 cases. J Am Vet Med Assoc. 1971;159: 1242–1256.

50. Caywood DD, Kramek BA, Feeney DA, Johnston GR. Hypertrophic osteopathy associated with a bronchial foreign body and lobar pneumonia in a dog. J Am Vet Med Assoc. 1985;186:698–700.

51. Stephens LC, Gleiser CA, Jardine JH. Primary pulmonary fibro-sarcoma associated with *Spirocerca lupi* infection in a dog with hypertrophic pulmonary osteoarthropathy. J Am Vet Med Assoc. 1983;182:496–498.

52. Vulgamott JC, Clark RG. Arterial hypertension and hypertrophic pulmonary osteopathy associated with aortic valvular endocarditis in a dog. J Am Vet Med Assoc. 1980;177:243–246.

53. Vanbrugghe B, Blond L, Carioto L, Carmel EN, Nadeau ME. Clinical and computed tomography features of secondary renal hyperparathyroidism. Can Vet J. 2011;52:177–180; quiz 180.

54. La Perle KMD, Capen CC. Endocrine System. In: McGavin MD, Zachary JF (eds): Pathologic Basis of Veterinary Disease. St. Louis: Mosby Elsevier, 2007;693–741.

6.2

Trauma

Fracture

Fractures of small size or in complex anatomic regions may not be appreciated on radiographs. CT and MR imaging both have the spatial resolution to depict these types of injuries in order to obtain a precise diagnosis and to aid in surgical planning.

Fractures of long bones and joints are common traumatic injuries (Figure 6.2.1). Fractures may also occur in sites predisposed to incomplete ossification, particularly the humeral condyle of Spaniels and other breeds. A region of sclerosis is present on CT images in one or both condyles, and a nondisplaced fissure or complete fracture of the condyle may occur (see also Figure 6.1.15).[1] MR imaging has detected a heterogeneous signal with central hyperintensity in the condyle on STIR images prior to fissure formation, and this may be an early sign of condylar disease.[2]

The carpus and tarsus are anatomically complex, and small fractures, multiple fractures, and comminuted fractures may be difficult to assess on radiographs (Figures 6.2.2, 6.2.3, 6.2.4). CT is most often used to image these regions and provides good interobserver agreement in complicated fractures.[3] Tarsal bone trauma is common in racing Greyhounds, and quantitative CT measures of volumetry and density have been developed to predict changes in the central tarsal bone in response to training.[4]

The pelvis is a frequent site of multiple traumatic fractures, which can be better appreciated on CT images in dogs and cats. The sites where CT is particularly valuable in accurate diagnosis include acetabular and sacral fractures.[5,6] Animals may be imaged under general anesthesia; however, sedated or fully conscious imaging has also been reported to provide satisfactory image quality.[4]

Soft tissue trauma

Muscle trauma can occur with or without accompanying skeletal injury. The CT and MR anatomy of pelvic limb musculature has been described previously.[7] Trauma to musculature, such as iliopsoas injury, causes muscular enlargement and heterogeneous contrast enhancement.[8] Injury of the iliopsoas muscle may also result in tendinitis and avulsion fracture of the lesser trochanter of the femur.[9] On STIR, T2, or contrast-enhanced T1 images, tissue hyperintensity is visible in the region of injury (Figure 6.2.5). Myotendinous strains to the gastrocnemius muscle have also been described in a group of herding dogs with similar MR imaging characteristics.[10] Myositis can occur secondary to trauma or infectious or noninfectious inflammatory disease (Figure 6.2.6).

Traumatic disorders of the shoulder and stifle joints

Because trauma to the shoulder and stifle are often evaluated using cross-sectional imaging, they are specifically addressed in the following two sections.

Shoulder disorders

Injuries of the shoulder joint or ligaments and tendons adjacent to the joint are common in active dogs and can be the result of either a single insult or repetitive trauma. Stability of the joint relies on active and passive stabilizers.

Atlas of Small Animal CT and MRI, First Edition. Erik R. Wisner and Allison L. Zwingenberger.

Passive stabilizers include the joint capsule and the lateral and medial glenohumeral ligaments. Active stabilizers, consist of the supraspinatus, infraspinatus, teres minor, subscapularis, biceps brachii, and deltoideus muscles, which are collectively referred to as the rotator cuff. Common traumatic disorders affecting the shoulder include supraspinatus insertional tendinopathy, bicipital tenosynovitis or rupture, infraspinatus tendinopathy, fibrotic infraspinatus muscle contracture, and medial shoulder instability, which involves changes of the medial glenohumeral ligament, joint capsule, and subscapularis tendon. Multiple disorders can occur simultaneously, and secondary degenerative joint disease is a common sequela.

One veterinary study comparing CT abnormalities with clinical findings in dogs with shoulder lameness concluded that although CT was useful for detecting osteochondrosis lesions and soft-tissue mineralization, correlation to the source of clinical lameness was questionable.[11] In our experience, MR is the preferred imaging modality when a specific diagnosis cannot be achieved using radiography and ultrasonography. MR is of particular value for diagnosis of medial joint disorders since the medial aspect of the shoulder joint (sometimes referred to as the medial compartment) is inaccessible with ultrasound. A standard protocol includes PD, T1, T2, STIR, and gadolinium arthrographic images in all three major anatomic planes with the shoulder in partial extension.[12–15] Fat-suppression and thinly collimated volume-acquisition sequences may be useful in some instances.

Supraspinatus tendinopathy is a common disorder of large-breed dogs. On MR images, affected tendons are enlarged and hyperintense on T2 and STIR images at the insertion on the greater tubercle (Figure 6.2.7).[16] Because it inserts on the craniomedial aspect of the greater tubercle, the supraspinatus tendon often encroaches on the bicipital bursa and biceps tendon when it becomes enlarged. Bicipital tenosynovitis has a similar appearance and can be readily detected on sagittal and transverse images (Figure 6.2.8).[17] Arthrography causes distension of the bicipital bursa, improving the visibility of the tendon and synovial lining. Bicipital tendon rupture appears as a discontinuity of the tendon in all imaging planes. Fibrotic subscapularis contracture appears as muscle volume loss with variable and heterogeneous T1 and T2 intensity. Infraspinatus myositis and tendinitis may also be a cause of shoulder lameness (Figures 6.2.9,6.2. 10). Medial shoulder instability causes thickening of the joint capsule, medial glenohumeral ligament, and subscapularis insertional tendon (Figure 6.2.11).[17,18] Distension of the joint on arthrographic images improves conspicuity of the joint capsule and glenohumeral ligaments.[12,13]

Stifle joint disorders

The most common stifle injury in dogs is rupture of the cranial cruciate ligament. Although diagnosis is often made after significant osteoarthrosis has occurred, early detection with CT and MR imaging could be advantageous for prevention of degenerative disease.

CT is particularly useful when osseous fragments are detected (Figure 6.2.12). CT arthrography has been used to detect cruciate ligament tears with good accuracy and meniscal tears with somewhat lesser accuracy. Meniscal tears appeared as vertical or semicircular accumulations of contrast in the plane of the soft-tissue attenuating meniscal cartilage. Submillimeter collimation is necessary to improve spatial resolution of small structures using multidetector CT scanners.[19] Osteoarthrosis is visible as marginal new bone formation on the femur, patella, trochlear ridges, and tibia as a secondary change.

MR is the gold standard of imaging the knee in people. Visualization of the small ligamentous and cartilaginous structures of the stifle is more challenging in dogs and cats because of the relatively smaller size of the joint. The normal cruciate ligaments are of low signal on MR images, with the cranial cruciate slightly smaller than the caudal cruciate ligament (Figure 6.2.13). Cruciate ligament injury may be seen as increased signal, discontinuity of the fibers, or absence of the ligament.[20]

MR arthrography has also been investigated for evaluating the cruciate ligaments and menisci.[21] Sagittal plane images were found to be useful for evaluating the cruciate ligaments, and dorsal plane images were optimal for visualizing the collateral ligaments and menisci. Three-dimensional FSPGR images were utilized for evaluating cartilage and erosions. Similar to CT arthrography, meniscal tears were seen as linear contrast accumulations within the low-signal region of the meniscus. Findings of cruciate ligament interruption and meniscal tears (Figure 6.2.14) have also been reported on nonarthrographic imaging with 1.5 T and 3 T magnets.[22,23] Heterogeneous signal intensity within the normally low-signal meniscus is indicative of degenerative disease (Figure 6.2.15).[24] A bucket-handle tear may have two linear regions of hyperintensity in the sagittal plane and one in the dorsal plane because of its curved shape.[24] Subchondral bone edema may be seen on T2 fat-suppressed images at the origin and insertion of the ruptured cruciate ligaments, or in the caudal tibia in the case of a meniscal tear.[24,25] Bone edema may also be associated with cartilage fractures or synovial invaginations in these regions (Figure 6.2.15).[20]

Figure 6.2.1 Humeral Condylar Fracture (Canine)

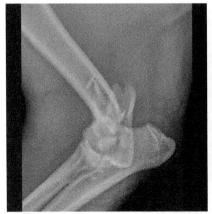

(a) DX, LAT

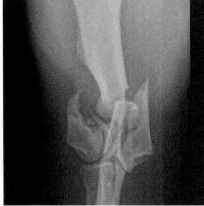

(b) DX, CC

2y M Boxer injured in a fight with another dog. On radiographs of the elbow, there is a bicondylar "Y" fracture of the left humerus with severe comminution (**a**,**b**). The 3D rendered CT images show the subluxation of the humeroulnar joint (**c**: arrow) and the displacement of the fragments of the condyle (**d**). The striation artifacts in the 3D rendered images are due to respiratory motion.

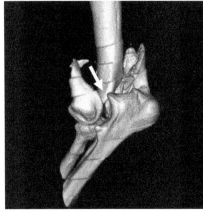

(c) CT, 3D, LLAT

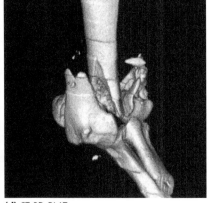

(d) CT, 3D, RLAT

Figure 6.2.2 Carpal Fracture (Canine)   CT

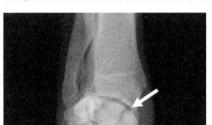

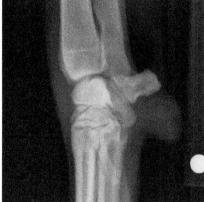

2y M Weimaraner with thoracic limb lameness of 6 weeks' duration. On carpal radiographs (**a,b**), there is a fracture with indistinct margins visible in the radiocarpal bone (**a**: arrow). The comparable dorsal plane CT image shows the fracture with surrounding sclerosis, indicating chronicity (**c**: arrow). There is moderate displacement of the fragment medially on the transverse image acquired at the level of the proximal row of carpal bones (**d**: arrowhead). The irregularity of the fracture margins and sclerosis are again visible.

(a) DX, DP   **(b)** DX, LAT

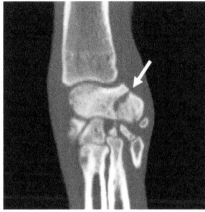

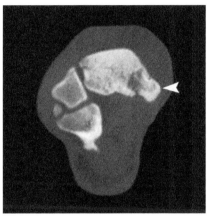

(c) CT, DP   **(d)** CT, TP

Figure 6.2.3 Tibial and Fibular Articular Fracture (Canine)   CT

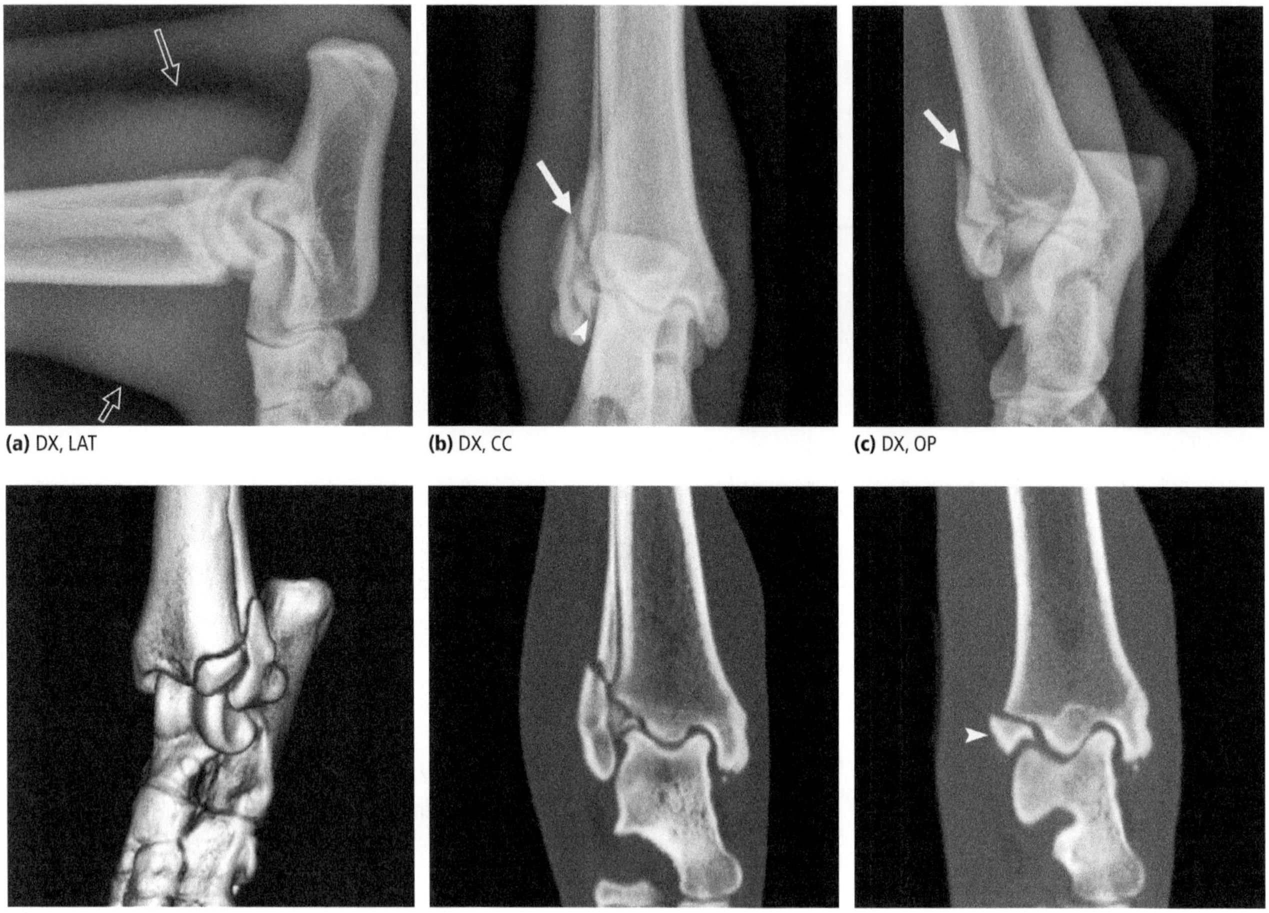

(a) DX, LAT

(b) DX, CC

(c) DX, OP

(d) CT, 3D, OP

(e) CT, DP

(f) CT, DP

2y M German Shepherd Dog with left pelvic limb lameness after jumping while playing ball. On radiographs of the left tarsus, there is soft-tissue swelling surrounding the distal tibia and fibula (a: open arrows). There is an oblique fracture through the distal fibula (b,c: arrows) and suspected fracture of the medial malleolus of the tibia (b: arrowhead). CT images are oriented in the dorsal plane (e,f). The fibular fracture is clearly defined. The tibial fracture is articular and moderately displaced (f: arrowhead). The 3D image depicts both fractures relative to the tarsus (d).

Figure 6.2.4 Monteggia Fracture (Canine)

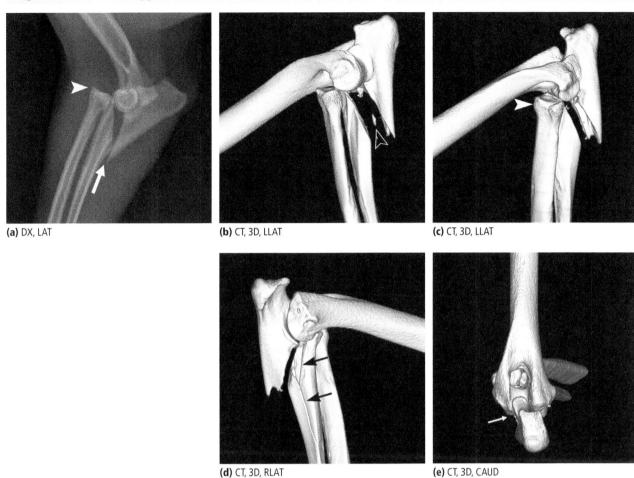

(a) DX, LAT   (b) CT, 3D, LLAT   (c) CT, 3D, LLAT

(d) CT, 3D, RLAT   (e) CT, 3D, CAUD

2y FS German Shepherd Dog with a history of vehicular trauma. There is an oblique fracture through the proximal third of the ulna with an articular component (a: arrow). The radial head is luxated cranially (a: arrowhead). The CT images show the comminution fragments within the fracture (b: open arrowhead). The luxation of the radial head (c: arrowhead) and subluxation of the humeroulnar joint (e: small arrow) are well visualized. Multiple longitudinal and oblique fissures are present in the proximal ulna (d: black arrows).

Figure 6.2.5 Iliopsoas Myositis (Canine)   MR

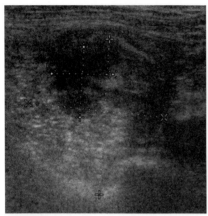

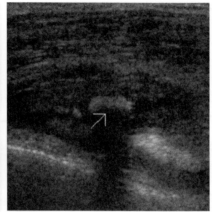

Adult MC mixed breed with acute right pelvic limb lameness. A transverse ultrasound image of the iliopsoas muscle shows enlargement of the muscle body and a hypoechoic region in the periphery (**a**: calipers). At the lesser trochanter of the femur, there is an avulsion fracture that is displaced from the cortical bone (**b**: arrow). Transverse MR images show enlargement and hyperintensity of the right iliopsoas muscle on T2 and STIR images (**c,d**: arrow). Reproduced with permission from Dr. Ryan Schultz, Seattle Veterinary Specialists, Kirkland, WA, 2014.

(a) US, TP

(b) US, SP

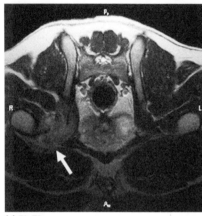

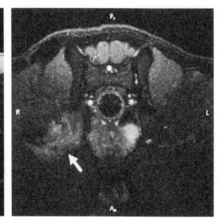

(c) T2, TP

(d) ST, TP

Figure 6.2.6   Gluteal Myositis (Feline)

MR

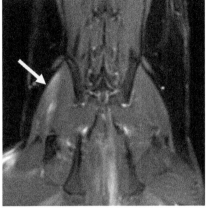

(a) T1+C, FS, DP

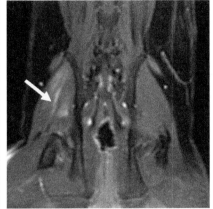

(b) T1+C, FS, DP

15y FS American Shorthair with acute para-paresis and lethargy. Dorsal plane images of the pelvic musculature were acquired during imaging of the spine. There is hyperintensity of the right gluteal muscles on the contrast-enhanced images (**a**,**b**: arrow). The striated, linear hyperintensities are also seen on the comparable dorsal plane STIR images (**c**,**d**). The cat was positive for *Cryptococcus* sp.; however, the lameness resolved within 2 weeks and was presumed to be traumatic.

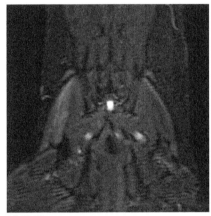

(c) ST, DP

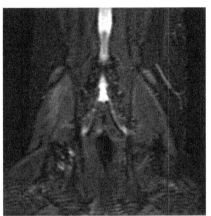

(d) ST, DP

Legend for Figures 6.2.7–6.2.11

Bib	Biceps brachii muscle	MGL	Medial glenohumeral Ligament
BT	Biceps tendon	SsT	Supraspinatus tendon
BB	Bicipital bursa	Ss	Supraspinatus muscle
IsT	Infraspinatus tendon	Su	Subscapularis muscle
Is	Infraspinatus muscle	SuT	Subscapularis tendon
LGL	Lateral glenohumeral ligament		

Figure 6.2.7 Supraspinatus Tendinopathy (Canine)   MR

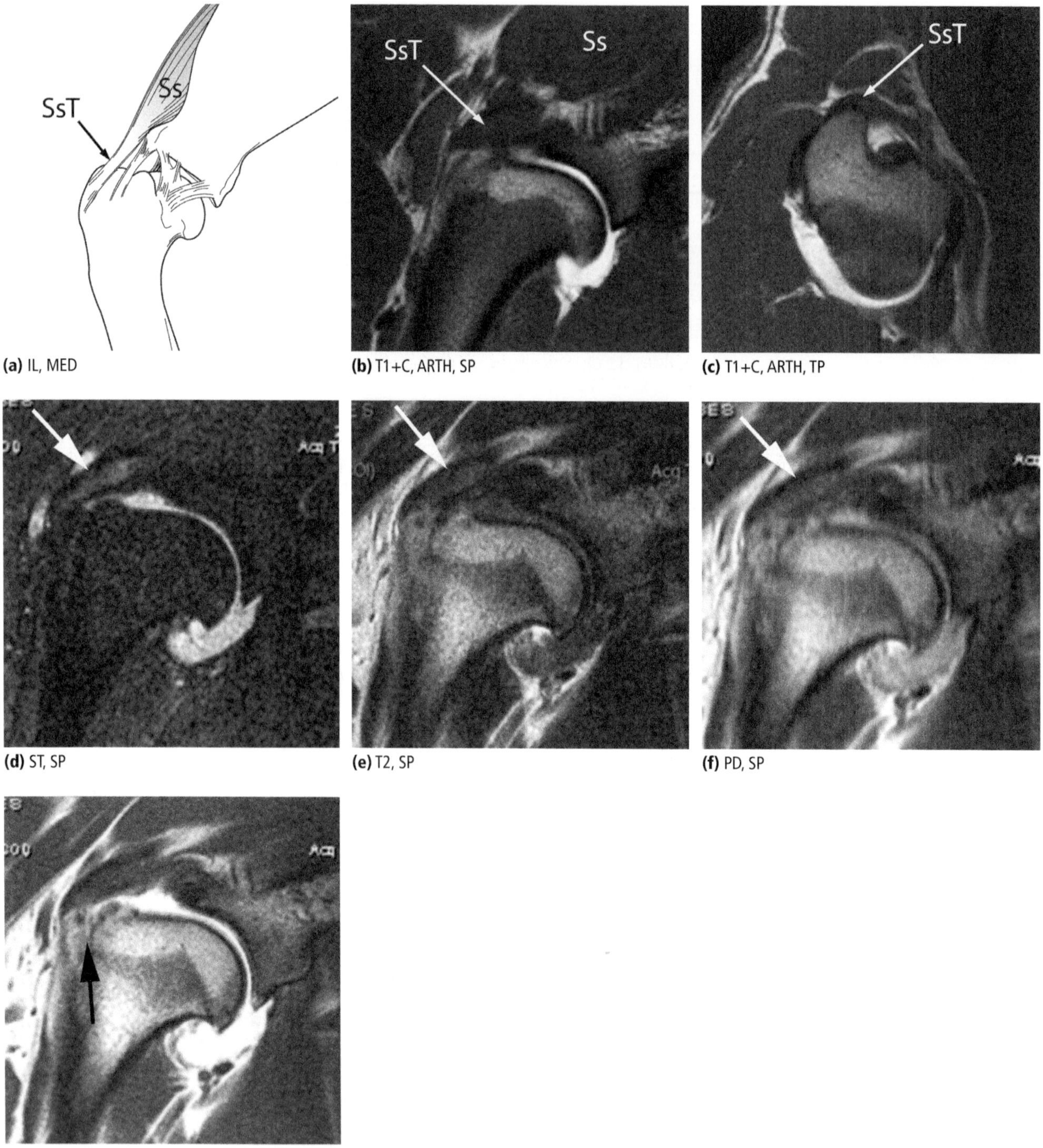

(a) IL, MED

(b) T1+C, ARTH, SP

(c) T1+C, ARTH, TP

(d) ST, SP

(e) T2, SP

(f) PD, SP

(g) T1+C, ARTH, SP

2y MC Labrador Retriever with acute-onset right thoracic limb lameness 1 month ago. Pain is elicited on shoulder flexion and extension. Image **a** shows the supraspinatus muscle (Ss) and its tendon of insertion (SsT) on the medial surface of the greater tubercle. Images **b** and **c** are arthrographic images of the normal supraspinatus muscle and tendon viewed in sagittal (**b**) and transverse (**c**) planes. Sagittal images of the patient (**d–g**) show STIR, T2, and PD hyperintensity of the supraspinatus tendon (**d–f**: arrow). Distension of the joint space on an arthrographic image highlights the remodeling of the medial aspect of the greater tubercle at the point of tendon insertion (**g**: arrow). See Legend for Figures 6.2.7–6.2.11. Agnello et al 2008.[12] Reproduced with permission from Wiley.

Figure 6.2.8 Chronic Bicipital Tendon Rupture (Canine)   MR

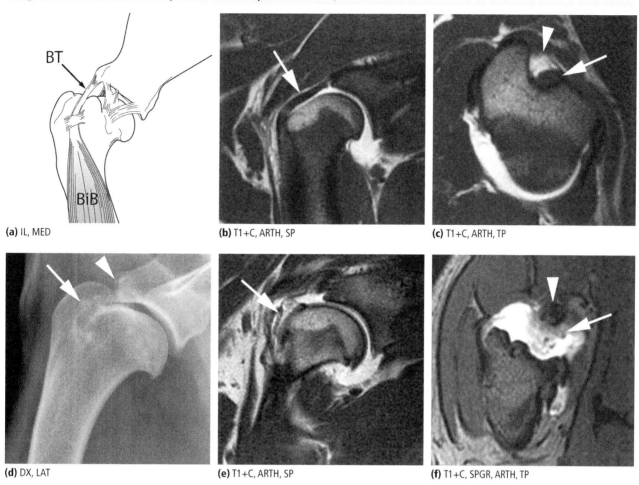

(a) IL, MED

(b) T1+C, ARTH, SP

(c) T1+C, ARTH, TP

(d) DX, LAT

(e) T1+C, ARTH, SP

(f) T1+C, SPGR, ARTH, TP

Same patient as in Figure 6.2.7. Image **a** shows the biceps brachii muscle (**a**: BiB) and its tendon of origin (**a**: BT) at its attachment to the supraglenoid tubercle. Images **b** and **c** are arthrographic images of a normal biceps tendon (**b,c**: arrow). Distension of the bicipital bursa (**c**: arrowhead) improves the conspicuity of the tendon. A lateral radiograph of the patient shows mineralization in the region of the bicipital bursa (**d**: arrow) and remodeling of the supraglenoid tubercle (**d**: arrowhead). The biceps tendon is irregularly shaped, T1 hyperintense, and discontinuous in the sagittal arthrographic image (**e**: arrow). T1 hyperintense remnants of the ruptured tendon (**f**: arrow) are seen adjacent to the cranial margin of the supraglenoid tubercle (**f**: arrowhead) on a transverse arthrographic image. Arthroscopic exploration confirmed rupture of the tendon. See Legend for Figures 6.2.7–6.2.11. Agnello et al 2008.[12] Reproduced with permission from Wiley.

Figure 6.2.9 Infraspinatus Traumatic Myositis (Canine)   MR

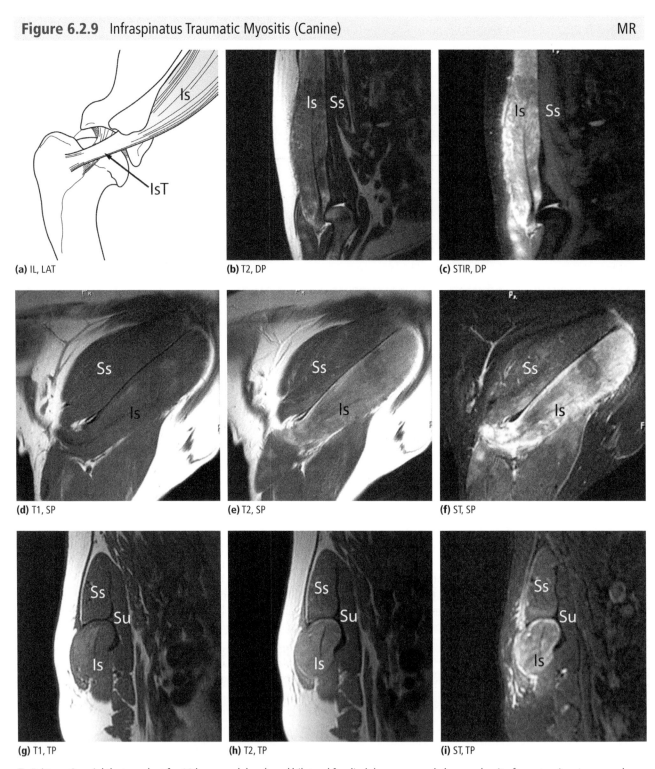

(a) IL, LAT   (b) T2, DP   (c) STIR, DP

(d) T1, SP   (e) T2, SP   (f) ST, SP

(g) T1, TP   (h) T2, TP   (i) ST, TP

7y Brittany Spaniel that was lost for 18 hours and developed bilateral forelimb lameness and abnormal gait after returning. Image **a** shows the infraspinatus muscle (Is) and its tendon of insertion (IsT). There is marked T2 and STIR hyperintensity throughout the infraspinatus muscle (**b,c,e,f,h,i**: Is), associated with increased muscle volume (**g–i**) due to muscle edema. There is also patchy muscle T1 hyperintensity (**e,g**: Is). Imaging features are consistent with traumatic myositis with early subacute intramuscular hemorrhage. This example may represent an early, active phase of trauma that can lead to fibrotic infraspinatus muscle contracture. See Legend for Figures 6.2.7–6.2.11. Reproduced with permission from Dr. Rob McLear, PetRad, LLC. Norristown, PA, 2014.

Figure 6.2.10   Infraspinatus Insertional Tendinopathy (Canine)   MR

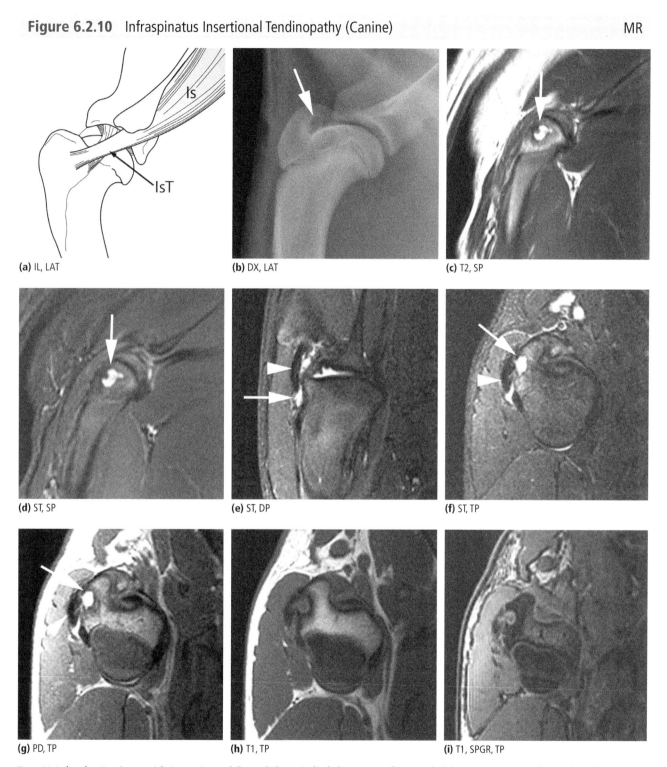

(a) IL, LAT

(b) DX, LAT

(c) T2, SP

(d) ST, SP

(e) ST, DP

(f) ST, TP

(g) PD, TP

(h) T1, TP

(i) T1, SPGR, TP

7mo M Labrador Retriever with intermittent bilateral thoracic limb lameness of 3 months' duration. Image **a** shows the infraspinatus muscle (Is) and its tendon of insertion (IsT) on the lateral surface of the greater tubercle. A radiograph of the right shoulder reveals a focal osteolytic defect in the region of the insertion of the infraspinatus muscle (**b**: arrow). MR imaging reveals the course of the infraspinatus tendon (**e–g**: arrowhead) and a focal cavitary defect at its insertion that appears STIR, T2, and PD hyperintense (**c–g**: arrow). T1 images show a hypointense rim surrounding the defect presumably due to sclerosis. Similar abnormalities were evident on radiographs and MR images of the contralateral limb. An extensive clinical and imaging evaluation of both thoracic limbs failed to identify any other cause for lameness. See Legend for Figures 6.2.7–6.2.11.

Figure 6.2.11   Medial Compartment Disorder (Canine)   MR

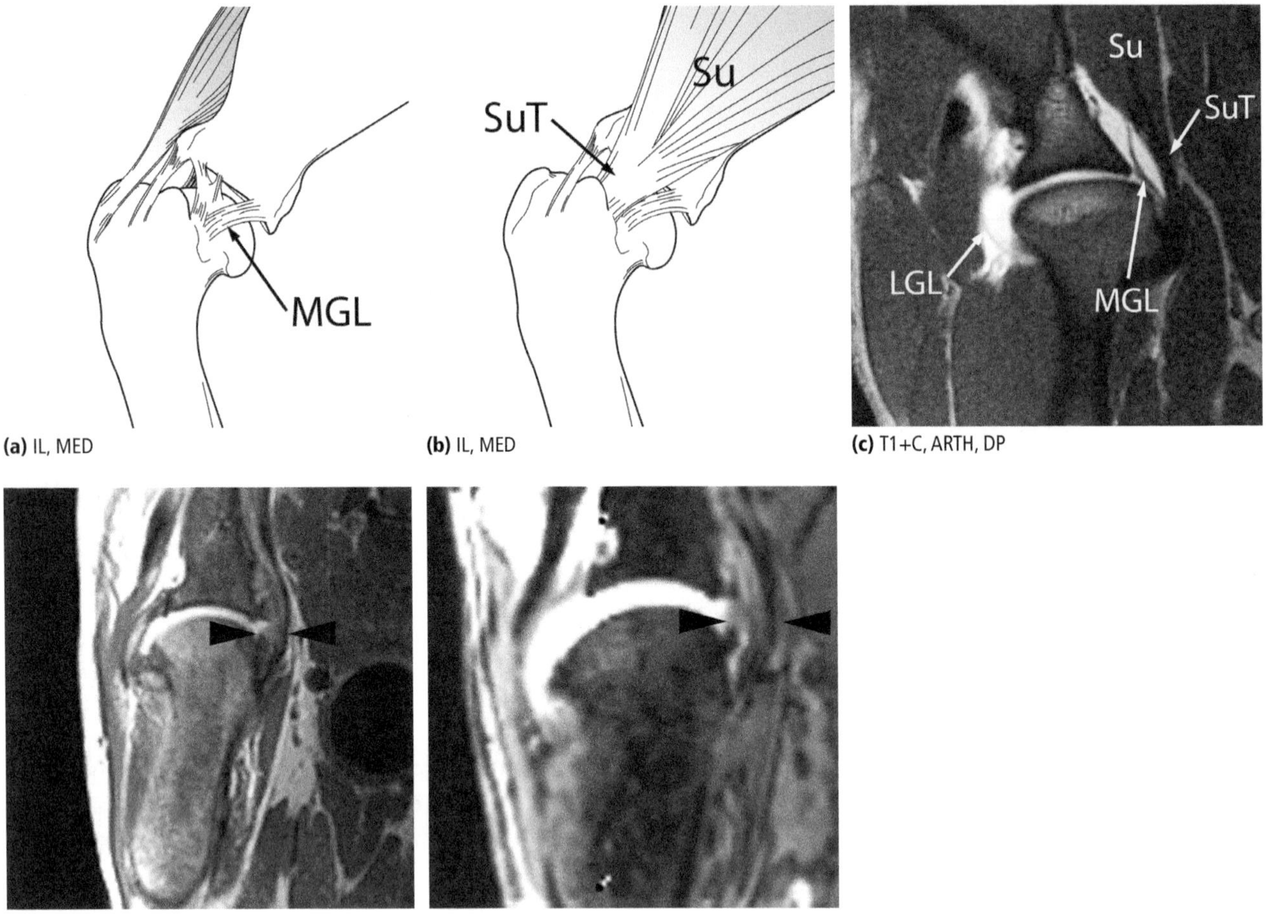

(a) IL, MED

(b) IL, MED

(c) T1+C, ARTH, DP

(d) T1+C, DP

(e) T1+C, SPGR, DP

8y MC Australian Shepherd with a history of left-sided bicipital tenosynovitis that was surgically treated previously with tendon transection. Lameness progressed following surgery. Images **a** and **b** show the medial glenohumeral ligament (**a**: MGL) and the overlying subscapularis muscle (**b**: Su) and subscapularis tendon of insertion (**b**: SuT) on the medial aspect of the humeral head. Image **c** is a dorsal plane arthrographic image of a normal shoulder in extension showing the lateral glenohumeral ligament (**c**: LGL), medial glenohumeral ligament (**c**: MGL), subscapularis muscle (**c**: Su), and subscapularis tendon of insertion (**c**: SuT). Image **e** is a magnification of **d**. Dorsal plane arthrographic images of the affected limb of the patient show marked muscle wasting. Although the medial glenohumeral ligament is not well delineated from the overlying subscapularis tendon of insertion, the combined width is markedly thicker than normal (**d,e**: arrowheads), indicative of medial compartment instability. See Legend for Figures 6.2.7–6.2.11. Agnello et al 2008.[12] Reproduced with permission from Wiley.

Figure 6.2.12 Cranial Cruciate Ligament Avulsion (Canine)

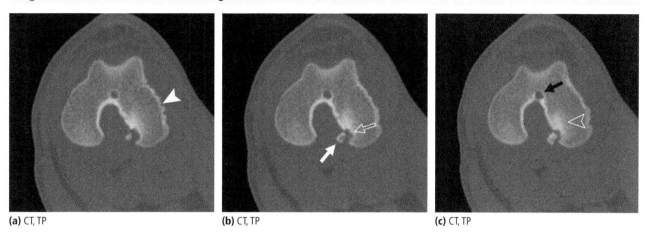

(a) CT, TP　　　　　　　**(b)** CT, TP　　　　　　　**(c)** CT, TP

6mo F Labrador Retriever with left pelvic limb lameness. Images **a–c** are ordered from proximal to distal through the distal femur. Irregular periosteal reaction is visible on the lateral femoral condyle (**a**: arrowhead), indicating degenerative joint disease. There is a well-defined osseous fragment (**b**: arrow) with an associated concavity in the medial aspect of the lateral femoral condyle (**b**: open arrow). The defect is surrounded by a rim of sclerosis (**c**: open arrowhead). There is an enlarged synovial invagination also associated with degenerative disease (**c**: black arrow).

Figure 6.2.13 Normal Stifle (Canine)

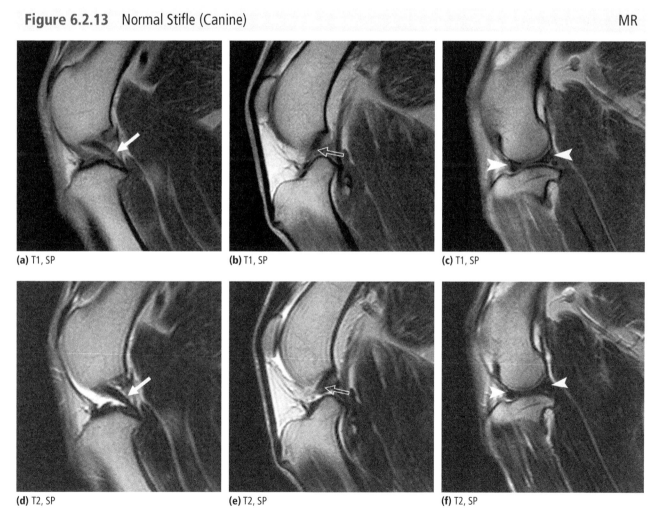

(a) T1, SP　　　　　　　**(b)** T1, SP　　　　　　　**(c)** T1, SP

(d) T2, SP　　　　　　　**(e)** T2, SP　　　　　　　**(f)** T2, SP

Adult Beagle. Sagittal T1 (**a–c**) and comparable T2 (**d–f**) MR images are ordered from medial to lateral. The caudal cruciate ligament spans the caudal tibia to the cranial femur in an oblique plane and is substantial in width with hypointense signal on T1 and T2 images (**a,d**: arrows). The cranial cruciate has the opposite orientation and is thinner (**b,e**: open arrows). The lateral meniscus has low signal on T1 and T2 images and appears as two triangular shapes contoured to the femoral condyles with a thin connecting isthmus (**c,f**: arrowheads). Reproduced with permission from Dr. Silke Hecht, University of Tennessee, Knoxville, TN, 2014.

Figure 6.2.14   Cranial Cruciate Ligament Rupture (Canine)   MR

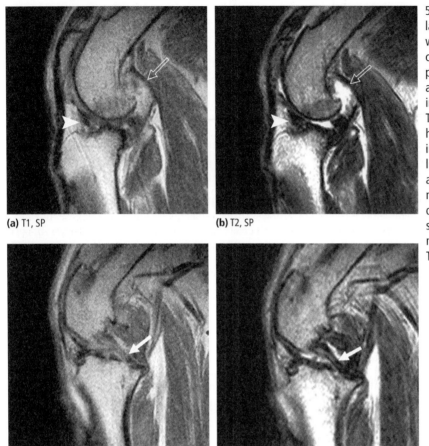

(a) T1, SP   (b) T2, SP

(c) T1, SP   (d) T2, SP

5y MC Boxer with history of left pelvic limb lameness. There is marked joint effusion within the stifle joint (**a,b**: open arrow). The cranial cruciate is not visible in its normal position (**a,c**). The caudal cruciate ligament appears intact with mixed signal intensity, indicating degenerative change (**c,d**: arrow). The menisci are ill defined and irregular with heterogeneous signal intensity on T1 and T2 images (**a,b**: arrowhead). A cranial cruciate ligament rupture, meniscal fragmentation, and degenerative joint disease were diagnosed. There is marked irregularity and osteophyte formation of the cortical bone surrounding the joint. Reproduced with permission from Dr. Silke Hecht, University of Tennessee, Knoxville, TN, 2014.

Figure 6.2.15   Partial Cruciate Ligament Rupture (Canine)   MR

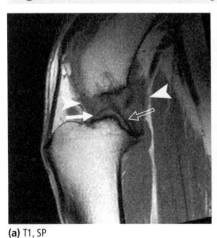   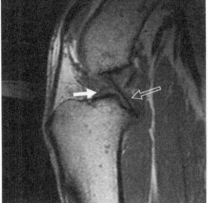   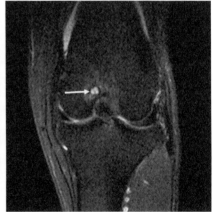

(a) T1, SP   (b) T2, SPGR, SP   (c) ST, DP

11y FS mixed breed with pelvic limb lameness. There is increased soft-tissue attenuating material within the joint capsule (**a**: arrowheads), representing synovial proliferation and effusion. The caudal cruciate ligament is intact (**a,b**: open arrow). The cranial cruciate is thinned (**a**: arrow) and has increased signal on T2 images (**b**: arrow). The caudal portion of the ligament (not shown) is out of plane but appeared intact. There is a STIR hyperintense subchondral cyst with surrounding bone edema in the lateral femoral condyle (**c**: small arrow). This was distant from the sites of cruciate ligament attachment and was presumed degenerative. A partial cranial cruciate ligament tear was diagnosed. Reproduced with permission from Dr. Silke Hecht, University of Tennessee, Knoxville, TN, 2014.

References

1. Carrera I, Hammond GJ, Sullivan M. Computed tomographic features of incomplete ossification of the canine humeral condyle. Vet Surg. 2008;37:226–231.
2. Piola V, Posch B, Radke H, Telintelo G, Herrtage ME. Magnetic resonance imaging features of canine incomplete humeral condyle ossification. Vet Radiol Ultrasound. 2012;53:560–565.
3. Hercock CA, Innes JF, McConnell F, Guilliard MJ, Ness MG, Hodson D, et al. Observer variation in the evaluation and classification of severe central tarsal bone fractures in racing Greyhounds. Vet Comp Orthop Traumatol. 2011;24:215–222.
4. Lee K, Heng HG, Jeong J, Naughton JF, Rohleder JJ. Feasibility of computed tomography in awake dogs with traumatic pelvic fracture. Vet Radiol Ultrasound. 2012;53:412–416.
5. Draffan D, Clements D, Farrell M, Heller J, Bennett D, Carmichael S. The role of computed tomography in the classification and management of pelvic fractures. Vet Comp Orthop Traumatol. 2009;22:190–197.
6. Crawford JT, Manley PA, Adams WM. Comparison of computed tomography, tangential view radiography, and conventional radiography in evaluation of canine pelvic trauma. Vet Radiol Ultrasound. 2003;44:619–628.
7. Sunico SK, Hamel C, Styner M, Robertson ID, Kornegay JN, Bettini C, et al. Two anatomic resources of canine pelvic limb muscles based on CT and MRI. Vet Radiol Ultrasound. 2012;53:266–272.
8. Rossmeisl JH, Jr., Rohleder JJ, Hancock R, Lanz OI. Computed tomographic features of suspected traumatic injury to the iliopsoas and pelvic limb musculature of a dog. Vet Radiol Ultrasound. 2004;45:388–392.
9. Vidoni B, Henninger W, Lorinson D, Mayrhofer E. Traumatic avulsion fracture of the lesser trochanter in a dog. Vet Comp Orthop Traumatol. 2005;18:105–109.
10. Stahl C, Wacker C, Weber U, Forterre F, Hecht P, Lang J, et al. MRI features of gastrocnemius musculotendinopathy in herding dogs. Vet Radiol Ultrasound. 2010;51:380–385.
11. Maddox TW, May C, Keeley BJ, McConnell JF. Comparison between shoulder computed tomography and clinical findings in 89 dogs presented for thoracic limb lameness. Vet Radiol Ultrasound. 2013;54:358–364.
12. Agnello KA, Puchalski SM, Wisner ER, Schulz KS, Kapatkin AS. Effect of positioning, scan plane, and arthrography on visibility of periarticular canine shoulder soft tissue structures on magnetic resonance images. Vet Radiol Ultrasound. 2008;49:529–539.
13. Schaefer SL, Baumel CA, Gerbig JR, Forrest LJ. Direct magnetic resonance arthrography of the canine shoulder. Vet Radiol Ultrasound. 2010;51:391–396.
14. Schaefer SL, Forrest LJ. Magnetic resonance imaging of the canine shoulder: an anatomic study. Vet Surg. 2006;35:721–728.
15. van Bree H, Degryse H, Van Ryssen B, Ramon F, Desmidt M. Pathologic correlations with magnetic resonance images of osteochondrosis lesions in canine shoulders. J Am Vet Med Assoc. 1993;202:1099–1105.
16. Lafuente MP, Fransson BA, Lincoln JD, Martinez SA, Gavin PR, Lahmers KK, et al. Surgical treatment of mineralized and non-mineralized supraspinatus tendinopathy in twenty-four dogs. Vet Surg. 2009;38:380–387.
17. Murphy SE, Ballegeer EA, Forrest LJ, Schaefer SL. Magnetic resonance imaging findings in dogs with confirmed shoulder pathology. Vet Surg. 2008;37:631–638.
18. Orellana-James NG, Ginja MM, Regueiro M, Oliveira P, Gama A, Rodriguez-Altonaga JA, et al. Sub-acute and chronic MRI findings in bilateral canine fibrotic contracture of the infraspinatus muscle. J Small Anim Pract. 2013;54:428–431.
19. Samii VF, Dyce J, Pozzi A, Drost WT, Mattoon JS, Green EM, et al. Computed tomographic arthrography of the stifle for detection of cranial and caudal cruciate ligament and meniscal tears in dogs. Vet Radiol Ultrasound. 2009;50:144–150.
20. Ho-Fung VM, Jaimes C, Jaramillo D. MR imaging of ACL injuries in pediatric and adolescent patients. Clin Sports Med. 2011;30:707–726.
21. Banfield CM, Morrison WB. Magnetic resonance arthrography of the canine stifle joint: technique and applications in eleven military dogs. Vet Radiol Ultrasound. 2000;41:200–213.
22. Galindo-Zamora V, Dziallas P, Ludwig DC, Nolte I, Wefstaedt P. Diagnostic accuracy of a short-duration 3 Tesla magnetic resonance protocol for diagnosing stifle joint lesions in dogs with non-traumatic cranial cruciate ligament rupture. BMC Vet Res. 2013;9:40.
23. Taylor-Brown F, Lamb CR, Tivers MS, Li A. Magnetic resonance imaging for detection of late meniscal tears in dogs following tibial tuberosity advancement for treatment of cranial cruciate ligament injury. Vet Comp Orthop Traumatol. 2014;27:141–146.
24. Olive J, d'Anjou MA, Cabassu J, Chailleux N, Blond L. Fast presurgical magnetic resonance imaging of meniscal tears and concurrent subchondral bone marrow lesions. Study of dogs with naturally occurring cranial cruciate ligament rupture. Vet Comp Orthop Traumatol. 2014;27:1–7.
25. Winegardner KR, Scrivani PV, Krotscheck U, Todhunter RJ. Magnetic resonance imaging of subarticular bone marrow lesions in dogs with stifle lameness. Vet Radiol Ultrasound. 2007;48:312–317.

6.3

Inflammatory disorders

Inflammatory disorders of bone

Osteomyelitis

Osteomyelitis is most often bacterial, with *Staphylococcus* the most common causative agent. Infection can also be due to other aerobic and anaerobic bacteria, and mixed infections are common. Bacterial osteomyelitis most frequently arises from penetrating injury or surgical contamination. Hematogenously disseminated bacterial osteomyelitis can occasionally occur as a consequence of septicemia, and immature and immunocompromised animals are more susceptible. Polyostotic osteomyelitis is more likely in these patients.

In certain geographic regions, systemic mycotic infection (*Coccidiodes, Blastomyces, Aspergillus, Histoplasma,* and *Cryptococcus* sp.) can also lead to hematogenously disseminated osteomyelitis. Protozoal agents, such as *Leishmania* sp., can also cause systemic disease with osteomyelitis as a component.

Although the imaging appearance and progression of bacterial and fungal osteomyelitis differ, both typically include mixed destructive and productive bone lesions. Acute bacterial osteomyelitis is often accompanied by regional cellulitis, and the initial destructive and periosteal productive responses are ill defined. Chronic bacterial osteomyelitis may appear more contained. A dense, sharply margined sequestrum, surrounding involucrum, peripheral bone sclerosis, and a cloaca leading to a draining open wound are classic features of chronic bacterial osteomyelitis but are not always present or easily detected. Fungal osteomyelitis often includes a poorly organized productive response that can sometimes mask significant underlying bone destruction.

In people, scintigraphy and MRI are considered sensitive imaging tests for early detection of osteomyelitis. CT and survey radiography are less useful, as results with these modalities are negative until bone destruction or reactivity occurs. CT features of osteomyelitis are similar to those described for conventional radiography (Figure 6.3.1; see also Figure 4.1.5). When present, a sequestrum will appear hyperattenuating to adjacent viable bone and will tend to have sharply delineated margins (Figure 6.3.2). Intravenous contrast administration can be useful to better characterize soft-tissue involvement. MR features as described in people include marrow T1 hypointensity, T2 and STIR hyperintensity, and enhancement following intravenous contrast administration (see Figure 3.3.5). Periosteal elevation with T2 hyperintense exudates can also be seen in acute infections. Cortical bone reactivity and cellulitis may also be detected, depending on the stage of the disease.[1-7]

Inflammatory disorders of joints

Arthritis is often designated as erosive or nonerosive and either infectious (septic) or immune-mediated. Immune-mediated arthritides can be either erosive or nonerosive, while infectious arthritides are typically erosive. Because immune-mediated inflammatory joint disease is a systemic disorder, it generally manifests as polyarthritis.[6,8-11]

Immune-mediated arthritis

Reports differ on the general signalment of dogs with immune-mediated arthritis. Some suggest that smaller breeds and females are overrepresented, while others indicate medium- to large-breed dogs may be more commonly affected and that there is no sex predilection. However, there is consensus that young to middle-aged dogs are predisposed to the disorder. Clinical signs include polyarthropathy, sometimes with intense pain. Dogs may also be febrile and have other signs referable to systemic disease.[8,9]

Nonerosive immune-mediated arthritis

This disorder is thought to be caused by articular inflammation that arises as a result of immune complex deposition within the synovium. Initiating causes include chronic systemic inflammatory diseases, systemic lupus erythematosus, neoplasia, and reactivity to certain drugs.[8] Imaging features are usually underwhelming, although joint effusion can manifest as joint space widening on CT images and prominent intraarticular T2 hyperintensity on MRI because of increased synovial fluid volume (Figure 6.3.3). Synovium and synovial fluid also enhance on T1 images following intravenous contrast administration. Chronically affected joints may show evidence of secondary degenerative disease, including periarticular remodeling, subchondral bone sclerosis, and enthesophyte formation.

Erosive immune-mediated arthritis

Erosive immune-mediated arthritis is similar to rheumatoid arthritis in people, in which antibodies specifically target synovium, initiating an inflammatory cascade. The inflammatory response leads to cartilage injury and underlying subchondral bone destruction. Joints of the distal extremities seem to be more significantly affected.[8,9] CT features can include joint effusion and surrounding soft-tissue swelling, multifocal subchondral osteolysis, and synovial contrast enhancement (Figure 6.3.4). MR features have not been described in the veterinary literature but would likely include prominent intraarticular T2 hyperintensity due

to increased synovial fluid volume, multifocal subchondral bone defects, T2 and STIR hyperintensity in subchondral bone, and enhancement of synovium and synovial fluid following intravenous contrast administration.[12] MR imaging criteria for rheumatoid arthritis diagnosis in people do not currently include direct assessment of articular cartilage, presumably because it is inconsistently seen, particularly in smaller joints.[13]

Infectious arthritis

Infectious (septic) arthritis is most often caused by penetrating injury or iatrogenic contamination although it can also be a sequela to septicemia. Septic arthritis has clinical features similar to those for immune-mediated polyarthritis but is most often limited to a single joint. Imaging features can be similar to those of erosive immune-mediated arthritis (described in the previous paragraph) and can also include features of osteomyelitis when subchondral bone involvement is extensive (Figure 6.3.5).[6,11,12]

Inflammatory disorders of soft tissues

Diffuse regional infections causing myositis and cellulitis result in increased soft-tissue volume, pitting edema, localized heat, and pain. CT imaging features include mild hypoattenuation of muscle associated with a loss of muscle margin definition. MR findings include T1 hypointensity and T2 hyperintensity from edema. Diffuse enhancement occurs because of increased vascular permeability following contrast administration with both modalities. CT imaging features of abscesses include central fluid attenuation with a surrounding thin to thick soft-tissue attenuating margin (Figures 6.3.6, 6.3.7; see also Figure 1.4.8). MR findings consist of central T1 hypointensity and T2 hyperintensity (see Figure 2.7.6). Peripheral enhancement occurs following contrast administration with both modalities.

Figure 6.3.1 Osteomyelitis (Canine)

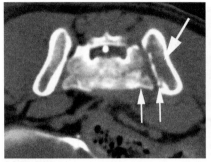

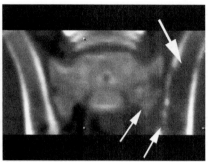

(a) CT+C, TP   **(b)** CT+C, DP

3mo M German Shepherd Dog with multifocal pain. Complete blood count revealed neutrophilia with a toxic left shift. There is ill-defined osteolysis of medullary bone of the left ilium (**a,b**: large arrow) as well as of left ilial and sacral cortical bone (**a,b**: small arrows). Widening of the left sacroiliac joint is indicative of septic arthritis. Blood culture was negative, but because there was no history or clinical evidence of a penetrating injury, this was thought to be hematogenously disseminated.

Figure 6.3.2   Chronic Osteomyelitis (Canine)   CT

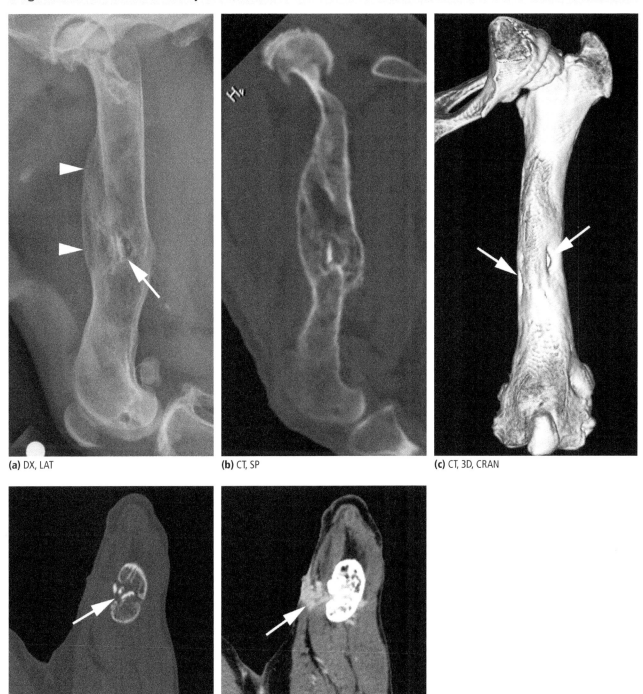

(a) DX, LAT   **(b)** CT, SP   **(c)** CT, 3D, CRAN

(d) CT, TP   **(e)** CT+C, TP

5y FS German Shepherd Dog with previous history of left femoral fracture that was repaired using internal fixation of unknown type. The dog currently has intermittent left pelvic limb lameness and a draining wound on the medial aspect of the limb, which resolves temporarily with antibiotic administration. A lateral radiograph shows a mid-diaphyseal malunion with exuberant smooth bony bridging of the fracture site (**a**: arrowheads). A central sequestrum with surrounding involucrum is also present (**a**: arrow). Similar features are seen on sagittal and transverse CT images (**b,d**) although multiple sequestra are now evident (**d**: arrow). A three-dimensional rendering shows defects in both the lateral and medial cortices (**c**: arrows). A contrast-enhancing tract is seen medial to the femur, which corresponds with the draining tract later identified clinically (**e**: arrow).

Figure 6.3.3 Nonerosive Immune-mediated Polyarthritis (Canine) MR

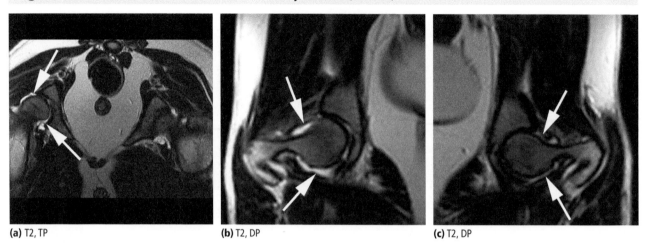

(a) T2, TP   **(b)** T2, DP   **(c)** T2, DP

5y MC German Shepherd cross with a 6-month history of decreased activity and suspected back pain. An MR examination of the caudal lumbar and lumbosacral regions was acquired. There is a mildly increased volume of synovial fluid in the right coxofemoral joint (**a,b**: arrows), which is more pronounced than that of the left (**c**: arrows). No other abnormalities were identified on the MR examination. Cytologic analysis of synovial fluid aspirated from multiple joints, including the right coxofemoral joint, yielded mild to moderate suppurative inflammation in all joints. Clinical signs and joint cytology improved with steroid and azathioprine administration.

Figure 6.3.4 Erosive Immune-mediated Polyarthritis (Canine)   CT

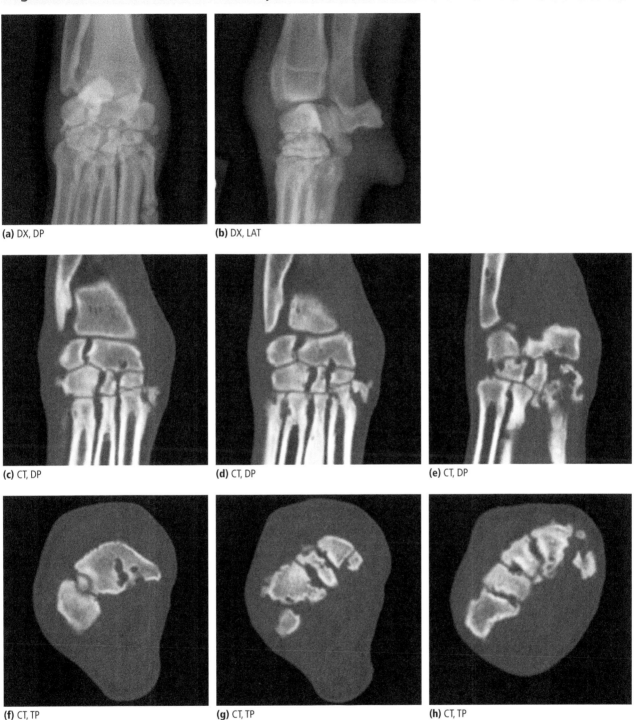

(a) DX, DP

(b) DX, LAT

(c) CT, DP

(d) CT, DP

(e) CT, DP

(f) CT, TP

(g) CT, TP

(h) CT, TP

8y MC Labrador Retriever cross with a 3-month history of pelvic limb discomfort and right carpal valgus deviation. A pain response was elicited on palpation of multiple joints. Images **c–e** are ordered from dorsal to palmar, and images **f–h** are ordered from proximal to distal. Radiographs of the right carpus reveal peri-arthrodial soft-tissue swelling and multiple osteolytic foci of the carpal and metacarpal bones. Similar radiographic abnormalities were seen on radiographs of the left carpus. CT images reveal pronounced widespread sub-chondral bone osteolysis. Cytology of synovial fluid from multiple joints revealed moderate suppurative inflammation. There was a marked improvement in clinical signs and joint fluid cytology following steroid administration.

Figure 6.3.5 Septic Arthritis (Canine) CT

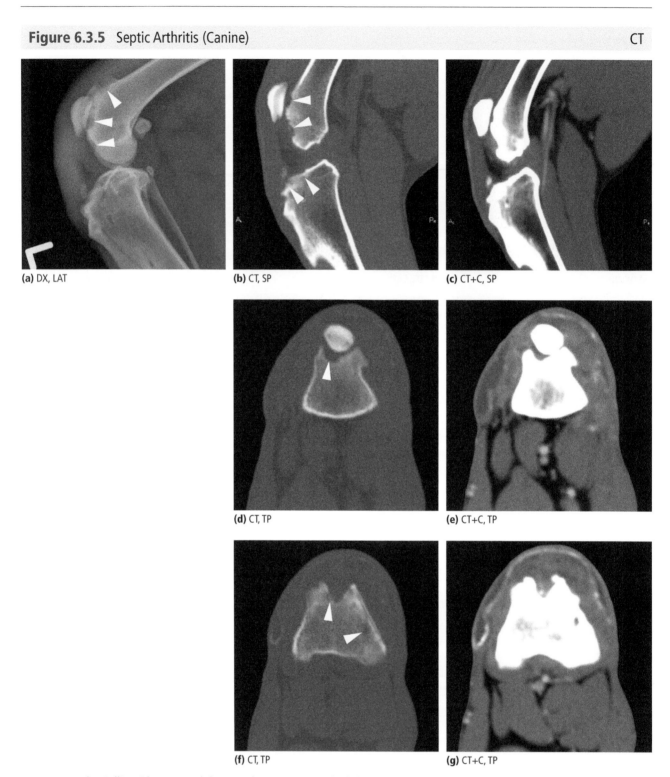

(a) DX, LAT

(b) CT, SP

(c) CT+C, SP

(d) CT, TP

(e) CT+C, TP

(f) CT, TP

(g) CT+C, TP

15mo M Border Collie with a 6-month history of open injury to the left stifle, which subsequently cultured positive with methicillin-resistant *Staphylococcus aureus*. Images **d** and **e** are proximal to images **f** and **g**. The injury was both surgically and medically managed. There is extensive extracapsular and intracapsular soft-tissue swelling/joint effusion on a survey radiographic image (**a**). Subchondral osteolytic foci involving the trochlear ridges of the femur are also evident (**a**: arrowheads). The extent of subchondral bone destruction is better appreciated on sagittal and transverse plane CT images (**b,d,f**: arrowheads). There is marked contrast enhancement of both the extracapsular and intracapsular soft tissues of the stifle due to cellulitis and synovitis, respectively (**c,e,g**).

Figure 6.3.6 Abscess (Canine)

CT

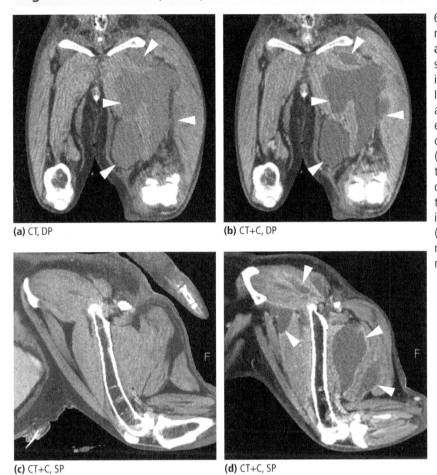

(a) CT, DP

(b) CT+C, DP

(c) CT+C, SP

(d) CT+C, SP

6y MC Mastiff with high fever and a swollen right pelvic limb with pitting edema. Images **a** and **b** were acquired with the dog positioned so that images show the proximal pelvic limbs in the dorsal plane caudal to the femurs. Image **c** represents the normal left pelvic limb as a comparison to image **d**. A large multicameral fluid-attenuating mass is present in the caudal aspect of the right proximal pelvic limb (**a**: arrowheads). Following intravenous contrast administration, the mass is more clearly defined as a thin-walled, multicameral abscess that extends into the semimembranosus, semitendinosus, gluteal, and quadriceps muscles (**b**,**d**: arrowheads). Aspiration cytology revealed marked neutrophilic inflammation with large numbers of gram-positive cocci.

Figure 6.3.7 Abscess and Osteomyelitis (Canine)   CT

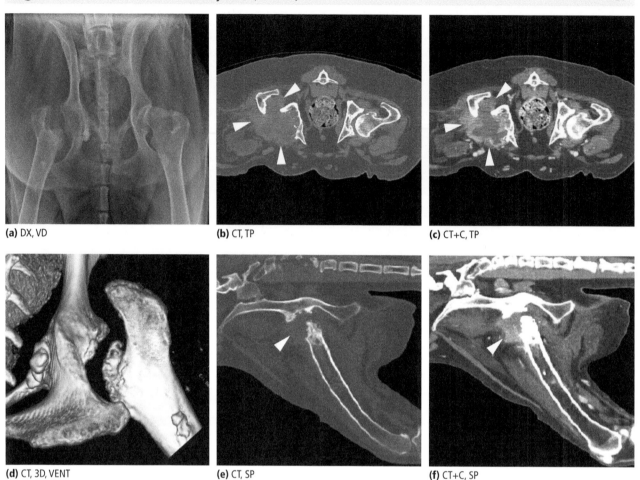

(a) DX, VD   **(b)** CT, TP   **(c)** CT+C, TP

(d) CT, 3D, VENT   **(e)** CT, SP   **(f)** CT+C, SP

3y FS Mastiff with a failed total hip implant that was recently removed. A radiograph and a 3D rendering of the right coxofemoral region reveals bone architectural change of the right proximal femur and acetabular remnant associated with previous total hip replacement (**a,d**). Altered bone margins are smooth but irregular, and bone density is heterogeneous. A small quantity of methyl methacrylate is present adjacent to the medial cortex of the right ilium. CT images show an irregularly shaped fluid and soft-tissue attenuating mass interposed between the proximal femur and acetabular remnant (**b,e**: arrowheads). Following intravenous contrast administration, the mass is clearly defined as a thick-walled abscess (**c,f**: arrowheads). The bone remodeling of the proximal femur and acetabular remnant is also indicative of concurrent osteomyelitis. The implant site was surgically drained and debrided. Bacterial culture of the abscess fluid was positive for *Enterobacter* sp. Biopsy of the proximal femur confirmed a diagnosis of osteomyelitis.

References

1. Bancroft LW. MR imaging of infectious processes of the knee. Radiol Clin North Am. 2007;45:931–941.
2. Eid AJ, Berbari EF. Osteomyelitis: review of pathophysiology, diagnostic modalities and therapeutic options. J Med Liban. 2012;60:51–60.
3. Karmazyn B. Imaging approach to acute hematogenous osteomyelitis in children: an update. Semin Ultrasound CT MR. 2010;31:100–106.
4. Lalam RK, Cassar-Pullicino VN, Tins BJ. Magnetic resonance imaging of appendicular musculoskeletal infection. Top Magn Reson Imaging. 2007;18:177–191.
5. Pineda C, Vargas A, Rodriguez AV. Imaging of osteomyelitis: current concepts. Infect Dis Clin North Am. 2006;20:789–825.
6. Stumpe KD, Strobel K. Osteomyelitis and arthritis. Semin Nucl Med. 2009;39:27–35.
7. Tehranzadeh J, Wong E, Wang F, Sadighpour M. Imaging of osteomyelitis in the mature skeleton. Radiol Clin North Am. 2001;39:223–250.
8. Johnson KC, Mackin A. Canine immune-mediated polyarthritis: part 1: pathophysiology. J Am Anim Hosp Assoc. 2012;48:12–17.
9. Johnson KC, Mackin A. Canine immune-mediated polyarthritis: part 2: diagnosis and treatment. J Am Anim Hosp Assoc. 2012;48:71–82.

10. Stull JW, Evason M, Carr AP, Waldner C. Canine immune-mediated polyarthritis: clinical and laboratory findings in 83 cases in western Canada (1991–2001). Can Vet J. 2008;49:1195–1203.

11. Weisbrode SE. Bone and Joints. In: McGavin MD, Zachary JF (eds): Pathologic Basis of Veterinary Disease. St. Louis: Mosby Elsevier, 2007;1041–1105.

12. Stoller DW, Tirman PFJ, Bredella MA. Elbow. In: Stoller DW, Tirman PFJ, Bredella MA (eds): Diagnostic Imaging: Orthpaedics. Salt Lake City: Amirsys, Inc., 2004;2:1–101.

13. Review: the utility of magnetic resonance imaging for assessing structural damage in randomized controlled trials in rheumatoid arthritis. Arthritis Rheum. 2013;65:2513–2523.

6.4

Neoplasia

Imaging features of axial musculoskeletal neoplasms are provided in Chapters 1.4 and 3.4. CT and MR imaging characteristics of appendicular musculoskeletal neoplasms are addressed in this chapter.

Primary bone tumors

Benign bone tumors

Benign neoplasms of the appendicular skeleton are uncommon but broadly include tumors of osteocytic, chondrocytic, mixed osteocytic/chondrocytic, and fibrocytic lineage. Although bone architecture can be significantly altered in these tumors, they tend be more localized with shorter zones of transition and do not have features of active osteolysis or aggressive productive reactivity (see Figure 1.4.10).[1]

Malignant bone tumors

Malignant bone tumors include osteosarcoma, chondrosarcoma, and fibrosarcoma. In some classification schemes, other tumors, such as hemangiosarcoma and liposarcoma, are also considered primary bone neoplasms if they arise from within bone. Osteosarcoma accounts for at least 85% of all canine bone tumors, and about 75% of those involve the appendicular skeleton. Older large- and giant-breed dogs are most commonly affected, with males overrepresented, and the distal radius, proximal humerus, distal femur, and proximal distal tibia are the most common anatomic sites. Chondrosarcomas comprise the majority of the remainder of primary malignant appendicular bone tumors, although they also have a propensity to arise from

within the axial skeleton. Primary bone tumors are locally aggressive, tend not to cross joints, and metastasize hematogenously to lungs, bone, visceral organs, and other tissues.[2-6]

Imaging characterization of distal limb osteosarcoma and other bone neoplasms is important when limb salvage or palliation with radiation therapy or other regional therapeutic techniques is contemplated. Accurate assessment of tumor distribution is also necessary for operative planning of proximal limb neoplasms.

CT features of osteosarcoma and other primary bone tumors are similar to those of survey radiography and include medullary and cortical bone destruction and periosteal reactive bone production. Tumors that have osteoblastic features may also produce amorphous, tumor-derived new bone. CT may also more clearly delineate internal and extracortical tumor margins compared to radiographs (Figures 6.4.1, 6.4.2, 6.4.3, 6.4.4). Intramedullary tumor invasion replaces normal fat-rich marrow, resulting in increased attenuation (Figure 6.4.3).

MR characteristics parallel CT features, with evidence of defects and remodeling of low-signal cortical bone. Mixed T1 and T2 or STIR intensity tumor soft-tissue replaces the normally uniformly T1 and T2 hyperintense, STIR hypointense medullary fat and can extend beyond the external cortical margins (Figure 6.4.5).[6-10]

Marked enhancement occurs with both CT and MR following intravenous contrast administration. Contrast uptake is typically heterogeneous because of regional hypovascularity or necrosis within the tumor volume.

Multiple comparisons of radiography, scintigraphy CT, and MR have been made to determine which

Atlas of Small Animal CT and MRI, First Edition. Erik R. Wisner and Allison L. Zwingenberger.
© 2015 John Wiley & Sons, Inc. Published 2015 by John Wiley & Sons, Inc.

modality is most accurate for defining tumor extent in long bones. Although results vary, a general trend is that imaging overestimates tumor extent in most instances as a result of bone reactivity and peripheral edema and hemorrhage.[7-10]

Metastatic bone tumors

Bone metastasis is uncommon but will likely increase in frequency as cancer therapies improve and survival times for primary neoplasms increase. Mammary carcinoma, urinary tract (transitional cell) carcinoma, prostatic carcinoma, osteosarcoma, hemangiosarcoma, melanoma, and round cell tumors, such as lymphoma and myeloma, have all been reported to have a predilection for bone metastasis, and the ribs, vertebrae, and metaphyses of long bones are the most common locations.[4,11-14]

Because bone metastasis is unpredictable, often multifocal, and sometimes not accompanied by clinical signs, bone scintigraphy and survey radiography are best used as screening tests. CT features include medullary and cortical osteolysis, with some lesions accompanied by peripheral productive reactivity (see Figure 4.1.9). MR features described for bone metastasis in people include reduced medullary T1 intensity and STIR hyperintensity compared to adjacent normal marrow signal and enhancement following intravenous contrast administration.[15]

Malignant neoplasia of joints

Synovial cell sarcoma

As the name implies, synovial cell sarcomas most often arise adjacent to synovial joints and tendon sheaths and have sarcomatous and epithelial morphometric forms, although most are classified as biphasic, having attributes of both cell types.[16,17]

CT features include a soft-tissue attenuating lobular mass that is centered on a joint and often associated with adjacent cortical osteolysis. Reactive new bone is usually minimal or absent. Masses heterogeneously enhance following intravenous contrast administration and can have a multicameral peripheral enhancement pattern (Figures 6.4.6, 6.4.7). MR features include a lobular mass that is mildly T1 hyperintense to adjacent muscle and heterogeneously T2 hyperintense (Figure 6.4.7). Invasion into bone can cause marrow to be T1 hypointense with STIR hyperintensity and T2 heterogeneity.[16,18-21]

Other neoplasms associated with synovium

Other reported synovial associated malignancies include histiocytic sarcoma, synovial myxoma, fibrosarcoma, and chondrosarcoma.[2,16,22] Imaging features in dogs and cats have not been widely reported, but some share characteristics seen with synovial cell sarcoma.

Other malignant soft-tissue neoplasms

Feline injection site sarcoma

Feline injection site sarcomas (FISS) are linked to vaccine administration, but the underlying cause for transformation is still under debate. Peak ages of onset are 6–7 and 10–11 years of age. Primary masses are rapid growing and unencapsulated although distant metastasis is considered relatively uncommon.[23-25] CT is frequently performed for surgical and radiation treatment planning since mass margins are difficult to define by clinical assessment alone. Masses are soft-tissue attenuating on unenhanced CT images and are intramuscular or subcutaneous. Subcutaneous masses often encroach on or overtly invade underlying muscle, resulting in loss of definition of the deep tumor margin (Figure 6.4.8). Large masses with central necrosis may have a fluid-attenuating core. FISS is T1 and T2 hyperintense in relation to adjacent muscle and may have regions of signal void when mineralization is present. With both modalities, depending on size and tissue perfusion, tumors uniformly, inhomogeneously, or peripherally enhance following intravenous contrast administration. Tumor margins defined by enhancement are typically indistinct.[26,27]

Other sarcomas

Other malignant soft-tissue sarcomas that can arise within or adjacent to muscle, tendons, and ligaments include, in approximate order of metastatic potential, malignant fibrous histiocytoma, malignant nerve sheath tumor, hemangiopericytoma, leiomyosarcoma, mesenchymoma, fibrosarcoma, myxosarcoma, rhabdomyosarcoma, spindle cell tumor, liposarcoma, hemangiosarcoma, and lymphangiosarcoma.[18] Imaging features vary depending on tumor type, but most produce a space-occupying mass with soft-tissue to fluid attenuation on unenhanced CT images (lower attenuation for liposarcoma) and variable enhancement following intravenous contrast administration (Figures 6.4.9, 6.4.10, 6.4.11, 6.4.12). Appearance on unenhanced MR images varies depending on the tissue properties of a given tumor type.[18,19,21]

Figure 6.4.1 Osteosarcoma (Canine)

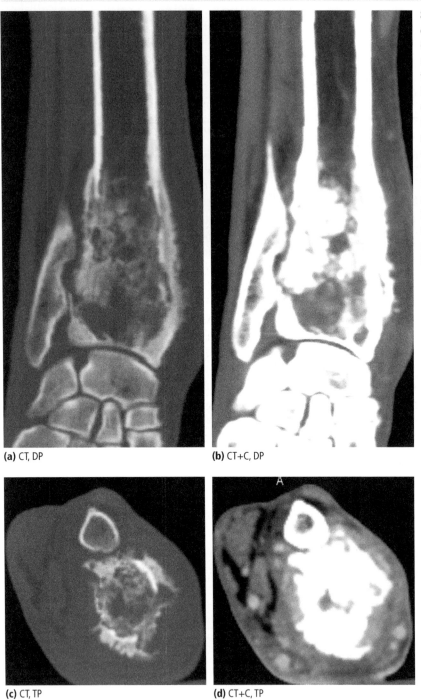

(a) CT, DP

(b) CT+C, DP

(c) CT, TP

(d) CT+C, TP

8y M German Shepherd Dog with recent onset of lameness in the left thoracic limb. CT images are of the distal aspect of the left radius, and transverse images are through the distal metaphyseal region. Unenhanced images (**a,c**) show a mixed productive and osteolytic bone lesion of the distal radial metaphysis. Contrast-enhanced images (**b,d**) show both intramedullary and extracortical enhancement of the soft-tissue component of the mass, which is unencapsulated. Despite the aggressive appearance of the mass, the distal ulna is relatively unaffected, and the integrity of the radiocarpal joint is uncompromised. The left thoracic limb was amputated, and the mass was confirmed to be an osteoblastic osteosarcoma.

Figure 6.4.2 Osteosarcoma (Canine) CT

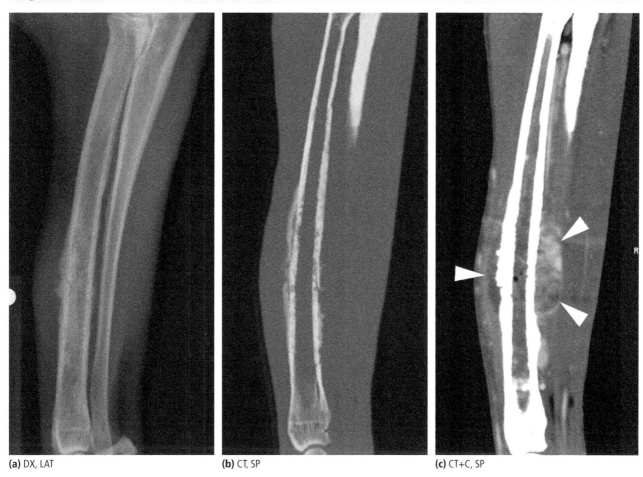

(a) DX, LAT   **(b)** CT, SP   **(c)** CT+C, SP

8y Great Dane cross with intermittent left thoracic limb lameness of 4 months' duration. A lateral radiograph of the left antebrachium shows mixed production and osteolysis of the radial diaphysis and distal metaphysis (**a**). There is also evidence of surrounding soft-tissue swelling. Similar findings are also present on a comparable unenhanced CT image (**b**), and the moth-eaten pattern of osteolysis is better appreciated. The highly vascular extracortical soft-tissue component of the mass is well visualized following intravenous contrast administration (**c**: arrowheads). The two small gas bubbles in the diaphyseal medullary cavity (**c**) are due to recent fine-needle aspiration biopsy. The left thoracic limb was amputated, and the mass was confirmed to be an osteoblastic osteosarcoma. The predominantly diaphyseal location of this primary bone tumor is atypical, but other imaging features support the diagnosis.

Figure 6.4.3 Osteosarcoma (Canine)   CT

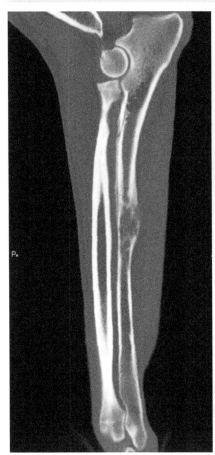

(a) CT, SP

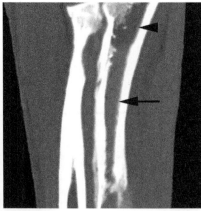

(b) CT, SP

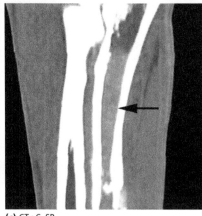

(c) CT+C, SP

10y M Belgian Tervuren with left thoracic limb lameness of 2 months' duration. There is an expansile mixed productive and osteolytic mass arising from the ulnar diaphysis (a). Image **b** is a magnification of image **a** centered on the ulna proximal to the primary lesion. There is a subtle increase in medullary attenuation (**b**: arrow) near the bone lesion as compared to the normal low attenuation seen more proximally (**b**: arrowhead). This region markedly and homogeneously enhances following contrast administration, indicative of proximal tumor extension (**c**: arrow). Fine-needle aspiration biopsy yielded a diagnosis of osteosarcoma.

Figure 6.4.4 Hemangiosarcoma (Canine)

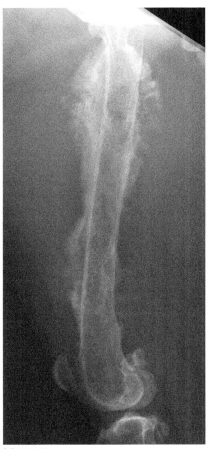

(a) DX, LAT

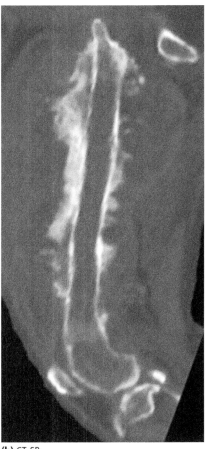

(b) CT, SP

11y FS Labrador Retriever with a 2-month history of left pelvic limb lameness. A lateral radiograph of the left femur shows aggressive mixed periosteal production and cortical osteolysis involving the entire femoral diaphysis (**a**). Similar findings are also present on an unenhanced CT image (**b**). An extensive extracortical, heterogeneously enhancing lobular soft-tissue mass is appreciated following intravenous contrast administration (**c**: arrowheads), which is documented on the pathology specimen (**d**: arrowheads). The mass was confirmed to be hemangiosarcoma and was considered to be of primary bone origin since no other masses were found on the staging evaluation of the patient.

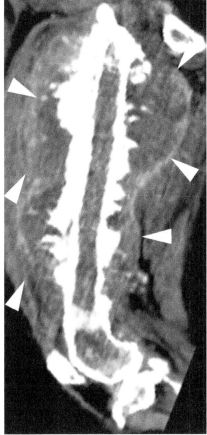

(c) CT+C, SP

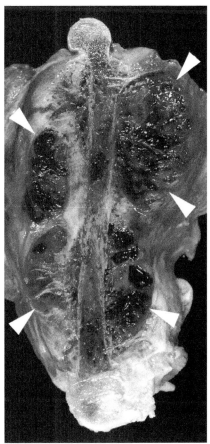

(d) GP, SP

Figure 6.4.5 Osteosarcoma (Canine)   MR

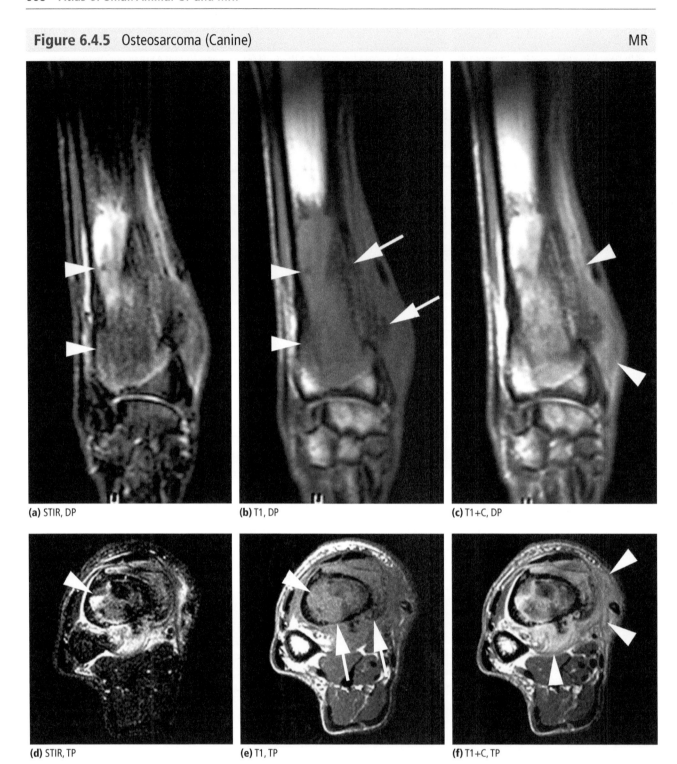

(a) STIR, DP

(b) T1, DP

(c) T1+C, DP

(d) STIR, TP

(e) T1, TP

(f) T1+C, TP

7y FS Rottweiler with recent-onset right thoracic limb lameness. Dorsal plane images (**a–c**) are through the distal radius. Transverse images (**d–f**) are through the distal radial metaphysis. There is STIR hyperintensity (**a,d**: arrowheads) and T1 hypointensity (**b,e**: arrowheads) in the distal radial medullary cavity compared to the intensity of adjacent fat-containing marrow seen more proximally. There is clear evidence of cortical osteolysis and associated periosteal reactive new bone formation, best seen on T1 images (**b,e**: arrows). There is marked enhancement of the soft-tissue components of the mass, which shows the extent of the extracortical distribution (**c,f**: arrowheads). Biopsy confirmed anaplastic osteosarcoma.

Figure 6.4.6 Synovial Cell Sarcoma (Canine)   CT

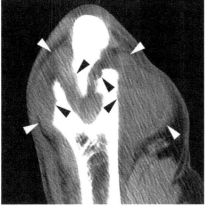

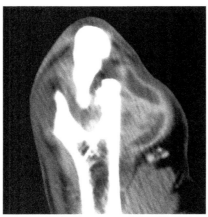

(a) CT, TP   **(b)** CT+C, TP

12y MC Rottweiler with a 3-month history of right thoracic limb lameness. A lobular soft-tissue attenuating mass is centered on the right elbow joint (**a**: white arrowheads). There is evidence of osteolysis of bone margins of both the ulna and the humerus (**a**: black arrowheads). The mass enhances nonuniformly following intravenous contrast administration and contains multiple relatively hypoattenuating cavitary regions (**b**). Biopsy confirmed a diagnosis of synovial cell sarcoma.

Figure 6.4.7 Synovial Cell Sarcoma (Canine)   CT & MR

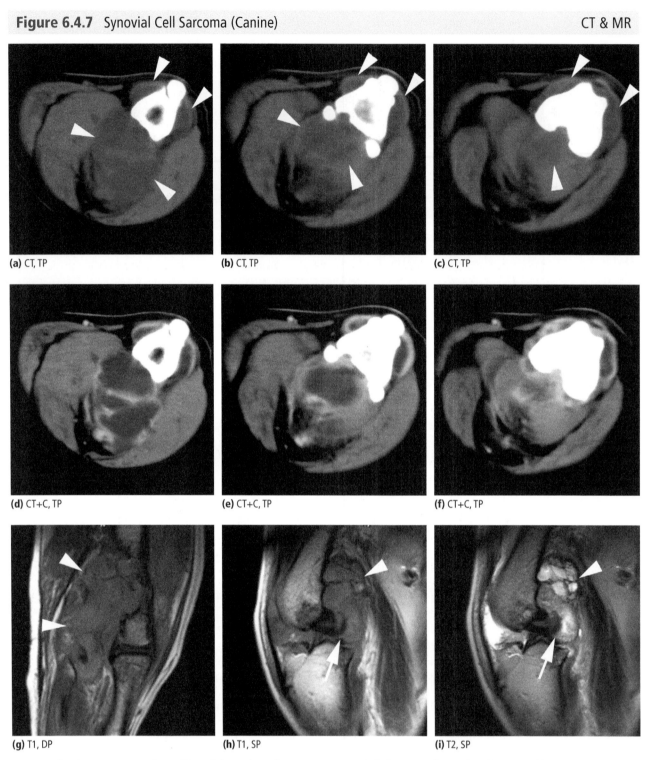

(a) CT, TP

(b) CT, TP

(c) CT, TP

(d) CT+C, TP

(e) CT+C, TP

(f) CT+C, TP

(g) T1, DP

(h) T1, SP

(i) T2, SP

12y FS Labrador Retriever with swelling of the right stifle. Images **a–c** and **d–f** are unenhanced and comparable contrast-enhanced transverse CT images, respectively, acquired at the level of the right stifle and ordered from proximal to distal. A lobular mass, which is hypoattenuating compared to adjacent muscle, surrounds the distal femur and encroaches on the femoropatellar joint (**a–c**: arrowheads). There is a multicameral, peripheral pattern of enhancement following intravenous contrast administration (**d–f**). The mass is heterogeneously T1 and T2 hyperintense to adjacent muscle (**g–i**: arrowheads), and MR images clearly show the tumor has an intra-articular component (**h,i**: arrow). Postmortem examination confirmed a diagnosis of low-grade synovial cell sarcoma.

Figure 6.4.8 Feline Injection Site Sarcoma (Feline)   CT

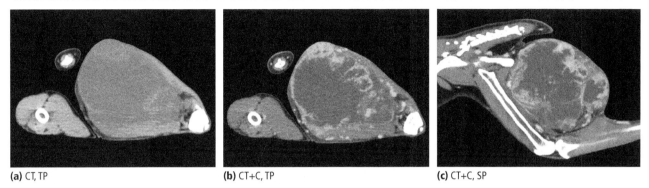

(a) CT, TP   **(b)** CT+C, TP   **(c)** CT+C, SP

6y MC Domestic Longhair with a large left pelvic limb mass. There is a large heterogeneously hypoattenuating mass arising from the proximocaudal aspect of the left pelvic limb, which is obliterating normal muscle anatomy (**a**). The mass heterogeneously and peripherally enhances following intravenous contrast administration (**b,c**). Microscopic evaluation showed a neoplastic cell population consistent with myxosarcoma, with small-caliber vessels surrounded by dense aggregates of lymphocytes and plasma cells. A diagnosis of feline injection site sarcoma was based on the combination of characteristic pathology findings, patient age, vaccination history, and lesion location.

Figure 6.4.9 Malignant Peripheral Nerve Sheath Tumor (Canine)   CT

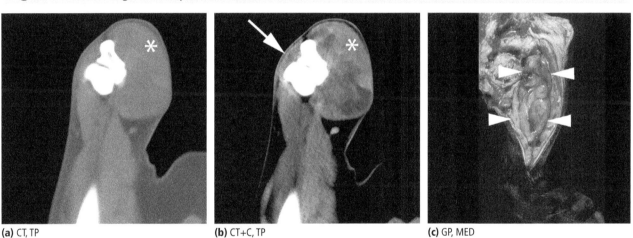

(a) CT, TP   **(b)** CT+C, TP   **(c)** GP, MED

6y FS Labrador Retriever with a 1.5-month history of right thoracic limb lameness. Images **a** and **b** are comparable unenhanced and contrast-enhanced CT images, respectively, acquired at the level of the radial head and olecranon near the proximal extent of the mass. There is a well-delineated globoid mass arising from the medial side of the limb and encroaching on the elbow joint (**a**: asterisk). The mass heterogeneously enhances following intravenous contrast administration (**b**: asterisk) and appears to encircle the elbow joint caudolaterally (**b**: arrow). The limb was amputated, and the mass was determined to be a malignant peripheral nerve sheath tumor that extended most of the length of the antebrachium (**c**: arrowheads). On gross inspection, the mass effaced adjacent musculature but did not invade the joint.

Figure 6.4.10 Malignant Peripheral Nerve Sheath Tumor (Canine) MR

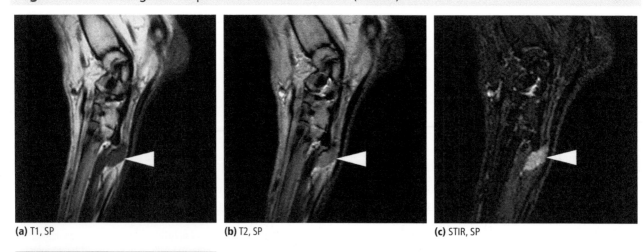

(a) T1, SP   **(b)** T2, SP   **(c)** STIR, SP

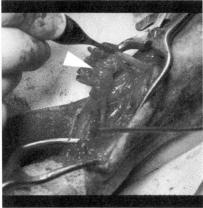

(d) GP

14y MC Akita cross with progressive right pelvic limb lameness. There is a small well-demarcated ovoid mass in the plantar aspect of the proximal metatarsus, which is T1 hypointense, T2 isointense, and STIR hyperintense compared to adjacent tissues (**a–c**: arrowhead). The mass is in the location of the superficial and deep digital flexor tendons. The mass, confirmed to be a grade II malignant peripheral nerve sheath tumor, was surgically excised (**d**: arrowhead), which required dissection away from the digital flexor tendons.

Figure 6.4.11 Fibrosarcoma (Canine) CT

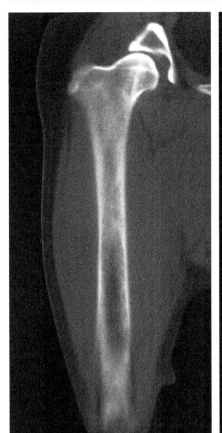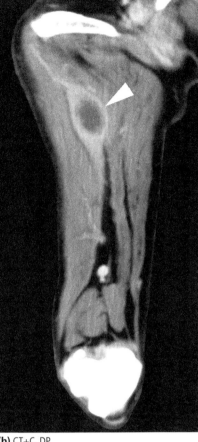

9y MC Dalmatian with a mass palpable in the proximocaudal aspect of the left pelvic limb. The patient was positioned with the left femur in the plane of the CT gantry to produce dorsal plane images. Image **a** is a MIP image at the level of the femur, and image **b** is in the same plane, caudal to the femur. An ovoid, peripherally contrast-enhancing mass is present within caudal thigh muscles (**b**: arrowhead). Excisional biopsy confirmed the mass to be a fibrosarcoma.

(a) CT, MIP, DP   **(b)** CT+C, DP

Figure 6.4.12 Hemangiosarcoma (Canine) CT

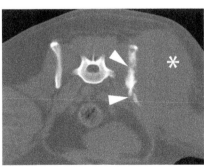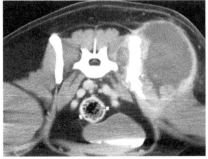

(a) CT, TP   **(b)** CT+C, TP

6y FS Labrador Retriever with a mass over the left hip, which is painful to palpation. There is a large soft-tissue attenuating, globoid mass arising lateral to the left ilium within the gluteal muscle group (**a**: asterisk). There is associated left ilial osteolysis and spiculated reactive new bone formation (**a**: arrowheads). The mass peripherally enhances following intravenous contrast administration, and extension medial to the ilium can now be appreciated (**b**). Margins are indistinct with no clear definition between the mass and adjacent muscle. Biopsy confirmed the mass to be a hemangiosarcoma.

References

1. Motamedi K, Seeger LL. Benign bone tumors. Radiol Clin North Am. 2011;49:1115–1134.
2. Chun R. Common malignant musculoskeletal neoplasms of dogs and cats. Vet Clin North Am Small Anim Pract. 2005;35:1155–1167.
3. Chun R, de Lorimier LP. Update on the biology and management of canine osteosarcoma. Vet Clin North Am Small Anim Pract. 2003;33:491–516.
4. Cooley DM, Waters DJ. Skeletal neoplasms of small dogs: a retrospective study and literature review. J Am Anim Hosp Assoc. 1997;33:11–23.
5. Morello E, Martano M, Buracco P. Biology, diagnosis and treatment of canine appendicular osteosarcoma: similarities and differences with human osteosarcoma. Vet J. 2011;189:268–277.
6. Vanel M, Blond L, Vanel D. Imaging of primary bone tumors in veterinary medicine: which differences? Eur J Radiol. 2013;82:2129–2139.
7. Davis GJ, Kapatkin AS, Craig LE, Heins GS, Wortman JA. Comparison of radiography, computed tomography, and magnetic resonance imaging for evaluation of appendicular osteosarcoma in dogs. J Am Vet Med Assoc. 2002;220:1171–1176.
8. Karnik KS, Samii VF, Weisbrode SE, London CA, Green EM. Accuracy of computed tomography in determining lesion size in canine appendicular osteosarcoma. Vet Radiol Ultrasound. 2012;53:273–279.
9. Leibman NF, Kuntz CA, Steyn PF, Fettman MJ, Powers BE, Withrow SJ, et al. Accuracy of radiography, nuclear scintigraphy, and histopathology for determining the proximal extent of distal radius osteosarcoma in dogs. Vet Surg. 2001;30:240–245.
10. Wallack ST, Wisner ER, Werner JA, Walsh PJ, Kent MS, Fairley RA, et al. Accuracy of magnetic resonance imaging for estimating intramedullary osteosarcoma extent in pre-operative planning of canine limb-salvage procedures. Vet Radiol Ultrasound. 2002;43:432–441.
11. Cooley DM, Waters DJ. Skeletal metastasis as the initial clinical manifestation of metastatic carcinoma in 19 dogs. J Vet Intern Med. 1998;12:288–293.
12. Goedegebuure SA. Secondary bone tumours in the dog. Vet Pathol. 1979;16:520–529.
13. McEntee MC. Radiation therapy in the management of bone tumors. Vet Clin North Am Small Anim Pract. 1997;27:131–138.
14. Trost ME, Inkelmann MA, Galiza GJ, Silva TM, Kommers GD. Occurrence of tumours metastatic to bones and multicentric tumours with skeletal involvement in dogs. J Comp Pathol. 2014;150:8–17.
15. Lecouvet FE, Larbi A, Pasoglou V, Omoumi P, Tombal B, Michoux N, et al. MRI for response assessment in metastatic bone disease. Eur Radiol. 2013;23:1986–1997.
16. Craig LE, Julian ME, Ferracone JD. The diagnosis and prognosis of synovial tumors in dogs: 35 cases. Vet Pathol. 2002;39:66–73.
17. Fisher C. Synovial sarcoma. Ann Diagn Pathol. 1998;2:401–421.
18. Ehrhart N. Soft-tissue sarcomas in dogs: a review. J Am Anim Hosp Assoc. 2005;41:241–246.
19. Kind M, Stock N, Coindre JM. Histology and imaging of soft tissue sarcomas. Eur J Radiol. 2009;72:6–15.
20. O'Sullivan PJ, Harris AC, Munk PL. Radiological features of synovial cell sarcoma. Br J Radiol. 2008;81:346–356.
21. Walker EA, Salesky JS, Fenton ME, Murphey MD. Magnetic resonance imaging of malignant soft tissue neoplasms in the adult. Radiol Clin North Am. 2011;49:1219–1234.
22. Moore PF. A review of histiocytic diseases of dogs and cats. Vet Pathol. 2014;51:167–184.
23. Ladlow J. Injection site-associated sarcoma in the cat: treatment recommendations and results to date. J Feline Med Surg. 2013;15:409–418.
24. Martano M, Morello E, Buracco P. Feline injection-site sarcoma: past, present and future perspectives. Vet J. 2011;188:136–141.
25. Seguin B. Feline injection site sarcomas. Vet Clin North Am Small Anim Pract. 2002;32:983–995.
26. Rousset N, Holmes MA, Caine A, Dobson J, Herrtage ME. Clinical and low-field MRI characteristics of injection site sarcoma in 19 cats. Vet Radiol Ultrasound. 2013;54:623–629.
27. Travetti O, di Giancamillo M, Stefanello D, Ferrari R, Giudice C, Grieco V, et al. Computed tomography characteristics of fibrosarcoma – a histological subtype of feline injection-site sarcoma. J Feline Med Surg. 2013;15:488–493.

6.5

Degenerative disorders

Many disorders of the musculoskeletal system lead to degenerative change and osteoarthritis. Many of these have been described in context of the inciting primary disorder in Chapters 6.1–6.4.

Soft tissues

The tendons and ligaments surrounding joints may be primary causes of degenerative change, because of instability, or may develop degenerative change in osteoarthritic joints. Expected imaging findings are enlargement, altered attenuation or signal intensity, partial tears, associated effusion, enthesiophyte formation, and dystrophic mineralization (see Figures 6.2.7, 6.2.8).

Joints

Terminology for degenerative joint disease has been inconsistent and has included the terms osteoarthritis, osteoarthrosis, and secondary degenerative joint disease. Since the larger body of human literature uses the term osteoarthritis, and there is evidence to support an underlying inflammatory process as part of the pathogenesis of the disorder, we have chosen to use the term osteoarthritis.

Osteoarthritis is defined on MR studies in people as the presence of osteophyte formation and full-thickness cartilage loss. Additional features may also be considered diagnostic in addition to one of the above changes, such as a subchondral bone marrow lesion or cyst not associated with meniscal or ligamentous attachments, meniscal subluxation or degenerative/horizontal tear, partial thickness cartilage loss, or bone attrition.[1] The smaller size of dogs and cats makes cartilage evaluation challenging because of limits of spatial resolution; however, joint space narrowing

may be present. Bone marrow edema in people is associated with trabecular thickening and increased remodeling and occurs in regions underlying cartilage degradation.[2] Bone marrow edema may be a more apparent indication of cartilage damage than cartilage lesions in small animals. Both CT and MR arthrography can be used to demonstrate cartilage loss and increase visualization of small structures.[3-6]

The primary finding of osteoarthritis on MR and CT imaging is marginal osteophyte formation surrounding the joint (Figures 6.5.1, 6.5.2). In most people, the increasing size of osteophyte formation correlates with the increasing severity of cartilage loss.[7] Osteophytes appear as low-signal irregular proliferations of bone in typical places, such as the distal patella, tibial plateau, trochlear ridges, and femoral condyles. In the nonsynovial joints of the spine, degenerative changes include narrowed intervertebral disc spaces and vertebral endplate sclerosis. While CT imaging can be useful in demonstrating the osseous changes at the margin of the joint or in subchondral bone (Figure 6.5.3), it is more limited in discriminating small soft-tissue structures.

Synovitis is often a component of degenerative change within the joint. On MR images, unenhanced images often fail to differentiate the proportion of joint effusion and synovial proliferation that is expanding the joint capsule. Contrast-enhanced images with fat saturation can more clearly define the degree of synovitis present, as the fluid appears as hypoattenuating signal surrounded by enhancing synovium (Figure 6.5.4).[1] Inflammation may extend to surrounding tendon sheaths or bursae depending on the joint anatomy.

Atlas of Small Animal CT and MRI, First Edition. Erik R. Wisner and Allison L. Zwingenberger.
© 2015 John Wiley & Sons, Inc. Published 2015 by John Wiley & Sons, Inc.

Figure 6.5.1 Osteoarthritis (Canine)   CT & MR

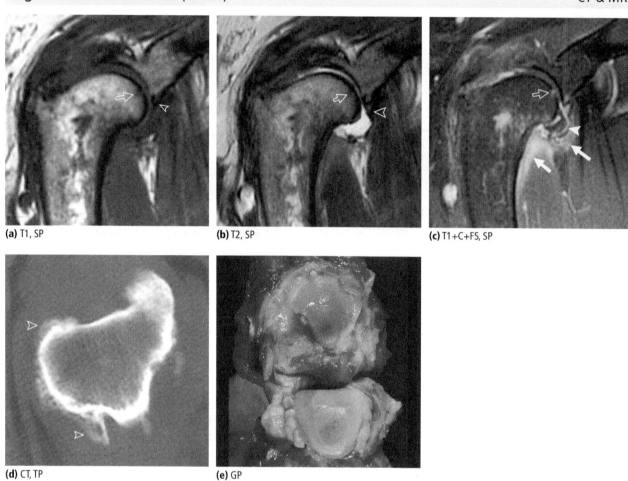

(a) T1, SP   **(b)** T2, SP   **(c)** T1+C+FS, SP

(d) CT, TP   **(e)** GP

10y MC Golden Retriever with chronic right thoracic limb lameness and previously performed biceps tenectomy. There is osteophyte formation surrounding the humerus and glenoid cavity (**a**,**b**: open arrowhead). This is better appreciated on the CT images surrounding the humeral head (**d**: open arrowheads). There is a focal T1 and T2 hypointense region in the subchondral bone of the humeral head (**a**,**b**: open arrow), which contrast enhances (**c**: open arrow). The soft tissues surrounding the humerus are enhancing (**c**: arrows), and the void in the caudal joint space (**c**: arrowhead) represents joint effusion with a rim of enhancing synovial tissue. The limb was amputated, and synovitis, cartilage erosion, and severe osteoarthritis were confirmed histologically.

Figure 6.5.2 Osteoarthritis (Canine)   CT

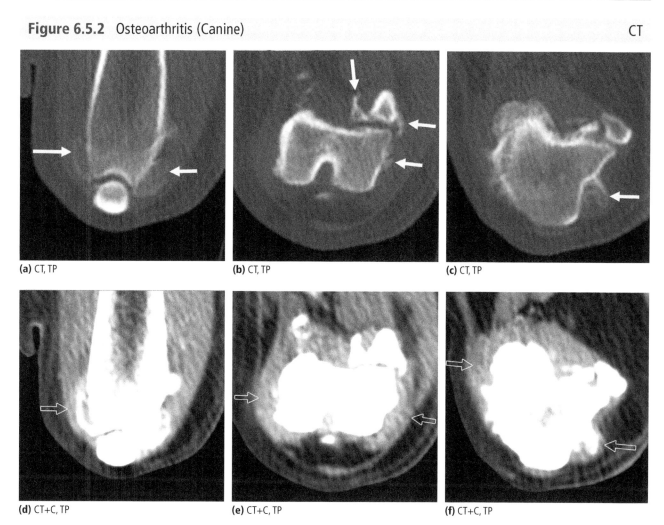

(a) CT, TP   **(b)** CT, TP   **(c)** CT, TP

(d) CT+C, TP   **(e)** CT+C, TP   **(f)** CT+C, TP

11y FS Labrador Retriever. Images of the stifle are ordered from proximal to distal. On unenhanced images, there is marginal osteophyte production at the level of the trochlear ridges (**a**: arrows), fabellae (**b**: arrows), and tibial plateau (**c**). There is a semicircular osteophyte surrounding the caudal portion of the long digital extensor tendon (**c**: arrow). Contrast-enhanced images show thickening of the synovium (**d–f**: open arrows).

Figure 6.5.3 Osteoarthritis (Canine)   CT

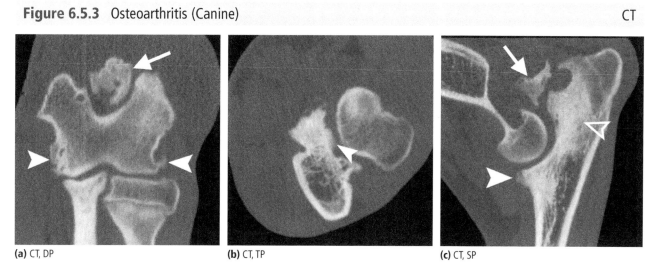

(a) CT, DP   **(b)** CT, TP   **(c)** CT, SP

8mo German Shepherd Dog with left thoracic limb lameness. There is an ununited anconeal process in the left elbow (**a,c**: arrow). There are marginal osteophytes surrounding the lateral and medial aspects of the joint (**a,b**: arrowheads). The medial coronoid process of the ulna is also fragmented (**c**: arrowhead). The subchondral bone of the ulna is sclerotic (**c**: open arrowhead).

Figure 6.5.4 Synovitis (Feline)

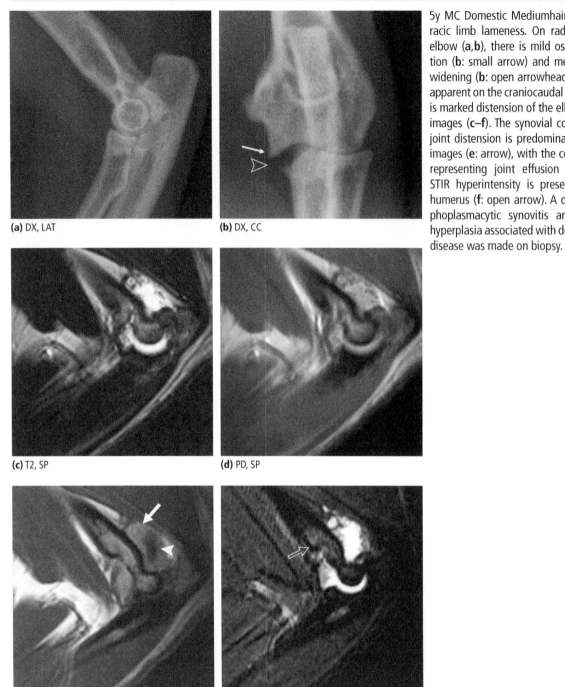

(a) DX, LAT

(b) DX, CC

(c) T2, SP

(d) PD, SP

(e) T1+C, SP

(f) ST, SP

5y MC Domestic Mediumhair with right thoracic limb lameness. On radiographs of the elbow (**a,b**), there is mild osteophyte formation (**b**: small arrow) and medial joint space widening (**b**: open arrowhead), which is most apparent on the craniocaudal projection. There is marked distension of the elbow joint on MR images (**c–f**). The synovial component of the joint distension is predominant on enhanced images (**e**: arrow), with the central low signal representing joint effusion (**e**: arrowhead). STIR hyperintensity is present in the distal humerus (**f**: open arrow). A diagnosis of lymphoplasmacytic synovitis and synovial cell hyperplasia associated with degenerative joint disease was made on biopsy.

References

1. Roemer FW, Eckstein F, Hayashi D, Guermazi A. The role of imaging in osteoarthritis. Best Pract Res Clin Rheumatol. 2014; 28:31–60.

2. Kazakia GJ, Kuo D, Schooler J, et al. Bone and cartilage demonstrate changes localized to bone marrow edema-like lesions within osteoarthritic knees. Osteoarthr Cartil. 2013;21:94–101.

3. Schaefer SL, Baumel CA, Gerbig JR, Forrest LJ. Direct magnetic resonance arthrography of the canine shoulder. Vet Radiol Ultrasound. 2010;51:391–396.

4. Tivers MS, Mahoney PN, Baines EA, Corr SA. Diagnostic accuracy of positive contrast computed tomography arthrography for the detection of injuries to the medial meniscus in dogs with naturally occurring cranial cruciate ligament insufficiency. J Small Anim Pract. 2009;50:324–332.

5. Samii VF, Dyce J, Pozzi A, et al. Computed tomographic arthrography of the stifle for detection of cranial and caudal cruciate ligament and meniscal tears in dogs. Vet Radiol Ultrasound. 2009; 50:144–150.

6. Samii VF, Dyce J. Computed tomographic arthrography of the normal canine stifle. Vet Radiol Ultrasound. 2004;402–406.

7. Roemer FW, Guermazi A, Niu J, Zhang Y, Mohr A, Felson DT. Prevalence of magnetic resonance imaging-defined atrophic and hypertrophic phenotypes of knee osteoarthritis in a population-based cohort. Arthritis Rheum. 2012;64:429–437.

Index

Page numbers in *italics* denote figures.

Atlas of Small Animal CT and MRI, First Edition. Erik R. Wisner and Allison L. Zwingenberger.
© 2015 John Wiley & Sons, Inc. Published 2015 by John Wiley & Sons, Inc.